BSAVA Manual of Canine and Feline Musculoskeletal Disorders

Editors:

John E.F. Houlton
MA VetMB DVR DSAO Diplomate ECVS MRCVS
Empshill, Robins Lane, Lolworth, Cambridge CB3 8HH

James L. Cook
DVM PhD ACVS
Comparative Orthopedic Laboratory, University of Missouri
379 East Campus Drive, Columbia, MO 65211, USA

John F. Innes
BVSc PhD CertVR DSAS (Orthopaedics) MRCVS
Small Animal Hospital, University of Liverpool
Crown Street, Liverpool L7 7EX

and

Sorrel J. Langley-Hobbs
MA BVetMed DSAS (Orthopaedics) Diplomate ECVS ILTM MRCVS
The Queens Veterinary School Hospital, Department of Veterinary Medicine
University of Cambridge, Madingley Road, Cambridge CB3 0ES

Series editor:

Gordon Brown
BVM&S CertSAO MRCVS
The Grove Veterinary Group, Grove House, Holt Road,
Fakenham, Norfolk NR21 8JG

Published by:

British Small Animal Veterinary Association
Woodrow House, 1 Telford Way, Waterwells
Business Park, Quedgeley, Gloucester GL2 2AB

A Company Limited by Guarantee in England.
Registered Company No. 2837793.
Registered as a Charity.

Copyright © 2006 BSAVA

All rights reserved. No part of this publication may be reproduced, stored in a retrieval system, or transmitted, in form or by any means, electronic, mechanical, photocopying, recording or otherwise without prior written permission of the copyright holder.

The colour illustrations in this book (excluding 3.1, 18.25, 20.1, 20.11a and 23.21) were drawn by S.J. Elmhurst BA Hons (www.living-art.org.uk) and are printed with her permission.

Figures 3.1, 18.25, 20.1, 20.11a and 23.21 were designed and drawn by Vicki Martin Design and are printed with their permission.

A catalogue record for this book is available from the British Library.

ISBN-10 0 905214 80 3
ISBN-13 978 0 905214 80 1

The publishers and contributors cannot take responsibility for information provided on dosages and methods of application of drugs mentioned in this publication. Details of this kind must be verified by individual users from the appropriate literature.

Typeset by: Fusion Design, Wareham, Dorset, UK
Printed by: Replika Press Pvt. Ltd, India

Other titles in the BSAVA Manuals series:

Manual of Advanced Veterinary Nursing
Manual of Canine & Feline Abdominal Surgery
Manual of Canine & Feline Behavioural Medicine
Manual of Canine & Feline Clinical Pathology
Manual of Canine & Feline Dentistry
Manual of Canine & Feline Emergency and Critical Care
Manual of Canine & Feline Endocrinology
Manual of Canine & Feline Gastroenterology
Manual of Canine & Feline Haematology and Transfusion Medicine
Manual of Canine & Feline Head, Neck and Thoracic Surgery
Manual of Canine & Feline Infectious Diseases
Manual of Canine & Feline Musculoskeletal Imaging
Manual of Canine & Feline Nephrology and Urology
Manual of Canine & Feline Neurology
Manual of Canine & Feline Oncology
Manual of Canine & Feline Wound Management and Reconstruction
Manual of Exotic Pets
Manual of Ornamental Fish
Manual of Psittacine Birds
Manual of Rabbit Medicine and Surgery
Manual of Raptors, Pigeons and Waterfowl
Manual of Reptiles
Manual of Small Animal Anaesthesia and Analgesia
Manual of Small Animal Cardiorespiratory Medicine and Surgery
Manual of Small Animal Dermatology
Manual of Small Animal Diagnostic Imaging
Manual of Small Animal Fracture Repair and Management
Manual of Small Animal Ophthalmology
Manual of Small Animal Reproduction and Neonatology
Manual of Veterinary Care
Manual of Veterinary Nursing
Manual of Wildlife Casualties

For information on these and all BSAVA publications please visit our website: www.bsava.com

Contents

List of contributors — v

Foreword — vii

Preface — viii

1 **An approach to the lame dog or cat** — 1
John E.F. Houlton

2 **Radiography** — 8
Jeremy V. Davies

3 **Laboratory investigations** — 21
Susan Bell and John E.F. Houlton

4 **Advanced diagnostic techniques** — 27
Steven C. Budsberg and Michael W. Thomas

5 **Diseases and disorders of the bone** — 34
Sorrel Langley-Hobbs

6 **Disturbances of growth and bone development** — 50
Sorrel Langley-Hobbs

7 **Arthritis** — 81
Ralph Abercromby, John Innes and Chris May

8 **Muscles and tendons**

    8a **Muscles and tendon injuries** — 110
    Angus Anderson

    8b **Diseases of muscle and the neuromuscular junction** — 120
    G. Diane Shelton

9 **Tumours of the musculoskeletal system** — 128
B. Duncan X. Lascelles

10 **Neurological causes of lameness** — 135
T. James Anderson

11 **Surgical biology of joints** — 144
Rory Todhunter

12 **Principles of articular surgery** — 151
Sorrel Langley-Hobbs

13	**Surgical instrumentation** *John Lapish*	161
14	**Biomaterials for joint surgery** *Derek B. Fox*	168
15	**Arthroscopy**	
	15a **Arthroscopic equipment** *John Lapish and Bernadette Van Ryssen*	177
	15b **Principles of arthroscopy** *Bernadette Van Ryssen*	184
16	**Postoperative management and rehabilitation** *Darryl L. Millis*	193
17	**The shoulder** *Steve Butterworth and James L. Cook*	212
18	**The elbow** *Geoff Robins and John Innes*	249
19	**The carpus** *Mike Guilliard*	281
20	**The distal limb** *Richard Eaton-Wells*	292
21	**The hip** *Carlos Macias, James L. Cook and John Innes*	309
22	**The stifle** *W. Malcolm McKee and James L. Cook*	350
23	**The tarsus** *Andrew Miller and Don Hulse*	396
24	**The temporomandibular joint** *Colin Stead*	418
Index		425

Contributors

Ralph H. Abercromby BVMS CertSAO MRCVS
Anderson Abercromby Veterinary Referrals, The 1870 Building, Jayes Park Courtyard,
Forest Green Road, Ockley, Surrey RH5 5RR, UK

Angus A. Anderson BVetMed PhD DSAS (Orthopaedics) MRCVS
Anderson Abercromby Veterinary Referrals, The 1870 Building, Jayes Park Courtyard,
Forest Green Road, Ockley, Surrey RH5 5RR, UK

T. James Anderson BVM&S MVM PhD MRCVS DSAO DipECVN ILTM
Division of Companion Animal Sciences, University of Glasgow, Veterinary School, Bearsden Road,
Bearsden, Glasgow G61 1QH, UK

Susan Bell LRCS PhD
The Veterinary Annexe, The Veterinary Science Building, University of Liverpool, Crown Street,
Liverpool L69 7ZJ, UK

Steven C. Budsberg DVM MS ACVS
Department of Small Animal Medicine, College of Veterinary Medicine, University of Georgia,
Athens, GA 30602, USA

Steven J. Butterworth MA VetMB CertVR DSAO MRCVS
Weighbridge Referrals, Kemys Way, Swansea Enterprise Park, Swansea SA6 8QF, UK

James L. Cook DVM PhD ACVS
Comparative Orthopedic Laboratory, University of Missouri, 379 East Campus Drive, Columbia,
MO 65211, USA

Jeremy V. Davies BVetMed PhD DVR Diplomate ECVS DipECVDI MRCVS
Davies Veterinary Specialists, Manor Farm Business Park, Higham Gobion, Hertfordshire SG5 3HR, UK

Richard Eaton-Wells BVSc MACVSc MRCVS
Queensland Veterinary Specialists, 263 Appleby Road, Stafford Heights, Brisbane, Qld 4053, Australia

Derek B. Fox DVM PhD
Comparative Orthopaedic Laboratory, University of Missouri, 379 East Campus Drive, Columbia,
MO 65211, USA

Mike Guilliard MA VetMB CertSAO MRCVS
Nantwich Veterinary Hospital, Crewe Road, Nantwich, Cheshire CW5 5SF, UK

John E.F. Houlton MA VetMB DVR DSAO Diplomate ECVS MRCVS
Empshill, Robins Lane, Lolworth, Cambridge CB3 8HH, UK

Don Hulse DVM Diplomate ACVS ECVS
Department of Small Animal Surgery, College of Veterinary Medicine, Texas A&M University,
College Station, TX 77843-4474, USA

John Innes BVSc PhD CertVR DSAS (Orthopaedics) MRCVS
Small Animal Hospital, University of Liverpool, Crown Street, Liverpool L7 7EX, UK

John P. Lapish BSc BVetMed MRCVS
Veterinary Instrumentation Ltd, Broadfield Road, Sheffield S8 0XL, UK

Sorrel Langley-Hobbs MA BVetMed DSAS (Orthopaedics) Diplomate ECVS ILTM MRCVS
The Queens Veterinary School Hospital, Department of Clinical Veterinary Medicine,
University of Cambridge, Madingley Road, Cambridge CB3 0ES, UK

B. Duncan X. Lascelles BSc BVSc PhD CertVA DSAS(Soft Tissue) Diplomate ECVS Diplomate ACVS MRCVS
Comparative Pain Research Laboratory and Surgery Section, Department of Clinical Sciences,
College of Veterinary Medicine, North Caroline State University, Raleigh, NC 27606, USA

Carlos Macias Ldo Vet DSAS (Orthopaedics) MRCVS
Centro Veterinario de Referencia 'Bahía de Málaga', Parque Empresarial Laurotorre,
25 Alhaurín de la Torre, 29130 Málaga, Spain

Christopher May MA VetMB PhD CertSAO MRCVS
Northwest Surgeons, Delamere House, Ashville Point, Sutton Weaver, Cheshire WA7 3FW, UK

W. Malcolm McKee BVMS MVS DSAO MACVSc MRCVS
Willows Referral Service, 78 Tanworth Lane, Solihull, West Midlands B90 4DF, UK

Andrew Miller BVMS DSAO MRCVS
Broadleys Veterinary Hospital, Craigleith Road, Stirling FK7 7LE, UK

Darryl Millis MS DVM Diplomate ACVS CCRP
University of Tennessee, College of Veterinary Medicine, Department of Small Animal Clinical Sciences,
C247, Veterinary Teaching Hospital, Knoxville, TN 37996, USA

Geoff Robins BVetMed (Hons) MRCVS FACVSc
St Lucia Surgical Services, 24 Tarcoola Street, St Lucia, Queensland 4067, Australia

G. Diane Shelton DVM PhD DipACVIM
Department of Pathology, University of California at San Diego, La Jolla, CA 92093-0612, USA

A. Colin Stead BVMS DVR DSAO FRCVS
Royal (Dick) School of Veterinary Studies, Hospital for Small Animals, Easter Bush Veterinary Centre,
Roslin, Midlothian EH25 9RG, UK

Rory Todhunter BVSc MS PhD
Cornell University, College of Veterinary Medicine, Department of Clinical Sciences, Ithaca, NY 14853, USA

Bernadette Van Ryssen DVM PhD
Department of Medical Imaging, Faculty of Veterinary Medicine, Ghent University, Salisburylaan,
133 9820 Merelbeke, Belgium

Foreword

This *BSAVA Manual of Canine and Feline Musculoskeletal Disorders* is another great addition to our ever-expanding range of Manuals. This new book and its sister manuals on Fracture management and Musculoskeletal imaging now cover the musculoskeletal system, its diseases and their modern management comprehensively for every practitioner.

The launch of this book and the inclusion of more specialized techniques exemplify how our knowledge is growing and how practitioners can now learn and attempt techniques hitherto considered outside their capabilities. Despite this, the Manual is easy to navigate, a pleasure to read and full of clear illustrations, tables and figures. Once bought, it will be well read and constantly referred to.

Without exception, the authors are the best in their field and are to be congratulated for finishing an excellent book. My thanks also go to the Publications Committee and staff. BSAVA is committed to keeping practitioners up to date in all aspects of veterinary medicine and surgery, and this book will certainly make a major contribution.

Carmel T. Mooney MVB MPhil PhD DipECVIM-CA MRCVS
BSAVA President 2005–2006

Preface

'Life is movement, movement is life'
Aristotle, 384–322 BC

This Manual is built upon the extremely successful *BSAVA Manual of Small Animal Arthrology*. However, in broadening the remit to cover *Canine and Feline Musculoskeletal Disorders*, we have been able to be more inclusive, such that conditions of bone, tendon and muscle are now incorporated. In this way we hope we have provided a ready reference for the small animal practitioner faced with a dog or cat showing lameness, stiffness or joint pain. We have excluded diagnosis and treatment of fractures from this manual because these are already covered in the excellent *BSAVA Manual of Small Animal Fracture Management and Repair*. Indeed, we have endeavoured to borrow some elements of style and presentation from that sister manual, so that the two manuals should complement each other and provide a rounded and up-to-date overview of orthopaedics and rheumatology in the dog and cat.

The early parts of this new Manual deal with generic issues related to the biology, diseases and treatment of bones, joints, muscles and tendons. There are also chapters on surgical instrumentation and biomaterials, to provide a theoretical basis for the more applied chapters that appear later in the book. This latter part embodies a systematic approach, focussed on each of the major synovial joints, including the temporomandibular joint. Each of these joint-specific chapters deals with basic anatomy and surgical approaches, before describing the conditions that affect the particular joint. The reader will note that we have covered common surgical procedures on joints with the use of Operative Techniques at the end of each chapter. We have tried to choose standard techniques that will prove useful to the reader. We hope therefore that this Manual will be both a source of theoretical information and will provide real practical guidance for the surgeon. Possible pitfalls and key points are highlighted throughout the Operative Techniques so as to make maximum use of the experience of our authors.

It goes without saying that development of surgical skill takes more than reading textbooks, and all surgeons need to attend practical training classes, discuss cases with experienced colleagues, and assist and learn from more experienced surgeons. In addition, some surgical techniques in this book are clearly more advanced than others. For example, we have included a description of total hip replacement, which is obviously not a procedure to be attempted lightly, nor by the inexperienced. However, within specialist centres this is now a relatively common technique and we felt it appropriate that this be reflected in a modern surgical Manual. Overall, practical surgical guides such as those contained in this book, can, we hope, provide a concise basis for sound clinical practice based on the experiences of the authors. We hope that this Manual will prove to be a handy and well thumbed companion to our clinical colleagues.

The editors owe the authors a huge debt of thanks. We have been lucky to assemble an enviable author list from around the world. They have all been extremely cooperative and responsive, as well as very understanding to our needs. During the course of this project there was a major change in direction and our authors accepted this without complaint (at least, not to us!) and we are very grateful for their forbearance and compliance. It has been easy to edit this manual with such great authors. Thank you to one and all.

In a Manual that includes so much artwork we are also very grateful for the skill, dedication and expertise of Samantha Elmhurst for the surgical drawings. We are also indebted to Fusion Design for their work on the layout of the book.

This has been a long and challenging project, which has taken a couple of twists and turns along the way. Throughout that process we have been helped greatly by Marion Jowett and her colleagues at the BSAVA publishing team and we are very grateful for their expertise, guidance and patience. We are also extremely grateful to the unsung hero of this manual, Gordon Brown, a fellow orthopaedic surgeon, who has spent a great deal of time providing external peer review of the material in this book; his insights, advice and overview were invaluable. He was able to raise our spirits at those low ebbs that occur throughout many projects such as this. Being a Scot, we know Gordon will appreciate the quote below. Thank you Gordon!

'What we can we will be,
Honest Englishmen.
Do the work that's nearest,
Though it's dull at whiles,
Helping when we meet them,
Lame dogs over stiles'
Charles Kingsley, 1819–1875

John Houlton
John Innes
James Cook
Sorrel Langley-Hobbs

February 2006

An approach to the lame dog or cat

John E.F. Houlton

Introduction

When asked to examine a lame animal, a number of approaches might be adopted. One might perform a complete physical examination, identify the seat of lameness, formulate a list of differential diagnoses, undertake additional tests to narrow that list and treat the most likely cause. Alternatively, one might locate the painful area or joint, work on the adage that common things happen commonly and treat accordingly. Finally, particularly when it is difficult to identify the painful area, the clinician might radiograph the entire limb in the hope of identifying a lesion.

Clearly the first approach is the one of choice. It can be further refined by making it problem-oriented in order to maximize the chances of diagnosing which lesions are clinically significant and which are incidental findings.

There may be some merit in the second approach but on occasions it will fail. Nevertheless, particularly where there are severe financial constraints, it is preferable to making an ill-informed guess. The last approach should be strictly discouraged, for even if a lesion is spotted, there is absolutely no indication as to its clinical significance.

The problem-oriented approach has three steps:

1. Sufficient data are collected to define the problem(s).
2. An initial plan is formulated, including tests required to establish a diagnosis and/or details of therapy.
3. The patient's progress is noted.

Data collection

Data collection can be conveniently divided into: background information; owner's complaint; patient's history; and the initial clinical findings.

Background information

Much of this may be gained by the receptionist or nursing staff prior to the consultation and recorded in a standard fashion. The animal's age, weight, sex and breed (signalment) should be entered as well as its vaccination status. Other information that may be relevant to record at this stage includes the animal's environment and its intended function. Whether it is a pet or used for working, showing, racing or breeding is particularly important with regard to prognosis. The amount and type of work expected of the animal should also be ascertained.

Enquiry should be made regarding any previous illness or injuries, and the length of time it has been in the current owner's possession. This may be of particular relevance if the animal has been bred by the owner, when questions can be asked about littermates. In working or racing dogs, the reason for their change in ownership should be sought, particularly if there has been a recent change in their 'form'.

Owner's complaint

A precise statement of the owner's complaint should be obtained. This may require considerable patience but, once established, serves as a useful basis for the rest of the history. If the problem is a gait abnormality, a description may be helpful, particularly if the signs are intermittent or of varying severity. On occasions, asking clients to provide a video of their animal displaying the perceived problem can be helpful, especially if it is intermittent.

History

The history must be accurate and sufficiently broad-based to identify all the significant problems. It should be taken by the clinician responsible for establishing the diagnosis, for it is he or she who must evaluate the information provided by the owner. Lay personnel and owners often pay insufficient attention to some problems, yet exaggerate the importance of others. For instance, undue emphasis is invariably placed on minor traumatic events, merely because they occurred at approximately the same time as the onset of lameness. Such events may be misleading if accepted as important. Equally, apparently trivial events may be underestimated by the owner. The person taking the history must determine the difference between owners' observations and their interpretation of these events. Frequently, owners' observations are accurate but their interpretation is flawed, and it is the veterinary surgeon who is best able to ascertain the true value of each.

Questions should be structured so that a clear difference between facts and opinions can be detected. Questions should be open, i.e. they should be structured so that the owner is given alternatives to

Chapter 1 An approach to the lame dog or cat

answer, rather than the answer being implied in the question. Many owners will provide the answer they think the clinician wants to hear, either because they are confused or because they want to help. Owners should feel able to say they don't know, or that they cannot remember, without feeling embarrassed or inadequate. Indeed, it may be that the animal is suffering from an intermittent or bilateral lameness when such hesitancy on the part of the owner may be helpful.

The onset of the problem should be ascertained; was it sudden or insidious? If it was traumatic, the details of the accident should be recorded. Many lameness cases are noticed suddenly even if their cause, when eventually established, would suggest a gradual onset of signs.

The duration of the lameness should be determined and its course recorded. It should be noted whether the problem is continuous or intermittent; whether it has deteriorated, remained static or is resolving. Any association with exercise or rest should be sought, particularly if the lameness is intermittent or it varies in severity. It should be ascertained whether the lameness alters during the day, particularly in the morning or evening, or with different types of weather.

Lameness due to osteoarthritis is often most noticeable after a period of rest, particularly if this follows strenuous exercise. Early morning stiffness is also a frequent sign and the condition is often more severe in cold, wet weather. Chronic pain may make it difficult for an animal to lie comfortably in its bed or basket, and owners may notice their pet constantly changing its position before going to sleep.

Attempts should be made to determine what causes or exacerbates the lameness and which limb(s) is involved. Questions to be asked include whether the owner has noticed swellings of joints and how severe the lameness is. Does it move from limb to limb; is it episodic or cyclic? Does the animal place the lame limb to the ground or is it carried? Does the severity of the lameness alter with the ground surface? Toe injuries may appear worse on hard or uneven ground whereas many upper limb joint problems are largely unaffected by the ground surface.

Details should be sought about the animal's usual exercise regime. Is the dog restricted to exercise on a lead or is it allowed to run freely? Does it exercise on its own or does it play with other dogs? It is important to determine both the quantity and the type of exercise.

It should be determined whether the animal's temperament has changed in any way or its performance has altered. Dogs may become bad tempered or aggressive when in pain. Changes in performance can be reflected in many different ways. A Greyhound may start to drift wide on corners; a working dog may fail to clear obstacles or appear to tire more quickly; a pet may find it increasingly difficult to jump into a car; all indicate reduced performance. Information relating to other body systems should also be sought, particularly where lameness is but one manifestation of a generalized problem.

Further general information may be helpful at this stage, including the animal's diet and housing, and the health of related or in-contact animals.

Initial clinical findings

Every physical examination must be performed in a routine and systematic fashion. This minimizes the chances of overlooking subtle changes, particularly when a very obvious problem exists. It also encourages the recording of the clinical findings in an orderly and meaningful fashion. Subtle changes will also be missed when the patient is anxious and tense. Slight alterations in the respiratory pattern, small changes in muscle tone, and little differences in range of pain-free joint movement will all be masked if the animal is not relaxed.

Large dogs are best examined on the floor and small dogs and cats on a table. However, most animals have been taught not to get on to tables and work surfaces, and their first reaction when placed on the consulting room table is to freeze or attempt to jump off. This is not conducive to performing a thorough clinical examination. Equally, it is confusing for a dog to be ordered to sit when it is unnatural for it to do so. Giant-breed dogs frequently prefer to be examined in lateral recumbency and Greyhounds are best examined standing.

It is generally helpful to have the owner present during the physical examination. They are frequently helpful in restraining the patient, although their personal safety must be considered. In general, most dogs are more relaxed in the presence of their regular handler. Moreover, if an unsuspected problem is discovered, there will be the opportunity to re-question the owner. Similarly, if the clinical signs do not seem to correlate with the history, a further attempt can be made to obtain additional information from the owner to determine the reason for the conflicting information.

A general clinical examination should precede the orthopaedic examination. Personal preference dictates how the latter is performed, but the author examines the thoracic limbs with the animal sitting or standing facing him, and the pelvic limbs with the animal standing facing away from him. It is important that the animal stands or sits squarely during this initial examination so that symmetry between limbs and joints can be assessed. Further detailed manipulation of the joints is generally performed with the animal in lateral recumbency, with the limb to be examined uppermost.

Restraint should be kept to a minimum as it is far easier to detect subtle changes in a relaxed animal. Sedation or general anaesthesia may be helpful for the final stages of the examination, as discussed later, but every attempt should be made to obtain as much clinical information as possible before important responses are masked.

The initial clinical findings will be obtained by observation, palpation, manipulation, gait analysis and, where appropriate, examination of the sedated or anaesthetized animal. A brief neurological examination will indicate whether a more detailed examination is necessary.

The aim of the initial physical examination should be to detect structural abnormalities first, evidence of pain second, and functional changes towards the end of the examination.

Observation

Observation of the patient should begin as soon as the animal is seen in the waiting room or consulting room. It should be noted whether the patient has difficulty and/or reluctance in getting up or walking. The veterinary surgeon should also observe whether it walks on all four limbs, whether it takes full or partial weight on its limb(s) or whether it carries a leg off the ground.

The animal should be observed as the history is taken and it should be noted whether it shifts its weight from the affected limb as it sits or stands. The posture of the limb should be noted. Is there obvious deformity, joint swelling or muscle atrophy? If the conformation of the dog is assessed at this stage it may help with questioning. For instance, dogs with chronic bilateral pelvic limb pain or low back pain may develop well muscled forequarters as a result of shifting their centre of gravity forwards. The associated hindquarter atrophy will contribute to the rather triangular appearance of the dog. In contrast, dogs with bilateral thoracic limb problems often appear to have a 'roached' back as they change their stance in an attempt to redistribute their weight.

Conformation and body type may predispose to certain injuries; for example, there appears be an association between straight tarsi and osteochondrosis of the talus. In general, each limb should be symmetrical about a vertical axis and aligned in the sagittal plane. However, gross deviations are considered normal for many breeds and comparison of the suspect limb with the contralateral one is a precept that should be followed throughout the clinical examination. It is generally assumed that the contralateral leg is normal, but it must be remembered that immature dogs may have bilateral developmental joint pathology. Similarly, bilateral ligamentous injuries, such as those seen in cruciate disease or with plantar ligament pathology, may also confuse the picture.

Observation should detect any change in limb shape, including hyperflexion or extension of joints if the animal is bearing weight on the affected limb. Hyperextension of the carpus may follow traumatic disruption of the palmar ligaments or occur as a developmental laxity in puppies. Hyperextension of the proximal interphalangeal joint, as a result of an avulsion of the insertion of the superficial digital flexor tendon, will result in a 'dropped toe' while avulsion of the deep digital flexor tendon will result in a 'knocked up' toe. Neither may be of clinical significance except in breeds where foot conformation is important in the show ring. Hyperflexion of the tarsus will occur after injury to the Achilles tendon, plantar ligament or fracture/subluxation of the intertarsal or tarsometatarsal joints, but the injury may not be immediately obvious as the limb may be carried.

Angular and rotational deformities are generally the result of physeal injuries but they may be seen following fractures and luxations. However, luxations tend to result in a characteristic posture for each dislocated joint. Observation may also reveal evidence of wounds or old scars, hair loss or discoloration of the skin. Inspection of the foot, including nails, pads and the interdigital skin, is mandatory as these are common sites of injury in the dog.

Palpation

Palpation of the axial and appendicular skeleton should follow a set sequence. Palpation of the spine should start at the head and finish at the tail. Each limb should be palpated from its top to toe, comparing each leg with its opposite.

Palpation should detect changes in muscles, anatomical deformities, swellings and pain.

Changes in muscles: By standing directly in front of, or behind the animal, one may palpate either both thoracic or both pelvic limbs simultaneously, checking for subtle asymmetries of shape due to swelling or atrophy, for spasm, contracture or weakness. Reduced muscle volume may be a result of neurogenic atrophy following lower motor neuron damage or due to disuse. Neurogenic atrophy is usually severe, develops rapidly and may be confined to those muscle groups normally innervated by a specific peripheral nerve.

In contrast, disuse atrophy usually reflects the degree and chronicity of the lameness rather than the cause or location of the problem. It is often most noticeable in those areas where muscle bulk is normally greatest, i.e. in the proximal third of the limb. Although disuse atrophy is not specific there are some occasions where it is possible to suspect the seat of lameness from the tissues involved. Thus, a dog that is reluctant to extend its shoulder will lose muscle bulk preferentially from its shoulder extensor muscles. Similarly, dogs with painful stifles will tend to develop atrophy of the quadriceps muscles. Since the latter dogs often just take weight on their toes, rather than putting their feet fully to the ground, they frequently also develop atrophy of their metatarsal pads.

Anatomical deformities: The spatial relationship of normal anatomical structures, particularly bony prominences, should be noted during palpation of the limbs. These may be altered in the presence of fractures and particularly luxations. For example, the palpable triangle formed by the greater trochanter of the femur, the tuber coxae and the tuber ischii will be distorted when the ipsilateral hip is luxated.

Swellings: These may involve bones, joints or the soft tissues. Swelling of the soft tissues may be due to bruising or haematoma formation and can be differentiated from oedema, which pits on pressure.

Acute joint injuries will result in synovial effusion. These are best appreciated where the joint capsule is least supported by the periarticular structures. Thus, effusions of the elbow are readily appreciated on the caudolateral aspect of the joint, whereas effusions of the shoulder are more difficult to palpate because of the overlying musculature. Effusions of the carpus are easily palpated on the dorsal aspect of the joint, where it is possible to push the synovial fluid under the tendon of extensor carpi radialis and the common digital extensor tendon from one side of the joint to the other. Effusions of the interphalangeal joints are similarly palpable on the dorsal aspect of the relevant joint. Effusions of both the carpus and the joints of the digits are best palpated when the joints are partially flexed.

Chapter 1 An approach to the lame dog or cat

Effusions of the hip must be gross before they are apparent, but quite mild effusions of the stifle are readily discernible. The swelling is best appreciated either side of the straight patellar ligament in the standing animal. The dog or cat should stand squarely, bearing weight equally on both limbs, to allow accurate comparison of both sides.

Persistent thickening of the joint capsule and retinaculum occurs as a result of fibrosis in chronic joint abnormalities. This periarticular fibrosis is readily differentiated from a joint effusion by its firm nature. It may be particularly noticeable at specific points around the joint, as in thickening of the medial aspect of the stifle with chronic cruciate disease.

Pain: Pain on palpation may be localized, diffuse, mild or severe. Both palpation and manipulation of the limb may be required to localize pain. This can be much the hardest part of the examination, requiring considerable discrimination and experience. Some animals will resent any attempt at handling while others are remarkably stoical. An assessment of the animal's temperament is therefore an important prerequisite.

Pain may arise from bone, muscle and tendons, neural tissue or joints. Bone and muscle pain may be apparent on simple palpation whereas joints may only be painful on manipulation. However, the standing dog that has painful hips frequently sits down when digital pressure is applied to the dorsum of its pelvis. Standing dogs should normally resist this force and remain standing. Nerve root pain is often particularly severe, resulting in the animal screaming when any attempt is made to palpate or manipulate the affected part.

Care should be exercised to differentiate between joint pain and pain from the adjacent bones. In particular, metaphyseal pain can be confused with joint pain in young dogs. Localization may be further hindered by the necessity to exert pressure on bones and muscles when manipulating joints.

Once pain is localized to an individual joint, efforts should be made to define the source yet further. This is not always possible but it should not deter a detailed examination. For instance, a metacarpophalangeal joint with reduced range of flexion may be painful because of palmar sesamoid disease or fracture. On the other hand the dorsal sesamoid may be painful, swollen or excessively mobile.

Careful palpation and manipulation should identify which structure is painful. Careful palpation may identify pain originating from a periarticular structure when it was first thought that the joint itself was painful. Thus, a lateral fabellar fracture may present as an apparently painful stifle, but a more detailed examination will reveal point pain over the fabella and an absence of articular pathology.

Manipulation

As with palpation, manipulation of the axial and appendicular skeleton should follow a routine sequence. The lower cervical spine is flexed and extended in the axial plane and to the left and right, and any pain response noted. Similarly, the lumbar spine should be flexed, extended and rotated. Limbs should be manipulated from their top to the foot to assess:

- Anatomical deformity or displacement, e.g. luxation, subluxation
- Pain
- Range of movement of the entire limb and of each joint
- Crepitus
- The integrity of the supporting structures of each joint, i.e. the collateral, dorsal, palmar and plantar ligaments, in addition to specialized structures, such as the cruciate ligaments.

Joints should, as far as possible, be manipulated one at a time. However, it is frequently difficult to be absolutely specific; for example, attempts at extension of the shoulder usually result in some degree of elbow extension. Joints should be manipulated throughout their normal range of motion to assess pain and crepitus, and also be moderately stressed at the extremes of flexion and extension. Abnormal joints are not necessarily always painful through their normal range of movement, but there is no simple answer to how much force needs to be exerted. Too little may fail to elicit a response crucial to the diagnosis; too much will produce a response in a normal joint and result in misdiagnosis. The aim is to start gently and then gradually increase the stress, always comparing with the contralateral limb. Significant responses should be consistent and reproducible.

Manipulation of the shoulder has always been a challenge, since it is difficult to determine the exact source of pain and the contribution that the articular and periarticular structures provide in terms of joint stability. Shoulder laxity associated with loss of integrity of the soft tissue supporting structures of the joint remains controversial. It has been suggested that insufficiency in the medial support (provided by the medial glenohumeral ligament and the subscapularis muscle tendon of insertion) can be evaluated by assessing the angle of abduction of the shoulder when compared with the normal limb or what is considered 'normal' (see Chapter 17). Although the interpretation of this test is still in question, it emphasizes the difficulty in localizing pathology of this area and in determining its clinical significance.

It is relatively easy to cause pain by over-extending the elbow and tarsus whereas over-flexion of the joints of the distal limb is usually resented more than hyperextension. If pain is suspected on the medial aspect of the elbow, pain on flexion can generally be exacerbated by simultaneous inward rotation (pronation) of the carpus.

It is important to differentiate between pain on hip extension and a painful lumbosacral joint. It is easier to flex and extend the spine while keeping the hips flexed rather than extending the hips without extending the lower spine. In this way, it is possible to differentiate between the two sites.

Range of motion: Range of joint movement should be assessed and compared to normal. Restricted range of movement may accompany acute injuries, such as sprains and luxations, as well as chronic conditions such as osteoarthritis.

In the thoracic limb, restriction of joint movement is often easier to detect in the distal joints than in the shoulder or elbow. Reduced shoulder extension may be overlooked unless pressure is kept on the scapular blade, since the animal's natural reaction is to shift its centre of gravity and sit back on its haunches. In doing so, it evades extending its shoulder fully.

It is easier to appreciate reduced extension of the elbow rather than a reduction in flexion. In most breeds of dog, the cranial aspect of the antebrachium should touch the biceps brachii region when the elbow is fully flexed. Nevertheless, over-extension of the elbow is frequently uncomfortable as the anconeal process is forced unnaturally between the lateral and medial parts of the humeral condyle.

Carpal swelling, deformity, deviation or abnormal joint posture is easily appreciable as there is little soft tissue surrounding the joint. The normal carpus can be flexed so that the digital pads contact the caudal surface of the antebrachium. Carpal extension is limited to approximately 10 degrees of hyperextension. Care must be exercised when manipulating the carpi of young dogs, as normal joints often appear extremely mobile. The dew claw should not be overlooked since it is easy to miss fractures and luxations of this digit.

Range of motion of each metacarpophalangeal joint should be assessed in turn, and each joint manipulated to assess its stability, both mediolaterally and rotationally. The palmar sesamoids should be carefully checked for pain, swelling or excess mobility. Similarly the dorsal sesamoid should be palpated for pain or instability. The metacarpophalangeal joints should flex to 90 degrees. However, decreased range of movement which is not accompanied by pain may not be clinically significant. In particular, the joints of older working dogs, or dogs that have habitually dug holes, may be thickened and have restricted flexion, but they are frequently not painful. Similarly, where painless, thickened metacarpophalangeal joints are identified in breeds known to suffer from osteochondrosis, careful examination of the elbow and shoulder should eliminate these joints as a source of pain before ascribing undue clinical significance to the foot.

Range of motion of each interphalangeal joint should be assessed, and each joint fully flexed and extended. Pain, or inability to extend the joint may indicate palmar joint capsule sprain, partial avulsion of the superficial digital flexor tendon, chronic subluxation or osteoarthritis. Each joint should be palpated to assess stability in a mediolateral direction and the integrity of the collateral ligaments. The interphalangeal collateral ligaments should always be assessed with the toe in extension, as slight laxity in the neutral or flexed position is normal. Rupture of a collateral ligament allows the joint to luxate when stressed; this may be accompanied by pain and/or crepitus.

Manipulation of the hip should assess flexion/extension and abduction/adduction. The normal range of flexion/extension is 110 degrees. With severe osteoarthritis and capsular fibrosis, this may be reduced to as little as 45 degrees. In the puppy, joint laxity is of more concern, particularly where hip dysplasia is suspected.

The stifle is a composite joint and there are several important structures which may be damaged. Patellar position should be evaluated in both the flexed and extended joint. Medial patellar instability is best assessed in the extended stifle while lateral instability is determined in the slightly flexed joint. Joint instability due to rupture of the cranial cruciate ligament is manifest by a positive cranial draw test or the tibial compression test (see Chapter 22). A positive cranial draw movement has a rather ill defined end to the movement whereas the normal stifle has a distinct end point. This is an important distinction in the young dog where normal joint laxity may be confused with a pathologically unstable joint. A further source of confusion may occur if inward rotation of the tibia is misinterpreted as a positive cranial draw movement. Inward rotation of the tibia is a normal finding when attempting a cranial draw movement in a healthy joint. In the joint with cranial cruciate deficiency, inward rotation is increased.

The normal tarsus should flex so that the dorsal aspect of the metatarsus touches the cranial aspect of the tibial region. In some of the well muscled, bow-legged breeds this is not always possible and due allowance should be made for their conformation. Joint movement may be enhanced, or movement occur in abnormal planes, if the joint is unstable through loss of its supporting ligaments or if the joint capsule is torn (see Chapter 23). Manipulation should assess joint stability both mediolaterally and rotationally. Collateral ligament stability should always be tested with the joint in a position such that the ligaments are taut.

Crepitus: Manipulation may reveal crepitus, a palpable or audible 'grating' of skeletal components as they move relative to each other. Crepitus following acute injury usually indicates fracture, while a somewhat smoother, but nevertheless abnormal, bone-to-bone contact might suggest luxation. Crepitus may also accompany chronic joint disease, particularly where extensive cartilage erosion has occurred and subchondral bone is exposed.

Crepitus is easily 'referred' along a bone leading to misdiagnosis of its origin. Care should therefore be taken to move only one joint at a time when attempting to localize crepitus. Crepitus can be mimicked by the presence of permanent suture materials used to repair a previous arthrotomy. Audible 'clicking' of joints during manipulation is not uncommon and does not necessarily indicate significant pathological change. However, 'clicking' of the stifle joint with cruciate pathology may suggest a medial meniscal tear. Crepitus will not be present in incomplete, undisplaced or some avulsion fractures. Thus a fracture should not be ruled out merely on the basis of the absence of crepitus.

Gait examination

A preliminary assessment may have been made while watching the dog walk into the consultation room, but before a detailed physical examination is performed its gait should be observed under more controlled conditions. In all but the smallest dogs this is best accomplished outdoors with the animal on a lead. It should be walked and trotted away and towards the veterinary surgeon on a firm level surface, and should be moved

Chapter 1 An approach to the lame dog or cat

in front of or around the veterinary surgeon to allow assessment of stride length and range of joint movement. Cats and very small dogs are best observed walking around the consulting room.

Supporting leg lameness, loosely defined as a reluctance or inability to place full weight on a limb, is most readily recognized in the thoracic limb as a downward nod of the head as the 'sound' limb is placed to the ground. Lifting of the head as the lame limb strikes the ground is seen in more severe cases. The dog may also show shortening of the stride.

Supporting leg lameness in the pelvic limb is characterized by a 'hiking up' of the gluteal region on the lame side during weightbearing. Bilateral pelvic limb abnormalities tend to result in a 'bunny hopping' gait.

Swinging leg lameness is seen while the affected limb is in flight. It tends to have a more characteristic pattern of movement depending upon the nature of the injury. Thus, hyperflexion and outward rotation of the tarsus, with inward rotation of the foot, is characteristic of gracilis contracture. In the thoracic limb, infraspinatus contracture will cause the foot to swing in a lateral arc during protraction. Neither contracture is painful and the lameness is due to mechanical reasons.

In practice, the majority of lame dogs have a mixed type of lameness. There is generally a degree of reduced weightbearing together with abnormal limb movement due to the animal's reluctance to move painful joints through a full range of motion. Thus, a dog with a painful hip has a shortened stride length due to its reluctance to extend the joint, and it will 'hike up' the ipsilateral gluteal region due to less weightbearing on that joint.

The dog's conformation may have a profound effect on its gait. Animals with medial (varus) or lateral (valgus) deviation of their distal limbs, or those that are knock-kneed (genu valgum) or bow-legged (genu varum) will have gait abnormalities that may be confused with a genuine lameness. For instance, a dog with a valgus deformity of the distal thoracic limb will flick its foot as it protracts the leg. Dogs with painful elbows (as in osteochondrosis for example), will flick their feet in a similar manner. However, the latter group do this since they circumduct their painful elbows rather than fully flexing and extending them. In doing so, there is a compensatory gait abnormality in the distal limb.

It must be remembered that not all limb deviations are due to genetic or traumatic physeal disturbances; some may be the result of articular problems. A good example is the dog with bilateral congenital medial patellar luxation, which often has a bow-legged appearance with internal rotation of the tibiae and medial deviation of its feet.

Gait abnormalities may also result from neurological problems leading to paresis (weakness), ataxia (incoordination), spasticity (stiffness) or hypermetria (often recognized as hyperflexion of the affected limb(s)). These should be distinguished from lameness due to orthopaedic disorders by performing a neurological examination.

The severity and the type of lameness should be recorded following gait analysis. Where an animal is presented unable or unwilling to place weight on a limb then fracture, luxation or severe ligamentous injury should be suspected. It may be necessary to re-question the owner following this part of the examination if a previously unsuspected problem is identified.

Examination of the anaesthetized or sedated animal
The aim should always be to generate as much information as possible from the examination of the dog or cat while it is conscious. However, additional information may be obtained when the part in question is re-examined in the sedated or anaesthetized animal. Additional information may be gained because:

- The joint may be too painful to allow assessment of its true range of movement or the existence of instability
- Some manipulations seem to be uncomfortable *per se* – whether or not the structures being manipulated are abnormal (e.g. the Barden and Ortolani tests – see Chapter 21)
- Muscle tension in the conscious dog may mask instability
- The instability is subtle, e.g. the assessment of cranial cruciate ligament injuries where the degree of cranial draw movement may be slight, as in partial tears of the ligament, or in chronic injuries, where periarticular fibrosis has partially stabilized the joint.

The area suspected of being painful should be examined last as the animal's cooperation will, not unnaturally, tend to lessen thereafter.

Detailed manipulation may be repeated when the animal is sedated or anaesthetized for radiography. This allows the clinician to confirm equivocal findings in the conscious dog and to make a more accurate assessment of joint stability.

Assessment of the nervous system
If neurological involvement is suspected from the gait analysis or initial general clinical examination, then a full neurological examination is indicated (see *BSAVA Manual of Canine and Feline Neurology*). The following procedures should be performed routinely in order to determine whether a more detailed examination is warranted as part of a routine orthopaedic investigation:

- Deep and superficial pain perception is assessed by squeezing the toes or pricking the skin. It is important to look for a response from the patient that indicates pain. In some cases the animal will look around or yelp; in others, the response is more subtle. Withdrawal of the limb in the absence of a cranial response is not evidence of pain perception
- Proprioception is assessed in the supported standing animal by turning the dorsum of the paw on to the ground. The normal response is an immediate return of the paw to a standing position. This assessment is repeated with each foot and it is noted whether the response is immediate, delayed or absent
- Myotatic reflexes are assessed. The patellar, sciatic, cranial tibial and triceps reflexes are the most easily evaluated and should be performed with the animal in lateral recumbency. The limb should be semi-flexed in a horizontal position.

Chapter 1 An approach to the lame dog or cat

The problem list

From the initial database, all the patient's problems are written down to form the initial problem list. Each problem should be defined as closely as possible so that diagnostic or therapeutic plans can be formulated for each one. A problem can be defined as anything that significantly affects the patient's well-being. It may concern either the owner or the clinician and is anything that does or could require treatment. The problem should be defined as closely as possible so that it can be treated with reasonable certainty. The list is not synonymous with a tentative diagnosis and the problem should not be overstated by trying to guess the underlying cause. For example, a problem can be defined as a clinical sign, such as a left pelvic limb lameness, or an abnormal radiographic finding, e.g. a luxated left femoral head.

The initial problem list should be drawn up to include all the problems. It should not be subdivided into major and minor problem lists, since apparently minor problems may turn out to be important once their aetiology is known.

Initial plans

Each problem should be analysed and given a diagnostic plan and/or a therapeutic plan. The possible causes of each problem are listed and the tests proposed to rule them in or rule them out are stated. The most probable causes should be evaluated first and the least probable last.

The specific cause of a clinical sign should only be determined by identifying the problem and determining its underlying disease mechanism. If the condition is life-threatening, e.g. the animal has been hit by a car and has a problem list of dyspnoea, epistaxis and a shear injury of its carpus, then the assessment of the relative importance of each problem is particularly important and suitable priority must be given to each. Constructing lists of problems in order of priority encourages a rapid but logical diagnostic plan, even in an emergency situation.

Further tests

Further tests are frequently required to establish a diagnosis. Once each problem has been investigated, the results should be evaluated to determine whether it requires treatment. Ideally, treatment should not be initiated until specific causes of all the problems have been defined. However, if treatment cannot be delayed, suitable samples should be collected (where possible) so that any outstanding problems can be evaluated at a later date. This information can then be added to the baseline data.

Imaging
Radiography remains the imaging modality most commonly employed (see Chapter 2). Additional imaging techniques include contrast arthrography (see Chapter 2), ultrasonography, computed tomography (CT), magnetic resonance imaging (MRI) (see Chapter 4) and arthroscopy (see Chapter 15).

Imaging has improved dramatically in recent years and the much greater access to advanced modalities such as CT and MRI has enabled previously unidentified pathology to be described. However, it is not always clear what the significance of 'pathology' is. The creation and/or identification of artefacts can be problematic and the interpretation of images requires experience. The clinician should also carefully consider the potential value of such images rather than obtaining them merely because it is possible to do so.

Evaluation of joint fluid
Evaluation of joint fluid is an underemployed technique in animals with joint disease (see Chapter 3). It is especially important when the cause of the disease is in doubt, in cases where multiple joints are involved or where an infective arthritis is suspected (see Chapter 7).

Synovial biopsy
Synovial biopsy may be indicated when a diagnosis of inflammatory arthritis is suspected from the history, physical examination, imaging and synovial fluid analysis, but the definitive diagnosis is lacking. Biopsy may be performed by open arthrotomy or arthroscopically (see Chapter 3).

Progress notes

Follow-up plans, or progress notes, are subsequently written at intervals determined by the nature and severity of the problem. These will be based on the data obtained from the initial plans and on any new information gathered during the management of each problem. Thus, the interpretation of every problem is continuously refined to the highest degree possible, and each problem is viewed in the context of all the others.

The notes may be structured under the headings Subjective, Objective, Assessment and Plan (SOAP). In the strictest form of problem-solving, a SOAP is written down separately for each problem. However, it is not unreasonable to record parameters common to all the problems first, and then deal with each problem separately.

Problems can be deactivated when their cause is known and they no longer require treatment. Problems may also be grouped when it is clear that they have a common cause. In doing this, it is important to be sure that each problem is fully assessed before amalgamating it with others.

Summary

This problem-oriented approach encourages a logical method of thinking. It ensures abnormal findings are not overlooked and the current status of each case is easily determined. Above all else, it offers the most reliable method of reaching an accurate diagnosis.

2

Radiography

Jeremy V. Davies

Introduction

Despite the advent of more complex imaging modalities, radiography remains the major diagnostic aid for most orthopaedic investigations of lameness. This chapter will consider the basic principles of radiographic technique, contrast studies, and special views that might be applied to the investigation of a lame dog or cat. For the most part the techniques for these two species are identical.

Equipment

As most orthopaedic radiography is carried out electively and/or on otherwise healthy patients, general anaesthesia or sedation is usually employed. This allows for accurate and consistent positioning. It also means that slower, high-detail film–screen combinations can be used. For the same reason, low-output X-ray sets are not necessarily a restricting factor. A fine focal spot, however, will improve detail and edge sharpness, and this is unlikely to be available in low-output equipment.

A fine grid (preferably a Potter–Bucky) should be used for any anatomy thicker than 10 cm, e.g. shoulder and pelvis/hip of medium- and large-sized dogs. The converse should be noted: the use of a grid on anatomy less than 10 cm in thickness will compromise image quality.

Rare earth film–screen combinations are standard equipment in veterinary practices. They are available in varying speeds. Relative speed (RS) 400 is standard, e.g. Fuji FG8. For higher-detail extremity imaging RS 100–200 may be preferred, e.g. Fuji FG3 (RS 120) or Fuji FG4 (RS 200). There is also the possibility of using single-side emulsion film with mammography screens, either in a rigid cassette or in a flexible re-usable envelope cassette. This will reduce the RS to about 100. Mammography systems have been popular with equine veterinary surgeons but it is debatable whether a film–screen combination designed for soft tissue/fat differentiation is ideally suited to orthopaedic radiography, although the images are pleasing to the eye and preferred by some. From a theoretical standpoint the author would reserve the use of mammography systems for extremity work in small-breed dogs and cats or for specific soft tissue use, e.g. the identification of foreign material in the pads of the feet.

On those occasions where a debilitated and therefore conscious patient needs to be radiographed, e.g. the dyspnoeic road traffic accident case, faster film–screen combinations (RS at least 400) are preferred so that short exposure times can be achieved.

There are few orthopaedic indications for diagnostic fluoroscopy but intraoperative image intensification systems can facilitate implant placement. Whilst this is common practice in human orthopaedic theatres, it is seldom used in veterinary surgery; the shape and size of the patients may be the major limiting factor.

Plain radiography

Vertical beam radiography, with or without a grid, is the predominant procedure. Occasionally, oblique or lesion-orientated views may be helpful. Horizontal beam views may be required to achieve useful caudocranial/craniocaudal (CdCr/CrCd) views of the femur and humerus if distorted by injury. In order to employ horizontal beams, an X-ray set with a tube suspension or stand that will allow the head to be lowered to tabletop level and rotated through 90 degrees is necessary (Figure 2.1). There are significant radiation safety implications: the horizontal beam will have to be directed at a suitable attenuating structure and personnel are required to be positioned appropriately and

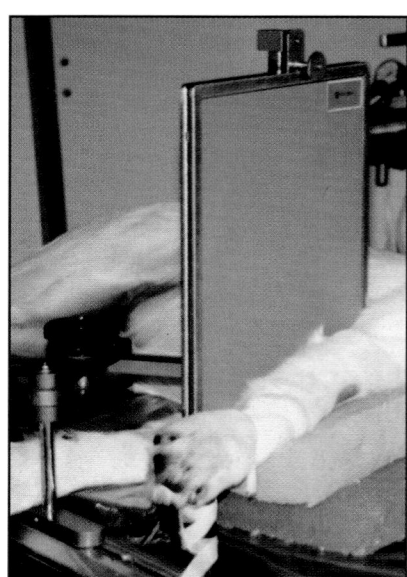

2.1 Horizontal beam views must take account of the path of the primary beam and utilize cassette-holding devices.

protected so as not to be exposed. The use of horizontal beams should only be authorized with the involvement of an approved radiation safety adviser (in the UK, the Radiation Protection Adviser).

Exposure factors should be selected to provide fine detail/good edge sharpness and minimal scatter. Selecting kVp settings that maximize the photoelectric effect is ideal for orthopaedic radiography. This means selecting kVp settings that are as low as possible but still afford adequate penetration of the subject area. Settings in the 50–75 kVp range are ideal. Edge sharpness is influenced by the penumbra effect. This can be reduced by using longer focus–film distances; ideally, 100 cm is selected. Small/fine focal spot settings will also improve sharpness. The object–film distance (OFD) also influences sharpness and should be kept to a minimum. It should be noted that as the OFD increases the image will be magnified; this could be important when using radiographs to measure lesions or select implants.

Contrast radiography

In the limbs, contrast radiography will be confined to arthrography, tendon sheath studies, sinography/fistulography, angiography and lymphangiography. Lameness may stem from spinal diseases that might be investigated using other contrast techniques (see Chapter 10).

Arthrography
Arthrography depends on the clinician's ability to penetrate the joint space accurately and deliver sufficient quantity of contrast medium to provide a useful image. In dogs and cats this is almost exclusively restricted to the shoulder joint and associated biceps tendon sheath. Contrast studies of other joints may be restricted to an assessment of the integrity of the synovial capsule and little else. Arthrographic studies require iodinated contrast media with a concentration of iodine of approximately 150 mg/ml. The media may be ionic or non-ionic; the latter are more expensive but arguably less irritant. It is possible to consider imaging the joint distended with air or using double contrast. For double contrast studies positive contrast medium previously instilled for an arthrogram is removed and the joint re-distended with air; any residual opaque contrast medium may highlight surface irregularities obscured by the positive arthrogram.

Sinography/fistulography
Sinography/fistulography also employs iodinated contrast agents. Cheaper ionic media are satisfactory and concentrations of iodine of approximately 200 mg/ml are appropriate.

Angiography and lymphangiography
Vascular studies may be useful when ischaemic or thrombotic injuries require investigation. In dogs and cats this will most often relate to the possible viability of a limb, e.g. following a road traffic accident. In cats, arterial studies may also be helpful in assessing the extent of thromboembolic disease.

Direct lymphangiography is a challenging procedure requiring the cannulation of a small lymphatic vessel in the distal limb and the administration of appropriate contrast medium. Indirect lymphangiography is less challenging and surprisingly effective. Large molecule (almost particulate) media are ideal. Ionic media, especially if they are dimers, are best. The agent (5–10 ml) is injected as an intra/subdermal bleb over the dorsum of the foot and immediately massaged to encourage its dispersal. Within seconds, the lymphatic tree and the local nodes from the distal limb to axilla or groin are highlighted.

Indications for skeletal (limb/joint) radiography

The indications for limb and joint radiography are listed in Figure 2.2.

Fractures: pre- and postoperative assessment
Acute or chronic lameness
Skeletal pain
Joint pain
Swelling around bones or joints
Limb deformity
Metabolic bone disease
Monitoring of inherited disorders
Evaluation of systemic disease that may affect bones or joints

2.2 Indications for limb and joint radiography.

Radiographic projections

At least two views at right angles are essential, and standard positioning will assist interpretation. In cases of fractures, the joint above and below the fracture must be included. The beam should be accurately centred and tightly collimated.

The following projections are generally used:

- Lateromedial (LM) (or mediolateral (ML))
- Craniocaudal (CrCd) (or caudocranial (CdCr)) – proximal to carpus and tarsus
- Dorsopalmar (DPa) or dorsoplantar (DPl) – distal to carpus and tarsus
- Skyline views may be employed as necessary
- Stressed views and weightbearing views may be used when examining ligamentous injuries, particularly when joint instability is suspected.

It is not within the remit of this chapter to discuss the routine projections used in limb radiography (see *BSAVA Manual of Canine and Feline Musculoskeletal Imaging*). However, it is pertinent to cover some aspects of safety, positioning aids and special views.

Radiation safety
Currently in the UK, veterinary radiography is carried out under the Ionising Radiation Regulations, 1999. These have been in force since January 2000. It

Chapter 2 Radiography

behoves each radiation employer (user) to appoint a Radiation Protection Adviser (RPA) to draw up Local Rules and Written Arrangements for each place of work. Under current legislation the RPA must be properly certificated from January 2005 onwards.

It should rarely be necessary to consider manual restraint of small animals for orthopaedic radiography. Despite this, it is essential that personal protective equipment (PPE) is available for such occurrences. These should include a minimum of two sets of PPE, consisting of gowns/aprons with a minimum lead equivalence (LE) of 0.25 mm and hand protectors with a minimum LE of 0.5 mm. The use of other PPE, e.g. thyroid shields, is at the discretion of the RPA. All those persons that work within the Controlled Area must be adequately trained and carry a personal dosemeter. Dosimetry is usually by way of a film badge or thermoluminescent dosemeter.

To facilitate positioning animals without the need for manual restraint, a number of positioning aids are essential. These are listed in Figure 2.3.

Table-top positioning pad
Lucent foam wedges and shapes
Long washable ties (e.g. football boot laces, calving ropes)
Floppy sandbags
Rigid positioning cradles

2.3 Positioning aids for radiography of dogs and cats.

Special views

There are a number of special views of the limbs that bear more detailed explanation.

Scapula: fractures

Because of superimposition shadows it can be difficult to demonstrate some scapular fractures. The standard lateral view aims to expose the scapula closest to the table/film, with the limb extended and the opposite limb retracted caudally. It can sometimes be worth deliberately reversing this situation, superimposing the scapula over the ribs/lungs. The air contrast in the lungs may enhance interruptions in the bony outline of the scapula (Figure 2.4).

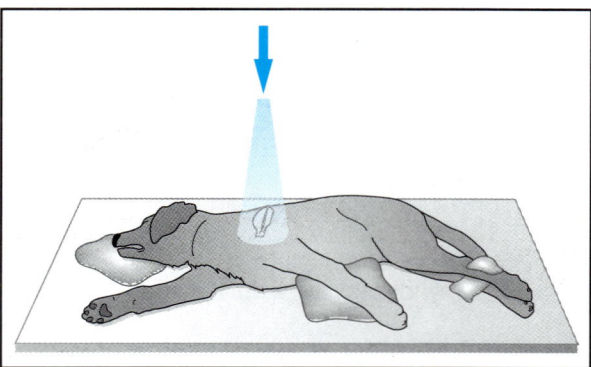

2.4 Positioning to project the uppermost scapula over the cranial thorax in an attempt to reveal occult scapular fractures.

Shoulder: skyline view of the intertubercular groove

Osteophytic reactions in the intertubercular groove may irritate the biceps tendon sheath. A skyline view may highlight such changes (Figure 2.5). It is also worth considering using this view once a shoulder/biceps tendon sheath arthrogram has been performed, as it may give further evidence of the state of the biceps tendon itself.

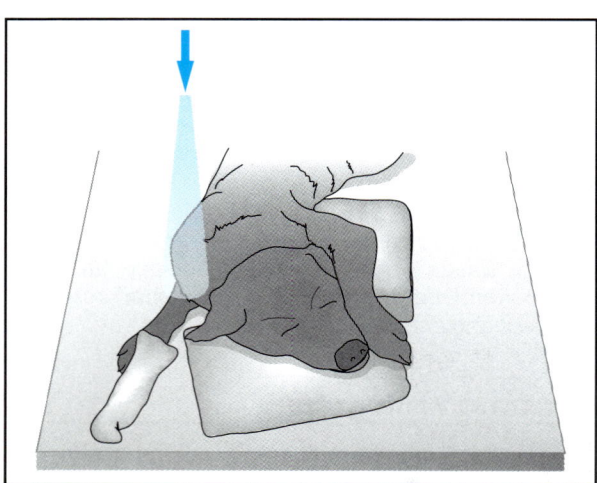

2.5 Positioning for a skyline view of the intertubercular (biceps) groove of the humerus, used to highlight osteophytes.

Humerus: horizontal beam view

Once the humerus has been fractured, particularly in the mid diaphysis to elbow segment, it can be difficult to extend the limb sufficiently to take CdCr/CrCd views. With the animal in lateral recumbency and the affected limb uppermost a horizontal beam view may overcome this problem.

Elbow

Flexed lateral view: This is not really a special view but rotational artefacts are common. Because the elbow is wider than the carpus, any restraining weight applied to the carpus will rotate the elbow. This can lead to overinterpretation of joint incongruity. Rotation can be minimized by use of a foam wedge (Figure 2.6).

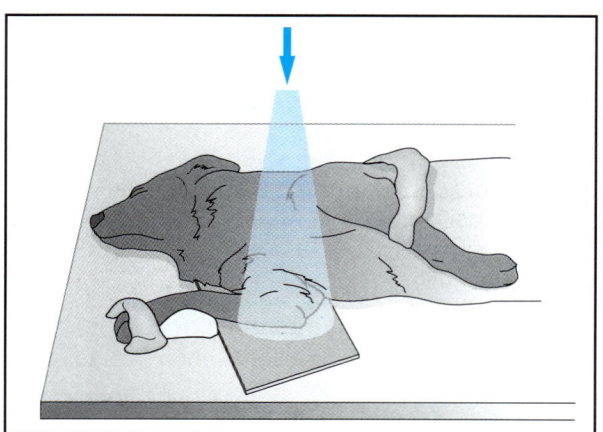

2.6 Positioning for flexed lateral elbow view. The carpus is elevated on a foam wedge to minimize rotation at the elbow.

Chapter 2 Radiography

CdCr/CrCd: This view is universally challenging and it is worth enumerating some practical tips that can improve technique. As there are at least five ways of achieving this projection it may be worth trying alternatives in an individual where the preferred technique seems to be failing (Figure 2.7).

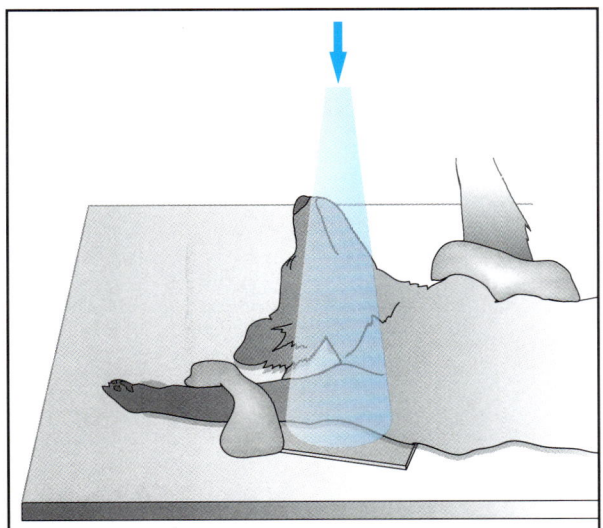

2.7 Positioning for 'frontal' view of the elbow with the dog in dorsal recumbency.

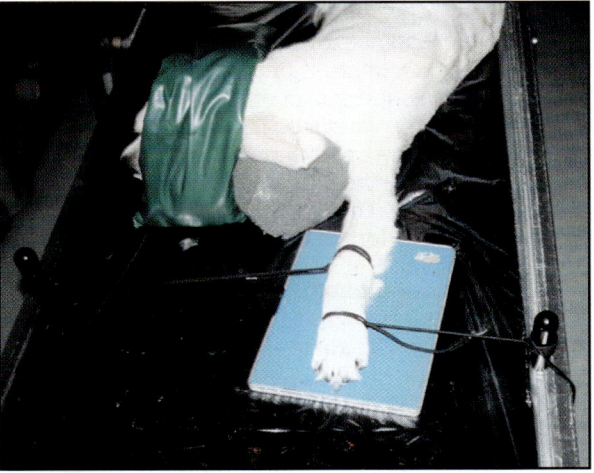

2.8 Positioning for stressed view of the carpus, using ties to avoid exposure of personnel.

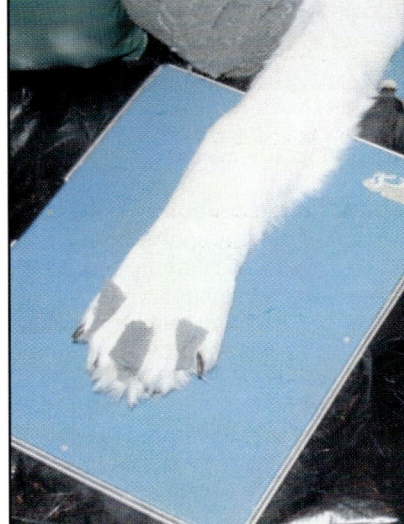

2.9 Positioning for dorsopalmar projection of the foot, with the toes separated by radiolucent foam.

Despite concentrating on the position of the elbow for this projection, gentle rotation of the caudal part of the animal may bring about the fine adjustment needed to position the elbow accurately. Where elbow fractures have resulted in some overriding or shortening, horizontal beam views in CrCd projection may be helpful. The author prefers the CdCr view with the animal in dorsal recumbency and the limb drawn cranially. Others may prefer the other options, i.e. CrCd in dorsal recumbency or CdCr/CrCd in sternal recumbency. In differently shaped animals, e.g. deep-chested or barrel-chested breeds, trying alternatives may provide the ideal image.

Carpus: stressed views
Ligamentous injuries to the carpus may disrupt intercarpal and collateral ligaments with no bony change and minimal soft tissue swelling. Stressed views will demonstrate the presence and location of any instability (Figure 2.8). These views are challenging in an environment where manual restraint is prohibited.

Digits: dorsopalmar/dorsoplantar views
Superimposition of surface debris and close proximity of adjacent digits can make interpretation difficult. Meticulous foot cleaning prior to radiography and spreading the digits with lucent foam improves images considerably (Figure 2.9).

Pelvis/hip

Dorsal acetabular rim view: The information gleaned from this view (Figure 2.10) is questionable. It may give some idea of 'femoral head coverage'. This may be of

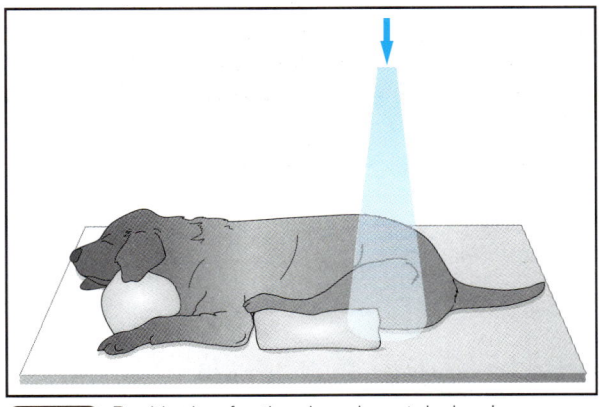

2.10 Positioning for the dorsal acetabular rim projection.

diagnostic benefit when deciding whether procedures such as triple pelvic osteotomy (TPO) might be of benefit and, thereafter, assessing the postoperative outcome of the procedure.

Chapter 2 Radiography

Distraction views for the assessment of hip dysplasia: Existing schemes for assessing hip dysplasia are based on a static impression of hip conformation. As joint laxity is an important component of hip dysplasia a dynamic study would be preferable. A real-time assessment is unrealistic and so a technique that attempts to demonstrate maximal subluxation might have added value. The Penn Hip Scheme (see Chapter 21) seeks to address this weakness.

Femur: horizontal beam view
A horizontal beam view can be helpful when investigating shaft fractures, as for the humerus and elbow (see above) (Figure 2.11).

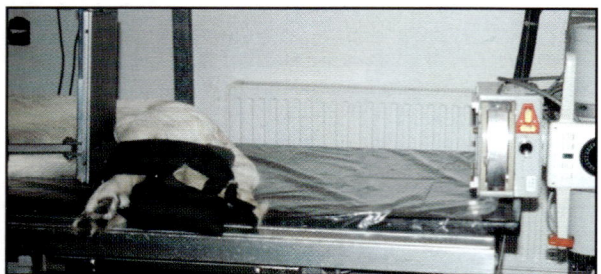

2.11 Horizontal beam view for imaging comminuted femoral fractures in a CdCr projection. A similar arrangement can be used for the humerus (see Figure 2.1).

Stifle: 'tibial plateau levelling osteotomy' views
The current trend in cruciate ligament surgery is to assess the tibial plateau angle and if appropriate alter it using a tibial plateau levelling osteotomy. Properly collimated stifle views may be diagnostic for cranial cruciate ligament damage but will not allow an accurate measurement of tibial plateau angle. For this, a long axis must be plotted through the length of the tibia against which the angle can be measured. This necessitates an exposure to include both the distal femur and the talocrural joint (Figure 2.12). Maintaining true mediolateral alignment becomes challenging. The optimal image will superimpose both femoral condyles accurately whilst allowing the long axis to be plotted.

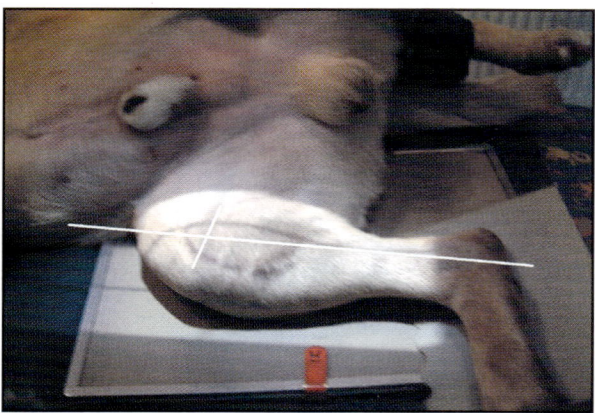

2.12 Tibial plateau angle measurements are made from reference points in the stifle and tarsus, which have to be exposed on the same cassette. The beam is centred on the stifle joint and the collimator opened to include the talocrural joint. The white lines show the long axis of the tibia and the tibial plateau axis, from which the plateau angle can be measured.

Tarsus
Ideally, plantarodorsal (PlD) views are preferred (Figure 2.13) but some workers will attempt the reverse, often as part of a ventrodorsal pelvis study. The dorsoplantar (DPl) projection tends to 'angle' the calcaneus across the joint, obscuring some important parts of the joint surfaces.

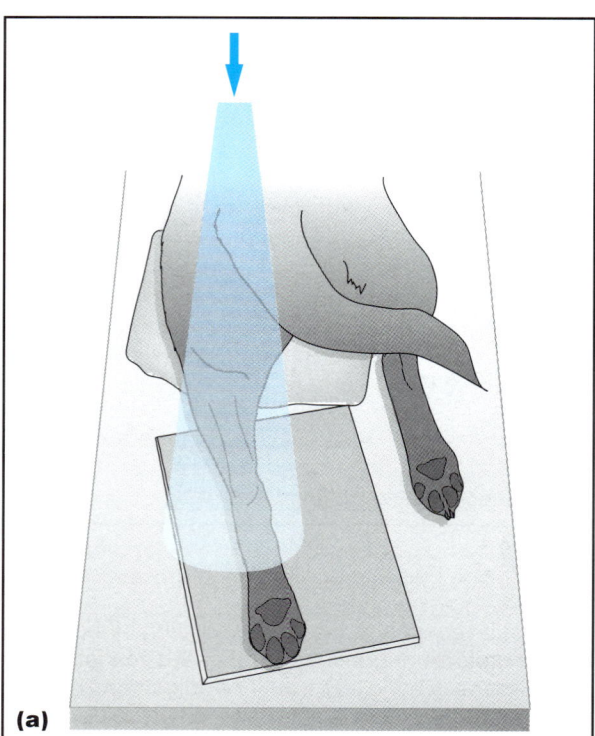

(a)

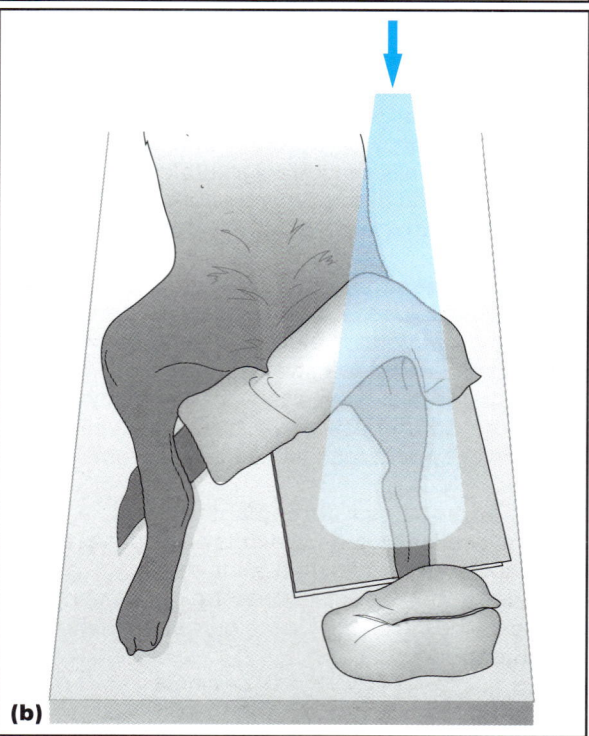

(b)

2.13 **(a)** The preferred projection for the tarsus is plantarodorsal (PlD). **(b)** The reverse projection (DPl) may superimpose the calcaneus obliquely across the joint.

12

Basic principles of interpretation

Viewing radiographs
The most perfectly exposed radiograph in the hands of the most experienced radiologist may well be interpreted poorly if the circumstances for viewing the film are substandard.

Viewing room
The ideal viewing room is quiet, warm and undisturbed. It should be able to be blacked out completely and there should be variable low-intensity illumination within the room. It is not a good idea to try and make use of the processing darkroom as a viewing room, as the potential sources of water and chemicals might spoil prepared films, and the chemical and fume hazards are unacceptable. A darkened room allows the eyes to become accustomed to the relatively low light intensity that is transmitted through the film and overcomes the effects of reflected light from the surface of the film. Ideally, the viewer should be able to sit at a desk or bench so that the films can be sorted into order and, if possible, displayed on a number of adjacent viewing boxes. A magnifying glass or goggles may be useful for examination of small details.

The film
Clinical decisions should, whenever possible, be made after examining a *dried* film. The increasing use of automatic processors ensures this. The film should be exposed, positioned and processed to a satisfactory standard; repeat films, altering the exposures or the positioning, may have to be made before a final opinion can be given.

Viewing boxes
Multiple viewing boxes are almost a prerequisite in orthopaedic radiography as multiple views are often typical of an orthopaedic radiographic investigation. The viewing boxes do not need to have variable light intensities; this is an expensive additional feature that often fails and is of little added benefit. The front screen of the viewing box should be made of even-surfaced opalescent plastic and should be clean and unscratched. The translucency of viewing boxes from different manufacturers may differ slightly and this can be disturbing when comparing films. The fluorescent tubes in the viewing box are also important: they should be of the same wattage and colour. Different colour tubes are available: 'Tropical Daylight' is the colour of choice.

> **WARNING**
> It is tempting to buy cheap models or even to attempt to self-build viewing boxes – this is, without doubt, a false economy.

Bright light source
It is sometimes necessary to examine a small part of a film under high-intensity light. To this end a 'bright light' is valuable. An angle-poise lamp will suffice but is poor in comparison to a proper high-intensity viewer. The heat from a domestic spotlight can damage the film. High-intensity lights incorporated into the viewing box are generally less useful than a separate unit. Such a light source will compensate for areas of the film that are relatively overexposed; they will not enhance an underexposed part of the film. They will also focus the attention to a small part of the subject whilst masking the rest of the film from vision.

Magnifying glass/goggles
A simple magnifying glass can be useful for examining small structures. The principles of lens use should be remembered. The lens should be held close to the eye and then one's head position adjusted to the focal length of the lens. Illustrations of the Sherlock Holmes' method of magnifying lens use are misleading! Magnifying goggles can also be used. These have the added advantage of collimating the field of vision to a small area of interest.

Problems associated with collimation
The safety constraints of modern radiographic practice dictate collimation of the beam to the smallest area possible. This will improve image sharpness but is counterproductive as far as viewing is concerned. For this reason it is necessary to have some dark card available so that a film can be masked off if necessary (Figure 2.14). Turning off adjacent viewing boxes when studying a particular film will also help, as will wearing viewing goggles (see above). Viewing boxes with adjustable shutters will assist masking but are usually very expensive and heavy.

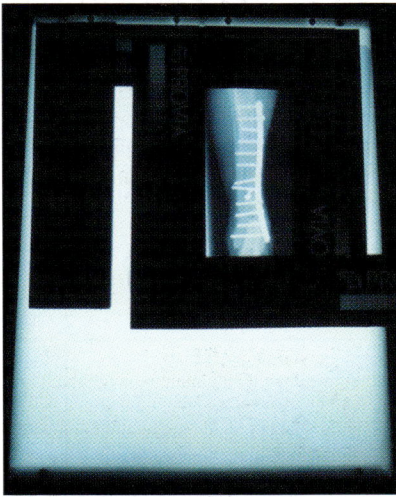

2.14 Collimating cards/strips for obliterating distracting white light from the viewer.

Reference sources
When viewing films it is often necessary to refer to both anatomical and clinical texts, so the ideal viewing room should have a small library immediately to hand. Of particular use are a standard anatomical text and a radiographic atlas of normal images. The practice can slowly generate a set of normal films for comparison.

Anatomical specimens
A set of anatomical specimens (Figure 2.15) is invaluable when considering radiographs, especially those taken at unusual degrees of obliquity. The availability of bone specimens to most practitioners should pose no problem.

Chapter 2 Radiography

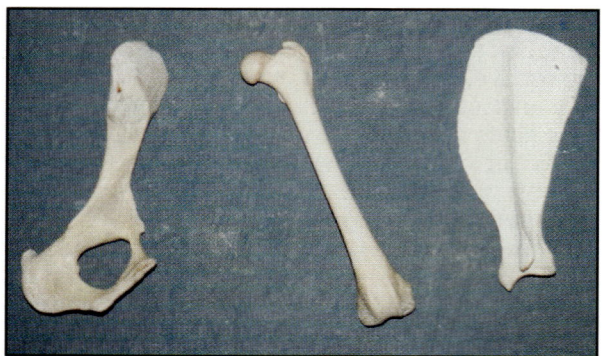

2.15 Anatomical specimens for reference when reporting films.

Reading the radiograph

Having considered all the above the viewer is ready to evaluate the film. Before this evaluation is undertaken it is important to consider the quality of the film. Technical faults can lead to erroneous diagnosis so note must be made of these at the outset. It would be wrong to arrive at a diagnosis of osteoporosis because the radiopacity of the bones on the film seemed diminished, when all that had happened was overexposure and/or overdevelopment of the film.

The full-time radiologist will usually be asked to study a film or films with little or no previous knowledge of the case. This overcomes the problem of only making observations that coincide with possibly ill-conceived clinical judgements. In veterinary medicine, even in larger practices or veterinary schools, the 'radiologist' often has 'prior knowledge' and in general practice the clinician, radiographer and radiologist are probably one and the same person. For this reason it is essential that a systematic approach is adopted for the evaluation of each film.

Each individual will develop his or her own protocol and, it is hoped, follow this consistently. The film can be viewed *geometrically*: the surface of the film can be scanned from the centre to the periphery or *vice versa*. A rectilinear scan, much as is used for viewing a blood smear, can also be used. Alternatively, the film can be viewed *anatomically;* this is the author's preferred method. The anatomical components of the film can be listed and considered one by one. For instance, if a lateral view of the antebrachium were being evaluated a protocol such as this might be adopted:

- General appearance of the limb (shape, position, etc.)
- Bones: shape, length, mineralization, trabecular pattern
- Joints: elbow, carpal, metacarpophalangeal, proximal interphalangeal, distal interphalangeal joints
- Soft tissues: skin, tendons, ligaments, joint capsules
- Miscellaneous: foreign bodies, gas shadows, contrast study if used.

For each anatomical structure a general system of radiological interpretation can be followed. Such lists appear in all textbooks of radiology and may be modified to personal taste.

Reporting the radiograph

Each film should be viewed and a report constructed following a specified format. This may be a mental exercise in most cases but it is important to adopt a regular protocol. The radiologist or primary clinician may be called upon to report films for a colleague or may be called as an expert in a legal or insurance dispute. Following such a protocol should ensure that all aspects of the film report have been covered. An example is given in Figure 2.16.

Step	Comments
1. Species, breed/type, sex, age, patient identification	These parameters will influence the differential list
2. Radiographic projections used, contrast studies undertaken with each film identified by its markings – date, time, contrast sequence, left/right etc.	Orthopaedic radiology often relies on sequential information so careful collation of films is essential
3. Radiographic quality	If there are defects in the quality of the film this may influence the observer's ability to make a diagnosis or could even create misleading results
4. Description of radiographic or Roentgen signs	Only descriptive terms such as the nomenclature illustrated in Figures 2.17 and 2.18 should be used. Diagnostic terms should be reserved for the conclusion/diagnosis section. E.g. a bone that shows a decrease in radiopacity could be described as radiolucent, transradiant or of decreased radiopacity or osteopenic. It is not appropriate to describe it as osteolysis, osteoporosis or osteoclastic neoplasia. This approach may seem pedantic but understanding the nature of the bone changes as a pathological process will increase the accuracy of the diagnostic conclusion
5. Conclusion	Based on the above description
6. Diagnosis/differential probability list	
7. Suggestions for further investigations	Radiographic, surgical, samples, etc.

2.16 Protocol for reporting a radiograph.

Basic radiological interpretation

It is tempting to view skeletal radiographs with an eye for the bony tissues only. Soft tissue changes may be important and may often modify the approach that needs to be adopted in the repair of the skeletal damage. The film should be considered for *all* the photographic evidence presented (Figure 2.17), not just the exciting fracture that might be obvious! A sound knowledge of radiographic anatomy and normal variants is an essential prerequisite. An algorithmic approach is advisable – a logical and sequential method of analysing a problem.

There are five radiographic opacities that may be discerned on radiographs. These are:

- Air/gas
- Fat
- Fluid or soft tissue
- Bone
- Mineral.

A radiograph shows not only the outline of an organ but also other body structures superimposed on it. The final image is a composite shadow of all structures through which radiation has passed. As the radiograph is a two-dimensional image of a three-dimensional structure, two views at 90 degrees must be taken for evaluation. More complex anatomical entities may require oblique views. Geometric rules apply in the formation of the radiograph. Magnification and distortion must be kept to a minimum. Consequently, the area of interest should be placed close to the film cassette and at a standard focal film distance. Radiographic technique must be standardized in order to ensure that the final radiograph is produced in a consistently standard manner and consequently produces a diagnostic image. Optical artefacts, inadequate care with radiographic technique and film processing, together with the fault of over-reading radiographs as a result of clinical bias, are just some of the contributory causes to inaccurate radiographic diagnosis.

The method of radiographic interpretation must incorporate the discipline of examining the whole radiograph. The various methods have already been described, i.e. reading the radiograph from the edges to the centre, from left to right or via the body systems. It is probably irrelevant as to which method is adopted provided that the method used is consistent.

An important first step is to place the films on the viewer in a standard manner, i.e. all lateral radiographs should be placed with the head or cranial aspect directed towards the left side of the viewer and all VD, DV, CrCd or CdCr studies should be interpreted with the right side of the animal on the left side of the screen and the head to the top. Limbs are positioned with the proximal parts to the top of the screen.

Radiographic nomenclature

Anatomical and radiological nomenclature, like units of measurement, has undergone many transformations during the last 20–30 years. The purpose of the modifications has been to simplify and standardize terminology. For those who have worked through these years at school, university and in practice it has been, to say the least, confusing. This section will explain the nomenclature as it was agreed by the American College of Veterinary Radiology in 1983 and published by Smallwood *et al.* (1985). An attempt will be made to correlate the 'new' terms with some of the older terminologies. Much of the early radiological and anatomical terminology was adapted from human texts. Terms such as anterior and posterior and superior and inferior were used with obvious potential to confuse. *Nomina Anatomica Veterinaria* (NAV) (Habel *et al.*, 1983) overcame these inaccuracies for veterinary anatomists but did not address the special needs of veterinary radiologists. At this stage cranial and caudal, dorsal and ventral became the norm and anterior and posterior, superior and inferior were dismissed:

Sign	Example
Size	The radius may be *shortened* in premature growth plate closure
Shape and contour	The distal radial metaphysis may *expand* and *lose its contour* if an osteosarcoma is present
Position	The radial head may be *displaced* in a Monteggia fracture
Radiopacity	The *mineralization* of all the bones in the skeleton may *diminish* in cases of hyperparathyroidism or soft tissues may *calcify* in response to the injection of depot steroids
Number	In cases of polydactyly *additional* bones may be present
Internal architecture/structure	The delicate *patterning* of long bones may be disturbed in cases of neoplasia or panosteitis
Foreign/abnormal material	May be present as a pathological finding but could be just the result of poor patient preparation
Function	It may not be possible to evaluate this except in fluoroscopic or contrast studies but if a flexed elbow radiograph shows a reduction in the degree of flexion it implies reduced elbow function
Progress of disease	Very subtle changes may be difficult to interpret but whether or not they progress or alter over a predetermined timescale may give further evidence to their origin and significance. This would be especially true in the conundrum that exists between osteomyelitis and bone neoplasia in the early stages

2.17 'Roentgen signs'. These possible changes may affect each anatomical structure.

Chapter 2 Radiography

- Cranial and caudal apply to the neck, trunk, tail and limbs proximal to the antebrachiocarpal (carpal or 'knee') and talocrural (tibiotarsal or 'hock') joints
- On the head, cranial is replaced by rostral
- In the thoracic limb distal to the antebrachiocarpal joint, cranial is replaced by dorsal and caudal is replaced by palmar
- In the pelvic limb distal to the talocrural joint, cranial is replaced by dorsal and caudal is replaced by plantar.

Occasionally, terminology used in human anatomy has been retained in veterinary descriptions of the head e.g. the superior maxillary sinus, the posterior clinoid process, but there seems little good reason for this.

Special terminology for radiology includes information as to the direction of the primary beam. For instance, a lateral view of the carpus would look much the same if taken from the medial or lateral aspect of the joint. However, it is usually more convenient in the standing horse to carry out a lateromedial (LM) view and in the recumbent dog a mediolateral (ML) view; thus, the terminology will enable the reader to understand exactly how the radiography was performed. When oblique views are considered, the information regarding the direction of the beam may be more important and the same principle must be adopted. Previously, nomenclature such as lateral oblique has been used; with the carpus, for example, this usually implied an oblique view of the carpus with the X-ray tube positioned cranial and lateral to the limb. This might then have been described as an APLMO or latterly a DPaLMO. Still, there is no indication of the direction of the beam. The current protocol would designate this view a DL-PaMO (dorsolateral to palmaromedial oblique).

The angle of obliquity is also of importance in some instances and can be added if the writer feels it necessary. The degrees of obliquity are inserted with reference to the movements of the tube head from the start position. Further information as to the position of the patient or its anatomy may be added, e.g. standing, erect, flexed and the direction of the beam (horizontal) if this deviates from the expected.

The following terms might be used:

- **Directional:** left (L) and right (R), dorsal (D) and ventral (V), cranial (Cr) and caudal (Cd), rostral (R) and caudal (Cd), medial (M) and lateral (L), proximal (Pr) and distal (Di), palmar (Pa) and Plantar (Pl), oblique (O)
- **Positional:** standing and recumbent, erect, flexed, open mouth, tilted with degrees of tilt (e.g. in myelography)
- **Radiographic:** horizontal (beam), intraoral (probably non–screen film), time (if part of a sequence, e.g. in a contrast study).

Construction of the radiographic description

This will involve a combination of all the terminology mentioned. Rules have been suggested for the systematic combination of these terms:

- Right and left are *not* used in combination and precede all other terms
- Medial and lateral are subservient when used in conjunction with other terms, e.g. dorsolateral, ventromedial, etc.
- On the head, neck, trunk and tail rostral, cranial and caudal take precedence, e.g. caudodorsal, rostroventral
- On the limbs, dorsal, palmar, plantar, cranial and caudal take precedence, e.g. palmarodistal, dorsodistal
- In bipartite terms the elements are not separated by a hyphen to denote point of entry and exit of the beam, i.e. dorsoventral (DV)
- In multipartite terms the point of entry and exit descriptions are separated by a hyphen, i.e. dorsolateral-palmaromedial oblique (DL-PaMO).

A glossary of terms is given in Figure 2.18.

Term	Meaning
Opacity/density	Density has been used for many years as the descriptive term denoting the degree of black or white on a film and refers to the amount of light transmitted through the film from a viewing box. This refers to optical density and is not to be confused with the structure's anatomical density. Because of this opacity is now preferred
Increased opacity	Denotes a lighter or whiter shadow on the X-ray film, as produced by substances of greater physical density or thickness
Decreased opacity	Denotes a darker or blacker shadow on the X-ray film. It is produced by substances of lower physical density or slight thickness
Increased radiolucency (hyperlucency, increased transradiancy)	Implies greater penetrability by the X-rays and has the same connotation as decreased opacity
Increased radiopacity	Implies diminished penetrability by the X-rays and has the same connotation as increased opacity
Laterality	In describing the laterality of the patient relative to the X-ray beam, one always names the lateral or oblique projection according to the side of the patient closer to the film. Thus a right lateral film is one taken with the right side of the patient next to the film. A left lateral is the reverse. Recumbency indicates that the animal is lying down when the film is taken. The animal may be either supine (on its back – ventrodorsal) or prone (on its abdomen – dorsoventral). The beam in these cases is vertical with respect to the patient

2.18 Glossary of terms with special radiological usage. (continues) ▶

Term	Meaning
Decubitus films	The animal is in the decubitus position when lying on either side while a ventrodorsal or dorsoventral film is taken. The beam in these cases is always horizontal. Thus, right lateral decubitus means that the left side of the patient is uppermost. Left lateral decubitus is the reverse. A more accurate terminology is desirable as follows: • Horizontal beam study, ventrodorsal, with the patient in right (or left) lateral recumbency • Horizontal beam study, dorsoventral, with the patient in right (or left) lateral recumbency • Horizontal beam study, with patient supine (or prone) and right (or left) side nearest film
Erect position	In this position the patient or the anatomical part is upright and the beam is horizontal
Filling defect	A space-occupying mass within a hollow organ especially with reference to contrast studies
Nidus/niche	In the wall of a hollow organ a recess that tends to retain contrast media. This term usually implies ulceration: the recess has a broad, wide neck fusing imperceptibly with the contour of the lumen of the organ, whereas a diverticulum has a narrow neck
Fluid level	The interface between fluid and air; it always assumes a horizontal appearance. The air above the fluid level is of diminished opacity, while the fluid itself is of intermediate opacity. This will only be appreciated with horizontal beam views
Bone sclerosis	An increase in the anatomical density of bone so that its radiographic appearance is much whiter than normal. Veterinary radiologists may use this term loosely for any increase in bone whitening. It may be important diagnostically to differentiate between true bone hardening and periosteal deposition on the surface of the bone. Both processes might have a 'sclerotic' appearance but have quite different diagnostic implications
Eburnation of bone	Wearing away of bone that usually provokes a hardening of the bearing surface leading to true sclerosis
Osteopenia	A descriptive yet non-diagnostic term for loss of mineral opacity within a bone. It does not indicate the type of disease bringing about that change
Osteoporosis	A pathological state in which there is a diminished number of ossified trabeculae, so that the bone appears more radiolucent. The trabeculae that remain are normal bone
Osteomalacia	A pathological state characterized by diminished bone density due to loss of bone mineral content. The protein content of the bone is less impaired or may not be impaired at all
New bone	Any deposition of bone that has been superimposed on normal anatomy at any site for any reason
Osteophyte	A small sharp projection of new bone often near a joint, sometimes referred to as spurs
Enthesophyte	A small sharp projection of bone arising at the point of origin or insertion of a tendon or ligament. These will mostly be periarticular and will follow the expected line of the soft tissue attachment
Hyperlucency of bone	A radiographic appearance of either osteoporotic or osteomalacic bone. This term should be used in the description of the radiographs unless the true pathological state is known
Lipping	A small osteophyte formation on the margins of the articular surfaces of bones. This is also called bony spur formation, although the latter term is commonly reserved for non-articular bone
Artefacts	Changes on the film which do not have an anatomical basis directly related to the part being radiographed but are introduced by some technical fault, such as dirt in the cassette or static electrical charge. Occasionally artefacts are introduced by collars, leads etc., immobilization devices or even hair braids projected over the part
Plain films/'scout' films	Films taken before a contrast study
Comparison films	Films taken of the side opposite to the one in question for comparison with the suspected abnormal side. These are very useful, particularly when the skeleton is immature, and should be taken whenever possible
Serial films	Films taken in sequence, either during a single study or after longer intervals of time, such as days or weeks
Normal variant	Recognized, occasional deviations from 'normal' anatomy that are of no clinical significance. These are often bilaterally symmetrical and so radiography of the contralateral limb may help establish the presence of such a variant

2.18 (continued) Glossary of terms with special radiological usage.

Interpretation of limb radiographs

A radiological assessment of the limbs in cases of lameness needs to follow a careful protocol.

Soft tissues
Potential changes in the soft tissues are summarized in Figure 2.19.

Change in size (mass)	
Increase	Any space-occupying lesion (neoplasm, haematoma, cellulitis)
Decrease	Muscle atrophy

2.19 Potential soft tissue changes. (continues) ▶

Chapter 2 Radiography

Change in density	
Gas	Post-surgical emphysema Penetrating wounds, open fractures Gas-forming bacterial cellulitis (uncommon in small animals, more likely in horses and farm animals)
Fat	Lipoma/liposarcoma Extruded fat from fractured medullary cavity
Radiopaque foreign material	Pellet or glass (lead content) Debris in hair coat Stray contrast medium on animal or equipment
Change in position	
• Fascial plane displacement (stifle effusion causes caudal displacement of a linear fat shadow that runs proximodistally in the line of the fabellae) • Soft tissue mass effect (displaces adjacent structures, e.g. popliteal lymphadenopathy shows well as surrounded by fat)	

2.19 (continued) Potential soft tissue changes.

Joints

Joints may be divided into:

- Diarthroses (those where a joint cavity is present)
- Synarthroses (those with no joint cavity):
    - Syndesmoses – bones are united by dense fibrous tissue, e.g. cranium, proximal and distal tibia and fibula, radius and ulna
    - Synchondroses – bones are united by hyaline cartilage (epiphyses and sternebrae)
    - Synostoses – united by connective tissue and bone as a result of ageing (old syndesmoses)
    - Symphyses – bones united by cartilage, fibrocartilage and fibrous connective tissue (intervertebral discs, pubic symphysis and mandibular symphysis).

Diarthroses allow the greatest range of movement and include all the appendicular joints, the articular facets of the vertebrae, the sacroiliac joints and the joints of the ribs with the thoracic vertebrae.

The signs of joint disease are listed in Figure 2.20, and types of joint disease are listed in Figure 2.21.

Increased synovial mass
Altered joint space
Subchondral osteolysis
Subchondral osteosclerosis
Subchondral bone cyst
Perichondral osteolysis
Perichondral bone proliferation
Mineralization of joint soft tissues
Joint mice – isolated and/or free bodies
Joint displacement
Joint malformation

2.20 Radiographic signs of joint disease.

Serous arthritis or synovitis
Osteoarthritis
Traumatic
Septic – haematogenous/direct penetration
Aseptic inflammatory (erosive/non-erosive)
Neoplastic (synovioma, synovial sarcoma)
Luxation/subluxation
Hypervitaminosis A
Mucopolysaccharidosis in Siamese cats
Craniomandibular osteopathy
Calcinosis circumscripta
Synovial osteochondromatosis in cats

2.21 Types of joint disease.

Abnormal alignment

Abnormal alignment of joints may be luxations or subluxations; those with a concomitant fracture are termed fracture luxations/subluxations (see the *BSAVA Manual of Small Animal Fracture Repair and Management*).

Bony structures

Potential changes to bony structures of joints include the following.

- Bone may remodel due to long-standing misalignment following fractures or angular deformities.
- Subchondral bone lucencies are seen with Legg–Calvé–Perthes disease and occasionally with osteochondritis dissecans.
- Periarticular new bone (osteophytes) may be seen as a result of trauma (associated instability) and arthroses (degenerative, infective, inflammatory, haemarthrosis). If associated with the origin or insertion of soft tissue elements then they are termed enthesophytes.

Sesamoids show a number of normal variations. They are inconsistently present, for instance in the tendon of the ulnaris lateralis muscle. They may be fragmented or multipartite, particularly the 2nd and 7th sesamoids in the manus and pes. Clavicular remnants (not a true sesamoid) occur in cats and some dogs. Occasionally, sesamoid bones are fractured. They may be displaced, as occurs when one of the heads of the gastrocnemius muscle is damaged. The small sesamoid in the head of the popliteal muscle caudolateral to stifle in larger-breed dogs may also be displaced.

Joint space

Weightbearing radiographs are necessary for critical assessment. These are rarely used in small animal radiography but are common in equine radiography.

Capsular distension may be noted in the distal limb as a change in the contour of the skin. In the stifle, it may be seen as a reduction in the size of the infrapatellar fat pad and caudal displacement of caudal fascial planes. In the elbow it is sometimes seen as a displacement of the fascial planes. Intracapsular gas is indicative of either an open wound or infective arthritis. Radiopaque isolated bodies may be fracture fragments, a mineralized osteochondritis dissecans flap or small separate ossification centres, e.g. as seen in the caudal glenoid of the scapula.

Joint involvement

The number of joints involved may provide useful information:

- Single joint involvement may indicate trauma, infection or neoplasia
- Bilaterally symmetrical involvement suggests congenital or developmental causes (e.g. elbow or hip dysplasia)
- Multiple involvement is more typical of systemic disease, e.g. infection, degenerative or autoimmune diseases.

Bones

Bone reacts to disease in a predictable and limited fashion. It may change its shape, its opacity (decreased, as in osteolysis/osteoporosis, or increased, as in osteoproliferation/sclerosis), or demonstrate different periosteal reactions.

Decreased size but normal conformation (reduced growth potential) is seen in pituitary dwarfism, hypothyroidism and arteriovenous shunts (e.g. portosystemic shunts). Decreased size and altered conformation (altered overall skeletal proportions) may be seen in chondrodystrophy and premature physeal closure.

Decreased bone opacity

It is useful to compare other bones and the surrounding soft tissues when evaluating decreased bone density. Decreased density may be due to *osteoporosis*, which is decreased bone mass due to failure of osteoblasts to lay down bone matrix (osteoid), or *osteomalacia*, which is decreased bone mass due to insufficient or abnormal mineralization of osteoid. It should be remembered that radiographic changes do not become evident until about 30% of mineral content is lost. Osteoporosis and osteomalacia cannot be distinguished radiologically and are better described under the general term osteopenia. The causes of osteopenia are listed in Figure 2.22.

Increased bone opacity

This is sometimes described as sclerosis. In histological terms, sclerosis implies hardening of the bone with an increase in the calcium content. Radiologically, increased radiopacity of a bony structure may result from true sclerosis or from the deposition of additional bone on the surface. This may seem a pedantic point but an ability to differentiate these two possibilities may alter the differential list significantly. Careful use of the term *sclerosis* is therefore advised.

Generalized increase in bone opacity is rare. It is seen in osteopetrosis (e.g. hypervitaminosis D, myelofibrosis, myelosclerosis) and in Basenji bone disease (hereditary anaemia). Polyostotic increase in bone opacity is much more common. Causes are listed in Figure 2.23.

Monostotic increase in bone opacity with multiple lesions is rarely seen but has been reported with sclerotic metastatic neoplasms. Monostotic increase in bone opacity as a solitary lesion may represent a primary neoplasm, metastatic neoplasia, a healed fracture, a sequestrum (this appears opaque due to the surrounding lucency), osteomyelitis (this may be surrounded by a zone of true sclerosis), periostitis (either traumatic or septic) or a periarticular osteophyte.

Cortical changes

Bone cortices may be thinned or thickened.

Bone thinning: This may be due to osteoporosis, which may be nutritional or due to disuse. Thinned cortices may also be evident on the non-weightbearing aspect of abnormally bent bones. Expansile intraosseous lesions with thinned cortices may represent cysts or cystic neoplasms.

Generalized

Hyperparathyroidism:
- Primary (rare)
- Adenoma/hyperplasia

Hyperparathyroidism: secondary, nutritional or renal. Reduced opacity, thin cortices and pathological fractures are seen

Atrophy: disuse, cachexia

Hypoplasia

Protein deprivation:
- Adrenocortical neoplasm
- Prolonged steroid therapy
- Dietary

Polyostotic – several bones in same limb or several bones throughout skeleton

Disuse atrophy
Multiple myeloma
Metastatic bone disease
Haematogenous osteomyelitis
Retained cartilaginous cores of distal ulnar metaphysis

Monostotic with multiple lesions

Haematogenous osteomyelitis
Metastatic neoplasia

Monostotic with single lesion

Osteomyelitis:
- Haematogenous
- Penetrating wound
- Direct spread from septic arthritis or soft tissue abscess

Primary (or secondary) bone neoplasia

2.22 Causes of osteopenia.

Inflammatory joint disease leading to:
- Subchondral sclerosis
- Periarticular osteophytes

Panosteitis (rarely symmetrical)
Metastatic bone neoplasia
Metaphyseal osteopathy
Healing folding fractures
Calcification of dead bone/infarcts
(Lead poisoning)
(Fungal osteomyelitis)
Myelosclerosis (associated with feline leukaemia virus infection)

2.23 Causes of polyostotic increase in bone opacity.

Chapter 2 Radiography

Bone thickening: If the periosteum is elevated, new bone will form beneath it. In the case of aggressive bone lesions (e.g. osteosarcoma or osteomyelitis) with cortical destruction and periosteal elevation, a triangle of solid bone is seen between the periosteum, the intact cortex and the lesion (Codman's Triangle). Periosteal reactions are seen about 7–10 days post-insult. They may be seen in metaphyseal osteopathy, chronic osteomyelitis, panosteitis, healing fractures, periostitis (inflammation/irritation), and angular limb deformities (weightbearing cortex). The pattern of periosteal new bone helps to define the lesion (Figure 2.24).

Appearance of periosteal reaction	Interpretation
Parallel (onion skin or lamellar)	Slow growing, non-aggressive lesions, e.g. trauma, infection, benign neoplasm
Smooth and well defined	Chronic but aggressive, e.g. old fracture, chronic infection
Irregular (lace-like)	Active, aggressive lesions, e.g. osteomyelitis, neoplasia, hypertrophic osteopathy, periostitis
Radiating or sunburst	Very aggressive lesion, e.g. osteosarcoma, severe osteomyelitis

2.24 Interpretation of periosteal reaction.

Focal cortical lesions are seen with greenstick, impacted or pathological fractures. They may also be seen with benign neoplasia and bone cysts.

Trabecular bone may be thickened in primary or metastatic neoplasia, osteomyelitis, late stage panosteitis, growth arrest lines and physeal scars. Endosteal new bone is seen in panosteitis, fracture callus, metastatic tumours and osteopetrosis.

Location of bony changes
The part of the bone affected aids in the differentiation of diseases:

- **Epiphysis**: conditions include primary bone neoplasia; haematogenous osteomyelitis; multiple epiphyseal dysplasia (occurs in Beagles and Poodles, characterized by irregular-shaped epiphyses with mixed punctate lucencies and opacities)
- **Physis**: conditions include haematogenous osteomyelitis, seen in young (rapidly growing) animals; enchondrodystrophy of the English Pointer; physeal injuries that result in premature closure of the affected physis
- **Metaphysis**: conditions include primary bone neoplasia (osteosarcoma, lymphosarcoma, reticular cell sarcoma); benign bone neoplasia; metaphyseal osteopathy
- **Diaphysis**: conditions include fractures; secondary (metastatic) neoplasia.

Aggressive or benign lesions
Aggressive or benign bone changes have a number of consistent features (Figure 2.25).

Change	Benign	Malignant
Zone of transition	Short and well defined	Long and poorly defined
Margin	Sharp	Indistinct
Border	Well defined and sclerotic	Ill defined and lytic
Cortex	Intact	Broken
Periosteum	Intact	Interrupted
Periosteal new bone	Well structured and smooth	Irregular
Rate of change	Slow	Rapid

2.25 Changes seen in benign and aggressive bone conditions.

There is a gradual change in appearance of new bone from benign to aggressive conditions. The transition in radiological appearance is as follows, with signs lower in the list indicating a more aggressive condition:

- Smooth
- Well defined
- Intact
- Irregular
- Scalloped
- Undulating
- Shell-like
- Lamellar
- Lace-like
- Velvet
- Broken
- Codman's triangle
- 'Hair-on-end'
- Brush-like
- Sunburst
- Amorphous

References and further reading

Barr F and Kirberger R (eds) (2006) *BSAVA Manual of Canine and Feline Musculoskeletal Imaging.* BSAVA Publications, Gloucester
Habel RE, Frewein J and Sack WO (1983) *Nomina Anatomica Veterinaria, 3rd edn.* World Association of Veterinary Anatomists, Ithaca
Sisson S and Grossman JD (1975) *Anatomy of the Domestic Animals (2 Vols), 5th edn.* WB Saunders, Philadelphia
Smallwood JE, Shively MJ, Rendano VT and Habel RE (1985) A standardised nomenclature for radiographic projections used in veterinary medicine. *Veterinary Radiology* **26**, 2–9

3

Laboratory investigations

Susan Bell and John E.F. Houlton

Synovial fluid collection and evaluation

Arthrocentesis and analysis of the synovial fluid obtained is a much under-employed technique in the investigation of joint disease. Dogs with persistent or cyclic pyrexia associated with a generalized stiffness or lameness are obvious candidates. In such cases, separate samples should be submitted from a minimum of three joints for cytology, since the smaller joints are generally involved and it can be difficult to obtain a sufficient volume. However, mono-articular effusions also frequently merit examination to establish the nature of the joint pathology.

Collection of synovial fluid

Equipment

Needles: The gauge and length of the needle should be determined by the size of the synovial cavity, the thickness of the tissues and the depth of the joint capsule from the surface of the skin. For any given joint, the shortest length and smallest diameter needle should be used but the needle should be of sufficient diameter to facilitate the flow of viscous synovial fluid. Sterile disposable needles of gauge 0.6–0.9 mm (20–23 G) are satisfactory for most dogs. Needles of length 16–25 mm ($5/_8$–1 inch) will be long enough to reach the distal joints, while 25–63 mm (1–2$1/_2$ inch) needles are necessary for the proximal joints. For small joints, a needle with a relatively short bevel should be used to ensure the entire lumen of the needle is within the synovial cavity. Rarely, a short-bevelled disposable spinal needle may be required in very small joints.

Syringes: A relatively small-capacity sterile syringe is recommended in order to maintain proper negative pressure during aspiration and to minimize the loss of synovial fluid within the syringe barrel. Typically, a 2.5 ml syringe is used in cats and small dogs, while a 5 ml syringe is used in larger dogs.

Miscellaneous equipment: Pre-cleaned microscope slides should be available for the preparation of smears of synovial fluid. Blood tubes containing ethylenediamine tetra-acetic acid (EDTA) or heparin are indicated for larger volumes. Blood culture bottles should also be available for those cases where sepsis is suspected.

Restraint

Arthrocentesis is most easily performed under general anaesthesia or heavy sedation.

Arthrocentesis of the carpus and stifle is tolerated relatively well and may be performed in a cooperative animal with a small amount of local anaesthetic. However, sampling is generally performed at the same time as diagnostic imaging and some form of chemical restraint is therefore used.

Patient preparation

The hair over the site should be clipped and the site prepared aseptically. It is not necessary to drape the area if a sufficiently wide margin of skin is prepared adequately. Sterile gloves should be worn if the clinician wishes to palpate the insertion site. A 'no touch' technique can be employed if the clinician is familiar with the local anatomy.

Site of puncture

The needle should avoid major neurovascular structures. Bony prominences should be selected as landmarks whenever possible, since they are easy to palpate and have the most consistent anatomical relationship to the adjacent joint. Soft tissues are more likely to be displaced by inflammatory or neoplastic processes. Insertion of the needle may be assisted by holding the limb flexed since this widens the joint spaces.

The needle is advanced through the soft tissues carefully until it enters the synovial cavity. If it encounters bone before entering the joint, it should be withdrawn a short distance and redirected. Care should be taken to avoid damaging the articular cartilage at all times. Once sufficient fluid has entered the syringe, suction is released to minimize the inadvertent aspiration of blood before the needle and syringe are withdrawn. Sites for needle insertion are illustrated in Figure 3.1.

Scapulohumeral joint: The animal is positioned in lateral recumbency with the shoulder joint partially flexed and the humerus slightly rotated externally. Distal traction can be applied to the limb by an assistant to open the joint space if required. The site for insertion of the needle is a few millimetres cranial and distal to the acromion and immediately caudal and proximal to the greater tubercle of the humerus. The needle should be directed caudally, slightly medially and slightly downward, medial to the acromial head of the deltoideus muscle.

Chapter 3 Laboratory investigations

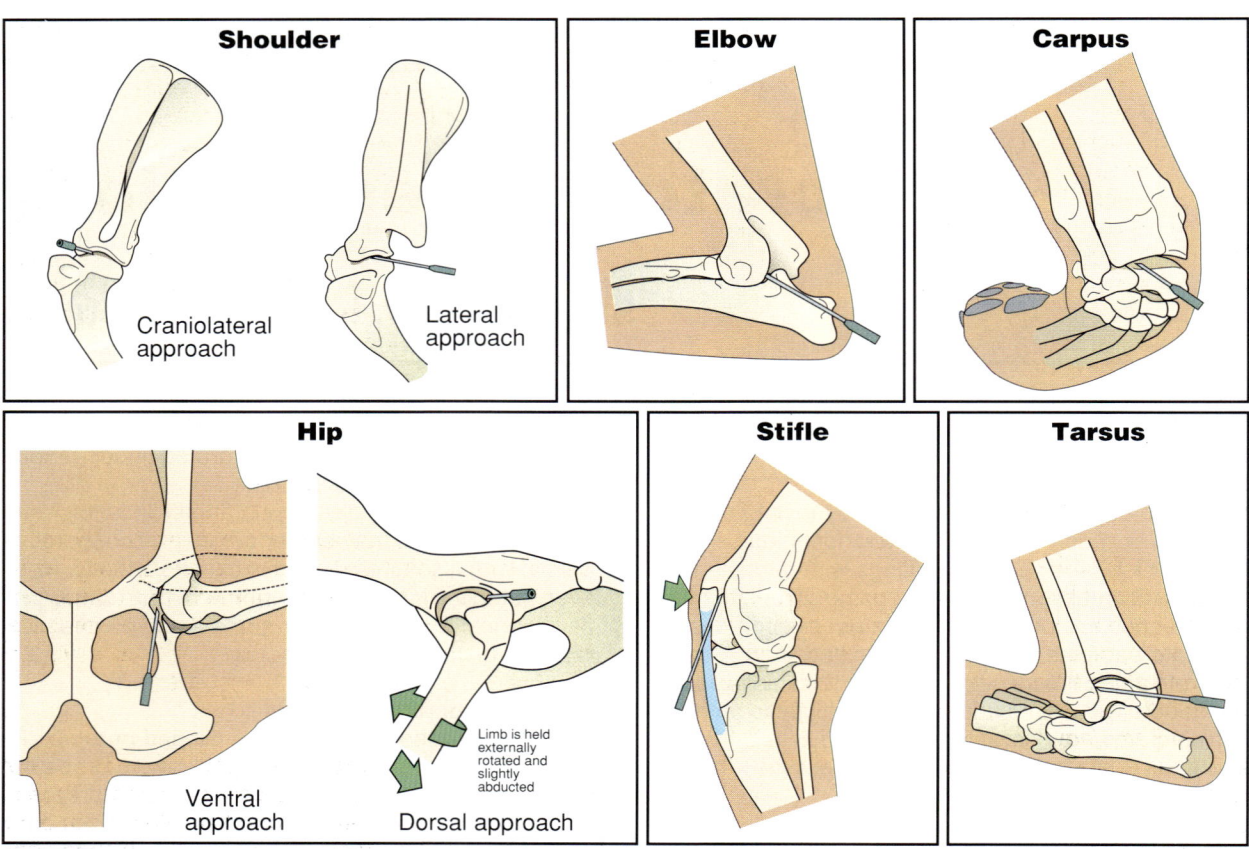

3.1 Sites for arthrocentesis. Reproduced from the *BSAVA Manual of Canine and Feline Clinical Pathology*, 2nd edition.

Alternatively, a more cranial approach can be used. The needle is directed into the cranial aspect of the joint starting at the most distal aspect of the scapular tuberosity. The needle is passed medial to the scapular tuberosity, in a caudal and slightly dorsal direction, so that it passes beneath the cranial lip of the glenoid cavity and above the humeral head.

Elbow: The caudolateral approach is the easiest. The animal is positioned in lateral recumbency with the elbow flexed to an angle of approximately 45 degrees. The lateral condyle of the humerus is palpated and the needle inserted between the prominence and the triceps tendon. The needle is advanced through the anconeus muscle in a downward and slightly medial direction along the craniolateral aspect of the olecranon and into the supratrochlear fossa of the humerus.

Carpus: The carpus is a composite joint consisting of the antebrachiocarpal, middle and carpometacarpal joints. The latter communicate, which is fortunate since it is difficult to penetrate the carpometacarpal joint. Thus, while arthrocentesis of all joints is possible, the antebrachiocarpal joint is generally chosen. The animal is positioned in lateral or sternal recumbency with the carpus fully flexed. The needle is inserted between the tendons of the extensor carpi radialis muscle and the common digital extensor tendon.

Metacarpo- (metatarso-) phalangeal joints: The animal is placed in lateral or sternal recumbency and the joint is fully flexed. The needle is inserted from the dorsal aspect, just to one side of the common digital extensor tendon. The dorsal sesamoid bone must be avoided.

Interphalangeal joints: The technique is as described for the metacarpo- (metatarso-) phalangeal joints.

Coxofemoral joint: Arthrocentesis may be performed via a lateral or ventral approach; the latter is generally easier and is recommended. The animal is positioned in dorsal recumbency. The femora are gently abducted until they are as near perpendicular to the midline as possible. The pectineus muscle is identified and traced to its origin at the iliopectineal eminence on the pelvis, and the ventral aspect of the acetabular fossa is identified immediately caudolateral to this bony landmark. The needle is inserted into the joint at a 45 degree angle in a caudocranial direction.

For the lateral approach, the animal is positioned in lateral recumbency with the pelvic limb at right angles to the long axis of the spine and parallel to the table surface. The greater trochanter is palpated and the needle introduced at its cranial aspect. It is directed into the lateral aspect of the joint immediately cranial to the dorsal margin of the greater trochanter in a medial and slightly ventral direction. If the needle strikes the femoral neck or acetabular rim it is redirected until the joint capsule is penetrated.

Stifle: The joint capsule of the stifle joint is the most extensive in the body and has three sacs, all of which communicate with each other. This makes arthrocentesis easy. The animal is positioned in lateral recumbency with the joint partially flexed. Digital pressure is applied to the joint capsule on the medial side of the straight patellar ligament to encourage it to bulge on the opposite side. The needle is directed into the cranial aspect of the joint immediately lateral to the straight patellar ligament, midway between the patella and the tibial tuberosity. The needle is directed into the joint space, through the fat pad, towards the intercondylar space.

Tarsus (hock): The talocrural joint can be penetrated from either the caudolateral or caudomedial aspect. The easier is the caudolateral approach with the animal in lateral recumbency and the affected limb uppermost. The space between the fibula and the distal tibia is palpated and the needle advanced in a distal direction with the joint in a flexed position.

Sample handling

The handling of the sample depends upon the volume obtained. If only a few drops are available for testing, the volume, colour, viscosity and turbidity should be recorded at the time of collection. Squash smears are then made (see *BSAVA Manual of Canine and Feline Clinical Pathology*) and rapidly air-dried to reduce cell shrinkage artefact. Delay can result in the large mononuclear cells undergoing vacuolation and nuclear degeneration (i.e. autolysis) (Fisher, 2001). If larger volumes are available, the fluid should be put into anticoagulant tubes. Normal synovial fluid does not clot since it lacks fibrinogen and most other clotting factors. However, clotting may occur if there has been iatrogenic blood contamination, intra-articular haemorrhage or protein exudation. EDTA is the preferred anticoagulant when cytological examination is proposed, while heparin is superior for the mucin precipitation test and measurement of viscosity.

Evaluation of synovial fluid

Gross appearance

Normal synovial fluid is a clear, viscous liquid, approximately 0.1–1.0 ml in volume, depending on the joint sampled. An increase in the volume indicates joint effusion, and is often accompanied by a reduction in the fluid's apparent viscosity. This reduction is caused by depolymerization of the long-chain polysaccharide hyaluronan and is usually associated with inflammatory changes within the joint.

Changes in colour generally reflect haemorrhage or inflammation. Red cells are normally absent in synovial fluid and their presence suggests haemarthrosis or blood contamination during arthrocentesis. Blood contamination is usually seen as a streak of blood within an otherwise clear fluid. In contrast, the red/pinkish colour is uniform in true haemarthrosis. Recent haemorrhage within the joint produces a bright red colour. This will become more orange or yellow over the next 2–4 weeks as the haemosiderin is gradually removed. Iatrogenic contamination can be assessed from the red cell count. Common causes of haemarthrosis are:

- Recent fractures
- Rupture of intra-articular ligaments
- Surgery
- Some haemostatic disorders.

Changes in the transparency of synovial fluid generally indicate inflammatory changes within the joint. In osteoarthritis and the immune-mediated arthritides, the fluid will be more yellow in colour. In infective arthritis, the fluid will be characterized by a visible turbidity due to increased cell numbers.

Cytology

The most useful test when investigating joint pathology is the estimation of its cytological properties. Whenever possible, a total and differential cell count should be performed. This generally means the involvement of a commercial laboratory, since the viscosity of synovial fluid demands an appropriate dilution of the sample, which is technically demanding and beyond the capability of most in-house facilities.

Normal synovial fluid has a low cellularity, containing <1.5 $\times 10^9$ cells/l. The nucleated cells of synovial fluid are a mixture of large mononuclear cells and lymphocytes, with <3% neutrophils. The large mononuclear cells are a mixture of synovial lining cells (synoviocytes) and macrophages and comprise 60–90% of the total cells. Synovial lining cells are round cells with a single round nucleus and a moderate amount of basophilic cytoplasm. Macrophages should comprise <10% of the large mononuclear cells while lymphocytes normally make up 3–30%. These characteristics change with differing arthropathies and their relative proportions will change, depending on the disease group (Figures 3.2 and 3.3). These cellular changes can be seen in smears treated with May–Grünwald–Giemsa stain or by using a Coulter counter.

Condition	Total cell count	Percentage of mononuclear cells	Percentage of neutrophils
Normal	<2 $\times 10^9$/l	94–100	0–6
Osteoarthritis	2–5 $\times 10^9$/l	88–100	0–12
Rheumatoid arthritis	8–38 $\times 10^9$/l	20–80	20–80
Non-erosive immune-mediated polyarthritis	4–370 $\times 10^9$/l	5–85	15–95
Infective arthritis	40–267 $\times 10^9$/l	1–10	90–100

3.2 Cellular composition of synovial fluids in canine arthropathies.

Chapter 3 Laboratory investigations

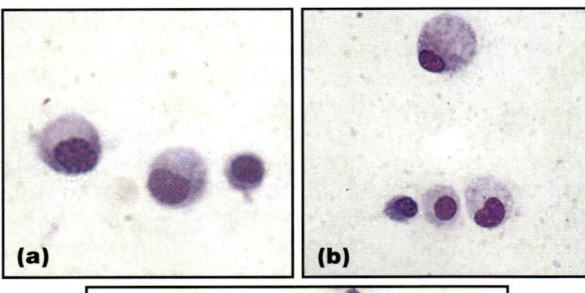
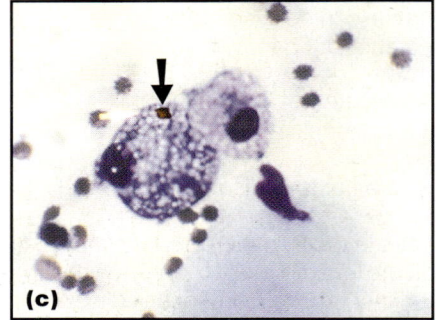
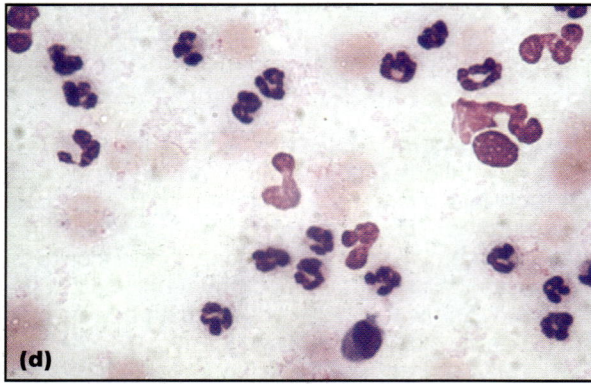
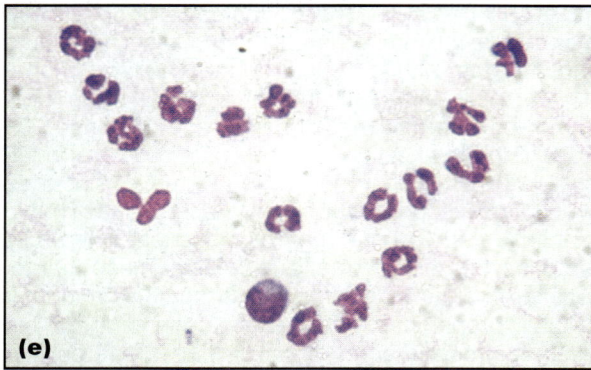

3.3 Synovial fluid cytology. **(a)** Normal canine synovial fluid showing a scant mononuclear population consisting of one lymphocyte and two larger mononuclear cells (synovial lining cells). **(b)** Synovial fluid from a stifle with OA. Some of the mononuclear cells have abundant foamy cytoplasm. **(c)** Synovial fluid from an elbow joint with haemarthrosis. A haematoidin crystal (arrowed) is present within a macrophage, reflecting erythrophagocytosis. **(d)** Synovial fluid smear from a dog with infective arthritis. Numerous neutrophils are present, some showing degenerative change. Red cells are present in the background. **(e)** Synovial fluid smear from a dog with immune-mediated arthritis, consisting predominantly of neutrophils with a small proportion of mononuclear cells. (Giemsa stain except (d) Wright's; original magnification X1000.) Reproduced from the *BSAVA Manual of Canine and Feline Clinical Pathology*, 2nd edition.

Since there is a significant overlap in the cytological changes between the different disease processes, they need to be interpreted in the light of the patient's history and clinical signs, and the results of imaging and other diagnostic tests.

Hydroxyapatite crystals may be deposited in peri-articular tissues, especially around the shoulder and sometimes in the hip, spine and peripheral joints. These can be detected by staining with alizarin red. However, crystal-induced arthropathies are exceedingly rare in the dog and the cat (Bennett, 1990).

Microbiology

Direct detection of infective agents by aerobic or anaerobic culture can confirm the diagnosis of bacterial infective arthritis. Most cases are associated with either staphylococci or β-haemolytic streptococci but not exclusively; indeed cultures are often negative. Usually there is more culture success using blood culture bottles or synovial membrane biopsy specimens (Montgomery *et al.*, 1989). Mycoplasmal arthritis is considered uncommon in cats (Earnst and Goggin, 1999) and rare in dogs (Barton *et al.*, 1985). However, polymerase chain reaction (PCR) assay may aid future positive identification, as it has done in human research.

Lyme disease: Antibodies to the spirochaete *Borrelia burgdorferi*, the causal agent of Lyme disease, can be detected in the serum of dogs and cats and are thus useful to support the diagnosis and to monitor subsequent treatment (May *et al.*, 1991, 1994). It is also possible to use PCR to identify the causal organism directly in synovial fluid or joint tissue, but false positives can be a problem as infection with *B. burgdorferi* does not always lead to clinical disease. In the cat, it was concluded that clinical signs were absent and lameness rarely reported (May *et al.*, 1994).

Biochemistry

Mucin clot test: This is a crude test used to evaluate the viscosity of synovial fluid. A small amount of fluid is dropped into a beaker of 5% acetic acid; normal fluid should form a tight clot, but fluid with depolymerized hyaluronan will fail to do this. The usefulness of the test is compromised, however, by variable results. The result is usually normal in osteoarthritis but clot formation is sometimes poor. The result is variable in inflammatory arthropathies, and fair to poor in acute haemarthroses.

Protein: Synovial fluid protein levels are normally low (20.0–40.0 g/l (2–4 x 10^4 μg/ml)). They can be measured by refractometer or by biochemical assay. Recent research has focused on the presence of specific proteins in synovial fluid as markers of disease. These can occur as a result of increased cartilage breakdown, as can be seen in osteoarthritis (OA) and rheumatoid arthritis (RA), compared with the dynamic equilibrium present in normal cartilage. Some examples are given in Figure 3.4.

Chapter 3 Laboratory investigations

Protein type	Protein concentration (µg/ml)			
	Normal	**Osteoarthritis**	**Rheumatoid arthritis**	**Infective arthritis**
COMP	298 ±124	401 ± 73	N/A	N/A
GAG	199 ± 41	282 ± 85	299 ± 273	N/A
KS	174 ± 70	132 ± 75	1148 ± 1091	N/A
C-4-S	0.9 ± 0.4	3.4 ± 3.0	49.4 ± 44.9	N/A
HA	2.1 ± 1.1	0.9 ± 0.4	0.1 ± 0.1	N/A

3.4 Specific cartilage proteins in synovial fluid of normal dogs and dogs with arthritis (C-4-S, chondroitin-4-sulphate (Arican et al., 1994b); COMP, cartilage oligomeric matrix protein (Misumi et al., 2002); GAG, glycosaminoglycans; HA, hyaluronan (Arican et al., 1994a); KS, keratan sulphate).

Matrix metalloproteinases (MMPs) are a group of serine proteinases that are active in synovial fluid, but some enzymes are altered in the arthropathies. For example, the gelatinase MMP9 is significantly increased in synovial fluid in RA but not in OA (Coughlan et al., 1998).

Immunology
The presence of autoantibodies in serum and synovial fluid is a feature of arthropathies with an inflammatory component. Rheumatoid factors (IgM and IgA) have been identified in both fluids (Bell et al., 1993) (Figure 3.5).

Serum antinuclear antibody (ANA) showed no specific disease association with the different arthropathies, but assay is still useful for systemic lupus erythematosus (SLE) in the dog in conjunction with a clinical examination (Bell et al., 1997). ANA can also be detected in cat serum, but the specificity is unclear (Bell, unpublished data).

Increased autoantibodies to collagen type II, the predominant collagen in cartilage extracellular matrix, have been detected in 52% of OA cases and in 72% of RA cases, but never in any radiographically normal dogs (Bari et al., 1989) and are thus indicative of matrix breakdown.

Antibodies to canine distemper virus (CDV) have been detected in synovial fluids of normal dogs and dogs with different joint diseases, but it was only the RA group that showed a significant increase in anti-CDV antibodies, indicating a possible role for CDV in inflammatory joint disease (Bell et al., 1991). It has been recommended that dogs with RA that have sufficiently high titres of circulating anti-CDV antibodies are not revaccinated whilst on therapy (May and Bennett, 1994).

Calicivirus, acquired either naturally or by vaccination, can cause a transient, self-limiting polyarthritis in cats and, more especially, kittens. Antibodies can be detected in serum and synovial fluid (Bennett et al., 1989). These cats also have high serum IgM rheumatoid factors (Bell, unpublished data).

Synovial membrane biopsy

Biopsy of synovial membrane can be performed using needles, arthrotomy or arthroscopy. Arthroscopy is the method of choice since the joint can be examined, and specimens taken from the most suitable area, with the minimum of trauma. Biopsy specimens should, in general, be 2–4 mm wide. Their length will depend upon the size of the joint. The specimen should be placed on a piece of cardboard, synovial membrane side uppermost, and pinned with a 25 gauge hypodermic needle at either end to prevent it from curling up. The specimen may then be fixed in 10% formalin solution for histopathology. Alternatively, synovial biopsy specimens may be submitted for microbiological culture or frozen immediately for immunohistopathology.

Histopathological examination of synovial membrane is an important part of the diagnostic protocol when investigating suspected inflammatory or chronic infective arthropathies (see Chapter 7). However, some caution must be exercised in the interpretation since there may be overlap between changes seen in OA and immune-mediated arthropathy. Canine OA may have an inflammatory component with moderate infiltrates of plasmacytes and lymphocytes in the synovial membrane which can appear similar to end-stage RA where the inflammatory process has largely burnt itself out.

Condition	IgM rheumatoid factor		IgA rheumatoid factor	
	Serum	**Synovial fluid**	**Serum**	**Synovial fluid**
Normal	3.42 ± 0.42	0.43 ± 0.05	1.13 ± 1.77	1.09 ± 0.27
Osteoarthritis	16.23 ± 1.5	7.85 ± 7.63	0.26 ± 0.42	0.75 ± 0.39
Rheumatoid arthritis	13.58 ± 1.17	5.50 ± 0.43	2.04 ± 1.38	2.10 ± 1.49
Infective arthritis	16.03 ± 1.81	8.07 ± 1.62	N/A	N/A

3.5 Presence of autoantibodies in synovial fluid. NB: IgM RF is not diagnostic for RA, as is the case for human RA, as it also occurs in some canine OA cases. IgA RF would appear to be associated with those dogs with RA that show erosive changes in their joints (Bell et al., 1993). (Units are ELISA arbitrary units.)

Other laboratory investigations

Other laboratory investigations, such as routine haematology and biochemical blood analysis, may be necessary. They will not be described here but the reader is referred to the *BSAVA Manual of Canine and Feline Clinical Pathology*. Pyruvate and lactate assays are occasionally employed in the investigation of muscle disorders (see Chapter 8b).

References and further reading

Arican M, Carter SD and Bennett D (1994a) Hyaluronan in canine arthropathies. *Journal of Comparative Pathology* **111**, 249–256

Arican M, Carter SD, Bennett D and May C (1994b) Measurement of glycosaminoglycans and keratan sulphate in canine arthropathies. *Research in Veterinary Science* **56**, 290–297

Bari ASM, Carter SD, Bell SC, Morgan K and Bennett D (1989) Anti type II collagen antibodies in naturally occurring canine joint diseases. *British Journal of Rheumatology* **28**, 480–486

Barton MD, Ireland L, Kirschner JL and Forbes C (1985) Isolation of *Mycoplasma spumans* from polyarthritis in a greyhound. *Australian Veterinary Journal* **62**, 206–207

Bell SC, Carter SD and Bennett D (1991) Canine distemper viral antigens and antibodies in dogs with rheumatoid arthritis. *Research in Veterinary Science* **50**, 64–68

Bell SC, Carter SD, May C and Bennett (1993) IgA and IgM rheumatoid factors in canine rheumatoid arthritis. *Journal of Small Animal Practice* **34**, 259–264

Bell SC, Hughes DE, Bennett D, Bari ASM, Kelly DF and Carter SD (1997) Analysis and significance of antinuclear antibodies in dogs. *Research in Veterinary Science* **62**, 83–84

Bennett D (1987) Immune-based non-erosive inflammatory joint disease of the dog. 1. Canine systemic lupus erythematosus. *Journal of Small Animal Practice* **28**, 871–879

Bennett D (1990) Joints and joint diseases. In: *Canine Orthopaedics*, 2nd edn, ed. WG Whittick, pp. 761–856. Lea and Febiger, Philadelphia

Bennett D, Gaskell RM, Mills A *et al.* (1989) Detection of feline calicivirus in the joints of infected cats. *Veterinary Record* **12**, 329–334

Coughlan AR, Robertson DH, Bennett D *et al.* (1998) Matrix metalloproteinases 2 and 9 in canine rheumatoid arthritis. *Veterinary Record* **143**, 219–223

Earnst S and Goggin JM (1999) What is your diagnosis? Mycoplasmal arthritis in a cat. *Journal of the American Veterinary Medical Association* **215**, 19–20

Innes JF (2005) Laboratory evaluation of joint disease. In: *BSAVA Manual of Canine and Feline Clinical Pathology*, 2nd edn, ed. E Villiers and L Blackwood, pp. 355–363. BSAVA Publications, Gloucester

Fisher D (2001) Musculoskeletal system. In: *Atlas of Canine and Feline Cytology*, ed. RE Raskin and DJ Meyer, pp. 313–324. WB Saunders, Philadelphia

May C and Bennett D (1994) Immune-mediated arthritides. In: *Manual of Small Animal Arthrology*, ed. JEF Houlton and RW Collinson, pp. 86–99. BSAVA Publications, Cheltenham

May C, Carter SD, Barnes A, Bell SC and Bennett D (1991) Serodiagnosis of Lyme disease in UK dogs. *Journal of Small Animal Practice* **32**, 170–174

May C, Carter SD, Barnes A *et al.* (1994) *Borrelia burgdorferi* infection in cats in the UK. *Journal of Small Animal Practice* **35**, 517–520

Misumi K, Vilim V, Carter SD *et al.* (2002) Concentrations of cartilage oligomeric matrix protein in dogs with naturally developing and experimentally induced arthropathy. *American Journal of Veterinary Research* **63**, 598–603

Montgomery RD, Long IR, Milton JL, DiPinto MN and Hunt J (1989) Comparison of aerobic culturette, synovial membrane biopsy, and blood culture medium in detection of canine bacterial arthritis. *Veterinary Surgery* **18(4)**, 300–303

Olby N (2005) Laboratory evaluation of muscle disorders. In: *BSAVA Manual of Canine and Feline Clinical Pathology*, 2nd edn, ed. E Villiers and L Blackwood, pp. 364–372. BSAVA Publications, Gloucester

4

Advanced diagnostic techniques

Steven C. Budsberg and Michael W. Thomas

Introduction

The range and sophistication of technologies available to the veterinary practitioner has dramatically increased over the past 15 years. While the complete history and physical examination remain the mainstay of lameness diagnosis, these new technologies offer the ability to gather new and far-ranging information. This can be beneficial not only in reaching the definitive diagnosis but it may also provide information about the degree of the injury and its prognosis. These technologies can be divided into two main categories: diagnostic imaging and quantitative gait analysis.

Advanced imaging

Advanced imaging with computed tomography (CT) and magnetic resonance imaging (MRI) has had a profound effect on the diagnosis and treatment of many musculoskeletal and joint disorders in dogs and cats over the last decade. Both these modalities provide cross-sectional images but use very different mechanisms of imaging. CT (first demonstrated by GN Hounsfield in 1972) is based on modulation of an X-ray beam as it traverses a subject. MRI is produced by resonance of polar molecules placed in a magnetic field. (Paul Lauterbur produced the first MRI images in 1972.) Both modalities require intensive computation and have advanced dramatically with the evolution of computer technology. The images have relatively low spatial resolution (lines per centimetre compared to lines per millimetre in conventional radiography) but excellent separation of tissue.

Computed tomography

CT measurements are in Hounsfield units, and each point in the image, a pixel, has a value related to the linear coefficient of absorption of water. Water has a value of 0, bone is >100, fat is −50 and air is 1000. CT scanning is therefore able to differentiate changes in soft tissues or bone that conventional radiographs are unable to delineate. Furthermore, CT allows for elimination of superimposed structures, which again aids in viewing specific structures. CT also has the capability to reformat the axial images in different planes, although the resolution is less than in the original cross-sectional image. These images are reformatted from cross-sectional images 1 mm in thickness with 1 mm overlap.

One of the most challenging lameness cases that faces the clinician involves the elbow. This complex joint has several conditions that cause lameness. Physical examination and conventional radiographs are often difficult to interpret but CT scanning can provide a diagnosis for both limbs without invasive surgery (Figure 4.1). While this technology is not required to diagnose every lameness, it can be very helpful in challenging cases.

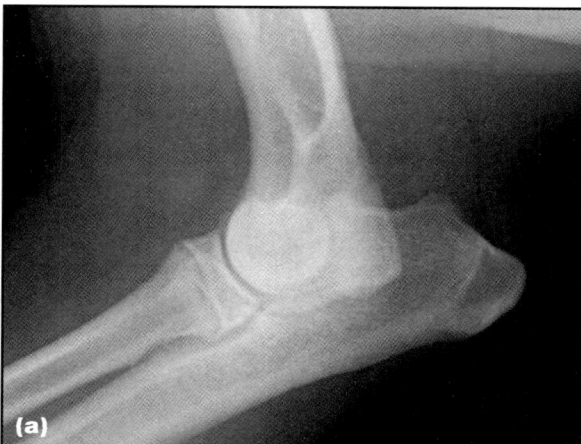
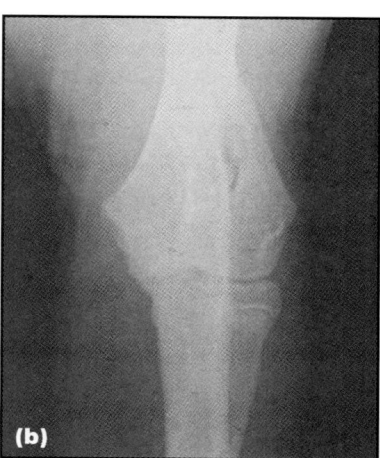
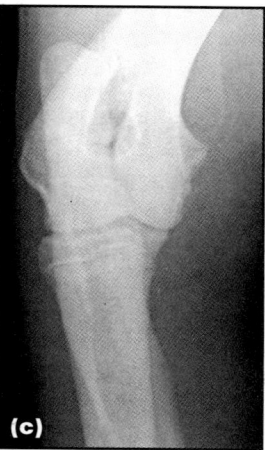

4.1 Images of the elbow of an immature dog with an intermittent shifting thoracic limb lameness. **(a)** Lateral radiographic view of the left elbow, showing very mild degenerative changes. **(b)** Craniocaudal radiographic view of the left elbow, showing mild changes in the region of the medial coronoid process of the ulna. **(c)** Oblique craniocaudal radiographic view of the right elbow of the same dog, showing mild degenerative changes. (continues) ▶

Chapter 4   Advanced diagnostic techniques

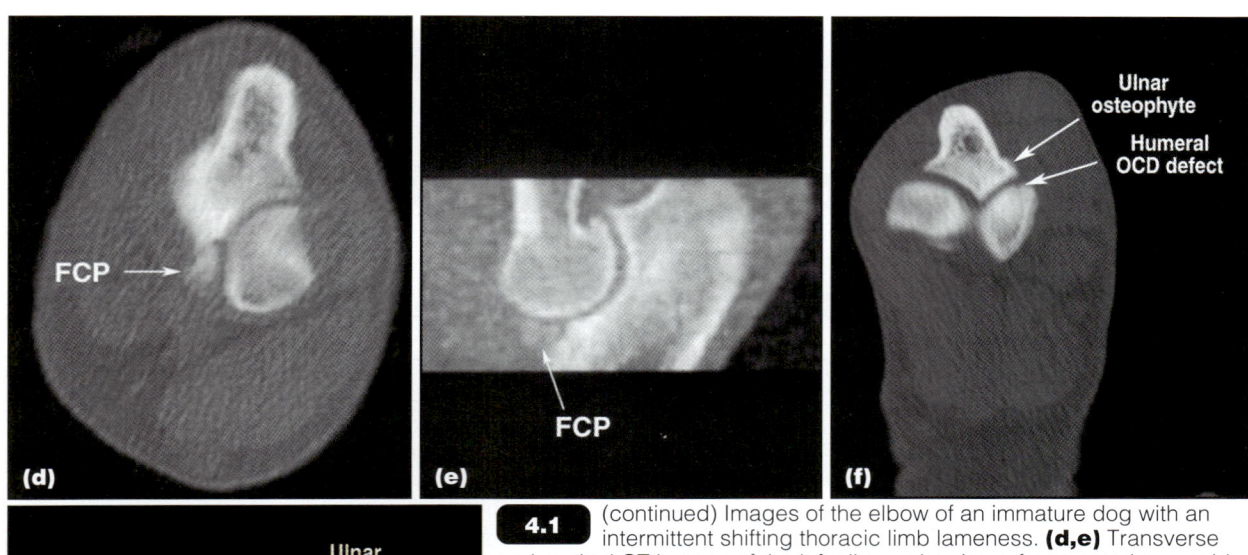

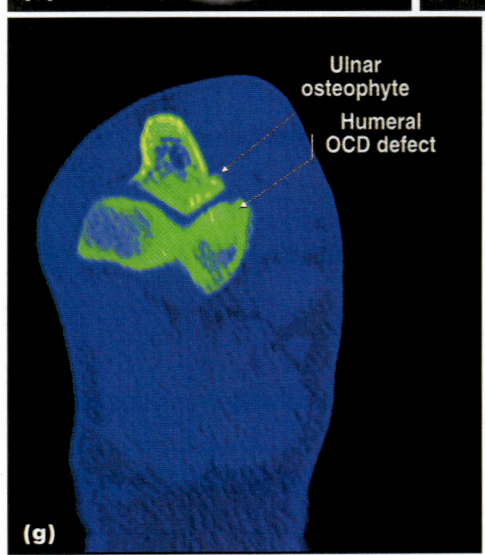

4.1 (continued) Images of the elbow of an immature dog with an intermittent shifting thoracic limb lameness. **(d,e)** Transverse and sagittal CT images of the left elbow, showing a fragmented coronoid process (FCP) of the ulna. **(f)** Transverse CT image of the right elbow, showing an osteochondritis dissecans (OCD) lesion in the humeral condyle and an associated osteophyte on the adjacent ulna. **(g)** A 'colorized' image of the OCD lesion in (f) highlights the pathological changes.

CT has been used to image bones of the spine and all the joints of the appendicular skeleton. Furthermore, the capability to reassemble (reconstruct) these cross-sectional images has progressed to a technique known as volume rendering, which can provide additional information about a joint in a non-invasive manner (Figure 4.2). With sufficient computing power, this volume image can be rotated in different planes. However, as it is a reformatted image, it has less resolution than the original cross-sectional images. While not commonly used in practice today due to resolution limitations, this may become a more important modality in the near future.

Magnetic resonance imaging

MRI has even greater tissue discrimination than CT, being able to detect 0.5% difference in water content. MRI also uses specific pulse/time sequences that

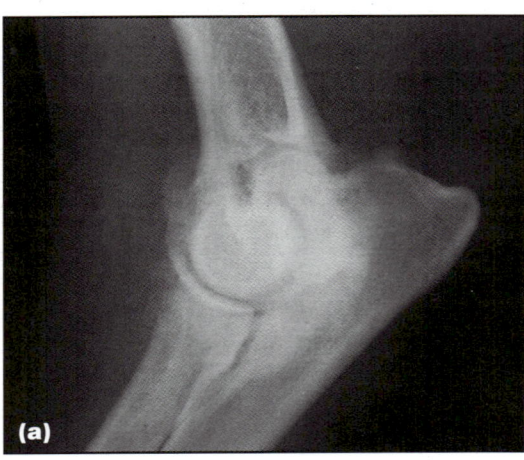

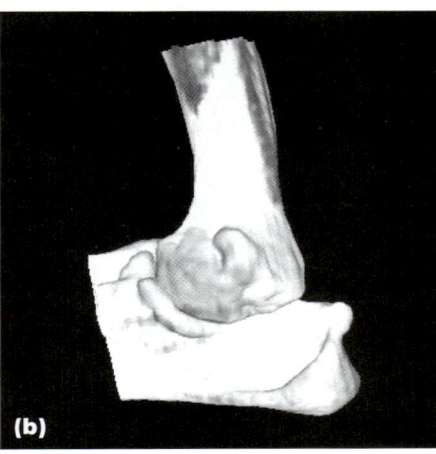

4.2 **(a)** Lateral radiograph of an elbow with severe degenerative changes. **(b)** Volume-rendered image of the same elbow, which provides a three-dimensional reconstruction of the joint.

Chapter 4 Advanced diagnostic techniques

differentiate between different tissue types. Bone, due to its relatively low water content, is almost always black on MRI. High water content and fat can have a relatively high signal return, resulting in a bright area. Other pulse sequences can suppress fat, accentuate proton density, and otherwise enhance separation of tissue. Thus, MRI has a superior ability to discriminate between soft tissues and bone components. The use of this modality is becoming more widespread in small animal practice and provides several advantages to the clinician.

MRI of the nervous system, including the brain, spinal cord and associated vertebral column is excellent (Figure 4.3). Thus, MRI can provide a rapid accurate and non-invasive diagnosis without the need for a myelogram, and allows for viewing of different planes from the same scan to assess lesion localization or lateralization.

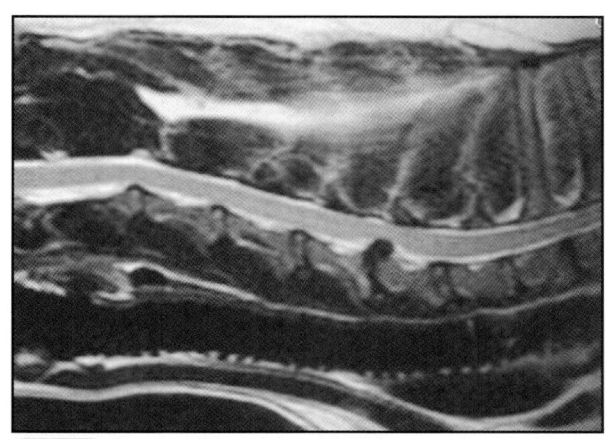

4.3 Sagittal T2-weighted MRI image of a C5–C6 intervertebral disc protrusion in a dog presented for a stiff gait and a right thoracic limb lameness.

In joints, the clinician is often faced with questions regarding the integrity of the intra-articular cartilage, the ligamentous structures and potential meniscal injuries. While MRI currently has a limited use in musculoskeletal disease, there are clearly unprecedented capabilities for it to evaluate joint pathology and tendon and ligamentous injuries. MRI provides excellent contrast and resolution, and provides the ability to differentiate between adjacent joint structures, such as subchondral bone lesions and intra-articular lesions. T1-weighted images provide excellent anatomical detail and high contrast between subchondral bone and cartilage. However, T1-weighted images are inappropriate where there is significant joint effusion as the amount of contrast between articular cartilage and joint fluid is limited and does not allow visualization of even quite significant chondral defects. T2-weighted images may provide additional important information in these cases as well as STIR (short tau inversion recovery), a fat suppression sequence. In evaluating osteoarthritis, MRI may provide more objective measures of disease progression and response to treatment than any other imaging modality.

Clinically in small animal practice, the majority of the work with MRI has been done in the stifle. This is due in part to the frequency of stifle lameness in the dog, as well as the relative ease of imaging this joint and the need to examine different tissues (subchondral bone, cartilage, menisci and cruciate or collateral ligaments; Figure 4.4). A disadvantage of these modalities is that the subject must remain near motionless during the acquisition of the images, i.e. general anaesthesia is required. Further disadvantages include the expense of purchasing and maintaining the equipment.

Nuclear scintigraphy

Nuclear scintigraphy uses radiopharmaceuticals to visualize a system or physiological process within the body. The radiopharmaceutical is given by intravenous injection and an external detector quantifies the radioactivity and location. The most common radionuclide used is technetium 99m (Tc99m). This man-made isotope decays with a gamma emission of 140 keV that is almost ideal for detection. For skeletal disease, Tc99m is coupled with either methylene diphosphonate (MDP) or hydroxymethylene diphosphonate (HDP). Immediately following intravenous injection, vascular/perfusion images can be acquired, detailing areas of increased blood flow. During the next 5–20 minutes, the radiopharmaceutical redistributes into the tissues; images at this time interval are of the 'pool phase'. Approximately 70% of the radioactivity is passed out in the urine during the next 2 hours. Skeletal images viewed after this interval have a good 'target (bone) to background (tissue) ratio'. The external detector of

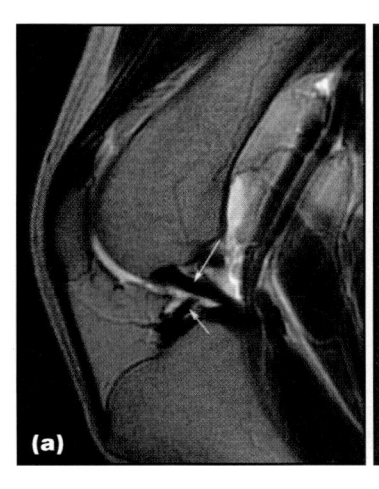

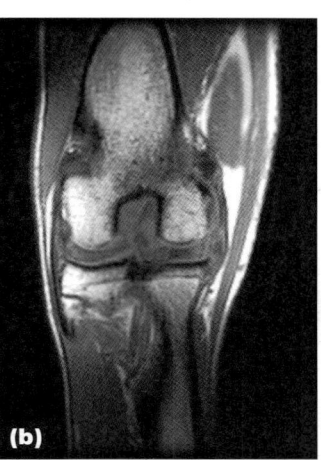

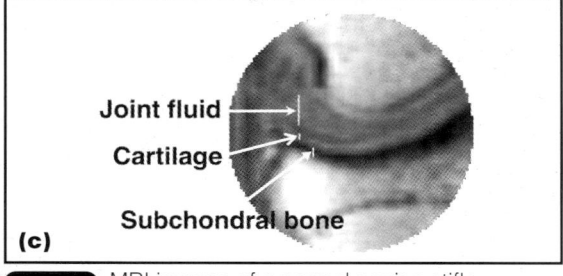

4.4 MRI images of a normal canine stifle. **(a)** Sagittal T2-weighted, with arrows identifying the cruciate ligaments (yellow, cranial cruciate; white, caudal cruciate). (Courtesy of Dr R Tucker.) **(b)** Transverse image. **(c)** Close-up view, showing joint fluid, articular cartilage and subchondral bone (arrowed). (Courtesy of Dr R Parks.)

Chapter 4 Advanced diagnostic techniques

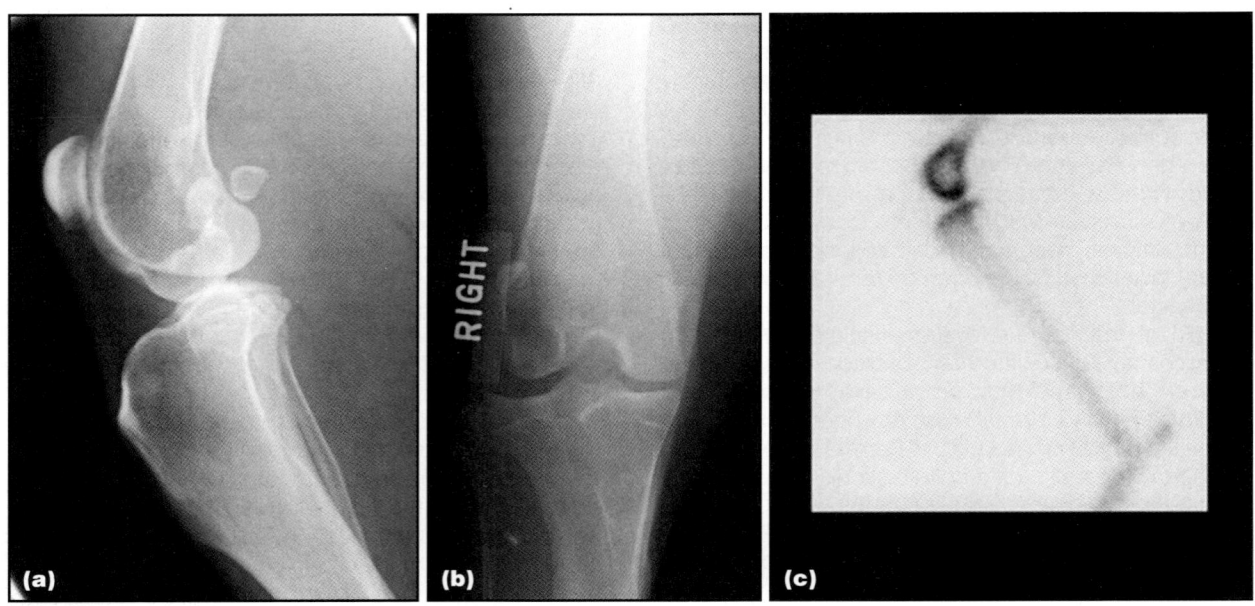

4.5 Images of the right stifle of a 10-year-old Greyhound with a history of a mild intermittent lameness that was followed by an acute non-weightbearing event. Lateral **(a)** and craniocaudal **(b)** radiographs show punctate subtle osteolysis in the distal femoral condyle. **(c)** Nuclear scintigraphic examination shows increased activity in the distal femur. In fact the activity in the central area is so intense that the scan is unable to count all the activity.

choice is a sodium iodide crystal coupled to photomultiplier tubes, called either an Anger or gamma camera. Electronic circuitry produces a planar image of small dots. Counting statistics require a certain number of these interactions to produce a useful image. Any motion by the subject will degrade the image. This matrix image is composed of picture elements, called pixels. The size of the matrix determines the resolution of the image. Each pixel has a limit of finite value and if this number is exceeded, the apparent counts in that pixel would be reset to zero. The radiographs in Figure 4.5 show only punctate osteolysis. Nuclear scintigraphy, however, reveals an increased area of activity in the distal femur (Figure 4.5c). The central region appears to have no radioactivity and is surrounded by areas of intense uptake. The area of increased radioactivity reflects increased metabolic activity. In fact, the activity is so intense centrally that the number of counts available per pixel was exceeded, giving the appearance of no uptake. Some software programmes 'reset' and begin counting again, others cease counting that pixel and it remains 'cold'. Unfortunately, while nuclear scintigraphy is very sensitive, it lacks specificity. However, scintigraphy can be very useful when a lameness has been isolated to a limb and radiographs show minimal or no change (Figure 4.6).

Ultrasonography

Ultrasonographic imaging of joints is currently very limited in small animal orthopaedics. Diagnostic high-frequency ultrasonography is commonly used in human medicine, offering superior spatial resolution and a dynamic examination in a comfortable, efficient and cost-effective manner. Ultrasonography offers a non-invasive technique to evaluate synovitis, periarticular masses, meniscal and ligamentous disease, as well as

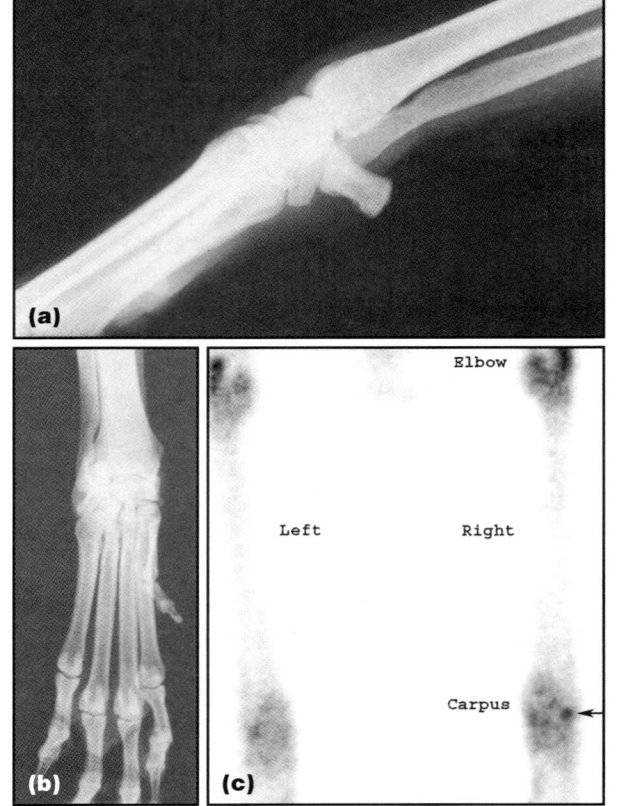

4.6 Images of a 2-year-old Collie with an intermittent lameness of the thoracic limb. Lateral **(a)** and dorsopalmar **(b)** radiographs show no changes. **(c)** Nuclear scintigraphic examination shows a subtle but significant area of increased activity in the right carpus (arrowed). While the scan identifies a potential site for the lameness, it does not provide any additional information about the anatomical or physiological cause; in this case, neither does radiography.

cartilage defects (Court-Payen, 2004). This modality, however, is still in its infancy in veterinary medicine. To date, canine studies have been mainly limited to identifying normal and pathological structures in the shoulder and stifle (Kramer *et al.*, 1999; Long and Nyland, 1999). Another study compared ultrasonographic evaluation of the coxofemoral joint to other commonly employed methods of hip evaluation, to determine the accuracy of diagnosing hip dysplasia and the development of secondary osteoarthritis (Adams *et al.*, 2000). More recently, ultrasonography has been reported to be advantageous in the non-invasive evaluation of the menisci and cruciate ligaments in dogs with stifle pathology (Mahn *et al.*, 2005). Given the potential to obtain accurate diagnostic information in a non-invasive manner, without sedation in most veterinary patients, there is a growing role for diagnostic ultrasonography in veterinary medicine. Clearly, more studies are needed to identify both normal and diseased structures, as well as optimizing transducer and frequency for each tissue.

Gait analysis

Use of kinetics (the study of the relationships of movement to the forces that create them) and kinematics (the description of movement, without regard of the influences of force and mass) is growing in small animal clinical medicine, both to establish a diagnosis and to assess the effectiveness of therapeutic agents (DeCamp, 1997; McLaughlin, 2001). Lameness is a variation of a normal gait; most of the lamenesses seen in clinical practice are due to musculoskeletal or neurological causes. In general, the majority of the musculoskeletal lamenesses are considered to be pain-induced, but the relationship or contribution of pain to lameness in many of the neurologically affected dogs and cats is less clear.

Kinetic gait analysis

Force platforms measure three orthogonal ground reaction forces (GRFs) resulting from limb placement during a gait (Figure 4.7). The forces represent the summation of the force transmitted to the ground from a single limb. The forces generated are vertical (F_z), craniocaudal (F_y) and mediolateral (F_x). Vertical force is most directly related to axial weightbearing and generates the waveform with the greatest magnitude. The craniocaudal force can be divided into the braking (or deceleration) phase and the propulsion (acceleration) phase. The mediolateral force measures the amount of limb side-to-side movement (Budsberg *et al.*, 1987).

Data are collected numerically but are often displayed in graphical form (Figure 4.8a). Data from three axes are measured as shown in Figure 4.8b, where the magnitude of the large vertical waveforms can be appreciated relative to the smaller craniocaudal waveform and the very small mediolateral waveform. Quantification of the waveforms includes measuring the maximum (peak) point of each waveform, the area under of the curve of each waveform (total force exerted on the ground during stance) and other variables, such as the slope of the waveform.

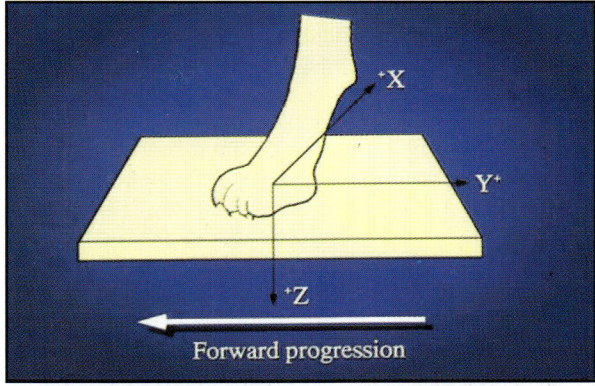

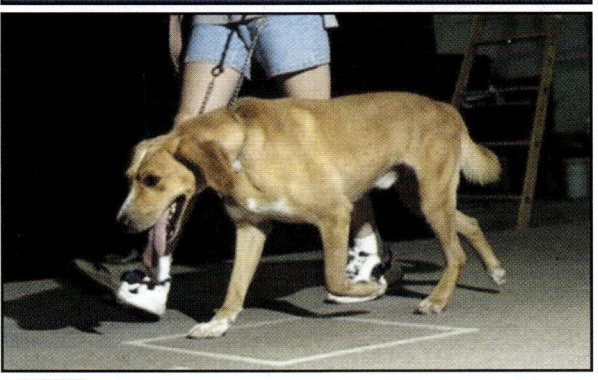

4.7 Kinetic gait analysis. A dog trots across a force plate embedded into a walkway. The force plate is outlined by tape on the carpet. The diagram shows a dog's limb striking a force plate and the axes measured by the plate.

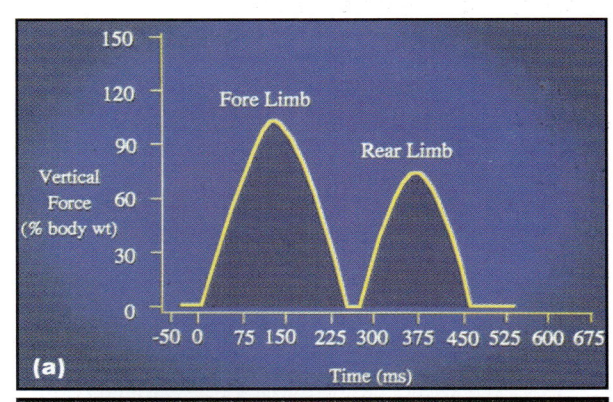

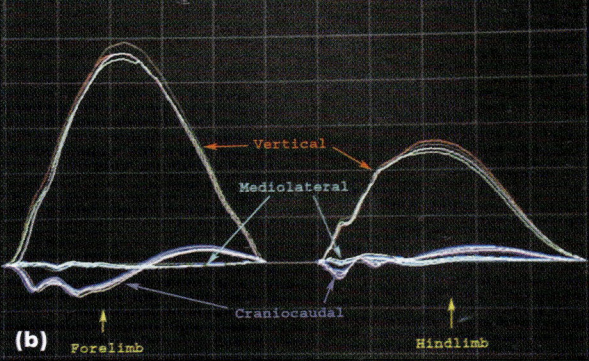

4.8 Kinetic gait analysis. **(a)** A single pass over a force plate by a dog at a trot produces this graphic information. **(b)** Multiple passes of a dog over a force plate, charted together to show the consistency and the repeatability of the data.

Chapter 4 Advanced diagnostic techniques

It is important to remember that GRFs measure general overall limb function and do not provide data specific to individual joints. There are data evaluating individual joint pathology but it is not possible at present to distinguish, for example, a hip lameness from a stifle lameness. Using repeated measurements between thoracic or pelvic limbs, or before and after treatment of a given limb, one can objectively quantify the improvement in the amount of force being placed on the ground. If specific collection protocols are followed, force plate data provide unbiased objective data with low variability, which is paramount in the clinical situation (McLaughlin *et al.*, 1991; Budsberg *et al.*, 1996, 1999; Cross *et al.* 1997; Johnson *et al.*, 2004). Force plates are usually embedded in the floor or a walkway where the animal traverses them. However, force plates can also be embedded in treadmills where they can be used to collect data continuously.

While force plates are the most common method of collecting kinetic data, pressure sensing systems have recently been used to assess gait data (including kinetic) in dogs and cats (Figure 4.9a). Although such pressure systems are limited to measuring vertical forces, and cannot measure mediolateral and craniocaudal forces during locomotion, they offer the advantage of being able to record from multiple foot strikes of all limbs during a single pass. They also have the advantages of being able to record data from a wide range of size of animals (including very small dogs and cats), and of being able to record static weight distribution across all the limbs in the standing animal (Figure 4.9b). However, the use of pressure mats is not without problems. The actual force measurements collected (in Newtons) from pressure mats are not identical to the measurements from force plates, although they are very consistent over time. Additionally, the amount of time required to process the data from the pressure mat system is significantly longer and the method is more labour-intensive. Importantly, both systems provide good objective and quantitative data that can be used in kinetic gait analysis.

Kinematic gait analysis

Use of kinematic gait analysis has dramatically increased over the last few years but it is still not commonly performed in the veterinary clinical setting due to the costs of equipment, the need for a laboratory setting, labour intensiveness and the expertise required. Data collection systems are either video- or optoelectronic-based, and use two to eight cameras depending on the particular system and its sophistication (Figure 4.10). These non-invasive methods provide information on individual joints which includes, but is not limited to, range of motion (flexion/extension: sagittal plane), speed of joint movement (angular velocity) and forces acting around the joint (joint moments). More sophisticated systems provide information about a joint in three dimensions (flexion/extension, abduction/adduction, internal/external rotation). Kinematic analysis can also be used to describe discrete temporal and spatial events from a given gait (walk, trot, pace, etc.) such as stride length and frequency, stance and swing phase duration and patient velocity (DeCamp *et al.*, 1993; Bennett *et al.*, 1996; Hottinger *et al.*, 1996; Tashman *et al.* 2004). As shown in Figure 4.11, the stifle joint of a dog with a ruptured cranial cruciate ligament remains more flexed throughout the stride. This difference from normal is most dramatic at the end of the stance phase where limb propulsion for the ensuing step should be generated. Other data from a study involving the extracapsular repair of induced rupture of the cranial cruciate ligament found that while kinetic data showed improvements to near normal state, the chosen kinematic descriptors did not improve, demonstrating that for specific joint function evaluations, kinematic data were vital to a complete assessment of the surgical intervention (Oakley *et al.*, 1996). Thus, kinematic data are very useful, particularly in assessing specific joint function.

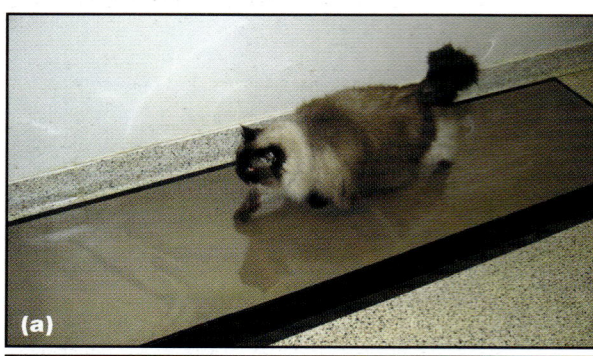

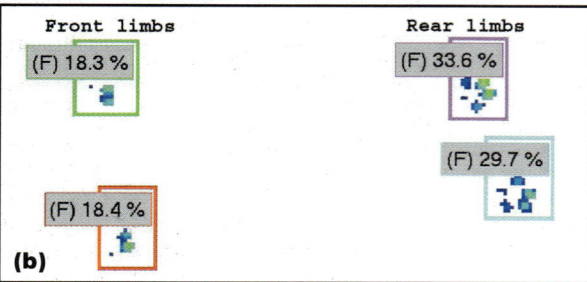

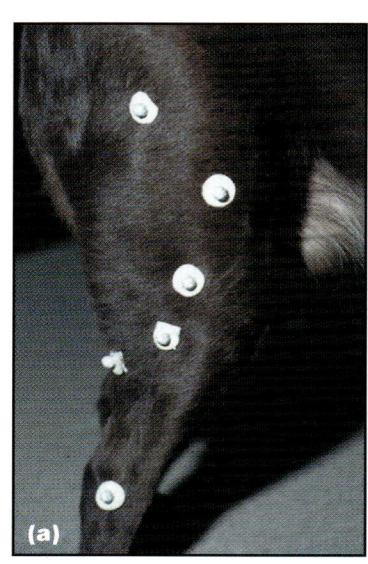

4.9 Kinetic gait analysis. **(a)** A cat walking on a pressure-sensitive mat. **(b)** Print out of weight distribution for an animal standing on the pressure-sensitive mat.

4.10 Kinematic gait analysis. **(a)** Dog with retroreflective markers placed over the femur and tibia to allow for the collection of kinematic data. (continues) ▶

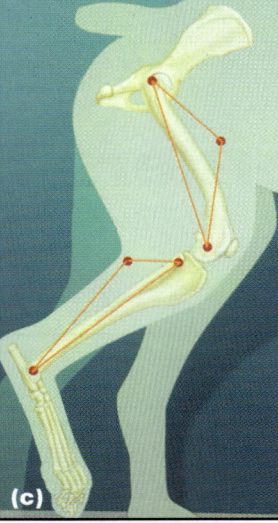

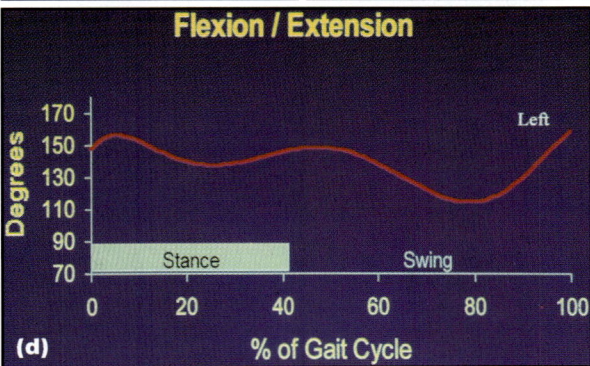

Chapter 4 Advanced diagnostic techniques

have limitations, but as the methodologies are better defined and redefined, the opportunity to improve our understanding of joint-specific problems in our patients will vastly improve. Thus, more precise description of musculoskeletal problems will result in better assessment of limb and joint function as well as improved therapeutic interventions.

References

Adams WM, Dueland RT, Daniels R, *et al.* (2000) Comparison of two palpation, four radiographic and three ultrasound methods for early detection of mild to moderate canine hip dysplasia. *Veterinary Radiology and Ultrasound* **411(4)**, 484–490

Assheuer J and Sager M (1997) *MRI and CT Atlas of the Dog.* Blackwell Science Ltd, Oxford

Bennett RL, DeCamp CE, Flo GL, Hauptman JG and Stajich M (1996) Kinematic gait analysis in dogs with hip dysplasia. *American Journal of Veterinary Research* **57**, 966–971

Bianchi S, Martinoli C, Bianchi-Zamorani M *et al.* (2002) Ultrasound of the joints. *European Radiology* **12**, 56–61

Budsberg SC, Chambers JN, Van Lue SL, Foutz TL and Reece L (1996) Prospective evaluation of ground reaction forces in dogs undergoing unilateral total hip replacement. *American Journal of Veterinary Research* **57**, 1781–1785

Budsberg SC, Johnston SA, Schwarz PD, DeCamp CE and Claxton R (1999) Efficacy of etodolac for the treatment of osteoarthritis of the hip joints in dogs. *Journal of the American Veterinary Medical Association* **214**, 1–5

Budsberg SC, Verstraete MC and Soutas-Little RW (1987) Force-plate analysis of walking gait in the healthy dog. *American Journal of Veterinary Research* **48**, 915–918

Chan WP, Lang P and Genant H (1994) *MRI of the Musculoskeletal System.* WB Saunders, Philadelphia

Court-Payen M (2004) Sonography of the knee: intra-articular pathology. *Journal of Clinical Ultrasound* **32**, 481–490

Cross AR, Budsberg SC and Keefe TJ (1997) Kinetic gait analysis assessment of meloxicam efficacy in a sodium urate-induced synovitis model in dogs. *American Journal of Veterinary Research* **58**, 626–631

Curry TS, Dowdey JE and Murry RE (1990) *Christensen's Physics of Diagnostic Radiology.* Lea & Febiger, Philadelphia

DeCamp CE (1997) Kinetic and kinematic gait analysis and the assessment of lameness in the dog. *Veterinary Clinics of North America* **27**, 825–840

DeCamp CE, Soutas-Little RW, Hauptman JG, *et al.* (1993) Kinematic gait analysis of the trot in healthy Greyhounds. *American Journal of Veterinary Research* **54**, 627–634

Hottinger HA, DeCamp CE, Olivier NB, *et al.* (1996) Noninvasive kinematic analysis of the walk in healthy large-breed dogs. *American Journal of Veterinary Research* **56**, 381–388

Johnson KA, Francis DJ, Manley PA, Chu Q and Caterson B (2004) Comparison of the effects of caudal pole hemi-meniscectomy and complete medial meniscectomy in the canine stifle joint. *American Journal of Veterinary Research* **65**, 1053–1060

Kramer M, Stengel H, Gerwing M, *et al.* (1999) Sonography of the canine stifle. *Veterinary Radiology and Ultrasound* **40(3)**, 282–293

Long CD and Nyland TG (1999) Ultrasonographic evaluation of the canine shoulder. *Veterinary Radiology and Ultrasound* **40(4)**, 372–379

Mahn MM, Cook JL, Cook CR and Balke MT (2005) Arthroscopic verification of ultrasonographic diagnosis of meniscal pathology in dogs. *Transactions of the Veterinary Orthopedic Society* **32**, 44

McLaughlin RM (2001) Kinetic and kinematic gait analysis in dogs. *Veterinary Clinics of North America* **31**, 193–201

McLaughlin RM, Miller CW, Taves CL, *et al.* (1991) Force plate analysis of triple pelvic osteotomy for the treatment of canine hip dysplasia. *Veterinary Surgery* **20**, 291–297

Oakley RE, Decamp CE, Flo GL, *et al.* (1995) Kinematic evaluation of two extracapsular surgical techniques for the treatment of cranial cruciate ligament rupture in dogs. *Veterinary Surgery* **25**, 435

Tashman S, Anderst W, Kolowich P, Havstad S and Arnoczky S (2004) Kinematics of the ACL-deficient canine knee during gait: serial changes over two years. *Journal of Orthopaedic Research* **22**, 931–941

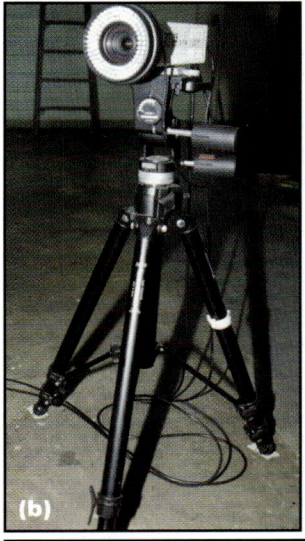

4.10 (continued) Kinematic gait analysis. **(b)** High-speed camera, which is connected to a dedicated computer, used to collect images from the markers. **(c)** Position of the markers on the pelvic limb. **(d)** Graph of the flexion/extension angles of the stifle of a normal dog at a trot.

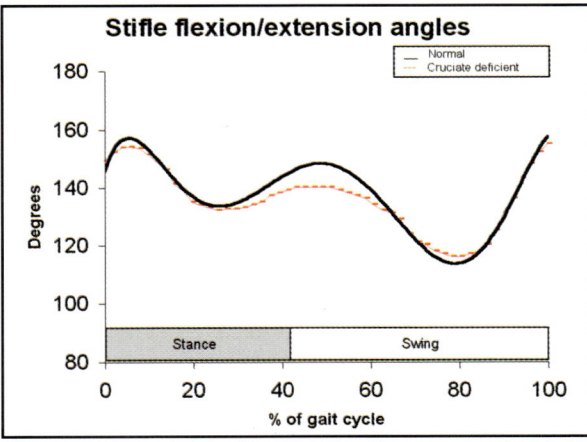

4.11 Graph of the flexion/extension angles of a cruciate-deficient stifle of a dog at a trot.

Kinematic assessment and evaluation of joint movement and function have been used to a limited degree in all the major appendicular joints of the thoracic and pelvic limbs in dogs. These data collection systems

5

Diseases and disorders of bone

Sorrel Langley-Hobbs

Introduction

This chapter will address a variety of metabolic bone diseases and some poorly categorized bone disorders, such as bone cysts and infarcts, that cause lameness in dogs and cats. There are numerous such bone conditions that have been reported in the literature but it is beyond the scope of this chapter to cover all of them. Conditions affecting the growth plates will be covered in Chapter 6, neoplastic bone disease in Chapter 9 and conditions specific to certain joints, such as ischaemic necrosis of the femoral head, will be covered in the appropriate chapters.

Metabolic bone diseases are conditions in which all parts of the skeleton are affected to a varying degree. Most conditions are characterized either by an increase in bone formation or by bone loss. They can therefore be classified into hyperostotic or osteopenic conditions.

Hyperostotic bone conditions

Panosteitis

Panosteitis is a self-limiting, episodic disease of the long bones, characterized by focal areas of endosteal bone proliferation. Synonyms include juvenile osteomyelitis, eosinophilic panosteitis and enostosis.

Signalment

Panosteitis is typically seen in young large-breed dogs, 6–18 months of age. Very occasionally middle-aged dogs are affected, and these are usually German Shepherd Dogs (Bohning *et al.*, 1970). There is a male:female ratio of 4:1 (Bohning *et al.*, 1970). When females are affected, the first episode is usually associated with the first oestrus. The most common breed affected is the German Shepherd Dog but panosteitis has also been reported in the Labrador Retriever, Bassett Hound, Dobermann, Great Dane, Golden Retriever and other large breeds.

Aetiology/pathogenesis

Canine panosteitis is a disease of the adipose bone marrow characterized by degeneration of medullary adipocytes. This is followed by stromal cell proliferation, intramembranous ossification, resorption and remodelling. Medullary vascular congestion and hyperaemia may account for the associated pain.

The precise aetiology of panosteitis has not been elucidated but there are many hypotheses. Bacterial osteomyelitis was originally thought to be the underlying cause but blood cultures are routinely negative and dogs have normal white blood cell counts; in one necropsy study of 18 affected dogs no bacteria were isolated (Zeskov, 1960).

Panosteitis has been successfully transmitted from affected dogs to healthy dogs by intramedullary inoculation of bone marrow (Zeskov, 1960), although the radiographic changes were equivocal. No bacteria were isolated from inocula and transmission was achieved with and without filtration to remove most bacteria. These findings may be consistent with a viral aetiology. Canine distemper virus, both the field and vaccination strain, has been implicated. However, when German Shepherd Dogs and Pointer puppies were reared together only the German Shepherd Dogs developed panosteitis. This would be unlikely to be the case if the cause were infectious, although breed susceptibilities may exist.

A hereditary cause is another possibility as the condition can be seen in whole litters of puppies. The incidence in German Shepherd Dogs might support this suggestion but it does not account for why the condition is also seen in so many other breeds, often sporadically. Other hypotheses include transient vascular anomalies, allergies, a metabolic phenomenon, hyperoestrogenism, parasite migration and an autoimmune reaction following a viral infection.

History and clinical signs

Lameness is usually acute in onset and severe, often progressing over the first few days to a non-weightbearing lameness. Bouts of lameness usually last 2–3 weeks. Lameness typically has a migratory pattern as the disease shifts from bone to bone. However bones in the same limb can be affected causing a prolonged single leg lameness. With age, the lameness usually becomes less pronounced and the interval between successive episodes increases.

Pain is elicited by deep palpation of the affected area of the bone. A normal dog can tolerate without signs of pain very firm bone palpation (pressure that causes blanching of the veterinary surgeon's fingernails). Care should be taken when palpating dogs with panosteitis as they can react unpredictably and aggressively, even with quite gentle bone palpation. Dogs with panosteitis can become systemically ill and exhibit pyrexia and tonsillitis with elevated white blood counts, but these signs are usually not present. Panosteitis may also be present with other common orthopaedic disorders, such as osteochondrosis and hip dysplasia, and these conditions may be detected on clinical examination.

Diagnostic imaging
Good quality radiographs are necessary to see the subtle radiographic changes (Figure 5.1). If changes are not apparent on the initial radiographs then further films should be taken 2–3 weeks later. It is generally recommended to take radiographs of multiple long bones if suspicious of panosteitis, as radiographic changes do not necessarily correlate with the dog's clinical signs or degree of pain exhibited on clinical examination. More obvious radiographic lesions may be found in bones that were not painful on palpation. The disease usually begins in the bones of the thoracic limb, with the proximal ulna most commonly affected (Figure 5.2), followed by the central radius, distal humerus, proximal and central femur and proximal tibia. Metacarpal bones and the pelvis can also be involved.

Scintigraphy has been found to be more sensitive than radiography in detecting early lesions of panosteitis. However, radiography is more sensitive and specific in the later stages of the disease and in establishing a definitive diagnosis (Turnier and Silverman, 1978).

Radiographic changes and pathological features of panosteitis are summarized in Figure 5.3.

Differential diagnoses
Differential diagnoses include all conditions causing lameness in the immature large-breed dog:

- Hip dysplasia
- Shoulder osteochondrosis
- Elbow dysplasia
- Cranial cruciate ligament rupture
- Metaphyseal osteopathy
- Osteomyelitis
- Nutritional secondary hyperparathyroidism.

5.1 An early and fairly subtle panosteitis lesion in the proximal humeral diaphysis.

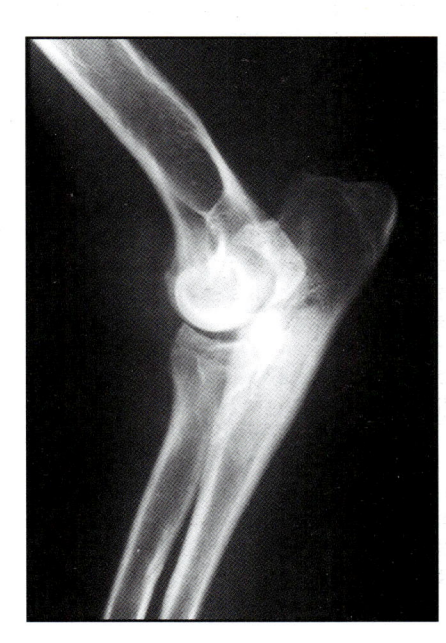

5.2 Radiograph of an elbow of a 10-month-old German Shepherd Dog with an area of increased medullary bone density characteristic of panosteitis in the proximal ulna. There is also marked incongruity of the humeroradial joint and flattening of the medial coronoid process.

Day of cycle	Radiographic phases	Pathogenesis
0	Very early – increased radiolucency to medullary bone	Degeneration of medullary adipocytes adjacent to nutrient foramen
10–14	Early – subtle poorly marginated and occasionally granular increased radiodensity evident in medullary canal. Medullary blurring and loss of corticomedullary contrast results	Proliferation of stromal and adventitial cells of bone marrow – intramembranous ossification starts
20–30	Middle – obvious patchy mottled increase in radiodensity, approaching that of cortical bone. Endosteal roughening and an accentuated coarsened trabecular pattern may be visible. Periosteal and endosteal new bone formation usually develops such that cortices may appear thickened and indistinct in affected areas – bone is usually smooth and laminar in appearance	Nidus enlarges, becoming attached to endosteal surface. Fibrous bone trabecular pattern replaced by laminar bone. Periosteal reaction appears secondary to medullary osseous reaction
70–90	Late – medullary canal regains normal appearance and patchy radiodensities disappear as lesions are gradually remodelled	Remodelling and re-establishment of vascularization. Osteolysis begins at area of initial nidus formation

5.3 Radiographic and pathological changes seen with panosteitis.

Chapter 5 Diseases and disorders of bone

Treatment and prognosis
Panosteitis is usually self-limiting, with a spontaneous recovery after several weeks, although lameness may persist or migrate from limb to limb in some dogs. Relapses are possible, usually occurring about 1 month apart (Bohning et al., 1970). Dogs with panosteitis are generally sound between bouts of lameness. In contrast, dogs with many other developmental orthopaedic diseases, such as osteochondrosis or hip dysplasia, often have a persistent lameness.

Treatment is supportive, with restriction of activity and anti-inflammatory medication. Corticosteroids can be effective but they should not be the first line of treatment. The prognosis is good for a complete recovery.

Metaphyseal osteopathy
Metaphyseal osteopathy (MO) is a condition seen in immature medium and large-breed dogs and is characterized by severe lameness, pyrexia, depression and bilaterally symmetrical distal metaphyseal bone changes. Synonyms include hypertrophic osteodystrophy, Möller Barlow's disease, skeletal scurvy, infantile scurvy, osteodystrophy II and metaphyseal dysplasia.

Signalment
The disease affects young, rapidly growing medium and large-breed dogs. Puppies present between the ages of 2 and 6 months, and males may be slightly predisposed. Many breeds are affected including the Boxer, Weimaraner, Great Dane, Irish Wolfhound, St Bernard and Border Collie. It is occasionally but rarely seen in smaller breeds.

Aetiology/pathogenesis
The cause of metaphyseal osteopathy is unknown but many hypotheses exist. Vitamin C levels have been described as being low in affected dogs. However, it is also known that these levels are dependent on exercise, food intake and stress. Since dogs suffering from MO are under stress and often anorexic, the finding may not, therefore, be unexpected. Additionally the results of vitamin C therapy have been disappointing. Dogs fed on diets with high levels of calcium and/or carbohydrates have also developed MO.

There is a history of prior illness in some dogs, so the possibility of an infectious cause has been cited. The multifocal perivascular infiltrations of neutrophils seen histologically may also be suggestive of osteomyelitis, but this histological picture is more typical of a bacterial rather than viral infection. Canine distemper virus has been isolated from bone samples from three dogs affected with MO (Mee et al., 1992). However, no convincing evidence has been found linking MO with canine distemper virus in the general population (Munjar et al., 1998). To attempt to fulfil Koch's postulates, blood from affected dogs was tranfused into 3-month-old puppies. Clinical signs of classical acute distemper developed 2 weeks later but the puppies died without signs of MO (Grondalen, 1979).

In Weimaraners, severe clinical signs and classic bone changes have developed following vaccination (Abeles et al., 1999; Harrus et al., 2002). It is likely that the development of MO in both Weimaraners and Irish Setters has a multifactorial aetiology, related to immunoincompetence, neutrophil dysfunction and canine distemper virus. The response to corticosteroids has been promising but dogs should be thoroughly evaluated first for bacterial infections.

History and clinical signs
Clinically the signs range from mild lameness to a severely affected collapsed animal. The latter dogs are often presented for the systemic manifestations of the disease, including pyrexia, anorexia, depression and collapse, rather than lameness. Dogs have swollen metaphyseal areas. Palpation and manipulation should distinguish this swelling from joint effusions (Figure 5.4). There may have been a history of diarrhoea prior to the first appearance of MO. Ocular and nasal discharge, tonsillitis and hyperkeratosis of footpads have also been reported in affected dogs.

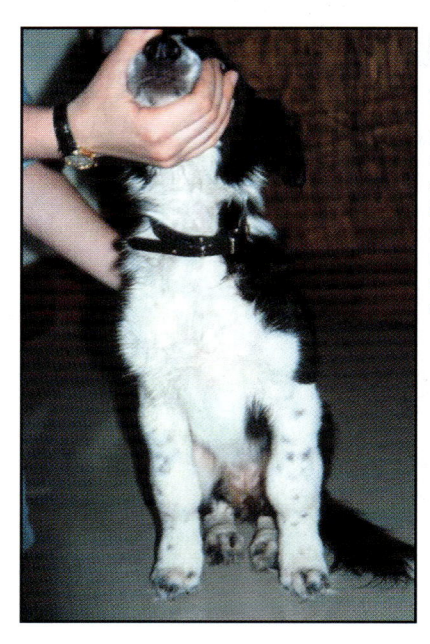

5.4 A 5-month-old Border Collie with metaphyseal osteopathy, showing marked swelling of the metaphyseal areas of the distal and proximal antebrachia.

Laboratory analysis
Mild decreases may be seen in the red blood cell count and in haemoglobin concentration, while the white blood cell count may be slightly increased. Bacteraemia has been reported in one dog. Bacterial culture of blood has been recommended in severely affected dogs (Schulz et al., 1991). However, the infection may represent a secondary manifestation in an immunocompromised dog rather than the primary cause.

Radiology
Changes are seen in the metaphyses of the long bones, most commonly the distal radius and ulna but also the distal tibia. In more chronic cases, the more proximal metaphyses may be involved. Other affected bones include the mandible, scapula, ribs and metacarpal bones. Changes are usually bilaterally symmetrical.

There is a linear area of increased radiodensity adjacent to the normal growth plate with a radiolucent zone in the metaphysis, parallel to the epiphysis (the Tummerfield zone). The epiphysis and growth plates appear normal or slightly widened. In the later phases of the disease calcification occurs proximal to the metaphysis (Figure 5.5). This probably represents mineralization of the subperiosteal haematoma and periosteum, and it may extend to involve the whole diaphysis. At this stage the radiolucent line may no longer be visible.

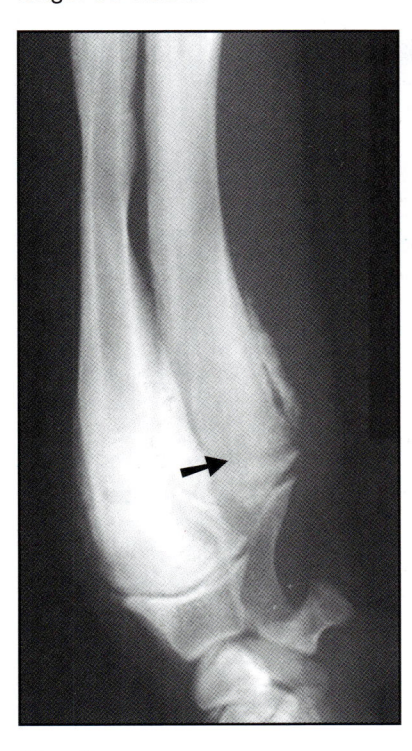

5.5 Radiograph of the distal radius and ulna from an Irish Wolfhound with metaphyseal osteopathy. There is periosteal new bone production in the metaphyseal regions; the classic radiolucent zone (arrowed) is just visible in the distal ulna.

Histology
Histologically the metaphyseal lesions are characterized by the following changes, progressing from the growth plate to the metaphysis:

- Normal or slightly widened growth plate, due to increased length of columns of hypertrophied chondrocytes
- Narrow zone of increased radiodensity immediately adjacent to the physis. This is a consequence of trabecular collapse and mineralization of trabecular haemorrhages
- Progressing towards the diaphysis the spongiosa becomes more disorganized, there is a broad band of cellular infiltration, while bone trabeculae become necrotic and more or less absent, reflecting the lucent zone seen radiographically
- Secondary trabeculae of woven bone deposited on pre-existing trabecular remnants, which are often necrotic
- Subperiosteal haemorrhage, thickened periosteum with subperiosteal fibrosis and inflammation and periosteal new bone formation.

Treatment
Treatment may not alter the outcome, although there are several aspects of management that can improve the dog's well-being. A suggested protocol is shown in Figure 5.6.

Analgesia	
Non steroidal anti-inflammatory drugs Injectable opioids if hospitalized or oral opioids by prescription (buprenorphine sublingual tablets)	
Antibiotics	
Broad-spectrum, to protect against osteomyelitis and secondary infections	
Intravenous fluids	
Given if dog is dehydrated, anorexic and pyrexic	
Physiotherapy and hydrotherapy	
Dogs are reluctant to move and bear weight because of pain, so gentle range-of-motion exercise and hydrotherapy should be performed to reduce joint stiffness and muscle atrophy	
Diet	
A balanced commercial diet should be fed. Mineral or vitamin supplements should not be given. Animal should be tempted with food if anorexic	
Nursing	
For recumbent animals, plenty of soft bedding should be provided and the animal should be turned every 2–4 hours to avoid pressure sores	
Cold packs	
Ice packs should be applied three or four times daily to reduce metaphyseal heat, alleviate pain and thus encourage movement	

5.6 A suggested treatment protocol for dogs with metaphyseal osteopathy.

Prognosis
Many dogs recover within a week, with no recurrence, but relapses are not uncommon. Death has been reported in 25–33% of cases and euthanasia may be requested, generally because of the distressing appearance of the puppy. Residual skeletal deformities have been seen in more severely affected animals related to the growth rate discrepancies, either within a given metaphysis or between metaphyses of paired bones (radius and ulna). Lateral patellar luxation has been seen secondary to bilateral premature closure of the lateral aspect of the distal femoral condyle, and puppies have been noted to be 'cow hocked' and to suffer from carpal valgus (Lenehan and Fetter, 1985).

Craniomandibular osteopathy
Craniomandibular osteopathy (CMO) is a non-inflammatory, non-neoplastic proliferative bone disease seen in immature dogs. The condition is most common in the bones of the skull, especially the occipital bone, tympanic bullae and mandibular body. Bone changes are usually bilaterally symmetrical. Synonyms include mandibular periostitis, temporomandibular osteodystrophy and lion jaw.

Signalment
The onset of signs is usually between 4 and 10 months of age. There is no reported sex predisposition. The breeds most commonly affected are the West Highland White and Scottish Terriers; however, it has

also been recognized in other breeds including the Boston Terrier, Cairn Terrier, Great Dane, Dobermann and Labrador Retriever (Alexander and Kallfelz, 1975). Irish Setters develop similar jaw changes associated with a more serious and ultimately fatal disease, canine leucocyte adhesion deficiency (Trowald-Wigh et al., 1995).

Aetiology
The condition is inherited in an autosomal recessive fashion in West Highland White Terriers (Padgett and Mostosky, 1986). Given its high prevalence in other breeds, such as Scottish Terriers, there may be other hereditary predispositions. There appears to be a lower but unproven risk of CMO after neutering, suggesting a possible hormonal influence (Watson et al., 1995). A viral aetiology, perhaps canine distemper virus, has been proposed, but there is no conclusive evidence to support this (Munjar et al., 1998).

Clinical signs
These include obvious mandibular swelling, inability to open the mouth completely, drooling, weight loss and intermittent pyrexia. Lymphadenopathy and temporal muscle atrophy may also be present.

Radiology
Changes are usually bilateral but can be asymmetrical. Proliferative palisading bone affects the mandible and petrous–tympanic area (Figure 5.7). The disease usually affects both regions but occasionally will just be confined to one area (Figure 5.8). Other bones that may be affected include the occipital, parietal, frontal, tentorium ossium, maxilla and, rarely, appendicular bones. Medullary cavity and cortices may be indistinguishable because of the superimposition of new bone.

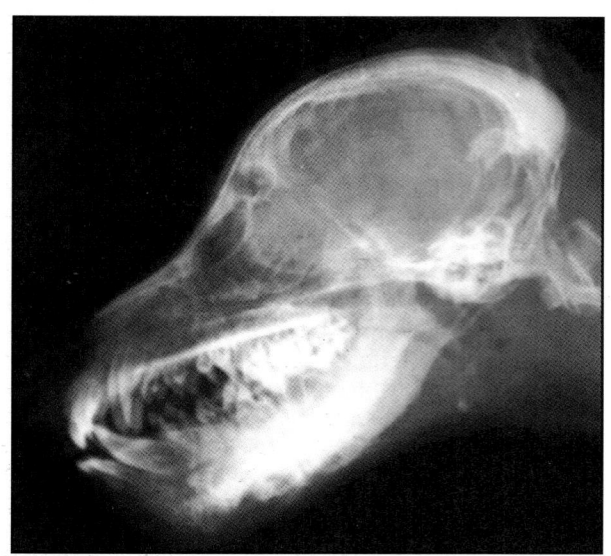

5.7 Skull radiograph showing proliferative palisading periosteal bone affecting the mandible of a dog with craniomandibular osteopathy. There is also smooth laminated bone production over the frontal and parietal bones.

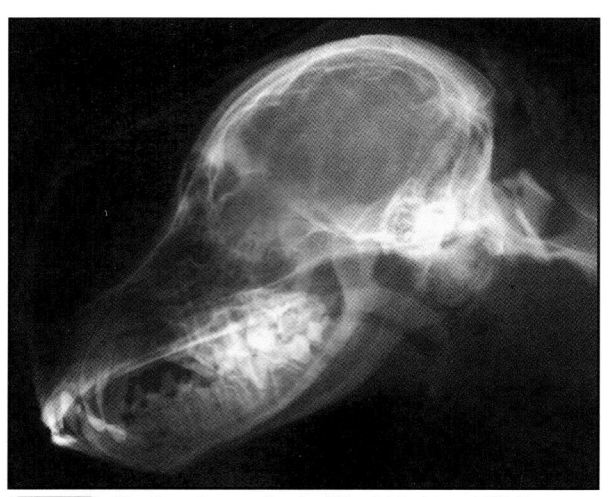

5.8 Skull radiograph of a West Highland White Terrier with craniomandibular osteopathy. Bone production is isolated to the petrous–tympanic area and there is some thickening of the frontal/parietal bones.

Laboratory analysis
No significant abnormalities have been found on haematological or biochemical analysis of blood. There may be mild elevations in alkaline phosphatase, phosphate, cholesterol and gamma-globulins. Multiple blood cultures from four West Highland White Terriers were all negative (Riser et al., 1967).

Histology
There is osteoclastic resorption of the original lamellar bone, followed by replacement with a primitive woven bone expanding beyond the normal periosteal boundaries. Normal bone marrow spaces are replaced with a highly vascular fibrous stroma and invaded by inflammatory cells (neutrophils, lymphocytes and plasma cells). The pattern of cement lines in the new bone is compatible with alternating periods of bone formation and resorption. Frontal and parietal bone changes show generalized thickening without disrupting the outer or inner surfaces.

Differential diagnoses
Differentials to consider, especially in atypical breeds or if changes are asymmetrical, include canine leucocyte adhesion deficiency, osteomyelitis, traumatic periostitis and neoplasia.

Treatment
Non-steroidal anti-inflammatory drugs should be prescribed initially but are often insufficient to alleviate the clinical signs. Corticosteroids frequently appear to be more beneficial. If food intake is impaired, liquefied food should be provided. In a few isolated and select cases, mandibulectomy may be necessary to allow oral intake of food when the bone deposition prevents or severely limits opening of the mouth. One attempt to remove excess bone surgically was unsuccessful (Pool and Leighton, 1969).

Prognosis
The prognosis depends on which bones are involved. New bone production slows after the patient is 7–8

months of age, becoming static and gradually resorbing with time (Alexander and Kallfelz, 1975). However, bone deposition can interfere with the temporomandibular joint, or even respiration; the poorest prognosis is associated with bone deposition around the temporomandibular joint. Some owners may request euthanasia because of a puppy's pain and/or inability to eat.

Hypervitaminosis A
This is a condition seen in cats, especially those fed a diet consisting largely of liver, and is characterized by extensive confluent exostoses of the cervicothoracic vertebrae and the appendicular skeleton.

Signalment
Affected cats are presented for treatment at ages ranging from 2 to 9 years.

Pathogenesis
Vitamin A causes increased sensitivity of the periosteum to trauma. The cervicothoracic region is particularly sensitive because of the grooming activity of cats. Vitamin A renders lysosomal membranes more labile, and susceptible to rupture and release of enzymes.

History and clinical findings
General signs consist of malaise, anorexia, lethargy, irritability, exophthalmos and a scurfy dull coat. Where there is encroachment of new bone on intervertebral foramina, signs can also include ataxia, paralysis and urinary problems.

Radiology
Confluent exostoses occur on the ventral aspect of the cervicothoracic spine producing ankylosis (Figure 5.9). Exostoses are also seen in the elbow, shoulder, hip, stifle, ribs and sternebrae.

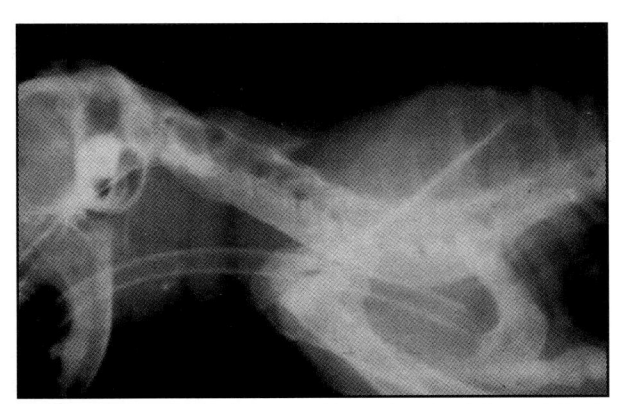

5.9 Spondylosis caused by extensive intervertebral exostoses in a 12-year-old cat with hypervitaminosis A. The first rib and sternum also show new bone deposition.

Histopathology
Subperiosteal proliferation of new woven bone occurs around the apophyseal joints. Proliferation of cartilage from the margins of articular hyaline cartilage overgrows the joint and replaces synovial membrane. Myeloid marrow becomes resorbed and replaced with fibrous marrow.

Treatment and prognosis
Removal of liver from the diet results in no further progression of the lesions and clinical signs improve markedly within a couple of weeks. However, there is little significant regression of the radiographic signs.

Hypertrophic osteopathy
This condition is characterized by lameness associated with swelling and periosteal new bone production affecting mainly the metacarpal and metatarsal bones. It is a paraneoplastic syndrome secondary to another disease process, usually thoracic neoplasia. Synonyms include hypertrophic pulmonary osteopathy, hypertrophic pulmonary osteoarthropathy and Marie's disease.

Signalment
This condition has been reported most frequently in humans and dogs, but it occurs in a variety of other species, including cats. As hypertrophic osteopathy occurs secondary to other disease processes, a wide variety of ages and breeds can be affected. Boxers may be over-represented, possibly reflecting their propensity to develop neoplasia. Affected animals are usually in middle to old age, again reflecting the incidence of neoplasia.

Primary causes
The most common underlying cause of hypertrophic osteopathy is pulmonary neoplasia (55 out of 60 in one report), both primary and metastatic (Brodey, 1971). Other thoracic causes include pulmonary granulomatous disease, pulmonary abscess, chronic bronchopneumonia, pulmonary tuberculosis, oesophageal *Spirocerca lupi*, dirofilariasis, rib tumours and bacterial endocarditis. Abdominal causes include liver adenocarcinoma, adrenocortical carcinoma and primary neoplasia of the bladder, with and without pulmonary metastases.

Pathogenesis
There are extensive and detailed discussions on the proposed pathophysiology of hypertrophic osteopathy reported in both the human and veterinary literature. Numerous hypotheses exist, the most accepted being a neurovascular mechanism whereby stimulation of the afferent fibres in the vagal or intercostal nerves causes stimulation of efferent fibres in the connective tissue and periosteum of the limbs. This results in an increase to the vascular supply to the limbs. Plethysmographic studies have revealed an increase in blood flow of two to three times normal in affected limbs (Holling *et al.*, 1961). The excess blood flow passes through arteriovenous shunts, bypassing the capillary bed. This produces local passive congestion and poor tissue oxygenation, stimulating proliferation of the connective tissues including the periosteum. It has been postulated that the afferent fibres originate in the thorax and join the vagus in the mediastinum; an alternative pathway might be from the parietal pleura and along the intercostal nerves. The extrapulmonary lesions are thought to exert their effects via the vasopharyngeal and vagus nerves, although release of humoral or toxic factors by the primary lesion may be a more plausible explanation in cases of hypertrophic osteopathy without thoracic involvement.

Chapter 5 Diseases and disorders of bone

Clinical signs
Animals usually present with acute or gradual onset lameness. Signs attributable to the primary lesion are rare at initial presentation. Affected animals may have palpably or visibly thickened non-oedematous limbs. The thickening is warm and pulsatile, and the normally loose skin over the distal limb region is taut.

Radiology
In very early cases only appendicular soft tissue swelling is seen. Bony changes consist of palisading proliferative new bone formation affecting the metacarpal and metatarsal bones and the bones of the distal limbs. The first bones to be affected are the abaxial aspects of the second and fifth metacarpal (Figure 5.10) and metatarsal bones. Changes are usually bilaterally symmetrical. In more advanced cases the bone lesions extend proximally to affect the tibia, radius and ulna, humerus and femur and occasionally the ribs, scapula and vertebrae.

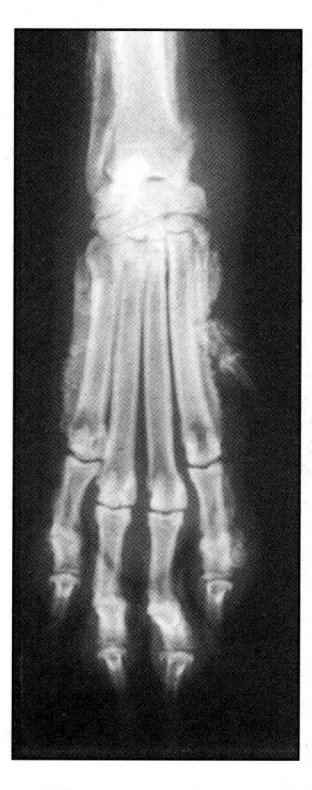

5.10 Palisading new bone formation, mainly affecting the abaxial aspects of metacarpal bones II and V, in a dog with hypertrophic osteopathy.

Thoracic radiographs often show a mass. In the absence of obvious thoracic disease, the abdomen should be scanned for a mass.

Treatment and prognosis
Treatment of hypertrophic osteopathy relies on treating the underlying disease. The bony lesions may resolve after mass resection (Becker *et al.*, 1999), thoracotomy, vagotomy and rib resection. Lameness gradually improves: the heat and pain diminish within a couple of weeks and all signs of lameness resolve within 3–4 months. Radiographic changes take longer to disappear completely but the periosteal bone gradually becomes smoother and less reactive. Long-term survival is often less than optimal because of the underlying disease.

Medullary bone infarcts
There are several reports in the literature of multifocal medullary bone infarcts associated with primary bone sarcomas, usually osteosarcomas (Ansari, 1991). Dogs are usually presented with signs attributable to the primary tumour and the infarcts are incidental radiographic findings.

Signalment
Infarcts tend to affect smaller breeds, with the Miniature Schnauzer being over-represented.

Histopathogenesis
Obliteration of intramedullary arteries with collagen leads to the production of poorly differentiated osteoid and necrosis of bone marrow as a result of hypoxia.

Clinical findings
Dogs may present with signs attributable to the primary bone tumour(s). These are more likely to affect the pelvic limb and multiple tumours may be present.

Radiology
Infarcts are characterized by irregularly demarcated areas of radiopacity in the medullary cavity (Figure 5.11). Bones distal to the elbow and stifle are more likely to be affected.

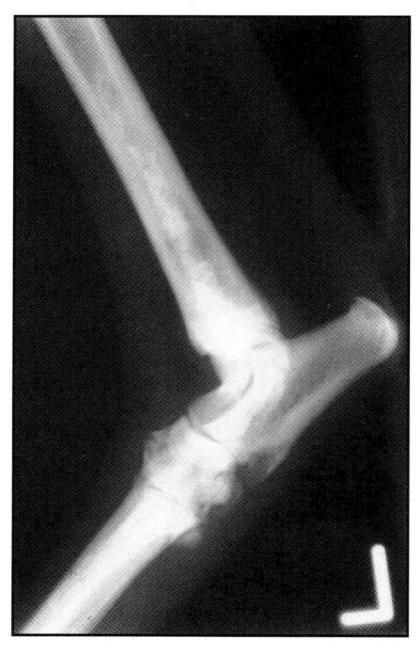

5.11 Infarcts in the distal tibia of an 11-year-old cross-bred dog. The contralateral tibia was affected by a poorly differentiated bone tumour.

Osteomyelitis
The term osteomyelitis implies inflammation of bone and marrow. The commonest causes are bacterial and fungal infections. There are three main forms of osteomyelitis: acute haematogenous, and acute and chronic post-traumatic forms.

Acute haematogenous osteomyelitis
This is an uncommon form of osteomyelitis in dogs and cats. It occurs most commonly in the neonate and may be confused with joint ill.

Chapter 5 Diseases and disorders of bone

Pathogenesis: Emboli of bacteria from septicaemia lodge in the metaphyseal region of bone. The initial focus of infection is frequently the umbilicus. Disruption to the metaphyseal vasculature causes necrosis, hyperaemia and migration of leucocytes. The infection can spread along the bone or break into the joint resulting in a septic arthritis.

Clinical signs: Pyrexia, malaise and lameness are usual. Several limbs or a single bone may be affected. The affected metaphyses are swollen and painful, and there may be evidence of a subsequent septic arthritis.

Radiology: In the early stages, only a soft tissue swelling may be appreciable. Later, irregular areas of bone lysis become apparent within the affected metaphysis. In severe cases, cortical lysis may be evident.

Culture: Blood samples or aspirated material from the swollen area should be submitted for culture and sensitivity testing, and a smear evaluated for the presence of bacteria.

Treatment and prognosis: Antibiotics should be administered *immediately after* collection of material for culture. High levels of bactericidal antibiotics should continue to be used for 3–4 weeks following the cessation of signs. If treatment is instituted quickly, the prognosis in the dog is good. Joint infections should be treated as a matter of urgency.

Acute post-traumatic osteomyelitis
Bacteria enter through a traumatic wound, a bite or gunshot wound, a foreign object such as a nail or, more commonly, through a surgical incision.

Clinical signs: The signs are classic for inflammation, i.e. heat, swelling, pain, redness and loss of function. There may well be wound disruption and a draining tract. If these signs occur and there has been a history of recent surgery or wounding then an infection should be suspected.

Radiology: Radiographs at this stage will only show soft tissue swelling. Nevertheless, they will be helpful in determining the status of any internal fixation device, if present, and to assess fracture stability. Radiographs should then be taken every 10–14 days to monitor progress and response to treatment. However radiographs record events that happened at least 10 days previously, so clinical progress is important in assessing response to treatment in the early stages.

Treatment: This should be instigated as soon as possible. Fracture stability is one of the most important means of controlling infection in bone. Therapy should consist of decompression, debridement, lavage and stabilization. All haematoma, fluid and necrotic material should be removed and samples should be submitted for culture and sensitivity. Following debridement and lavage, the wound can be primarily closed or a closed-suction drain placed. Antibiotics should be given at high levels and for a sufficient length of time, usually for a minimum of 6 weeks.

Chronic post-traumatic osteomyelitis
Following inadequate treatment of acute post-traumatic osteomyelitis the condition may become chronic. Chronic osteomyelitis can become apparent weeks, months or even years later, particularly if implants are present; the condition is rarely cured until these are removed.

Clinical signs: Lameness may or may not be present. There is usually pain, disuse atrophy and tenderness around the affected limb or bone. Discharging sinuses, which drain intermittently, often respond to antibiotic therapy but recur once therapy ceases. The patient is generally well systemically.

Radiology: Sequestra are dead pieces of bone which appear radiographically as dense pieces of bone, with sharp margins. The sequestra can be surrounded by a radiolucent zone and a sclerotic bony margin, the involucrum (Figure 5.12). They are not common in small animals and the more frequent radiographic appearance of chronic osteomyelitis is a lytic area with a sclerotic margin. If a periosteal reaction is present, it is irregular and may extend the length of the diaphysis. This can be differentiated from a healing callus, which will be localized in the area of the fracture.

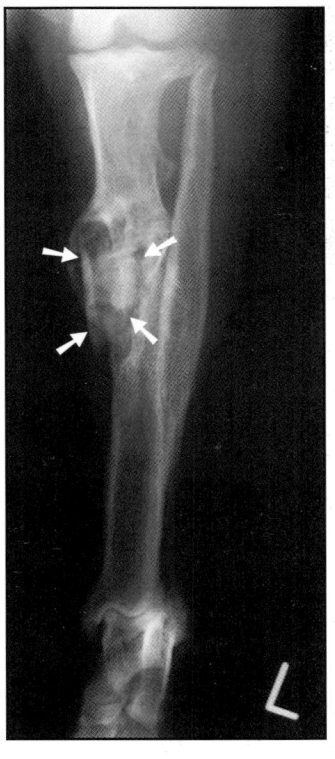

5.12 Radiograph of the tibia of a mature dog presenting with a history of discharging sinuses. A sequestrum is present (arrowed) surrounded by an involucrum. There is massive hypertrophy of the fibula.

Treatment: Chronic osteomyelitis is a surgical disease. The underlying cause should be established and addressed. Instability of a fracture needs to be corrected both to resolve the infection and to allow fracture healing (see *BSAVA Manual of Small Animal Fracture Repair and Management*). If the fracture has healed *completely* then implants should be removed. A treatment regimen is given in Figure 5.13.

Chapter 5 Diseases and disorders of bone

1. Identification of underlying cause: often motion at the fracture site or sequestra.
2. Assessment of the likelihood of successful treatment; amputation is considered if there is loss of joint function, neurological defects or severe muscle or soft tissue loss.
3. Addressing underlying cause:
   - Removal of loose or broken implants
   - Debridement of sequestra and avascular tissue
   - Restoration of stability (external skeletal fixator/plate and screw fixation/interlocking nail); ultimately the stability achieved is more important than the choice of implant.
4. Placement of an autogenous cancellous bone graft?
5. Closure of incision and placement of either a
   - Closed-suction drain
   - Ingress/egress system
   Or initial primary closure.
6. Submission of samples for culture and sensitivity prior to starting on antibiotics.
7. Treatment with broad-spectrum bactericidal antibiotics whilst awaiting sensitivity results.
8. Treatment for 4–6 weeks after cessation of clinical signs with appropriate antibiotics.
9. If implants are still present, these may need removal once fracture has healed and if infection persists.

5.13 Principles of treatment of post-traumatic osteomyelitis.

Fungal osteomyelitis

This is very rare in temperate climes, though more common in hot wet regions. Young animals and immunosuppressed patients seem to be more at risk. Clinical signs are often non-specific and may include general malaise, anorexia, weight loss, respiratory signs, ocular signs and diarrhoea. Abnormalities may be detectable on haematological and biochemical blood analysis. It is always advisable to take thoracic radiographs, as the route of infection is often by inhalation of spores and respiratory tract signs are common. Pulmonary granulomas may be mistaken for lung metastases in association with bone lesions, which themselves can be misdiagnosed as being neoplastic without thorough investigations. When osteomyelitis is present, animals may present with lameness and obvious limb swelling or palpable bony nodules. A summary of the fungal osteomyelitides is given in Figure 5.14.

Species	Distribution	Route of infection	Common clinical signs	Radiographic signs	Diagnostic tests	Treatment options
Coccidioides immitis	South-western USA and South America	Inhalation of spores	Dry non-productive cough, pyrexia	Areas of increased bone density, periosteal elevation and joint involvement	Cytology, culture, serology	Ketoconazole or itraconazole
Blastomyces dermatitidis	USA and Canada	Inhalation of yeast	Respiratory signs, lymphadenopathy, skin papules, ocular signs	Bone destruction or production; often multiple appendicular lesions	Direct microscopic examination of pus	Itraconazole or amphotericin B
Histoplasma capsulatum	Temperate and subtropical areas of the world	Inhalation or ingestion of macroconidia	Variable – multisystemic disease	Mixed bone production and destruction; joints may be involved	Cytology, histopathology, culture	Itraconazole or amphotericin B
Actinomycetes: *Actinomyces bovis* – commensal; *Nocardia* – soil saprophyte	Worldwide	Invades penetrating wound	Jaw and scapular enlargement. Thick mucoid tenacious greenish yellow non-odorous pus with sulphur granules	Bone destruction without formation – early, reaction pronounced	Direct microscopic examination of pus	Iodine solution and systemic antibiotics
	Worldwide	Inhalation, ingestion or direct inoculation into tissue	Mass with numerous sinuses, pyothorax (respiratory signs)	Chronic suppurative osteomyelitis – vertebral, nasal, hock	Culture, direct Gram stain of pus	Penicillin and streptomycin or sulfadiazine 6–12 weeks. Surgical excision of masses

5.14 Summary of the characteristics of selected fungal osteomyelitides. (continues) ▶

Chapter 5 Diseases and disorders of bone

Species	Distribution	Route of infection	Common clinical signs	Radiographic signs	Diagnostic tests	Treatment options
Cryptococcus neoformans (see Figure 5.15)	Worldwide – avian habitats, especially USA and Australia	Inhalation, bird droppings	Sinusitis, nasopharyngeal and pulmonary granulomas. Neural and ocular involvement	Skeletal lesions seen in diaphyses (25% of cases have musculoskeletal involvement)	Cytology, histopathology, culture, serology	Amphotericin B or flucytosine
Aspergillus fumigatus	Worldwide	Inhalation	Nasal: nasal discharge, epistaxis, nasal pain	Loss of nasal turbinates with radiolucency and opacity	Radiology, cytology, histopathology, serology	Topical clotrimazole or enilconazole
			Disseminated: vertebral pain, paraparesis/lameness	Focal bone lucencies and soft tissue mineralization	Urinalysis, serology	Itraconazole

5.14 (continued) Summary of the characteristics of selected fungal osteomyelitides.

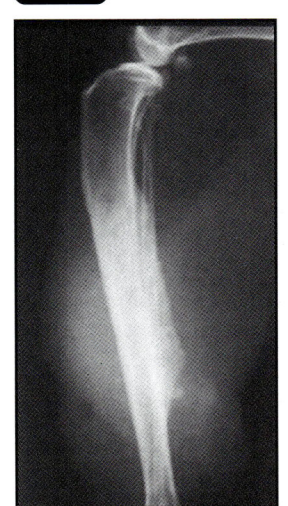

5.15 Proliferative osteomyelitic skeletal lesion in a cat with *Cryptococcus neoformans* infection. A pulmonary granulomatous lesion was also present in the caudal lung lobes (arrowed).

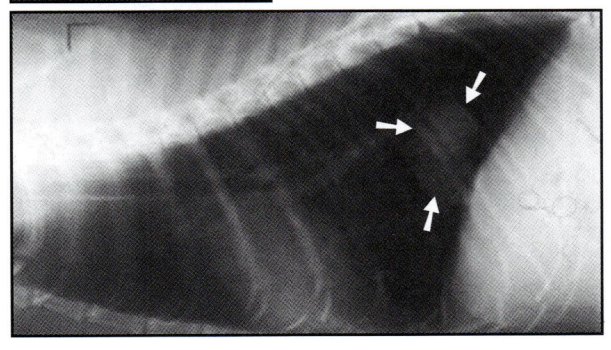

Osteopenic bone conditions

Nutritional secondary hyperparathyroidism

Nutritional secondary hyperparathyroidism (NSH) is usually associated with an absolute deficiency of dietary calcium, most commonly attributed to an all-meat diet. As a multitude of balanced commercial diets are widely available, dietary deficiency diseases are now rare. However, there are still pet owners and breeders who may feed an imbalanced diet through ignorance or misguidance. Therefore NSH should still be considered as a differential diagnosis, particularly in growing dogs or cats with spontaneous fractures or seizures. Other causes of this disease include an inability to absorb dietary calcium or excessive dietary phosphate. Synonyms include osteitis fibrosa, juvenile osteoporosis and paper bone.

Signalment
NSH is primarily a disease of growing animals because of their increased calcium demand for bone growth. Adult animals still develop osteoporosis but more slowly.

Pathogenesis
When the serum calcium level drops, parathyroid hormone (PTH) secretion and synthesis is stimulated. Increased PTH leads to accelerated bone resorption and increased renal calcium resorption, phosphorus excretion and renal synthesis of active vitamin D (calcitriol). Calcitriol stimulates intestinal absorption of calcium and phosphorus through increased synthesis of intestinal calcium-binding protein. Hyperphosphataemia does not stimulate the parathyroid gland directly but does so indirectly by virtue of its ability to lower blood calcium levels.

Clinical signs
Predominant signs are a reluctance to move and play, and lameness. Affected animals may exhibit a plantigrade/palmigrade stance (Figure 5.16) and carpal

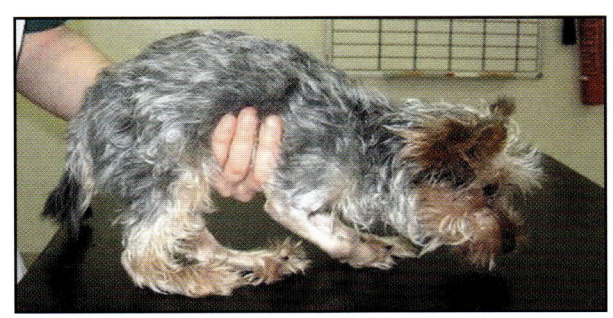

5.16 Nutritional secondary hyperparathyroidism in a 6-month-old Yorkshire Terrier. The dog had recent bilateral radial and ulnar fractures, healed femoral, humeral and pelvic fractures, a fused cervical spine and a plantigrade stance.

Chapter 5 Diseases and disorders of bone

valgus. Affected kittens may present with lordosis subsequent to spinal fractures. Other neurological signs include ataxia, paraparesis, paraplegia and seizures. Acute deterioration may occur after pathological fractures, and tooth eruption and development can be abnormal.

Laboratory investigations
Abnormalities detectable on laboratory analysis of dogs and cats suffering from NSH are listed in Figure 5.17.

Parameter	Finding in NSH
Calcium	Normal or low
PTH	Elevated
Phosphorus	Usually elevated but can be low
Alkaline phosphatase	Increased
25(OH)D$_3$	Low/normal
1,25(OH)$_2$Vitamin D$_3$ (calcitriol)	Normal/elevated
Urine	Decreased urinary calcium

5.17 Abnormalities detectable on laboratory analysis of dogs and cats with nutritional secondary hyperparathyroidism.

Radiology
There is extensive osteopenia of the diaphyses of the long bones and vertebrae. Bone mineralization must be decreased by at least 50% before it is recognized radiographically and in NSH the resulting thinned cortical bone develops a similar radiodensity to medullary bone. A good descriptive term is 'ghost-like' (Figure 5.18). A double cortical line may also be seen (Lamb 1990), reflecting intracortical resorption of bone.

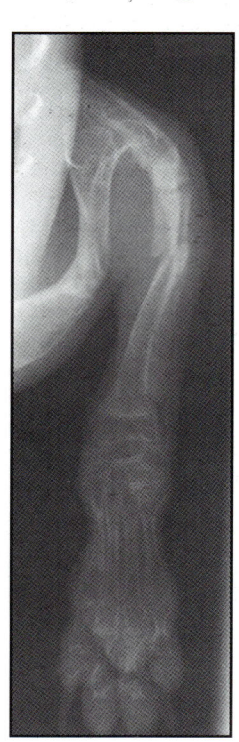

5.18 'Ghost-like' bones of a dog with nutritional secondary hyperparathyroidism. The density of the bone is similar to that of the soft tissue density of the pads. There are radial and ulnar fractures and a healed mid-diaphyseal humeral fracture.

The epiphyses are normal but there may be an area in the metaphysis with an increased density. This probably represents an area of preferential mineralization. Pathological fractures may occur. They are often compression fractures occurring in regions of metaphyseal bone in the vertebrae, pelvis, scapula and proximal humerus.

Histology
Resorption of bone proceeds at a faster rate than repair by fibrous connective tissue proliferation. This results in a decreased bone volume and is called hypostotic fibrous osteodystrophy.

Treatment
The diet should be corrected. This is best achieved by using a commercial puppy or kitten diet. Supplements should not be necessary. Parenteral calcium should be administered if seizuring occurs. Cage rest is necessary to allow the fractures to heal. Internal fixation should be avoided as implants do not hold well in osteopenic bone.

Prognosis
The prognosis is good for uncomplicated cases. Improvement in demeanour should be seen within a week of initiating therapy. The prognosis is guarded if neurological signs are present secondary to vertebral fractures. Healed pelvic fractures can lead to constipation and megacolon.

Renal secondary hyperparathyroidism
Secondary hyperparathyroidism can occur as a complication of chronic renal failure. The jaw seems to be particularly affected.

Pathogenesis
When renal disease is sufficiently advanced to result in phosphorus retention and hyperphosphataemia, PTH is released as a result of the relative hypocalcaemia. This causes secondary hyperparathyroidism and excessive bone resorption. The cancellous bone of the skull is particularly affected and resorption of alveolar socket bone may result in loose teeth.

In chronic renal disease there is also reduced production of vitamin D, and therefore impaired intestinal absorption of calcium, resulting in elements of rickets/osteomalacia due to the impaired mineralization of osteoid. Mandibular bone becomes softened and pliable (fibrous osteodystrophy). Extraosseous calcification, with deposition of mineral in periarticular, visceral and vascular tissues, occurs subsequent to the disordered mineral metabolism.

Clinical signs
The predominant clinical signs relate to the renal disease, and include vomiting, polyuria, polydipsia and depression. Signs relating to the osteopenia/osteomalacia include loose teeth, a pliable mandible and failure to close the jaw properly. This results in drooling of saliva and protrusion of the tongue. Mandibular fractures can occur after minimal trauma such as dental extractions or dog fights. With such presentations, the

possibility of underlying renal secondary hyperparathyroidism should be suspected and investigated. Signs can be more severe in puppies with congenital renal disease, particularly swelling of the jaw and disruption of tooth eruption.

Laboratory investigations
Laboratory findings include elevations in phosphate, urea, creatinine and alkaline phosphatase. Calcium is normal or low (elevated in 5–10% of cases). PTH levels are elevated, often to a level above that in primary hyperparathyroidism.

Diagnostic imaging
Generalized osteopenia of the skull and soft tissue mineralization is evident. Teeth may apparently float in the osteopenic skull (Figure 5.19). All parathyroid glands will appear evenly enlarged on ultrasonography.

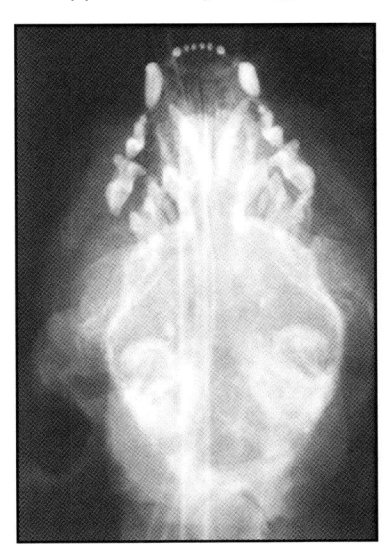

5.19 An osteopenic skull and the appearance of 'floating teeth' in a cat with renal secondary hyperparathyroidism.

Histology
A high percentage of bone has generalized fibrous osteodystrophy. In adults the volume of bones is usually normal (isostotic fibrous osteodystrophy); in immature dogs hyperostotic lesions can be seen, often as facial swellings.

Treatment
The aim must be to treat the renal disease with a reduction in dietary phosphate intake, phosphate bonders and erythropoietin injections, if anaemia exists. If fractures are present, traditional methods of fracture stabilization may not be effective as implants are unlikely to hold well in such osteopenic bone. Thus, salvage options such as hemimandibulectomy should be considered.

Primary hyperparathyroidism
Primary hyperparathyroidism occurs when PTH is produced in excess of normal by functional tumours of the parathyroid glands. These are generally adenomas, but adenocarcinomas may occur. The excess PTH causes increased calcium retention and phosphate excretion by the kidneys. There is accelerated bone resorption and bone is replaced by fibrous tissue. The cancellous bone of the skull is particularly affected.

Clinical signs
These are often attributable to the hypercalcaemia rather than the bone demineralization. Signs include polyuria, polydipsia, anorexia, vomiting, constipation and muscle weakness. Occasionally animals may present with fractures of long bones or vertebrae. Other bony changes include facial hyperostosis due to the deposition of excess woven bone.

Laboratory investigations
Laboratory findings include elevations in calcium, alkaline phosphatase and PTH, and low or normal phosphate levels.

Diagnostic imaging
Radiographic changes in primary hyperparathyroidism include subperiosteal cortical resorption, loss of lamina dura dentes, soft tissue mineralization, bone cysts and a generalized decrease in bone density. In advanced cases fractures may be present, particularly in cancellous bone. There may be nephrocalcinosis and urolithiasis.

Ultrasound examination of the parathyroid glands may show enlargement of one or more glands. All four glands should be assessed and if there is no obvious enlargement the anterior mediastinal area near the base of the heart should be assessed for ectopic tissue.

Treatment
The aim of therapy is to eliminate the source of PTH production. Surgical excision of the parathyroid adenoma or adenocarcinoma is the treatment of choice. The dog should be prepared for surgery by addressing the negative effects of hypercalcaemia preoperatively. Diuresis and the use of bisphosphonates can usefully decrease the hypercalcaemia. Surgical excision of affected tissue should result in a rapid resolution of the problem. As PTH has a half-life of approximately 20 minutes, serological assessment can be a useful indicator of the success of therapy. The calcium levels may drop precipitously after surgery and the dog should be monitored for signs of hypocalcaemia. If calcium levels remain elevated for a week or more after surgery, the presence of a second adenoma or metastases should be suspected.

Rickets
Rickets is an extremely rare bone disease in dogs and cats, characterized by defective mineralization.

Pathogenesis
The metabolic pathway for vitamin D is illustrated in Figure 5.20. Rickets has been recognized in dogs and cats as being secondary to dietary deficiency or as a hereditary defect in either the vitamin D pathway, the vitamin D receptors or renal tubular resorption of phosphate. Summaries of the different forms are listed in Figure 5.21. A diet deficient in either calcium and/or phosphorus and a lack of vitamin D are necessary to produce the disease in normal animals. An absence of exposure to sunlight may also be a significant part of the history, as dogs and cats need sunlight to metabolize vitamin D (Malik et al., 1997).

Chapter 5 Diseases and disorders of bone

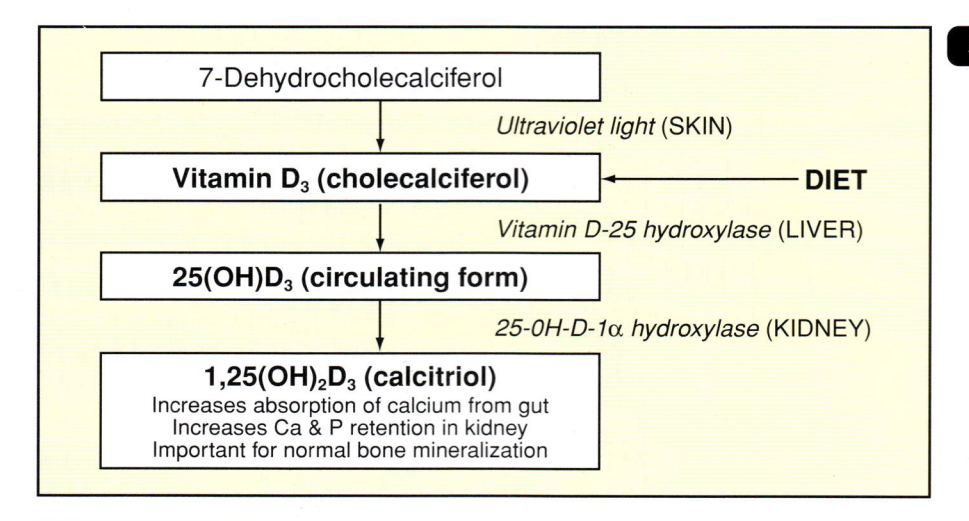

```
┌─────────────────────────────────────────────┐
│         7-Dehydrocholecalciferol            │
│                    │                        │
│                    │ Ultraviolet light (SKIN)│
│                    ▼                        │
│     Vitamin D₃ (cholecalciferol) ◄── DIET   │
│                    │                        │
│                    │ Vitamin D-25 hydroxylase (LIVER)
│                    ▼                        │
│         25(OH)D₃ (circulating form)         │
│                    │                        │
│                    │ 25-OH-D-1α hydroxylase (KIDNEY)
│                    ▼                        │
│         1,25(OH)₂D₃ (calcitriol)            │
│    Increases absorption of calcium from gut │
│    Increases Ca & P retention in kidney     │
│    Important for normal bone mineralization │
└─────────────────────────────────────────────┘
```

5.20 The metabolic pathway of vitamin D.

Type of rickets	Laboratory analysis	Treatment	Reference
Nutritional: vitamin D deficiency. Diet deficient in vitamin D, calcium and/or phosphate	Low 1,25(OH)₂D₃ Hypophosphataemia and/or hypocalcaemia Secondary hyperparathyroidism	Balanced diet, exposure to sunlight	Malik et al., 1997
Hereditary: X-linked hypophosphataemic rickets. Defect in renal tubular resorption of phosphate	Hypophosphataemia High urinary fractional clearance of phosphorus Normocalcaemia Normal 25(OH)D₃ *(high in reference) Normal to low 1,25(OH)₂D₃ Secondary hyperparathyroidism	Phosphate salts	Henik et al., 1999
Hereditary: Vitamin D-dependent rickets type I: defect in calcitriol production	Very low 1,25(OH)₂D₃ Hypocalcaemia Secondary hyperparathyroidism	Calcitriol supplementation	Johnson et al., 1988
Hereditary: Vitamin D-dependent rickets type II: impaired responsiveness of target organs to calcitriol because of defects in vitamin D receptors	Normal 25(OH)D₃ Elevated 1,25(OH)₂D₃ Hypocalcaemia Secondary hyperparathyroidism	Oral calcium supplementation Additional calcitriol	Schreiner and Nagode, 2003

5.21 The different forms of rickets recognized in dogs and cats.

Deficiency of vitamin D causes the production of a cartilage matrix that is highly stable and therefore uncalcifiable and difficult to resorb. In the young animal this results in cartilage cells that fail to degenerate and capillaries from the metaphysis that are unable to penetrate the cartilage. Epiphyseal lines become thickened and irregular.

In adults, osteomalacia occurs, as vitamin D is needed for osteoclasts and osteocytes to respond to PTH and allow bone resorption.

Clinical signs
Affected animals are often young, severely stunted, bowlegged and plantigrade. Metaphyseal areas and costochondral junctions (the so-called 'rachitic rosary') are prominent. Signs can be attributable to the systemic effects of hypocalcaemia rather than the effects on bone. Thus, muscle weakness, tremors or seizures may be the predominant features (Schreiner and Nagode, 2003).

Radiology
Puppies and kittens with rickets show characteristic cup-shaped growth plates due to the accumulation of cartilage at the epiphyses (Figure 5.22). In adults, the bones appear osteopenic and folding fractures may be present.

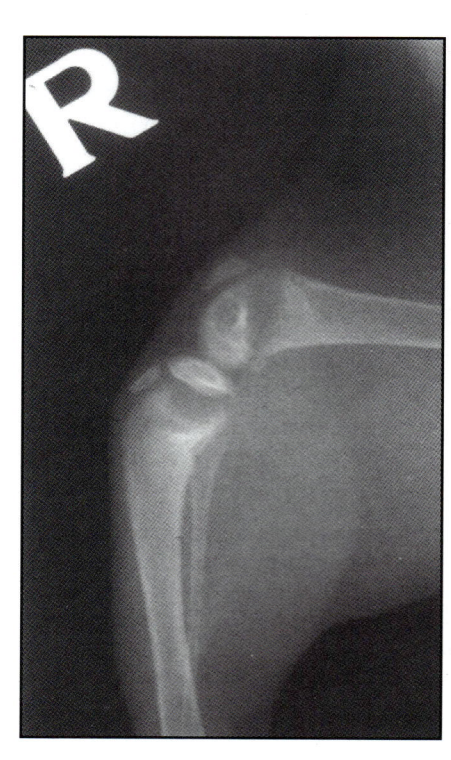

5.22 Epiphyseal widening, or cup-shaped growth plates, in a kitten with congenital rickets (vitamin D-dependent type II) caused by a deficiency or lack of binding to vitamin D receptors.

Treatment and prognosis
If rickets is due to dietary deficiency then providing a balanced diet and exposure to sunlight should be adequate treatment. However, there may be permanent growth plate damage (Malik *et al.*, 1997). The prognosis for the hereditary forms is more guarded for a complete resolution of signs and return to normality.

Bone cysts
Three types of bone cyst are recognized in dogs: unicameral bone cysts; aneurysmal bone cysts; and subchondral cysts associated with osteoarthritis. Subchondral cysts are extremely rare and are believed to form as a result of invagination of the synovial membrane (Basher *et al.*, 1988).

Unicameral bone cysts
Unicameral bone cysts are found in young large-breed dogs in the metaphyses of long bones (Figure 5.23). Such lesions are also classified as monostotic fibrous dysplasia and polyostotic fibrous dysplasia. The term 'fibrous dysplasia' emphasizes the one feature that all these conditions have in common, namely the replacement of bone by fibrous tissue that may contain areas of cystic degeneration.

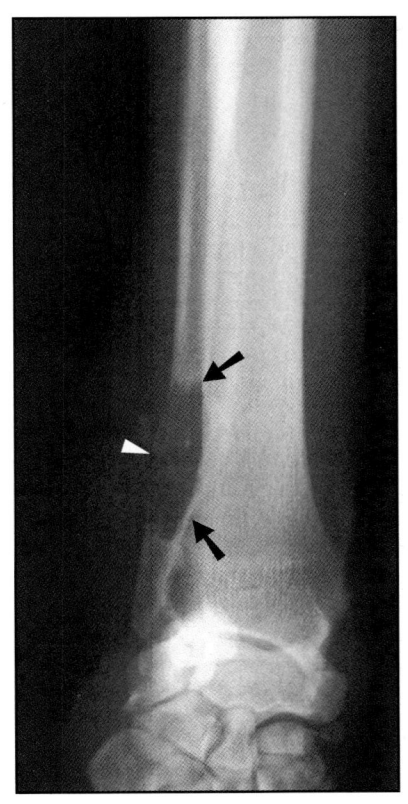

5.23 A bone cyst (arrowed) in the distal ulna of a 3-year-old Boxer. The dog presented lame after fracture of the cyst wall (arrowhead).

5.24 Polyostotic multicameral bone cysts (fibrous dysplasia) (arrowed) affecting the distal radius and ulna in a Dobermann. A pathological fracture is present (arrowhead).

Signalment: Polyostotic (several bones affected) cystic bone lesions (Figure 5.24) have been reported in families of Dobermanns, and a genetic aetiology has been suggested in this breed. Monostotic (one bone affected) lesions have been reported in Great Danes, Weimaraners, Irish Wolfhounds, German Shepherd Dogs and other large breeds.

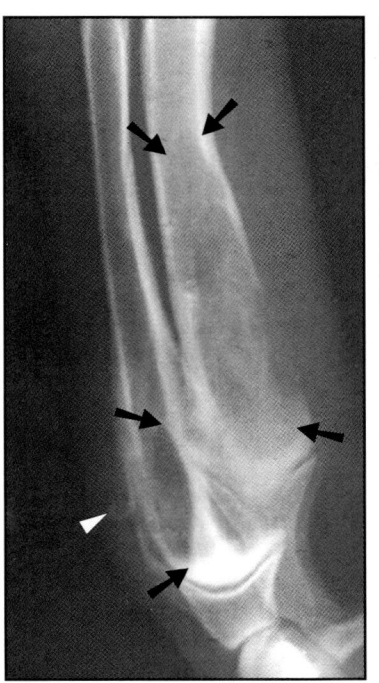

Histopathogenesis: Lesions are lytic and expansile and may be divided by fibro-osseous septa lined by fibrous connective tissue. Cysts usually contain straw-coloured fluid or fibrous tissue. If fractures are present they may be blood-filled. The only purely cystic lesion is seen at the ends of the large cylindrical bones of the extremities of the growing skeleton. Other cyst-like lesions should be designated as areas of liquefaction necrosis rather than cysts because they are merely areas of degeneration in proliferative processes.

Clinical signs: Most bone cysts do not produce clinical signs until they reach a fairly large size or they fracture, when acute lameness can occur. Pain, swelling and stiffness of the adjacent joint may be noted with large cysts.

Radiology: A bone cyst appears as an expansile radiolucent area in the metaphysis, near to, but not affecting, the physis or epiphysis. The expanding cyst often thins the cortex. Cysts may be unicameral, with one cavity, or multicameral, when the cavity is divided by osseous septa.

Treatment: Drainage, curettage and packing with cancellous bone graft is the described method of treatment, if necessary. Fractures can be challenging to repair given the metaphyseal location and tremendously thin cortices (Dueland and VanEnkevort, 1995).

Aneurysmal bone cysts
Aneurysmal bone cysts are expansile solitary lytic bone lesions. The name, aneurysmal, comes from the cyst's gross resemblance to the true aortic aneurysm seen in humans.

Signalment: A summary of the cases in which this lesion has been reported is shown in Figure 5.25.

Chapter 5 Diseases and disorders of bone

Signalment		Bone affected	Treatment/outcome	Reference
Dogs:	Dalmatian, 11 y, FN, 26 kg	Tibia – pathological fracture (osteosarcoma)	Euthanasia	Renegar *et al.*, 1979
	Crossbred, 12 y, F	Tibia – pathological fracture	Unreported	Cited in Pernell *et al.*, 1992
	Crossbred, 13 y, MN, 25 kg	Pelvis – previous fracture	Euthanasia	Bowles and Freeman, 1987
	Crossbreed	Metatarsal (osteosarcoma)	Unknown	Liu and Thacher, 1991
	Yorkshire Terrier, 6 m, FE, 4 kg	Distal humerus – fracture	Amputation	Pernell *et al.*, 1992
	Shetland Sheepdog, 4 y, M	Tibia – distal	Curettage and cancellous bone graft	Duval *et al.*, 1995
	Crossbred, 8 y, MN	Lumbar vertebrae	Euthanasia	Shiroma *et al.*, 1993
Cats:	DSH, 1y 3m, ME	Scapula	Amputation	Walker *et al.*, 1975
	DSH, 2 y, F	Sacrum	Euthanasia	Liu *et al.*, 1974
	DSH, 2 y, F	Coccygeal vertebrae	Euthanasia	Liu *et al.*, 1974
	DSH, 14 y, F	Wing of ilium	Euthanasia	Liu *et al.*, 1974
	DSH, 3y 6m, FN	Rib	Surgical resection	Biller *et al.*, 1987

5.25 Summary of clinical details of cats and dogs affected with aneurysmal bone cysts. (DSH, domestic shorthair; E, entire; F, female; m, months; M, male; N, neutered; y, years)

There are probably too few reports to be able to make any specific comments. In dogs, aneurysmal cysts were diagnosed in animals ranging from 6 months to 13 years and in a variety of breeds and sizes. Also in dogs, aneurysmal bone cysts were more commonly reported in the appendicular skeleton, particularly the tibia. In cats the cysts were generally seen in younger animals and they mainly affected the axial skeleton. In both dogs and cats females were over-represented but again the limited number of cases makes it difficult to attach much significance to this.

Pathogenesis: Aneurysmal bone cysts are purported to develop secondary to haemodynamic alterations in bone marrow. Venous obstruction or arteriovenous fistula formation results in haemorrhage, lysis and subperiosteal expansion. However, no evidence for this has been found in any of the reported canine or feline cases. The periosteum lays down new bone as it expands creating the eggshell-like appearance. Benign and malignant neoplasia, fibrous dysplasia, unicameral bone cysts and trauma have also been proposed as inciting factors for aneurysmal cyst formation.

Clinical signs: Swelling over the cysts and pain and tenderness are commonly reported clinical findings. Some animals are presented with signs attributable to an obstructive lesion and others present when the cyst acutely fractures.

Radiology: The cysts are usually thin-walled non-reactive and expansile bone lesions. When affecting the appendicular skeleton, they are often eccentric in the metaphysis. They can have a characteristic soap bubble appearance.

Histopathology: The cyst consists of a thin bony shell divided by bony and fibrous septa. The septa are lined with fibroblasts and multinucleated giant cells. Lytic areas of bone contain extensive zones of haemorrhage and dilated coalescent spaces filled with blood. Blood clots are rare. Differential diagnoses include telangiectatic osteosarcoma, haemangiosarcoma and giant cell tumours.

Treatment: Therapy is dependent on location. As lesions can develop secondary to malignancy, multiple representative biopsy specimens from various areas are mandatory. There is a distinct paucity of reports in the veterinary literature, and treatment protocols are taken from those reported for humans. Treatment of axial lesions is traditionally by curettage, bone grafting, local excision and irradiation. Treatment of appendicular lesions is similar but also includes the option of amputation. Superselective embolization using cyanoacrylate can provide definitive therapy in humans.

References and further reading

Abeles V, Harrus S, Angles JM *et al.* (1999) Hypertrophic osteodystrophy in six Weimaraner puppies associated with clinical signs. *Veterinary Record* **145**, 130–134

Alexander JW and Kallfelz FA (1975) A case of craniomandibular osteopathy in a Labrador retriever. *Veterinary Medicine: Small Animal Clinician* **70**, 560–563

Ansari MM (1991) Bone infarcts associated with malignant sarcomas. *Compendium on Continuing Education for the Practicing Veterinarian* **13(3)**, 367–370

Barrett RB, Schall WD and Lewis RE (1968) Clinical and radiographic features of eosinophilic panosteitis. *Journal of the American Animal Hospital Association* **4**, 94–104

Basher AWP, Doige CE and Presnell KR (1988) Subchondral bone cysts in a dog with osteochondrosis. *Journal of the American Animal Hospital Association* **24**, 321–326

Becker TJ, Perry RL and Watson GL (1999) Regression of hypertrophic osteopathy in a cat after surgical excision of an adrenocortical carcinoma. *Journal of the American Animal Hospital Association* **35**, 499–505

Biller DS, Johnson GC, Birchard SJ, Fingland RB (1987) Aneurysmal bone cyst in a rib of a cat. *Journal of the American Veterinary Medical Association* **190**, 1193–1195

Bohning RH, Suter PF, Hohn RB and Marshall J (1970) Clinical and radiologic survey of canine panosteitis. *Journal of the American Veterinary Medical Association* **156**, 870–883

Chapter 5   Diseases and disorders of bone

Bowles MH and Freeman K (1987) Aneurysmal bone cyst in the ischia and pubes of a dog: a case report and literature review. *Journal of the American Animal Hospital Association* **23**, 423–427

Brodey R (1971) Hypertrophic osteoarthropathy in the dog. A clinicopathological study of 60 cases. *Journal of the American Veterinary Medical Association* **159**, 1242–1256

Capen CC (1985) Calcium-regulating hormones and metabolic bone disease. In: *Textbook of Small Animal Orthopaedics*, ed. CD Newton and DM Nunamaker, pp. 690–693. JB Lippincott, Philadelphia

Dubielzig RR (1985) Medullary bone infarction in dogs. In: *Textbook of Small Animal Orthopaedics*, ed. CD Newton and DM Nunamaker, pp. 615–619. JB Lippincott, Philadelphia

Dueland RT and VanEnkevort B (1995) Lateral tibial head buttress plate: use in a pathological femoral fracture secondary to a bone cyst in a dog. *Veterinary Comparative Orthopaedics and Traumatology* **8**, 196–199

Duval JM, Chambers JN and Newell SM (1995) Surgical treatment of an aneurysmal bone cyst in a dog. *Veterinary Comparative Orthopaedics and Traumatology* **8**, 213–217

Goldschmidt MH and Biery DN (1985) Bone cysts in the dog. In: *Textbook of Small Animal Orthopaedics*, ed. CD Newton and DM Nunamaker, pp. 611–613. JB Lippincott, Philadelphia

Grondalen J (1976) Metaphyseal osteopathy (hypertrophic osteodystrophy) in growing dogs. A clinical study. *Journal of Small Animal Practice* **17**, 721–735

Grondalen J (1979) Letter to the editor re: metaphyseal osteopathy. *Journal of Small Animal Practice* **20**, 124

Harrus S, Waner T, Aizenberg I *et al.* (2002) Development of hypertrophic osteodystrophy and antibody response in a litter of vaccinated Weimaraner puppies. *Journal of Small Animal Practice* **43**, 27–31

Henik RA, Forrest LJ and Friedman AL (1999) Rickets caused by excessive renal phosphate loss and apparent abnormal vitamin D metabolism in a cat. *Journal of the American Veterinary Medical Association* **215**, 1644–1649

Holling H, Brodey R and Boland C (1961) Pulmonary hypertrophic osteoarthropathy. *Lancet* **2**, 1269–1274

Johnson KA, Church DB, Barton RJ and Wood AKW (1988) Vitamin-D dependent rickets in a Saint Bernard dog. *Journal of Small Animal Practice* **29**, 657–666

Lamb CR (1990) The double cortical line: a sign of osteopenia. *Journal of Small Animal Practice* **31**, 189–192

Lenehan TM and Fetter AW (1985) Hypertrophic osteodystrophy. In: *Textbook of Small Animal Orthopaedics*, ed. CD Newton and DM Nunamaker, pp. 597–602. JB Lippincott, Philadelphia

Lenehan TM and Fetter AW (1985) Metaphyseal Osteopathy. In: *Textbook of Small Animal Orthopaedics*, ed. CD Newton and DM Nunamaker, pp. 603–607. JB Lippincott, Philadelphia

Lenehan TM, Van Sickle DC and Biery DN (1985) Canine Panosteitis. In: *Textbook of Small Animal Orthopaedics*, ed. CD Newton and DM Nunamaker, pp. 591–596. JB Lippincott, Philadelphia

Liu S, Dorfman HD and Patnaik AK (1974) Primary and secondary bone tumours in the cat. *Journal of Small Animal Practice* **15**, 141–156

Liu S and Thacher C (1991) Case report 673. *Skeletal Radiology* **20**, 311–334

Malik R, Laing C and Alan GS (1997) Rickets in a litter of racing greyhounds. *Journal of Small Animal Practice* **38**, 109–114

Mee A, Bennett D and May C (1992) Canine distemper virus in bone. *Veterinary Record* **131**, 496

Muir P, Dubielzig RR and Johnson KA (1996) Panosteitis. *Compendium on Continuing Education for the Practicing Veterinarian* **18**, 29–33

Muir P, Dubielzig RR, Johnson KA and Shelton GD (1996) Hypertrophic osteodystrophy and calvarial hyperostosis. *Compendium on Continuing Education for the Practicing Veterinarian* **18**, 143–151

Munjar TA, Austin CC and Breur GJ (1998) Comparison of risk factors for hypertrophic osteodystrophy, craniomandibular osteopathy and canine distemper virus infection. *Veterinary Comparative Orthopaedics and Traumatology* **11**, 37–43

Nunamaker DM (1985) Osteomyelitis. In: *Textbook of Small Animal Orthopaedics*, ed. CD Newton and DM Nunamaker, pp. 499–510. JB Lippincott, Philadelphia

Padgett GA and Mostosky UV (1986) Animal model: the mode of inheritance of craniomandibular osteopathy in West Highland white terriers. *American Journal of Medical Genetics* **25**, 9–13

Pernell RT, Dunstan RW and DeCamp CE (1992) Aneurysmal bone cyst in a six-month-old dog. *Journal of the American Veterinary Medical Association* **201**, 1897–1899

Pool RR and Leighton RL (1969) Craniomandibular osteopathy in a dog. *Journal of the American Veterinary Medical Association* **154**, 657–660

Renegar WR, Thornburg LP, Burk RL and Stoll SG (1979) Aneurysmal bone cyst in the dog. A case report. *Journal of the American Animal Hospital Association* **15**, 191–195

Riser WH, Parkes LJ and Shirer JF (1967) Canine craniomandibular osteopathy. *Journal of the American Veterinary Radiological Society* **8**, 23–29

Riser WH and Newton CD (1985) Craniomandibular Osteopathy. In: *Textbook of Small Animal Orthopaedics*, ed. CD Newton and DM Nunamaker, pp. 621–626. JB Lippincott, Philadelphia

Seawright AA, English PB and Gartner RJW (1970) Hypervitaminosis A of the cat. *Advances in Veterinary Science and Comparative Medicine* **14**, 1–27

Schreiner CA and Nagode LA (2003) Vitamin D-dependent rickets type 2 in a four-month-old cat. *Journal of the American Veterinary Medical Association* **3**, 337–339

Schulz KS, Payne JT and Aronson E (1991) *Escherichia coli* bacteraemia associated with hypertrophic osteodystrophy in a dog. *Journal of the American Veterinary Medical Association* **199**, 1170–1173

Shiroma JT, Weisbrode SE, Biller DS and Olmstead ML (1993) Pathological fracture of an aneurysmal bone cyst in the lumbar vertebra of a dog. *Journal of the American Animal Hospital Association* **29**, 434–437

Tabaoda J (2000) Systemic mycoses. In: *Textbook of Veterinary Internal Medicine: Diseases of the Dog and Cat, 5th edn*, ed. SJ Ettinger and EC Feldman, pp. 453–476. WB Saunders, Philadelphia

Tomsa K, Glaus T, Hauser B *et al.* (1999) Nutritional secondary hyperparathyroidism in six cats. *Journal of Small Animal Practice* **40**, 533–539

Trostel CT, Pool RR and McLaughlin RM (2003) Canine lameness caused by developmental orthopaedic diseases: panosteitis, Legg-Calve-Perthes disease and hypertrophic osteodystrophy. *Compendium on Continuing Education for the Practicing Veterinarian* **25**, 282–294

Trowald-Wigh G, Ekman S, Hannsson K *et al.* (1995) Clinical, radiological and pathological features of 12 Irish Setters with canine leucocyte adhesion deficiency. *Journal of Small Animal Practice* **41**, 211–217

Turnier JC and Silverman S (1978) A case study of canine panosteitis: comparison of radiographic and radioisotope studies. *American Journal of Veterinary Research* **39**, 1550–1552

Van Sickle D (1975) Canine panosteitis. In: *Selected Orthopaedic Problems in the Growing Dog*, pp. 20–28. Monograph, American Animal Hospital Association, South Bend

Walker MA, Duncan JR, Shaw JW and Chapman MD (1975) Aneurysmal bone cyst in a cat. *Journal of the American Veterinary Medical Association* **167**, 933–935

Watson ADJ, Adams WM and Thomas CB (1995) Craniomandibular osteopathy in dogs. *Compendium on Continuing Education* **17**, 911–922

Zeskov B (1960) A contribution to 'eosinophilic panosteitis' in dogs. *Zentralblatt für Veterinarmedizin* **7**, 671–680

6

Disturbances of growth and bone development

Sorrel Langley-Hobbs

Introduction

A wide variety of diseases in dogs and cats can affect bone growth and development. Problems affecting growth plates tend to affect cartilage formation (chondrogenesis), cartilage transformation or bone formation (ossification). Underlying causes may be hormonal (including excess or lack of growth hormone, thyroid hormones and steroid hormones), congenital, nutritional, metabolic or traumatic.

Dogs experience a rapid growth spurt between approximately 4 and 5 months of age. The rate of growth then slows considerably from the age of about 6 months and is 95% complete by 7 months (in Greyhounds). The time of closure of the growth plate is dependent on many factors, including the bone, species, genetics and the size of the animal. The stimulus for closure is an alteration in secretion of a variety of hormones. This results in an arrest in cartilage proliferation, allowing multiple bony bridges to traverse the metaphyseal growth plate. Diseases or conditions that affect the growth plate generally cause premature closure and a decrease in length of the affected bone. An increase in length or delay in physeal closure is much less common but has been reported in association with neutering (May *et al.*, 1991) and with fractures (Denny, 1989).

Angular limb deformities as a result of growth plate injuries

The growth plate or physis is the weak link in the skeleton of the growing animal, being only 20–50% as strong as adjacent bone or ligamentous insertions. Thus trauma in immature animals is more likely to result in a physeal fracture than a dislocation. The majority of physeal fractures involve the metaphyseal growth plate. The management and diagnosis of traumatic physeal fractures (epiphysiolysis) is covered in the *BSAVA Manual of Small Animal Fracture Repair and Management*. Premature growth plate arrest occurs if there is injury to the germinal cells or blood supply. This chapter will deal with the secondary effects of growth plate closure. The potential for problems after premature closure is dependent on a wide variety of factors, including age and bone affected (Figure 6.1).

- **Age of the animal at time of injury:** How much potential is there for further growth? (95% of growth is complete by 7 months of age in Greyhounds)
- **Which bone is affected?** Complete closure of a growth plate in a single bone, such as the femur, is less likely to be a problem than closure of a growth plate of a paired bone such as the radius, ulna tibia or fibula
- **Is the closure complete or partial?** Complete closure may cause shortening, which may be compensated for by alteration in joint angles. Partial closure is likely to cause angulation of the affected bone as the unaffected part of the growth plate continues to grow
- **Is there joint subluxation?** This is likely to be the cause of lameness and is the most important aspect to address. Is there secondary osteoarthritis?
- **Shortening** (Leg length discrepancy, LLD): Generally, shortening is not a problem if it is less than 20% of the total length of the mature bone
- **Rotational deformity:** often a significant problem
- **Angular deformity:** may be less serious than rotational deformity. Mediolateral deviation is more of a problem than craniocaudal deviation

6.1 Factors to consider after premature growth plate closure.

Investigation

When an animal is presented with an angular limb deformity, the history taken should include: whether it has suffered any previous trauma; its diet; and, if known, whether any siblings are affected. A general physical and full orthopaedic examination should be performed. Orthopaedic examination of the affected leg and contralateral limb should particularly include assessment for joint pain, rotational and angular deformity, and limb length discrepancy (LLD).

Investigations should include radiography. Some general principles apply when radiographing an animal with angular deformity secondary to growth plate closure (Figure 6.2).

General approach to premature growth plate closure

Some general principles apply when correcting deformity that has occurred after premature growth plate closure (Figure 6.3). However, the major aim is total restoration of bone geometry by correction of angular, rotational and length deformities.

Chapter 6 Disturbances of growth and bone development

- Both the affected and unaffected contralateral limb are radiographed
- The whole bone is radiographed, including the joints above and below the affected bone, and as much of the adjacent bones as possible is included on the films in order to assess deviation
- The leg is positioned so the most proximal joint is 'normal' or straight. The distal joints can then be assessed for rotational deformity by comparison with the proximal limb. For example, when taking craniocaudal views of the antebrachium, the elbow is positioned so it is in a true craniocaudal position and then rotation can be assessed or estimated from the carpal rotation
- If there is concern or suspicion of joint subluxation, specific films are taken centred on the affected joints
- Adjacent bones in the limbs are radiographed to enable measurement for compensatory overgrowth; if present this should be taken into account when estimating the LLD

6.2 Diagnostic imaging for premature growth plate closure.

Restoration of joint congruity
Restoration of paw to a functional position
Correction of rotational deformity
Correction of angular deformity
Restoration of limb length

6.3 Principles of corrective surgery for premature growth plate closure.

Many deformities can be corrected by division and repositioning of the bone (Piermattei and Flo, 1997). An osteotomy is an elective surgical division of a bone; an ostectomy is resection of a piece of bone. These can be classified into a variety of types:

- **Transverse.** A transverse cut is made through the bone. It is used for correction of rotational, angular or combination deformities. Kirschner wires can be inserted into each piece of bone prior to making the cut so the amount of derotation can be determined (e.g. intertrochanteric osteotomy for hip dysplasia) (Figure 6.4a)
- **Opening wedge.** This is a transverse osteotomy used to correct angular deformity and the bone length is maintained. Rotation can also be corrected. Muscle tension can limit the amount of opening possible (Figure 6.4b)
- **Cuneiform ostectomy.** A predetermined piece of bone is removed from the point of maximal deformity (e.g. in the closed wedge procedure) (Figure 6.4c). This is simpler to reduce than the opening wedge and gives good stability postoperatively, but it will shorten the limb further unless distraction osteogenesis is performed postoperatively
- **Oblique osteotomy.** An oblique cut is made parallel to the distal articular surface. The proximal part is inserted in the medullary canal of the distal fragment. This procedure usually increases length slightly and can be used to correct rotation and valgus or varus deformity. It is most frequently used in corrective surgery for radius curvus (Figure 6.4d)

- **Segmental (partial) ostectomy.** Part of a bone is removed, usually after two parallel cuts. This is to allow overall bone shortening or to prevent or delay healing (Figure 6.4e).

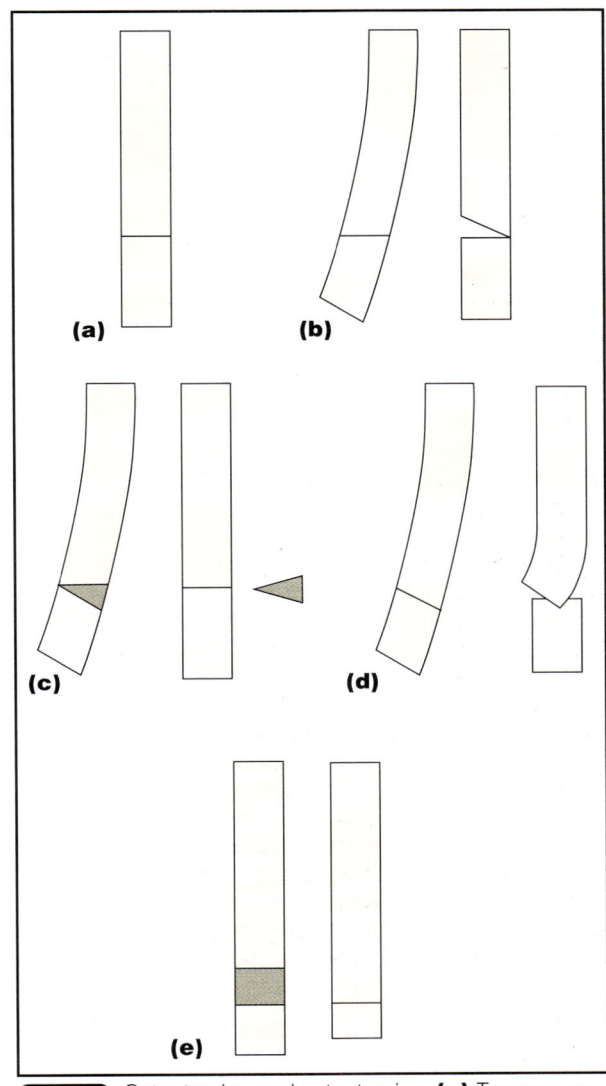

6.4 Osteotomies and ostectomies. **(a)** Transverse. **(b)** Opening wedge. **(c)** Closing wedge after cuneiform ostectomy. **(d)** Oblique cut. **(e)** Segmental ostectomy.

Corrective surgery should be carried out early to avoid or minimize irreversible pathological changes in adjacent joints. It is, however, an elective procedure, not an emergency, and *planning is essential.* When examining the patient, the whole limb and the rest of the animal must be examined thoroughly. Non-traumatic growth plate closure is often bilateral. Radiographs should be taken in two planes (orthogonal views) and include the joint above and below the affected limb segment (see Figure 6.2). Tracings of the bones from the radiographs allow some preplanning of the osteotomy. However, it must be realized that the rotational changes are not always adequately appreciated from conventional radiography, and muscle tension contracture and fibrosis may affect the ability to reduce the bone intraoperatively.

Chapter 6　Disturbances of growth and bone development

Deciding which is the optimal surgical technique to perform will depend mainly on the degree of deformity and the age of the dog. When determining skeletal maturity, Figure 6.5 should provide a useful guide.

Breed type	Skeletally immature: 2–3 months' growth potential remains	Skeletally mature: growth plates not necessarily completely closed but little potential for further growth remaining
Giant breed	<7–8 months	>8 months
Large breed	<5–6 months	>7 months
Small breed	<3 months	>4 months

6.5 Approximate age ranges at which differently sized dog breeds achieve skeletal maturity. (Modified from Piermattei and Flo, 1997.)

For angular deformity, the osteotomy should be performed as close to the point of maximal deformity as possible, whilst avoiding ending up with too small a fragment of bone to stabilize adequately. If it is necessary to cut the bone proximal to the point of maximum deformity, an S-shaped curve will result in the bone (Figure 6.6). However this is acceptable as long as the joints above and below the bone segment are parallel. Final limb alignment is done visually, using joint manipulation, particularly flexion and extension. It is, therefore, important to be able to assess this intraoperatively.

A small surgical approach is made to cut the bone. Periosteum is incised longitudinally and elevated using a periosteal elevator. The bone can then be cut in the appropriate preplanned direction using an oscillating saw, Gigli wire or osteotome and mallet. Care is needed if an osteotome and mallet are being used as the sole method for cutting diaphyseal bone, as the brittle nature of the bone makes it liable to fissure or crack in the wrong direction. Pre-drilling small holes first and then linking them with the osteotome is a safer technique. Autogenous cancellous bone grafts should be used around the osteotomy site in mature animals. Stabilization needs to be appropriate for the fracture created (see *BSAVA Manual of Small Animal Fracture Repair and Management*). Radiographs should be taken approximately every 4 weeks until healing is documented.

Radius and ulna

The distal radial and ulnar growth plates are the most commonly affected physes in the dog, either singly or both together. They are in a location where they are susceptible to damage. Also, the bones have to develop in synchrony and their distal growth plates contribute greatly to overall length. The distal radial physis is responsible for 60% of total radial length, while the distal ulnar physis is responsible for 85% of total ulnar length. Since the distal radial and ulnar growth plates are both very active, they are good areas to evaluate if a generalized physeal disorder is suspected.

Premature closure of the distal ulnar growth plate
This is the commonest cause of canine thoracic limb angular deformity. It is especially seen in large-breed dogs and may be bilateral. There is often no confirmed history of trauma. Causes of premature closure, aside from trauma, may be retained cartilaginous cores in the distal ulna (Johnson, 1981), metaphyseal osteopathy, or a form of dwarfism seen in dogs such as the Skye Terrier (Lau, 1977).

Dogs may be presented because of visible deformity or lameness. Clinical signs of lameness are often due to joint pain from elbow or carpal subluxation. Animals should be assessed carefully for angular and rotational deformity, joint pain and LLD.

Radiography: The whole antebrachium should be radiographed to include the elbow and carpal joints (see Figure 6.2). If there is a suspicion of elbow subluxation, views centred on this joint should also be taken. Radiographs must be taken of both thoracic limbs.

Radiographic changes and clinical signs are related to the continued growth of the radius against a short ulna, which acts as a limiting factor or bowstring (Carrig *et al.*, 1975). This results in the classical signs of radius curvus (Figure 6.7); all or some of these changes may be present in an individual case.

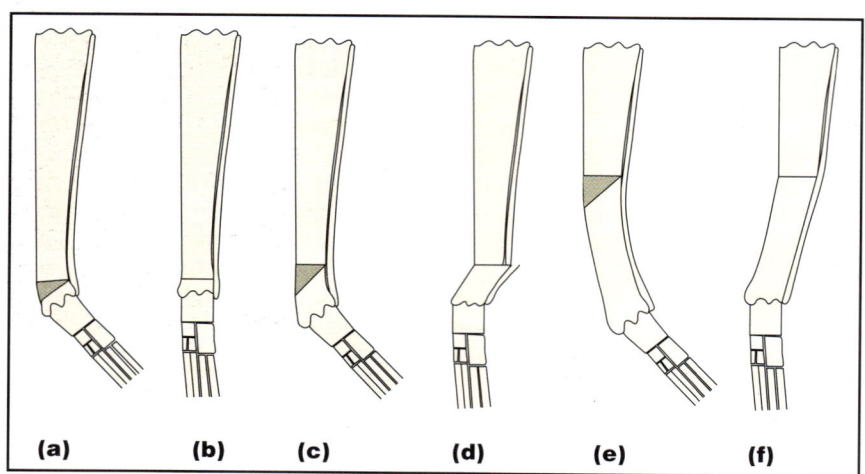

6.6 The importance of preoperative planning. **(a)** An osteotomy performed at the level of maximal deformity results in a very small epiphyseal fragment in the distal tibia. **(b)** A small epiphyseal fragment can be difficult to stabilize adequately. **(c)** Making the cut proximal to the level of maximal deformity results in a larger piece of bone that is easier to stabilize. **(d)** When reduced, the bone in (c) will not be straight; however, this is not usually a problem as long as the joints are parallel. **(e,f)** Making the cut too far from the point of maximal deformity will cause a significant deformity of the bone once reduced.

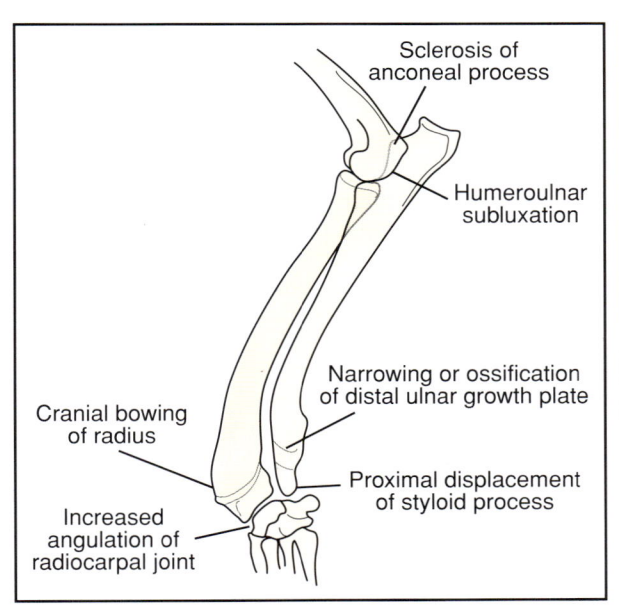

Chapter 6 Disturbances of growth and bone development

Bowing: cranial bowing of the radius followed by medial bowing
Carpal valgus: lateral angulation of the foot
Supination: radius rotates externally around a short ulna leading to external rotation of the paw

Elbow:
  Subluxation of the humeroulnar joint
  Possible ununited anconeal process

Carpus: Caudolateral subluxation of antebrachiocarpal joint

6.7 Radiographic changes associated with premature closure of the distal ulnar growth plate (radius curvus).

Longer limbed dogs, such as the Irish Wolfhound and Great Dane, may be more prone to angular deformity, and shorter limbed breeds, such as the Jack Russell Terrier and Bassett Hound, more prone to joint subluxation (Figure 6.8).

Growth plates are generally discoid; an important exception is the distal ulnar growth plate in the dog, which is conical or V-shaped. This is reflected in the high percentage of bone that the growth plate provides, as the conical shape increases the surface area of the physis by 50% compared to that of a flat plate of similar diameter. The shape of the canine distal ulnar physis means that shear forces are generally transformed into compressive forces, resulting in premature closure in immature animals (Figure 6.9).

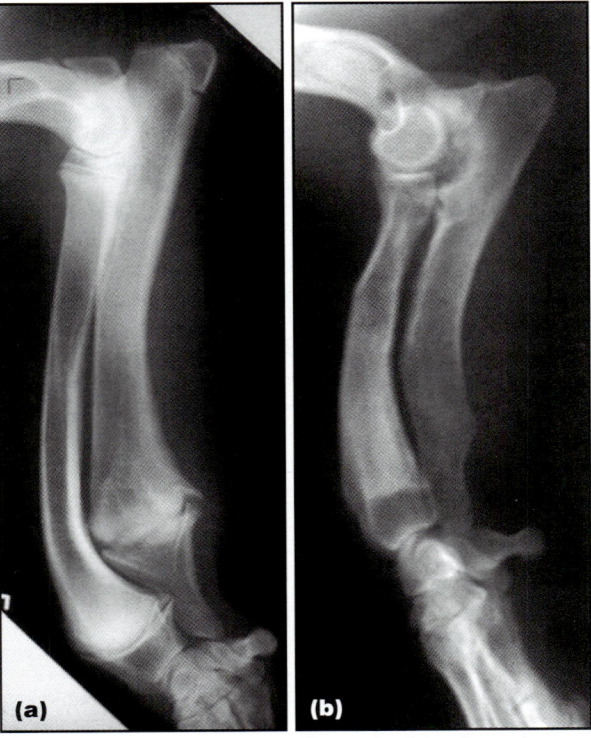

6.8 **(a)** Mediolateral radiograph of the thoracic limb of a Great Dane with carpal valgus, showing premature closure of the distal ulnar growth plate and radius curvus but no elbow joint subluxation. **(b)** Mediolateral radiograph of the thoracic limb of a Bassett Hound with carpal valgus, showing premature closure of the distal ulnar growth plate, radius curvus and a humeroulnar subluxation. The dog also had panosteitis.

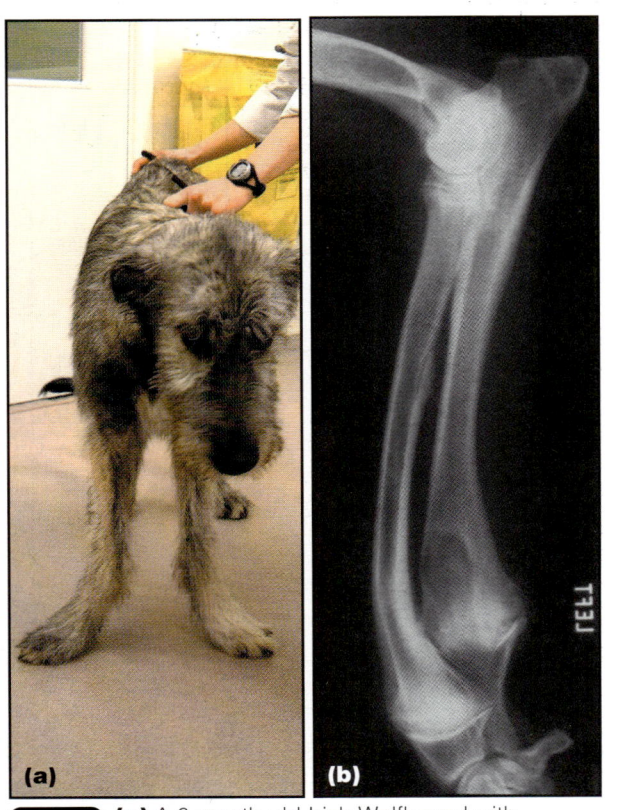

6.9 **(a)** A 6-month-old Irish Wolfhound with bilateral carpal valgus secondary to metaphyseal osteopathy. **(b)** Mediolateral radiograph of the antebrachium of a 7-month-old Irish Wolfhound with radius curvus and a retained cartilaginous core in the distal ulna.

Chapter 6 Disturbances of growth and bone development

Treatment: The options depend on the nature of the physeal closure, the type and degree of deformity, the presence of joint subluxation, and the age of the animal (Figure 6.10).

Skeletally immature animals: Early surgery is indicated to minimize further deformity, muscle shortening or contracture, and degenerative joint changes. For mild carpal valgus in a dog with potential for further growth, a partial ulnar ostectomy (see Operative Technique 6.1) and possibly distal radial stapling (see Operative Technique 6.2) may be sufficient. One study reported that partial ulnar ostectomy alone was only effective in young dogs (median age 5 months) with <25 degrees of carpal valgus or in older animals (median age 6.5 months) with <13 degrees of valgus (Sheilds and Gambardella, 1989). If carpal valgus is >25 degrees in an immature dog, segmental ulnar ostectomy combined with temporary stapling of the medial radial physis or corrective osteotomies of both radius and ulna are necessary (see Operative Technique 6.3). If elbow subluxation (humeroulnar) is marked, a proximal osteotomy rather than, or in addition to, a distal ulnar ostectomy should be performed; this should allow the triceps to 'pull' the proximal ulna proximally and improve elbow congruency (see Operative Technique 6.4).

Skeletally mature animals: Corrective radial and ulnar osteotomies are necessary (see Operative Technique 6.3).

Although the commonest cause of carpal valgus is premature closure of the distal ulnar growth plate, partial closure of the caudolateral aspect of the distal radial growth plate may also result in carpal valgus. It is important to differentiate as therapeutic options differ (see Figure 6.10). Careful radiographic evaluation of the distal radial physis and distal ulnar physis is essential, as premature closure of both growth plates can occur concurrently.

Correction needs to address the partial closure of the distal radius and distal ulnar physeal closure if it is also present. In immature animals a distal segmental ulnar ostectomy can be combined with an attempt to remove the bony bridge (see Operative Technique 6.5). Prognosis for recovery must be guarded, but in one report in the literature the dog returned to normal (Vandewater and Olmstead, 1983). In mature animals corrective osteotomies of the radius and ulna are normally necessary (see Operative Technique 6.3).

Retained cartilaginous cores

Retained cartilaginous cores can affect the distal ulna and are a reflection of the very active growth rate that occurs at around 5 months of age. They are generally of little clinical significance, but they can cause slower growth or premature physeal closure. In these cases the cores are often irregular, with ill-defined borders; cartilage cores in dogs without a growth disturbance have smooth well defined borders (Fox, 1984). The core is composed of columns of

Deformity	Growth plate affected	Age and severity	Corrective surgery	Comments
Carpal valgus	Distal ulnar	Skeletally immature; <25 degrees	Segmental ulnar ostectomy distally	Moderate humeroulnar subluxation of the elbow will correct following distal ostectomy but more severe disease requires proximal ulnar osteotomy
	Distal ulnar	Skeletally immature; >25 degrees	Segmental ulnar ostectomy and wedge ostectomy of radius	
	Distal ulnar	Skeletally mature; >13 degrees	Segmental ulnar ostectomy and wedge ostectomy of radius	
	Radial – caudolateral aspect	Skeletally immature	Ulnar ostectomy and resect bony bridge and apply fat graft	Guarded prognosis for success
	Radial – caudolateral aspect	Skeletally mature	Segmental ulnar ostectomy and wedge ostectomy of radius	
	Retained cartilaginous cores	Skeletally immature	Try a decreased plane of nutrition initially	
	Retained cartilaginous cores	Skeletally mature	Segmental ulnar ostectomy and wedge ostectomy of radius	
Humeroulnar subluxation	Distal ulnar	Skeletally mature	Dynamic proximal ulnar osteotomy	
Humeroradial subluxation	Distal or proximal radial	Skeletally immature	Segmental ulnar ostectomy OR proximal radial osteotomy and dynamic fixation	Distraction ostegenesis to increase limb length using an Ilizarov or ring fixator may be necessary
Distal tibial valgus/varus	Distal tibial	Skeletally mature	Opening or closing wedge ostectomy of distal tibia and ESF application	

6.10 Procedures for surgical correction of angular deformity.

Chapter 6 Disturbances of growth and bone development

hypertrophic cartilage cells that fail to develop normally. The matrix septa in the hypertrophic zone fail to calcify, and vascularization is impeded. There are various speculations about the aetiology. As the condition is seen in giant breeds, nutrition may play a role in its development, and it has also been classified as a form of metaphyseal osteochondrosis.

Decreasing the plane of nutrition to slow growth is recommended in the 3–4-month-old puppy. In the older, though still skeletally immature, puppy a segmental ulnar ostectomy (see Operative Technique 6.1) and transphyseal stapling (see Operative Technique 6.2) can be successful. Corrective osteotomy is occasionally indicated in a mature dog with functional problems due to deformity (see Operative Technique 6.3).

Premature closure of the distal radial growth plate
Closure of the distal radial growth plate is less common than closure of the distal ulnar plate. Closure may be symmetrical or asymmetrical. Symmetrical premature closure results in a short bone and the leg is usually straight. A varus deformity of the foot is rare, as continued growth in the ulna is generally not strong enough to force the foot in a medial direction (Figure 6.11). Asymmetrical closure may, however, result in angular deformity and cause either a valgus or varus deviation, depending on which part of the growth plate is affected. Premature closure of the caudolateral part of the distal radial growth plate tends to be most common and results in carpal valgus, mimicking premature closure of the distal ulnar growth plate (Figure 6.12).

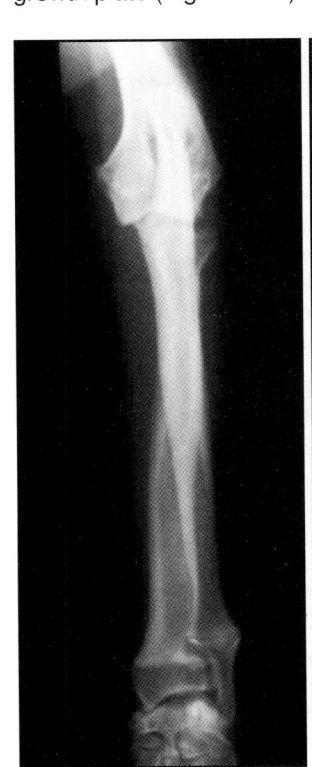

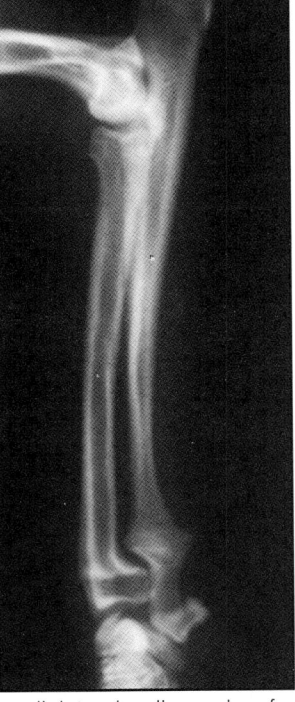

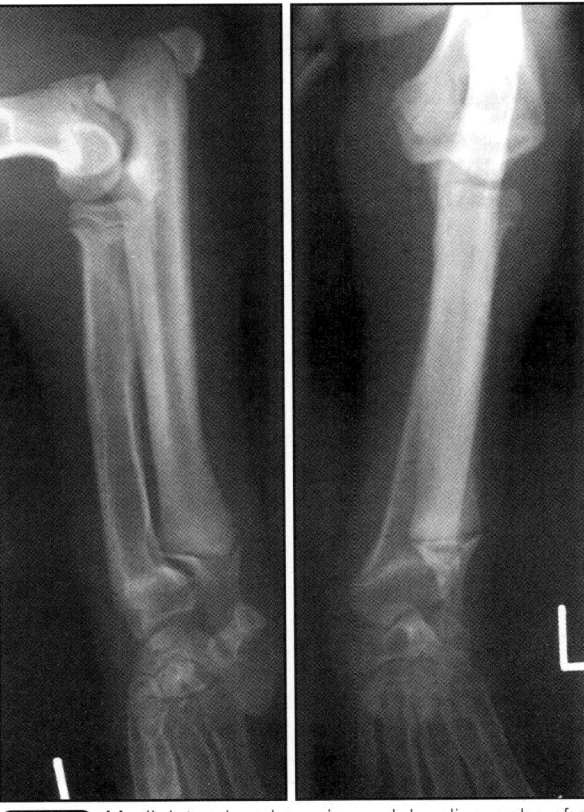

6.12 Mediolateral and craniocaudal radiographs of a 5-month-old crossbreed with partial closure of the caudolateral aspect of the distal radial growth plate combined with an abnormal appearance of the distal ulnar growth plate probably associated with delayed growth. There is humeroradial and humeroulnar subluxation. The radius has lost its normal cranial bow and has a straight appearance. There is a carpal valgoid deformity induced by the partial growth plate closure.

6.11 Craniocaudal and mediolateral radiographs of a 9-month-old Cavalier King Charles Spaniel with premature closure of the distal radial growth plate. The radius has lost its normal cranial bowing, there is a marked humeroradial subluxation and secondary humeroulnar subluxation. There is no significant angular deformity.

Lameness is often attributable to luxation of the humeroradial joint (Olson *et al.*, 1979). As the ulna continues to grow, the shortened radius is pulled distally by the interosseous ligament in the middle third of the bones, thus increasing the joint space between the radial head and humeral condyle. The medial and lateral collateral ligaments impinge the humeral condyle on the medial coronoid process, which may result in fragmentation of this area of the ulna and a secondary humeroulnar subluxation (Macpherson *et al.*, 1992).

The presenting complaint is usually one of lameness. If partial closure is present then the complaint may be one of deformity. Affected animals should be assessed particularly for LLD, angular and rotational deformity and joint pain.

Radiography: The radiographic changes associated with premature closure of the distal radial growth plate are summarized in Figure 6.13. At the other end of the antebrachium there is overgrowth of the styloid process of the ulna and an increase in the width of the antebrachiocarpal joint space (Vandewater and Olmstead, 1983).

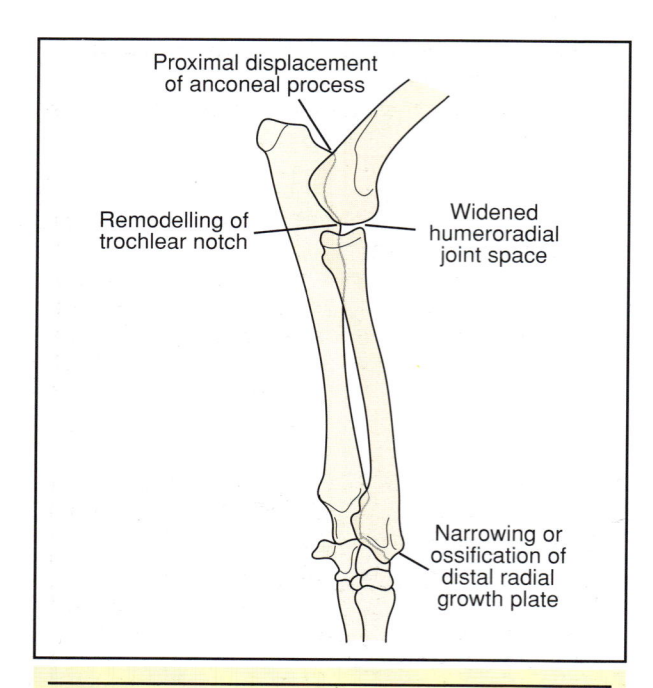

Chapter 6 Disturbances of growth and bone development

Proximal displacement of anconeal process

Remodelling of trochlear notch

Widened humeroradial joint space

Narrowing or ossification of distal radial growth plate

Elbow joint:
  Increase in width of the humeroradial joint
  Abnormal development of the trochlear notch
  Fragmentation of the medial coronoid process of ulna
Secondary humeroulnar subluxation
Short radius or short antebrachium
Straight radius: loss of normal cranial bow
Reduction of cortical thickness and bone diameter
Antebrachiocarpal joint: subluxation and secondary osteoarthritis

6.13 Radiographic changes associated with premature closure of the distal radial growth plate.

Treatment: The major problem with this condition is usually the humeroradial subluxation and the main decision is whether to reduce this by shortening the ulna or by lengthening the radius. Shortening the ulna is a simpler procedure and postoperative stabilization is easier, but it will cause further antebrachial shortening in an already short limb. Lengthening the radius has the advantage of increasing (or at least not decreasing) overall limb length but postoperative stabilization of the radius is required. The decision is usually made considering many factors including age, LLD, and economic and technical factors. As previously mentioned, fragmentation of the medial coronoid process can occur and the elbow joint should be inspected for this (see Chapter 18).

For ulnar shortening, a proximal segmental osteotomy is performed, removing a piece of bone equal or greater in size to the humeroradial gap (see Operative Technique 6.4). No postoperative stabilization is necessary. An ulnar intramedullary pin is sometimes used; it increases stability and decreases patient morbidity, but it may restrict dynamic reduction of the joint. This procedure can also be combined with distal radial and ulnar osteotomies to correct angular and rotational defects (see Operative Technique 6.3).

Radial lengthening, and hence reduction of the humeroradial subluxation, can be achieved by a variety of techniques involving a proximal or mid radial osteotomy. The osteotomy can be progressively stretched either using pins and elastic bands (see Operative Technique 18.11) or by use of a circular or linear external skeletal fixator designed for distraction osteogenesis (see Operative Technique 6.6). Alternatively, static lengthening can be achieved in a 'one off' using plate and screw fixation. The latter technique has the disadvantage that it may need repeating if there is the potential for further growth, and if the humeroradial joint is incongruent on the postoperative radiograph further alteration is not easily achieved.

Premature closure of the distal radial and ulnar growth plates
Partial or complete premature closure of both the distal radial and ulnar physes can occur in the same limb. Both the radius and ulna will be shortened and this is often the major concern, particularly in a very young puppy. Humeroulnar subluxation may be present due to continued growth of the proximal radial growth plate (the proximal ulnar growth plate, although unaffected, is only responsible for growth of the olecranon or the ulna above the elbow joint). Treatment involves radial and ulnar osteotomies to correct angular and rotational deformities (see Operative Technique 6.3). If the LLD is large, or has the potential to be large, then distraction osteogenesis can be considered.

Synostosis
A synostosis is a fusion between two bones not normally fused. The radius and ulna can form a synostosis secondary to a fracture or surgery. In the immature dog, synchronous growth and joint congruity is dependent on the two bones being able to grow, independently or separately from each other, and being able to 'slide' past one another. Synostosis of the two bones in a young dog can therefore result in humeroulnar subluxation due to continued growth in the proximal radial growth plate (Figure 6.14) (Alexander *et al.*, 1978). Overgrowth of the styloid process may also occur at the carpus, but this is less likely to cause a clinical problem.

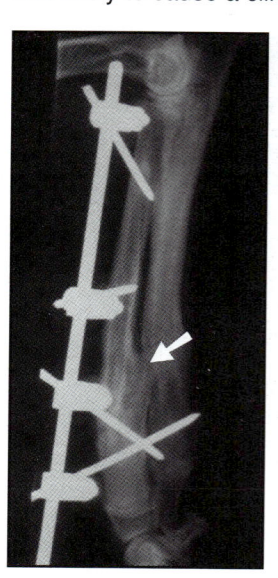

6.14 Synostosis (arrowed) between the radius and ulna in a 6-month-old Pointer after a mid diaphyseal fracture was stabilized with external skeletal fixation. Continued growth of the proximal radial growth plate in this immature dog may result in a humeroulnar subluxation.

Chapter 6 Disturbances of growth and bone development

The humeroulnar subluxation can be treated in most cases with a dynamic proximal ulnar osteotomy (Operative Technique 6.4).

Pelvic limb

Premature closure of the distal femoral and/or proximal tibial growth plate

Genu valgum ('knock-knees') is diagnosed sporadically in certain large breeds, such as the Great Dane, St Bernard and Mastiff, at 4–6 months of age (Newton, 1985b). It is frequently a bilateral problem. Clinical signs include:

- Genu valgum due to medial bowing of the distal femur and proximal tibia
- Lateral luxation of the patella; lameness can be severe
- Progressive femoral bowing may cause coxa valga and anteversion, leading to hip subluxation
- There may be external rotation of the distal tibia and foot.

The abnormal bone development probably occurs during the rapid growth phase and has been associated with retained cartilaginous cores (Newton, 1985b). There is overgrowth of the medial femoral condyle and medial tibia and the lateral aspects of the bones of the stifle joints tend to be hypoplastic. Other deformities may also be present in the thoracic limbs, such as carpal valgus secondary to distal ulnar growth plate closure. These animals need thorough assessment prior to contemplating or performing any surgical intervention.

Genu varum ('bow legs') is most often associated with medial patellar luxation in both small- and large-breed dogs. Affected dogs often have mild medial bowing of the distal femur and a compensatory bend or S shape to the tibia. Patellar luxation is usually the cause of lameness, and it is this that will need addressing (see Chapter 22).

Premature closure of the caudal aspect of the proximal tibial growth plate

This results in an altered craniocaudal angle of the tibial plateau, which can cause altered stifle mechanics and can predispose to rupture of the cranial cruciate ligament. In affected dogs the results of conventional treatment for cranial cruciate ligament rupture have been poor, and corrective osteotomy is needed (Read and Robins, 1982). The problem may occur secondary to the combined fracture of the tibial plateau and tibial tuberosity (Pratt, 2001). A significant increase in tibial plateau angle has also been recognized in both large and small breeds (e.g. West Highland White Terrier) without any history of trauma. The corrective surgery for this physeal closure or deformity is described in Chapter 22.

Premature closure of the tibial tuberosity

This can result in 'tibial drift': the tibial plateau continues to grow, but if the tibial tuberosity is fused to the tibial diaphysis it will remain distal to the stifle. This has the potential to cause problems in athletic breeds, such as Greyhounds, due to the more distal insertion point of the patellar ligament compared to normal.

Premature closure of the distal tibial or distal fibular growth plate

Tarsal varus (pes varus) has been recognized in Dachshunds (Johnson et al., 1989). In reported cases there was no history of trauma and, as the condition is often bilateral, a hereditary cause was suspected. Clinical signs first appear at 5–6 months of age and surgical correction is recommended.

Tarsal valgus has been recognized in Shetland Sheepdogs (Figure 6.15). This is thought to arise from premature closure of the distal fibular growth plate. With continuing growth of the tibia against a short fibula there is lateral deviation of the distal tibia (Vaughan, 1987; Jevens and DeCamp, 1993).

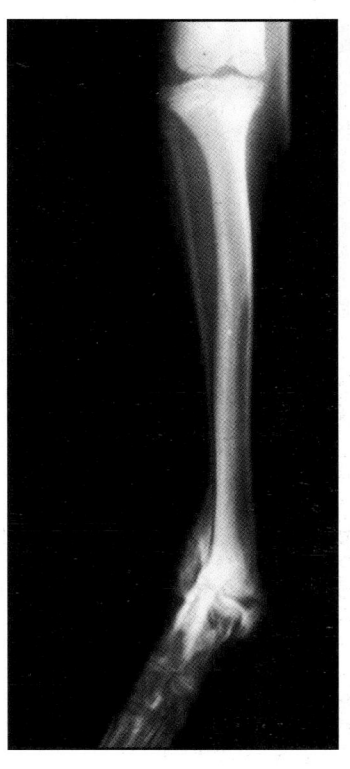

6.15 Radiograph of a Shetland Sheepdog with a valgoid deformity of the tibia. The deformity has developed subsequent to premature closure of the distal fibular growth plate, either alone or combined with partial closure of the lateral aspect of the distal tibial growth plate.

Surgical treatment for both tarsal valgus and tarsal varus involves corrective osteotomy and realignment (see Operative Technique 6.7). In the Dachshund, opening wedge osteotomy and stabilization with external skeletal fixation has been described (Johnson et al., 1989). In other breeds, if the LLD is minimal then a closing wedge osteotomy after removing a predetermined cuneiform piece of bone is easier and the repair is more stable (see Operative Technique 6.7).

Genu recurvatum

Genu recurvatum literally translated means 'stifle bent backwards' (Figure 6.16). It is seen in puppies and kittens as a congenital abnormality. Affected animals present with a hyperextended pelvic limb. It is possible to flex the stifle partially in early cases, which differentiates it from quadriceps contracture, but the flexor muscles or hamstrings seem to be weak and inadequate to maintain the stifle in a normal slightly flexed position. As the animal ages the stifle becomes fixed in extension.

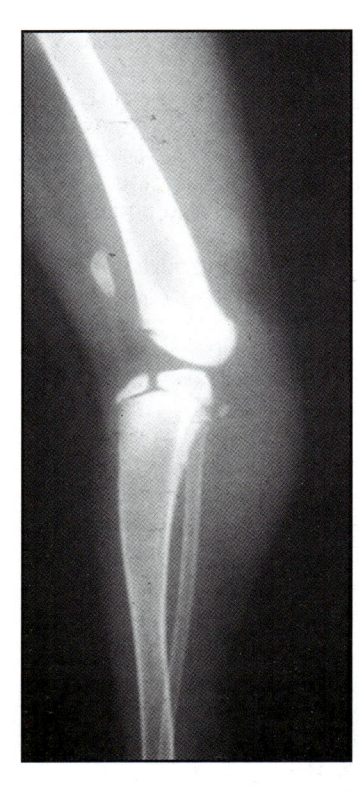

Chapter 6 Disturbances of growth and bone development

6.16 Lateral radiograph of the stifle of a kitten with genu recurvatum. (Courtesy of Matthew Pead.)

Radiographically, the distal femur and proximal tibia develop abnormally and the stifle is also abnormal with an increased angle of extension. Treatment can be attempted in early cases, for example using transarticular external skeletal fixators in an attempt to maintain stifle flexion, but the prognosis is guarded.

Genetically determined bone disorders

Many genetically determined disorders of the osseous skeleton, or bone dysplasias, that occur in dogs and cats have been selected for by breeders and have become considered 'normal' for the breed. In humans a system of classification is used for constitutional (intrinsic) disorders of bone (Figure 6.17). Not all the disorders can be covered in detail in this chapter; many of the common conditions are dealt with in detail in other chapters. In addition, this is a human classification system and animal examples do not exist for all categories.

Osteochondrodysplasias

Osteochondrodysplasias are inherited abnormalities of development of cartilage and bone. The deformity may not always be obvious at birth and may only become apparent as the animal develops. They are all associated with varying degrees and types of dwarfism.

Defects of growth of tubular bones and/or spine

Chondrodysplasia: Chondrodysplastic dwarfs have been developed by selective breeding and include the Dachshund and Basset Hound. They are disproportionate dwarfs with short bent legs but dolichocephalic or mesocephalic heads. This form of dwarfism, with

Osteochondrodysplasias
Abnormalities of cartilage or bone growth and development of both
Defects of growth of tubular bones and/or spine
Disorganized development of cartilage and fibrous components of skeleton
Abnormalities of density of cortical diaphyseal structure and/or metaphyseal modelling
Dysostoses
Malformation of individual bones, singly or in combination
Dysostoses with cranial and facial involvement
Dysostoses with predominant axial involvement
Dysostoses with predominant involvement of extremities
Idiopathic osteolysis
Phalangeal
Tarsocarpal
Multicentric
Chromosomal aberrations
Specific disorders; primary metabolic abnormalities
Calcium and/or phosphorus
Complex carbohydrates
Lipids
Nucleic acids
Amino acids
Metals

6.17 Summary of the international nomenclature of constitutional disorders of bone in humans. (Adapted from Jezyk, 1985.)

reduced limb length relative to the trunk, is also known as rhizomelic or micromelic disproportionate dwarfism. They have radiographic features that would be considered abnormal in other breeds. These features include:

- Short thick limb bones
- Short vertebrae
- Wide physes with delayed closure
- Accentuated shape of bones due to prominent tuberosities and flared epiphyses.

Thoracic limb lameness can occur secondary to extremes of the conformational abnormalities, such as humeroulnar subluxation, shoulder dysplasia or an ununited anconeal process. Hip dysplasia, tarsal varus and patellar luxation are all recognized problems in the pelvic limbs.

Osteochondrodysplastic dwarfism: Chondrodystrophic puppies are occasionally recognized in breeds that are not usually overtly chondrodystrophic but often have mild chondrodystrophic traits. This type of dwarfism has been reported in a variety of breeds including the Labrador Retriever, Alaskan Malamute, Norwegian Elkhound, Great Pyrenees, Miniature Poodle, Newfoundland, German Shepherd Dog, St Bernard, Clumber Spaniel and Scottish Deerhound (Breur et al., 1989; Bingel and Sande, 1994). Osteochondrodysplastic dwarfs have short bowed thoracic limbs with carpal valgus, cubital varus and external rotation of the feet (Figure 6.18). Radiographic features include humeroulnar subluxation and caudolateral subluxation of the

Chapter 6 Disturbances of growth and bone development

radial head. The distal ulnar metaphysis is wide and ragged, with an obliquely running depression and radiolucent insertion groove seen cranially. The condition is not usually recognized until puppies are aged between 4 and 5 months of age and males may be predisposed. Heritability may be due to a single autosomal recessive gene with complete penetration but with variable phenotypic expression (Fletch et al., 1973; Bingel and Sande, 1994). Surgery can be attempted to correct the elbow incongruity and straighten the limbs.

Concurrent abnormalities have been recognized in specific breeds (Figure 6.19) including macrocytic anaemia in Alaskan Malamutes (Fletch et al., 1973), retinal abnormalities and cataracts in the Samoyed (Meyers et al., 1983), glucosuria in Norwegian Elkhounds and ocular anomalies in Labrador Retrievers (Carrig et al., 1977). A breeding colony was established to investigate the inheritance of associated ocular and skeletal dysplasia in Labrador Retrievers (Carrig et al., 1988); 124 pups were examined for the presence of ocular lesions,

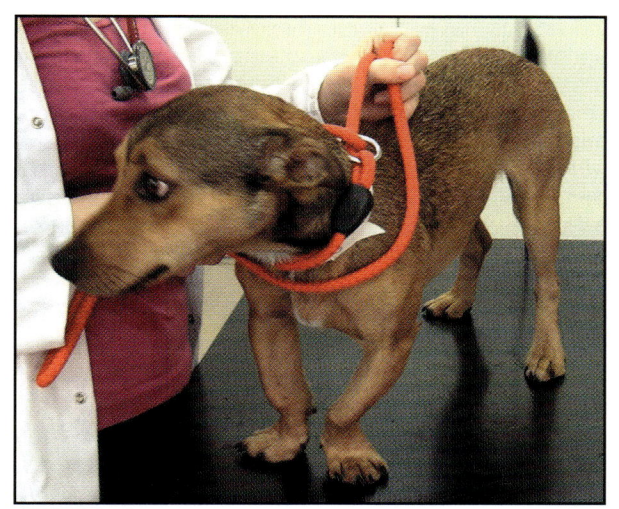

6.18 Osteochondrodysplastic dwarfism in a crossbreed. The dog has marked curvature of the antebrachium with cubital varus, carpal valgus and external rotation of the foot. The pelvic limbs are relatively straight.

Disorder	Synonyms	Breeds affected	Radiographic changes	Other	Genetics
Chondrodysplasia punctata	Multiple epiphyseal dysplasia	Beagle, Miniature Poodle	Short limbs, enlarged joints, stippled epiphyses. May be dysplastic hips	Present from birth or develops in late puppyhood	Autosomal recessive (Beagle)
Achondroplasia		Shih Tzu, Pekingese, Pug	Limb shortening, flared metaphyses, depressed nasal bridge, short maxilla, small foramen magnum, wedge/hemivertebrae	Soft tissue airway problems, medial patellar luxation, elbow luxation	Autosomal dominant
Hypochondroplasia		Dachshund, Welsh Corgi, Scottish Terrier, Irish Setter	Limb shortening	Disc disease, elbow dysplasia	Autosomal dominant
Metaphyseal chondrodysplasia		Small breeds	Medial patellar luxation, hypoplasia of medial femoral condyle		
		Dachshund	Tarsal varus due to distal medial tibial dysplasia		
		Giant breeds	Retained cartilaginous cores	Carpal valgus, osteochondrosis	
Osteochondrodysplastic dwarfism	Arthro-ophthalmopathy, dyschondrosteosis	Labrador Retriever, Samoyed	Short radius and ulna: mesomelic dwarfism	Cataract, detached retina	Autosomal recessive
	Alaskan Malamute chondrodysplasia	Alaskan Malamute, Norwegian Elkhound	Short radius and ulna: mesomelic dwarfism	Anaemia (Alaskan Malamute)	Autosomal recessive (Alaskan Malamute)
Pseudochondroplasia		Miniature Poodle	Enlarged joints, stippling and patchy densities of epiphyses in young animals, in older bones short and deformed	Stiff joints	
Enchondrodystrophy		English Pointer	Flared metaphyses, wide growth plates	Cystic degeneration of articular cartilage	Autosomal recessive

6.19 Osteochondrodysplasias: abnormalities of cartilage and/or bone growth and development.

Chapter 6 Disturbances of growth and bone development

including cataracts, retinal dysplasia, folds or detachments and skeletal abnormalities. Affected dogs had shorter than normal thoracic limbs and an abnormal morphological appearance of the radius and ulna (osteochondrodysplastic dwarfism). The conclusion was that the syndrome was caused by one abnormal gene with recessive effects on the skeleton and incompletely dominant effects on the eye. Carrier dogs could be identified by a test mating with a known homozygote. Heterozygotes had a clinically normal skeleton and mild ocular deformities, whereas the homozygotes had skeletal abnormalities and severe ocular abnormalities.

Achondroplasia: Achondroplastic dwarfs have also been developed by selective breeding. Failure of cartilaginous growth results in proportionate short-limbed dwarfs. The dwarfism is present at birth. It is an autosomal dominant condition and is seen in breeds such as the Bulldog, Shi Tzu, Lhaso Apso and Pekingese. These breeds have short limbs, flared metaphyses, brachycephalic skulls, a depressed nasal bridge and short maxilla. Numerous defects are seen, including mandibular prognathism (lower jaw overshot), stenotic nares, overlong soft palate, hemivertebrae and cardiac defects. Lameness can occur secondary to congenital elbow luxation and patellar luxation (Jezyk, 1985). Histologically there is evidence of retarded endochondral ossification.

Enchondrodystrophy: This is an inherited dwarfism seen in the English Pointer (see Figure 6.19) (Whitbread, 1983). Signs of growth plate deformity appear before weaning. Clinically, the pups have a stiff, stilted gait and experience difficulty in turning. They may exhibit a 'bunny-hopping' motion when moving at speed. The affected animals remain considerably smaller than their normal littermates.

Radiographically, there is widening of the growth plates (not dissimilar to the appearance of rickets) with flaring of the metaphyses and periosteal bone production around the growth plates. The distal ulnar, radial and tibial growth plates are worst affected. Late changes include limb deviation, and elbow or hip deformity with secondary osteoarthritic changes. The vertebral bodies are also affected.

Histological examination of the growth plates reveals an increased zone of hypertrophic chondrocytes with the columns of cells regularly aligned (very different to rickets). Cystic degeneration of articular cartilage can affect several joints. There seems to be a homozygous recessive mode of inheritance (Whitbread, 1983).

Rickets is a differential diagnosis but it does not occur in suckling animals and histologically there is usually a disorderly appearance of the chondrocytes.

Scottish Fold osteodystrophy: The Scottish Fold breed of cat originated in Scotland from breeding naturally occurring spontaneously mutated farm cats having folded ears with British and American shorthaired cats. The breed has since been banned in the United Kingdom because of the strong association with both ear mites and deafness. In addition to the folded ears autosomal dominant individuals in the breed can suffer from skeletal deformities or osteodystrophy. These individuals have a short, thick, inflexible tail, which usually precedes other problems. Breeders use the presence or absence of the deformed tail to assess whether the cats are affected with osteodystrophy but this is not a completely reliable indicator (Mathews *et al.*, 1995). Exostoses affect the tarsal and metatarsal bones and can cause severe lameness. Carpi can also be affected. The pathogenesis is related to disordered endochondral ossification in the epiphysis.

Disorganized development of cartilage and fibrous components of skeleton

Canine osteochondromatosis: This condition is characterized by ossified protuberances arising from the metaphyseal cortical surfaces of long bones, ribs and vertebrae. They can occur singly or as multiple lesions. In the latter case they may be referred to as hereditary multiple exostoses. There may be a familial tendency. Dogs are first affected from 4–6 months of age. The osseous nodules are trophic, ceasing growth at maturity. They are asymptomatic unless the bone enlargement encroaches on neurovascular, tendinous or ligamentous structures. Malignant transformation to osteosarcomas or chondrosarcomas has been recognized. Signs vary from discomfort and lameness to paralysis depending on the location.

It is suspected that the lesions develop from chondrocytes displaced from the growth plate which undergo osseous differentiation in a juxtacortical position. On palpation they are firm swellings. Radiographically, lesions appear as pedunculated sessile excrescences with smooth or irregular outline arising from multiple cortical surfaces. Histopathologically there is a layer of cartilage overlying trabecular bone.

Feline osteochondromas: In cats this condition has been reported to affect an older age group than in dogs; animals tend to be between 2 and 4 years. Siamese cats were over-represented in the early literature. The prognosis was guarded as cats often tested positive for feline leukaemia virus (FeLV). The lesions recurred after excision and most cats were euthanased.

Solitary osteochondromas have also been reported in cats. The Burmese may be over-represented and the elbow is a site of predilection (Figure 6.20). The

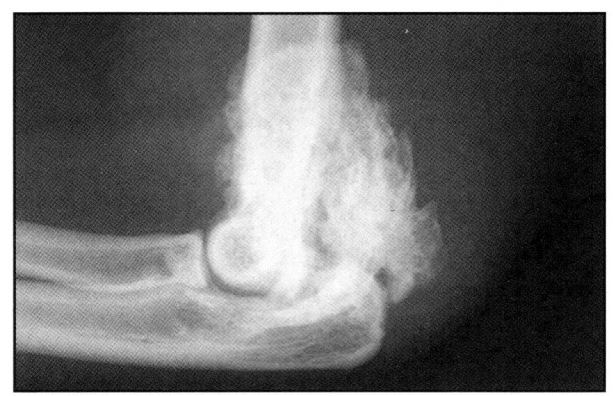

6.20 Radiograph of the elbow of a Burmese cat with an osteochondroma. The cat was sound for 6 months after local excision; however, the lesion recurred and a sarcoma developed. Amputation was curative.

Chapter 6 Disturbances of growth and bone development

prognosis is better than when multiple lesions occur, although metaplastic change is possible.

Multiple enchondromatosis: This is a rare polyostotic disease with chondroma-like proliferations in the metaphyseal and diaphyseal region of cartilaginous bones. It has been reported in Toy Poodles (Krauser *et al.*, 1989) and a Bull Terrier (Watson *et al.*, 1991). Dogs presented with pathological fractures or lameness between 4 months of age and adulthood. Multiple bones can be affected and the Poodles were also chondrodysplastic. Radiological characteristics included rounded or oval eccentrically situated metaphyseal areas of increased radiolucency. The areas were usually sharply defined and extended into the diaphysis or epiphysis. They were only found in bones that develop by endochondral ossification. The lesions are thought to develop as a result of internal remodelling disorders from the remains of the epiphyseal growth plates or due to a metaplastic process with formation of cartilage instead of bone in the ossification zone.

Abnormalities of density of cortical diaphyseal structure and/or metaphyseal modelling

Osteogenesis imperfecta: This is an inherited bone disease characterized by poor mineralization and excessive bone fragility. Clinically the disease mimics nutritional secondary hyperthyroidism and both conditions occur in kittens and puppies. Osteogenesis imperfecta should be suspected in young animals presenting with osteopenia, but where a normal diet is being fed.

Affected animals are very susceptible to pathological fractures and often have deformed limbs subsequent to malunion or folding fractures. Radiography usually (but not always) reveals poor mineralization or osteopenia of the skeleton and pathological fractures (Figure 6.21).

Blue sclerae may be seen. The teeth may have a translucent appearance and tooth fractures are also reported. The skin may be thin and hernias are common.

Histologically, cortical bone quantity is reduced; the bone is woven and has increased porosity. These diseases probably result from an abnormality of collagen metabolism. In one series of three dogs, analysis of type I collagen from cultured skin fibroblasts was used to confirm the suspected diagnosis of osteogenesis imperfecta (Campbell *et al.*, 1997). Collagen type I constitutes more than 85% of the organic matrix of bone and provides the structural framework for mineralization. Deficiency or abnormal collagen type I results in brittle bones.

Osteopetrosis: This is a rare congenital and familial developmental abnormality of skeletal growth. Synonyms include osteosclerosis fragilis, chalk bones and marble bones. Physeal formation is normal and bone development and shape is relatively normal. There is, however, marked retardation of the remainder of the endochondral ossification cycle, which includes bone maturation, resorption of immature bone, bone remodelling and cortex formation. There is an accumulation and persistence of cores of calcified cartilage, osteoid and primitive bone in the medullary cavities, resulting in abnormally dense bone. There is a paucity of reports in the dog. Riser and Fankhauser (1970) reported the post-mortem results of three Dachshund puppies and there is a single case report in an Australian Shepherd Dog (Lees and Sautter, 1979), which presented at 1 year of age with anaemia. The basic defect in osteopetrosis relates to osteoclastic function. There may be decreased activity of lysosomal and oxidative enzymes or an absolute decrease in osteoclasts.

Clinical signs can be either related to pathological fracture of the brittle bone or obliteration of normal marrow spaces that can result in aplastic anaemia. The condition may also be detected as an incidental finding (Figure 6.22).

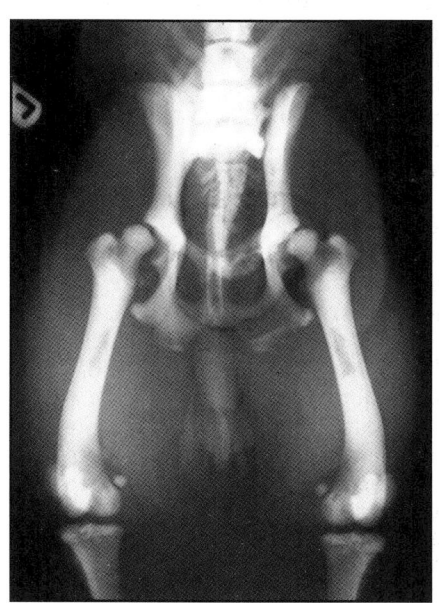

6.21 Osteogenesis imperfecta in an 11-month-old cat that was presented with a tibial fracture. Radiographs showed **(a)** the presence of healed fractures in the same bone (and in the opposite tibia). **(b)** The cat suffered spontaneous bilateral humeral fractures whilst being caged during hospitalization. Bone density in this cat was not grossly reduced radiographically.

6.22 Osteopetrosis. This 1-year-old male entire Bulldog presented because of lameness secondary to hip dysplasia. (Courtesy of George Papadopoulos)

Idiopathic acquired osteopetrosis of adult cats is characterized by thickened cortices and vertebrae. It has also been seen in cats associated with FeLV, probably through infection of haematopoietic cells.

Dysostoses

Malformation of individual bones, singularly or in combination

The cause of these dysostoses may be either hereditary spontaneous mutations or exposure to teratogens, usually in the first trimester of gestation. Dysostoses with cranial and facial involvement are common in certain dog breeds. Mandibular hypoplasia (undershot lower jaw or brachygnathism) is seen in mesocephalic and dolichocephalic breeds, such as Cocker Spaniels, Poodles, Greyhounds and Whippets. This abnormality can cause dental occlusion problems. Axial dysostoses are also common and include hemivertebrae and fused or block vertebrae (Figure 6.23). Such abnormalities are often incidental findings although they can occasionally cause spinal cord compression.

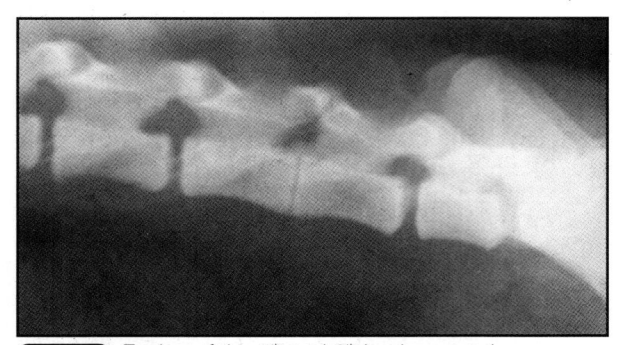

6.23 Fusion of the 5th and 6th lumbar vertebrae. Block vertebrae are examples of axial dysostoses and are often incidental findings.

Limb development commences with a projection of mesoderm covered by ectoderm that has an inductive ectodermal ridge. Subsequently the individual bones form from a cartilage anlage. Three mesodermal rays, ulnar, radial and central, contribute to pectoral limb formation. Disturbances of one or more 'rays' results in abnormal formation of the soft tissues and corresponding bones. Most appendicular dysostoses in cats and dogs occur sporadically.

Apodia is incomplete absence of either the thoracic or pelvic limbs. It is seen occasionally especially in the cat. Defects include **hemimelia**, which can be either paraxial or transverse. Paraxial hemimelia occurs when one of a paired bone is absent (*melia* – limb, *hemi* – half). Radial agenesis is one of the commonest defects (Winterbotham *et al.*, 1985); agenesis of the tibia has also been reported (Jezyk, 1985). In cases of radial hemimelia, the affected limb or limbs are shortened with a varus deformity. They are not functional for weightbearing. In transverse hemimelia the distal portion of the limb is absent. Causes can be hereditary, from strangulation by a restrictive band of tissue or from an accident in utero.

In **phocomelia** an intercalary segment of limb is missing. The radius and ulna may be absent with the paw attached to the trunk like a seal flipper. The proximal aspect of the femur was absent in a Dalmatian in one report.

Segmental **hemiatrophy** has been reported in a dog (Hardie *et al.*, 1985). One limb was significantly smaller and shorter than the other one. Limb hypoplasia may be a more accurate descriptive term than atrophy, which suggests the limb was once a normal size (Johnson and Watson, 2000). The cause may be an uneven blood supply. In humans, an enlargement or increase in length is more commonly termed hemihypertrophy.

Ectrodactyly: The literal translation of ectrodactyly is 'lack of digits'. However, in the veterinary literature the term is used to describe splitting of extremities, even when the full requirement of digits is present (Barrand, 2004). Usually only one foot is affected and the site of splitting is variable. The splitting results from failure of fusion of the embryonic precursors of the bones of the thoracic limb. There is separation of the medial and lateral aspects of the limb, occurring between any of the metacarpal bones and extending proximally between the radius and ulna. There may also be absence or hypoplasia of carpal and metacarpal bones (Figure 6.24). The necessity for treatment is dependent on the severity of the deformity, which may just be cosmetic. The condition occurs sporadically in dogs but may be hereditary in cats.

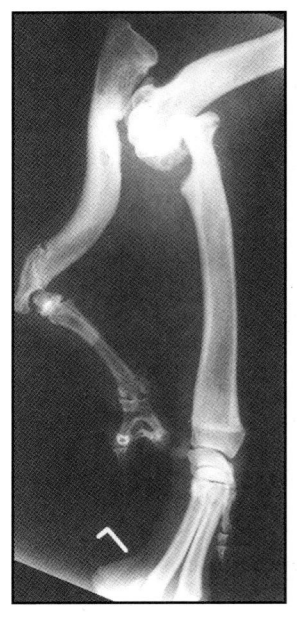

6.24 Ectrodactyly in a dog with associated elbow deformity and luxation. (Courtesy of John Innes)

If the deformity continues proximally, elbow luxation or subluxation may be present (Montgomery and Tomlinson, 1985). It is therefore recommended that the elbow joint is carefully examined and radiographed in dogs affected with ectrodactyly.

Polydactyly: This is the presence of one or more extra digits. It is thought to be inherited as an autosomal dominant trait with variable expressivity, and is seen most commonly in cats (Jezyk, 1985). A similar inheritance pattern appears to apply to the occurrence of multiple dewclaws in the dog, such as in the Pyrenean

Mountain Dog. In some giant breeds there may also be anomalous tarsal bones. Some have a large curved bone that seems to be an extension of the central tarsal bone on the medial side of the proximal row of tarsal bones. These tarsal anomalies are often bilateral and incidental findings.

Syndactyly: This is bony and/or soft tissue union of two or more digits. Cases may be unilateral or bilateral. Simple syndactyly is a lack of cutaneous separation between the digits. Lameness may result from stretching of the skin as digits attempt to spread during weightbearing (Richardson *et al.*, 1994).

Chromosomal aberrations: lysosomal storage diseases

Mucopolysaccharidoses

The mucopolysaccharidoses are conditions that occur as a result of inborn errors of glycosaminoglycan (mucopolysaccharide) metabolism. They are lysosomal storage diseases typified by a deficiency of a specific enzyme involved in the degradation of glycosaminoglycans. Numerous different types have been described in humans. Types I, II, VI and VII have been reported in the cat, and I, II, IIIA and IV in the dog. Typical clinical signs associated with mucopolysaccharidosis (MPS) include dwarfism, facial abnormalities and multifocal neurological deficits. There may be severe skeletal deformities with bony proliferation around the joints and the spine.

Mucopolysaccharidosis VI: Feline MPS VI is an inherited autosomal recessive disease that occurs in Siamese and Siamese-cross cats. It is not reported in the dog. Clinical signs begin at an early age, although affected animals may not be presented until they are young adults. Clinical features include broadening of the maxilla, corneal clouding, pectus excavatum and diffuse neurological abnormalities. The animals often have a crouching gait with abduction of the stifles, and pain and crepitus in several joints. The epiphyseal and metaphyseal areas of the long bones are enlarged and irregularly shaped. Neck manipulation is painful, and there is increased muscle tone in the limbs. Most cats have a chronic mucoid ocular discharge and chronic upper respiratory tract infection. Chronic diarrhoea occurs in some cases. Cats may suffer bilateral coxofemoral luxation at an early age.

The radiographic features include bilateral hip luxation/subluxation, coxa valga, fusion of the cervical vertebrae, flaring of the ribs at the costochondral junctions and irregular osseous proliferation of the ends of the long bones (Figure 6.25).

Diagnosis is confirmed by the demonstration of urinary glycosaminoglycans, identification of excessive amounts of dermatan sulphate and confirmation of decreased arylsulphatase B activity. Urinary glycosaminoglycans can be demonstrated with a urine spot test using toluidine blue stain or a commercial reagent. The examination of a blood smear, stained with Wright–Giemsa stain, will demonstrate coarse granular material in over 90% of neutrophils. The granules stain metachromatically blue with toluidine blue.

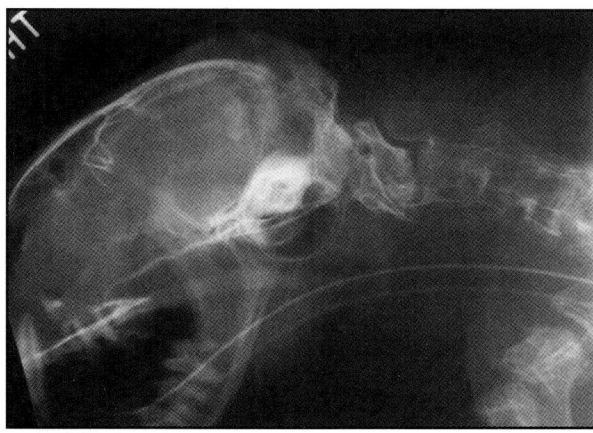

6.25 Cervical spine, skull and shoulder of a cat with mucopolysaccharidosis. There is vertebral fusion, with widened intervertebral disc spaces and abnormally shaped vertebral bodies. The shoulder joint shows irregular bone proliferation on the humeral head.

Mucopolysaccharidosis I: This has been recognized in cats and dogs. It is thought to be an autosomal recessive disease. It has been described in white DSH cats. The clinical and radiographic features are similar to type VI disease, except that long bone epiphyseal dysplasia is not a feature and cats are of normal or larger than normal size. Cats excrete increased amounts of dermatan and heparin sulphate in the urine, associated with a deficiency of L-iduronidase. Metachromatic granules are not present in the circulating neutrophils. Affected cats can survive comfortably for several years.

Mucopolysaccharidosis VII: This is associated with a deficiency of β-glucuronidase and has been reported in a family of mixed breed dogs (Jezyk, 1985) and a cat (Gitzelmann *et al.*, 1994). The affected animals had a large head with a shortened maxilla and a protruding mandible. Clinical findings included glossoptosis, peg-shaped and wide-spaced teeth, corneal clouding, pelvic limb paresis, a dorsoventrally compressed rib cage and short, curved limbs. Joints were lax, swollen and crepitant. Radiographic changes included platyspondyly (flattened vetrebrae), caudal beaking of vertebrae and generalized epiphyseal dysplasia. There were radiolucent areas within the femoral heads, irregular acetabula and bilateral coxofemoral luxation. Femoral diaphyses were widened. Peripheral lymphocytes and granulocytes contained cytoplasmic granules that stained metachromatically with toluidine blue. β-Glucuronidase was deficient in cultured fibroblasts and chondroitin sulphates were excreted in excess in the urine (positive toluidine blue test).

Mucopolysaccharidosis II: This has been identified in a 7-month-old female DSH cat (Hubler, 1996). Characteristics included abnormal facial features, retarded growth and progressive pelvic limb paresis and thickened skin. Radiography revealed a severely deformed spinal column, fused vertebrae, bilateral hip luxation and dysplasia, abnormally shaped skull and decreased bone opacity. A toluidine blue test on urine was negative for glycosaminoglycans. Further biochemical tests revealed deficiency of the enzyme

Chapter 6 Disturbances of growth and bone development

N-acetylglucosamine-1-phosphotransferase in peripheral leucocytes and an elevation of many lysosomal enzymes in serum, which is diagnostic for MPS II. A Labrador Retriever (Wilkerson *et al.*, 1998) with MPS type II had coarse facial features, macrodactyly (long toes), generalized osteopenia, progressive neurological deterioration and a positive urine test for glycosaminoglycan. Iduronate-2-sulphatase activity was deficient in cultured dermal fibroblasts.

Mucopolysaccharidosis IIIA: This has been recognized in two Wirehaired Dachshund littermates. It is caused by decreased sulphanilamide activity and is principally associated with neurological signs.

Mannosidoses
Another form of lysosomal storage disease is typified by intralysosomal accumulation of mannose-rich oligosaccharide due to deficient activity of acidic α-mannosidase. This has been recognised in a litter of Persians and a DSH cat (Blakemore, 1986). Characteristics included dwarfism, limb deformity, ataxia and an intention tremor. Radiographs showed osteolytic lesions in the vertebrae and generalized osteopenia. Corneas were clear but suture line cataracts were present.

Mucolipidoses
Mucolipidosis has been recognized in a 7-month-old female cat with abnormal facial features and gait (Hubler *et al.*, 1996). It had a deficiency of N-acetylglucosamine-1-phosphotransferase. Inclusion bodies in lysosomes contained oligosaccharides, mucopolysaccharides and lipids. A urine test was negative.

Bone abnormalities due to disturbances of extraskeletal systems

Congenital hypothyroidism
Congenital hypothyroidism has been reported in a Boxer, Scottish Deerhounds, Giant Schnauzers, Abyssinian cats and Japanese cats (Jezyk, 1985; Greco *et al.*, 1991; Jones *et al.*, 1992; Mooney and Anderson, 1993). The lack of thyroxine does not allow the developing bone to respond normally to growth hormone in a similar manner to hypopituitarism. Pedigree analysis is consistent with a simple autosomal recessive mode of inheritance.

The animals are disproportionately dwarfed with a large head and short limbs and spine. Muscle weakness, lethargy and apathy are seen. The hair coat is thin and juvenile and there may be myxoedematous facial features. Kyphosis may be present and radiography may show lack of epiphyseal ossification, metaphyseal flaring, shortened facial bones and open suture lines in the skull. Exophthalmos, strabismus and glossoptosis, constipation and hydrocephalus are also reported (Jezyk, 1985).

The clinical signs of stunted growth are due to a decrease in rate of growth in the proliferative zone and decreased maturation in the hypertrophic and ossification zones of the physis. There is decreased vascular invasion and premature formation of lamellar bone. Secondary centres of ossification are abnormal (multiple rather than single) and delayed in formation or missing. Radiographically there is delayed growth plate closure and epiphyses have a ragged appearance.

Definitive diagnosis is by thyroid stimulation tests. There is low basal serum thyroxine that fails to increase following administration of thyroid stimulating hormone (TSH). In one dog repeated administration of TSH resulted in reactivation of the thyroid gland, suggesting a central rather than primary problem (Mooney and Anderson, 1993). This dog also had consistently low basal plasma cortisol, suggestive of concurrent secondary or tertiary hypoadrenocorticism. Plasma growth hormone levels were also elevated but decreased once therapy with thyroid hormone had commenced.

Panhypopituitarism or growth hormone deficiency (pituitary dwarfism)
Pituitary dwarfism (proportionate) is a rare congenital (autosomal recessive) condition most commonly recognized in German Shepherd Dogs (Allan *et al.*, 1978). It has also been recognized in the Carnelian Bear Dog, Weimaraner, Spitz, Toy Pinscher and cats. Lack of growth hormone production occurs following cystic or abnormal development of the pituitary gland. Other hormones can be deficient, including thyroxine, androgens and antidiuretic hormone.

Affected animals are usually recognizable by 2–3 months of age. The appendicular skeleton shows retarded growth, although radiographically the physes remain open longer but are inactive. Epiphyses may show disordered ossification suggestive of hypothyroidism. Animals are usually proportionate dwarfs (Figure 6.26). Affected dogs retain deciduous dentition, often have an undershot mandible, shrill puppy bark, puppy hair coat and a 'rat tail'. As they mature they develop hyperpigmentation and bilateral symmetrical

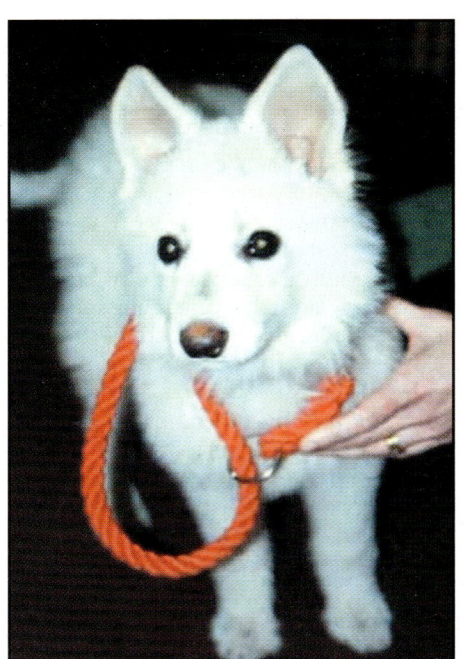

6.26 A 6-month-old German Shepherd Dog with pituitary dwarfism. The dog is a proportionate dwarf with a retained puppy coat and 'rat tail'.

alopecia. The os penis has delayed mineralization. This normally occurs at 4–5 months but may be delayed to 15 months. Other abnormalities include behavioural and cardiac disorders, cryptorchidism and megaoesphagus. Diagnosis is by hormonal testing.

References and further reading

Alexander JW, Walker TL, Roberts RE and Dueland R (1978) Malformation of canine forelimb due to synostosis between the radius and ulna. *Journal of the American Veterinary Medical Association* **173**, 1328–1330

Allan GS, Huxtable CR, Howlett CR *et al*. (1978) Pituitary dwarfism in German shepherd dogs. *Journal of Small Animal Practice* **19**, 711–727

Barrand KR (2004) Ectrodactyly in a West Highland white terrier. *Journal of Small Animal Practice* **45**, 315–318

Bingel SA and Sande RD (1982) Chondrodysplasia in the Norwegian elkhound. *American Journal of Veterinary Pathology* **107**, 219–229

Bingel SA and Sande RD (1994) Chondrodysplasia in five Great Pyrenees. *Journal of the American Veterinary Medical Association* **205**, 845–848

Blakemore WF (1986) A case of mannosidosis in the cat: clinical and histopathological findings. *Journal of Small Animal Practice* **27**, 447–455

Breur GJ, Zerbe CA, Slocombe RF, Padgett GA and Braden TD (1989) Clinical, radiographic and pathologic and genetic features of osteochondrodysplasia in Scottish Deerhounds. *Journal of the American Veterinary Medical Association* **195**, 606–612

Campbell BG, Wootton JAM, Krook L, DeMarco J and Minor RR (1997) Clinical signs and diagnosis of osteogenesis imperfecta in three dogs. *Journal of the American Veterinary Medical Association* **21**, 183–187

Carrig CB, MacMillan A, Brundage S, Pool RR and Morgan JP (1977) Retinal dysplasia associated with skeletal abnormalities in Labrador retrievers. *Journal of the American Veterinary Medical Association* **170**, 49–57

Carrig CB, Morgan JP and Pool RR (1975) Effects of asynchronous growth of the radius and ulna on the canine elbow joint following experimental retardation of longitudinal growth of the ulna. *Journal of the American Animal Hospital Association* **11**, 560–567

Carrig CB, Sponenburg DP, Schmidt GM and Tvedten HW (1988) Inheritance of associated ocular and skeletal dysplasia in Labrador retrievers. *Journal of the American Veterinary Medical Association* **193**, 1269–1272

Chastain CB, McNeel SV, Graham CL and Pezzanite SC (1983) Congenital hypothyroidism in a dog due to an iodide organification defect. *American Journal of Veterinary Research* **44**, 1257–1265

Cohn LA and Meuten DJ (1990) Bone fragility in a kitten: an osteogenesis imperfecta-like syndrome. *Journal of the American Veterinary Medical Association* **197**, 98–100

Cowell KR, Jezyk PF, Haskins ME and Patterson DF (1976) Mucopolysaccharidosis in a cat. *Journal of the American Veterinary Medical Association* **169**, 334–339

Denny H (1989) Femoral overgrowth to compensate for tibial shortening in the dog. *Veterinary Comparative Orthopaedics and Traumatology* **1**, 47–48

Fetter AW, Siemering GH and Riser WH (1985) Osteoporosis and osteopetrosis. In: *Textbook of Small Animal Orthopaedics*, ed. CD Newton and DM Nunamaker, pp. 627–631. Lippincott, Philadelphia

Fletch SM, Smart ME, Pennock PW and Subden RE (1973) Clinical and pathologic features of chondrodysplasia (dwarfism) in the Alaskan Malamute. *Journal of the American Veterinary Medical Association* **162**, 357–361

Fox SM (1984) Premature closure distal radial and ulnar physes in the dog: Part 1 pathogenesis and diagnosis. *Compendium of Continuing Education, Small Animal Practice* **6**, 128–144

Franczuszki D, Chalman JA, Butler HC, DeBowes RM and Leipold H (1987) Postoperative effects of experimental shortening in the immature dog. *Journal of the American Animal Hospital Association* **23**, 429–437

Gitzelmann R, Bosshard NU, Superti-Furga A *et al*. (1994) Feline mucopolysaccharidosis VII due to β-glucuronidase deficiency. *Veterinary Pathology* **31**, 435–443

Greco DS, Feldman EC, Peterson ME *et al*. (1991) Congenital hypothyroid dwarfism in a family of giant schnauzers. *Journal of Veterinary Internal Medicine* **5**, 57–65

Hansen JS (1968) Historical evidence of an unusual deformity in dogs ('short-spine dog'). *Journal of Small Animal Practice* **9**, 103–107

Hanssen I, Falck G, Grammeltvedt AT, Haug E and Isaksen CV (1998) Hypochondrodysplastic dwarfism in the Irish Setter. *Journal of Small Animal Practice* **39**, 10–14

Hardie EM, Chambers JM and Mahaffey MB (1985) Segmental hemiatrophy in a dog. *Journal of the American Veterinary Medical Association* **186**, 1315–1317

Hubler M, Haskins ME, Arnold S *et al*. (1996) Mucolipidosis type II in a domestic shorthaired cat. *Journal of Small Animal Practice* **37**, 435–441

Jevens DJ and DeCamp CE (1993) Bilateral distal fibular growth abnormalities in a dog. *Journal of the American Veterinary Medical Association* **202**, 421–422

Jezyk PF (1985) Constitutional disorders of the skeleton in dogs and cats. In: *Textbook of Small Animal Orthopaedics*, ed. CD Newton and DM Nunamaker, pp. 637–654. Lippincott, Philadelphia

Johnson KA (1981) Retardation of endochondral ossification at the distal ulnar growth plate in dogs. *Australian Veterinary Journal* **57**, 474–478

Johnson KA and Watson ADJ (2000) Skeletal diseases. In: *Textbook of Veterinary Internal Medicine – Diseases of the Dog and Cat, 5th edition*, ed. SJ Ettinger, pp. 1887–1916. WB Saunders, Philadelphia

Johnson SG, Hulse DA, Vangundy TE and Green RW (1989) Corrective osteotomy for pes varus in the dachshund. *Veterinary Surgery* **18**, 373–379

Jones BR, Gruffydd TJ, Sparkes AH and Lucke VM (1992) Preliminary studies on congenital hypothyroidism in a family of Abyssinian cats. *Veterinary Record* **131**, 145–148

Kene ROC, Lee R and Bennett D (1982) The radiological features of congenital elbow luxation/subluxation in the dog. *Journal of Small Animal Practice* **23**, 621–630

Krauser K, Matis U, Schwartz-Porsche D and Putzer-Brenig AV (1989) Multiple enchondromatosis in the dog. Clinical findings. *Veterinary Comparative Orthopaedics and Traumatology* **4**, 144–151

Langweiler M, Haskins ME and Jezyk PF (1978) Mucopolysaccharidosis in a litter of cats. *Journal of the American Animal Hospital Association* **14**, 748–751

Lau RE (1977) Inherited premature closure of the distal ulna physis. *Journal of the American Animal Hospital Association* **13**, 609–612

Lees GE and Sautter HJH (1979) Anaemia and osteopetrosis in a dog. *Journal of the American Veterinary Medical Association* **175**, 820–824

Lodge D (1966) Two cases of epiphyseal dysplasia. *Veterinary Record* **79**, 136–138

Macpherson GC, Lewis DD, Johnson KA, Allen GS and Yovich JC (1992) Fragmented coronoid process associated with premature distal radial physeal closure in four dogs. *Veterinary Comparative Orthopaedics and Traumatology* **5**, 93–99

Mathews KG, Koblik PD, Knoeckel MJ, Pool RR and Fyfe JL (1995) Resolution of lameness associated with Scottish fold osteodystrophy following bilateral ostectomies and pantarsal arthrodeses: a case report. *Journal of the American Animal Hospital Association* **31**, 280–288

May C, Bennett D and Downham DY (1991) Delayed physeal closure associated with castration in cats. *Journal of Small Animal Practice* **32**, 326–328

Meyers VN, Jezyk PF, Aguirre GD and Patterson DF (1983) Short-limbed dwarfism and ocular defects in the Samoyed dog. *Journal of the American Veterinary Medical Association* **183**, 975–979

Mooney CT and Anderson TJ (1993) Congenital hypothyroidism in a boxer dog. *Journal of Small Animal Practice* **34**, 31–35

Montgomery M and Tomlinson JL (1985) Two cases of ectrodactyly and congenital elbow luxation in the dog. *Journal of the American Animal Hospital Association* **21**, 781–785

Newton CD (1985a) Radial and ulna osteotomy. In: *Textbook of Small Animal Orthopaedics*, ed. CD Newton and DM Nunamaker, pp. 533–544. JB Lippincott, Philadelphia

Newton CD (1985b) Genu valgum. In: *Textbook of Small Animal Orthopaedics*, ed. CD Newton and DM Nunamaker, pp. 633–636. JB Lippincott, Philadelphia

Olson NC, Carrig CB and Brinker WO (1979) Asynchronous growth of the canine radius and ulna: effects of retardation of longitudinal growth of the radius. *American Journal of Veterinary Research* **40**, 351–355

Piermattei DL and Flo G (1997) Correction of abnormal bone growth and healing. In: *Brinker, Piermattei & Flo's Handbook of Small Animal Orthopaedics and Fracture Repair, 3rd edn*, pp. 686–714. WB Saunders, Philadelphia

Pratt JN (2001) Avulsion of the tibial tuberosity with separation of the proximal tibial physis in seven dogs. *Veterinary Record* **149**, 352–356

Rasmussen PG (1971) Multiple epiphyseal dysplasia in a litter of beagle puppies. *Journal of Small Animal Practice* **12**, 91–97

Read RA and Robins GM (1982) Deformity of the proximal tibia in dogs. *Veterinary Record* **111**, 295–298

Chapter 6   Disturbances of growth and bone development

Richardson EF, Wey PD and Hoffman LA (1994) Surgical management of syndactyly in a dog. *Journal of the American Veterinary Medical Association* **205**, 1149–1151

Riser WH and Fankhauser R (1970) Osteopetrosis in the dog. A report of three cases. *Journal of the American Veterinary Radiology Society* **11**, 29–34

Riser WH, Haskins ME, Jezyk PF and Patteson DF (1980) Pseudoachondroplastic dysplasia in Miniature Poodles: clinical, radiologic, and pathologic features. *Journal of the American Veterinary Medical Association* **176**, 335–341

Sande RD and Bingel SA (1982) Animal models of dwarfism. *Veterinary Clinics of North America: Small Animal Practice* **13**, 71–89

Sheilds LH and Gambardella PC (1989) Premature closure of the ulnar physis in the dog: a retrospective clinical study. *Journal of the American Animal Hospital Association* **25**, 573–581

Vandewater AL and Olmstead ML (1983) Premature closure of the distal radial physis in the dog – a review of 11 cases. *Veterinary Surgery* **12**, 7–12

Van Vechten BJ and Vasseur PB (1993) Complications of mid-diaphyseal radial ostectomy performed for treatment of premature closure of the distal radial physis in two dogs. *Journal of the American Veterinary Medical Association* **202**, 97–100

Vaughan LC (1987) Disorders of the tarsus in the dog II. *British Veterinary Journal* **143**, 498–505

Watson AFJ, Miller AC, Allan GC, Davis PE and Howlett PE (1991) Osteochondrodysplasia in bull terrier littermates. *Journal of Small Animal Practice* **32**, 312–317

Whitbread TJ (1983) An inherited endochondrodystrophy in the English Pointer dog. *Journal of Small Animal Practice* **24**, 399–411

Wilkerson MJ Lewis DC, Marks SL and Prieur DJ (1998) Clinical and morphologic features of mucopolysaccharidosis type II in a dog: naturally occurring model of Hunters syndrome. *Veterinary Pathology* **35**, 230–233

Winterbotham EJ, Johnson KA and Francis DJ (1985) Radial agenesis in a cat. *Journal of Small Animal Practice* **26**, 393–398

Chapter 6 Disturbances of growth and bone development

OPERATIVE TECHNIQUE 6.1
Distal ulnar osteotomy/segmental ostectomy

Positioning
Lateral recumbency with affected leg uppermost.

Assistant
Useful

Tray extras
Hohmann retractors (two); oscillating saw, or Gigli saw, or mallet and osteotome.

Surgical approach
A skin incision is made over the lateral aspect of the ulna, extending from the distal third of the antebrachium proximally to the ulnar styloid process distally (Figure 6.27).

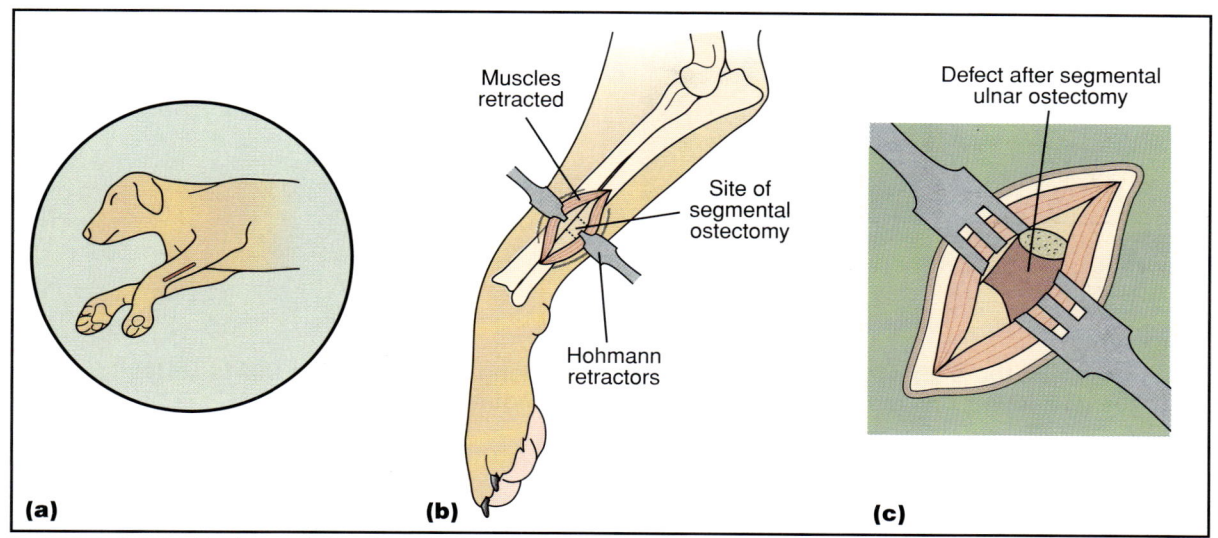

6.27 (a) Positioning and site of surgical incision. (b) Hohmann retractors are used to retract muscles prior to cutting the ulna. (c) The length of ulna resected, when performing a segmental ulnar ostectomy, should approximate 1.5–2 times the diameter of the bone.

Surgical technique
Dissection is performed between the ulnaris lateralis caudally and the lateral digital extensor cranially. A longitudinal incision is made through the periosteum and an area (length approximately equal to twice the diameter of the bone) is elevated cranially and caudally. Hohmann retractors are used cranially and caudally to protect and elevate the soft tissues and to prevent the inadvertent cutting of the radius. The ulna is then cut using a Gigli wire, oscillating saw, or mallet and osteotome. The length of the excised ulnar segment should be approximately 1.5 times the diameter of the bone (Figure 6.28).

Chapter 6 Disturbances of growth and bone development

OPERATIVE TECHNIQUE 6.1 *continued*
Distal ulnar osteotomy/segmental ostectomy

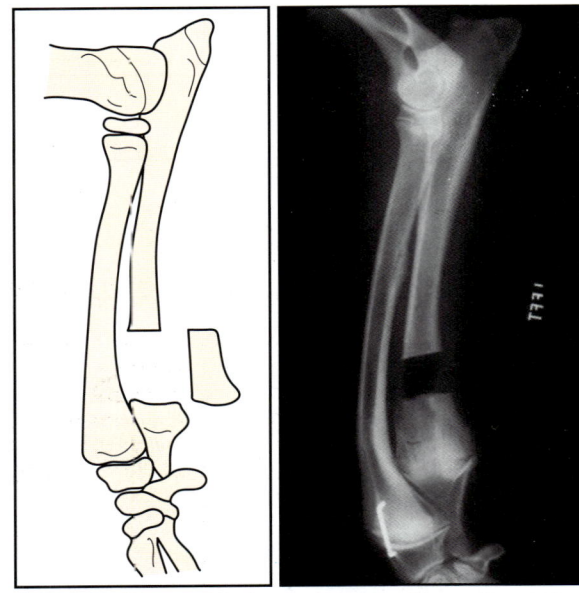

6.28 Segmental ulnar ostectomy. The radiograph shows a transphyseal staple across the distal radial growth plate.

> **WARNING**
> **With Gigli wire there should be no risk of cutting or 'nicking' the radius, but this is certainly a risk with the oscillating saw or mallet and osteotome, and should be avoided.**

The periosteum should be removed to avoid premature fusion of the segmental ulnar ostectomy. Bleeding may occur when dissecting the periosteum off the radius.
This technique can be combined with radial stapling (see Operative Technique 6.2).

Closure
Soft tissues should be apposed to minimize the dead space. Skin closure is routine.

Postoperative care
A firm padded support bandage is applied for 7–10 days postoperatively.

Chapter 6 Disturbances of growth and bone development

OPERATIVE TECHNIQUE 6.2
Stapling the distal radial growth plate

Positioning
Lateral recumbency with the medial aspect of affected leg exposed.

Assistant
Optional.

Tray extras
Smooth bone staples; hypodermic needle; mallet.

Surgical approach
A craniomedial skin incision is made, centred on the radial physis, a prominent bony protrusion proximal to the antebrachiocarpal joint.

Surgical technique
A hypodermic needle is used to locate the physis (Figure 6.29). A bone staple is placed medially, with the tines positioned halfway between the joint and the physis. A second staple can be placed in a craniomedial position (Figure 6.30).

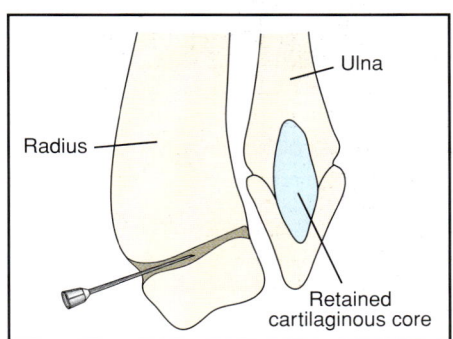

6.29 A hypodermic needle is used to locate the physis.

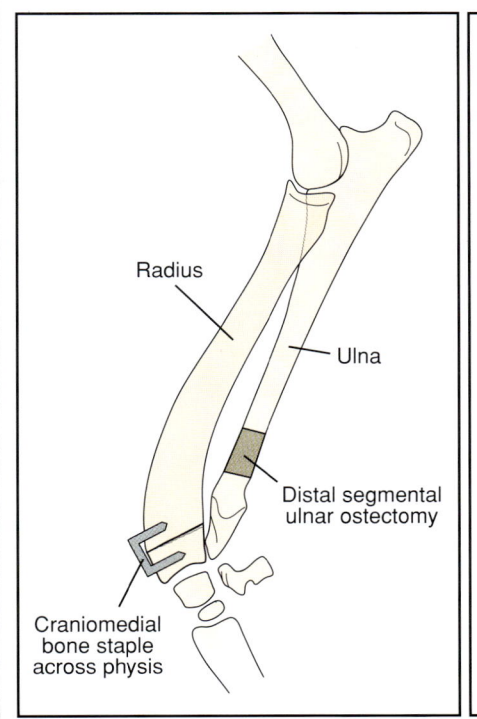

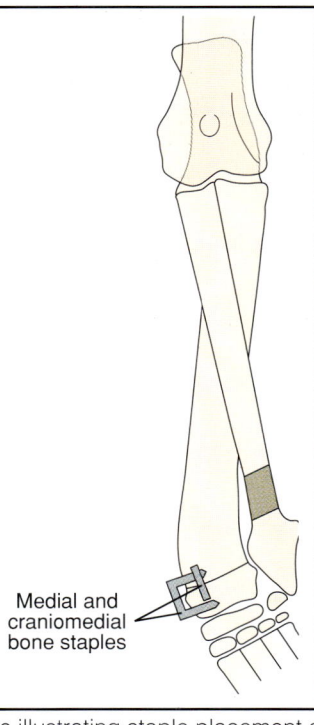

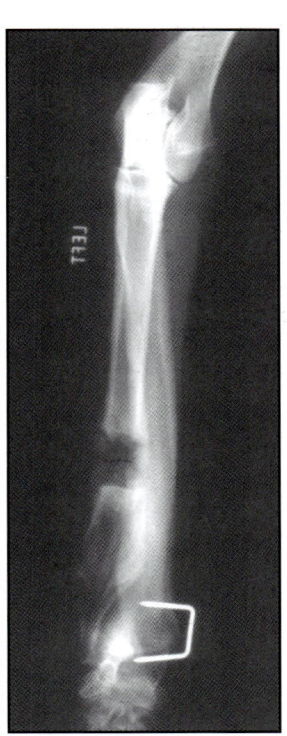

6.30 Mediolateral and craniocaudal views illustrating staple placement and distal segmental ulnar ostectomy. The radiograph showing distal ulnar ostectomy and single staple placement 4 weeks after carpal valgus correction in an Irish Wolfhound. The ostectomy is showing evidence of healing and the staple tines have bent from the force of attempted continued growth by the physis.

69

Chapter 6 Disturbances of growth and bone development

OPERATIVE TECHNIQUE 6.2 *continued*
Stapling the distal radial growth plate

Stapling the radius can be combined with a distal ulnar osteotomy/ostectomy (see Operative Technique 6.1) (Figure 6.31).

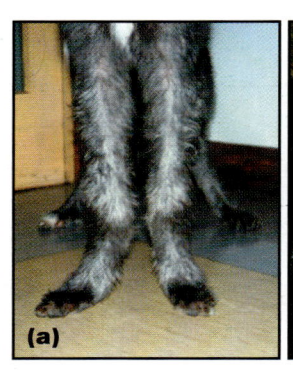

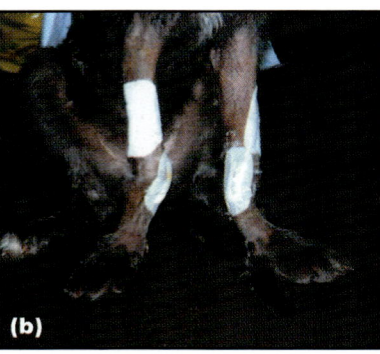

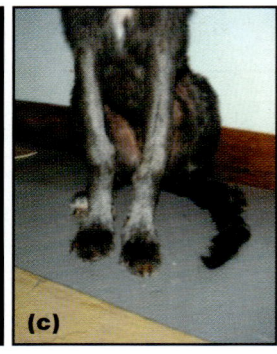

6.31
(a) Bilateral carpal valgus in a 4-month-old Deerhound.
(b) Immediately after bilateral double staple application and bilateral distal segmental ulnar ostectomy.
(c) 4 weeks after surgery: carpal valgus has corrected and the dog is due for staple removal.

Closure
The subcutaneous tissues are closed over the staples, followed by routine skin closure.

Postoperative care
A padded support bandage is applied for 3–7 days postoperatively. Radiographs are taken at 4 weeks. Staples may need to be removed to prevent valgus overcorrection and a varus deviation.

Chapter 6 Disturbances of growth and bone development

OPERATIVE TECHNIQUE 6.3
Radial and ulnar osteotomy

Indications
This technique is indicated for carpal valgus in a mature animal or for an immature animal with valgus >25 degrees.

Planning
Orthogonal radiographs are taken of the antebrachium, including the elbow and carpus. The radiographs are traced. The angle of maximal deformity is calculated using the lining or bisection technique (Figures 6.32, 6.33). The level of cut is adjusted if necessary to ensure an adequate size of the distal fragment for stabilization. The proposed wedge ostectomy is drawn on the diagram. Correct alignment is checked by 'cutting out' the wedge. External skeletal fixator pin placement is preplanned on the diagram.

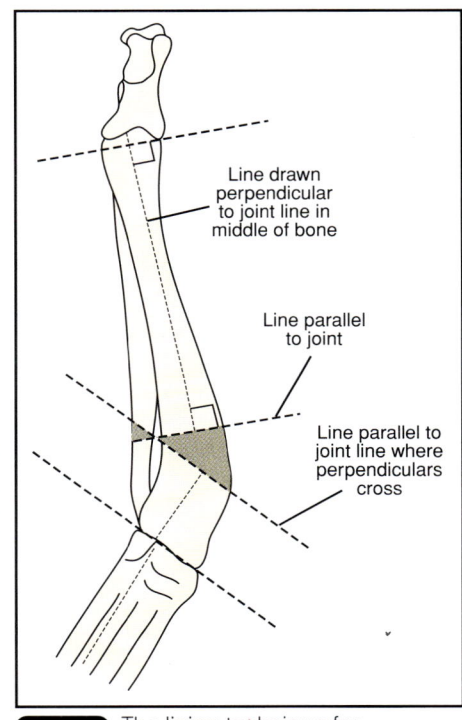

6.32 The lining technique for calculating the point of maximal deformity and the size of the cuneiform (wedge) ostectomy.

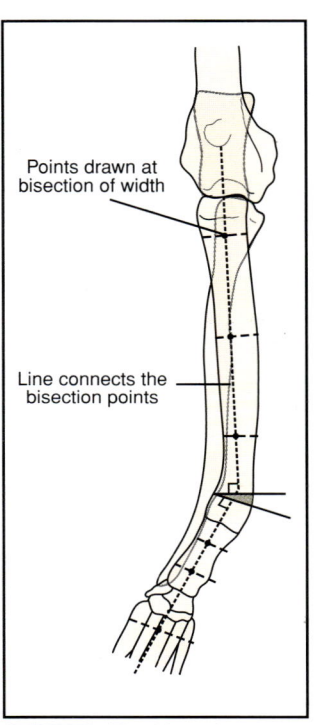

6.33 The bisection technique for calculating the point of maximal deformity and the size of the cuneiform (wedge) ostectomy.

Positioning
Dorsal recumbency with leg suspended or lateral recumbency with access to the medial and lateral aspects of limb.

Assistant
Useful.

Tray extras
Oscillating saw (or mallet and osteotome or Gigli wire); external fixator pins; bars and clamps; periosteal elevator; two Hohmann retractors; Gelpi retractors; slow speed drill and drill bits.

→

Chapter 6 Disturbances of growth and bone development

OPERATIVE TECHNIQUE 6.3 continued
Radial and ulnar osteotomy

Surgical approach and technique
A centrally threaded, positive profile ESF pin is placed across the proximal radius, perpendicular to the radius and parallel to the proximal articular surface – estimated by limb manipulation (flexion and extension of elbow). A similar type of pin is placed across the distal radius, parallel to the articular surface and perpendicular to its axis. A hypodermic needle can be used to identify the joint.

A skin incision is made over the lateral aspect of the ulna, extending proximally from the distal third of the antebrachium to the ulnar styloid process distally.

Ulnar osteotomy
Dissection is performed between the ulnaris lateralis and the lateral digital extensor. A longitudinal incision is made through the periosteum and an area (length approximately equal to twice the diameter of the bone) is elevated cranially and caudally. Hohmann retractors are used cranially and caudally to protect and elevate the soft tissues, and to prevent the inadvertent cutting of the radius. The bone is cut using a Gigli wire, oscillating saw, or mallet and osteotome level to or distal to the proposed radial cut. The length of the excised ulnar segment should be approximately 1.5 times the diameter of the bone.

> **WARNING**
> **With Gigli wire there should be no risk of cutting or 'nicking' the radius, but this is certainly a risk with the oscillating saw or mallet and osteotome, and should be avoided.**

To avoid premature fusion of the segmental ulnar osteotomy, the periosteum should be removed. Bleeding may occur when dissecting the periosteum off the radius.

Radial osteotomy
It may be possible for both osteotomies to be performed through a craniolateral skin incision, depending on the size of the dog. Otherwise a separate skin incision is made craniomedially at the level of the proposed radial cut. Using the prepared diagrams a wedge of bone is removed according to the preoperative calculations. The distal cut should be parallel to the distal articular surface and the proximal one parallel to the proximal radial articular surface. These are estimated by flexion and extension of the appropriate joints. The craniocaudal direction of the cut is angled to correct cranial bowing, with more bone being removed from the cranial aspect of the limb.

External skeletal fixator placement
ESF bars with preplaced ESF clamps are connected according to the preoperative plan (Figure 6.34). A minimum of two pins should be placed in each bone fragment. The limb should be aligned by careful visual assessment and evaluation of flexion and extension of the limb. The paw should be in line with the humerus (Figure 6.35). The carpal pad should be in line with the olecranon when viewed caudally. When the elbow and carpus are flexed there should not be any rotation or deviation of the paw medially or laterally. It is often difficult to fully reduce the cranial bowing due to contracture of the flexor muscles. Clamps are tightened and alignment checked again. A minimum of one half pin is then placed into the distal fragment and two half pins into the proximal fragment.

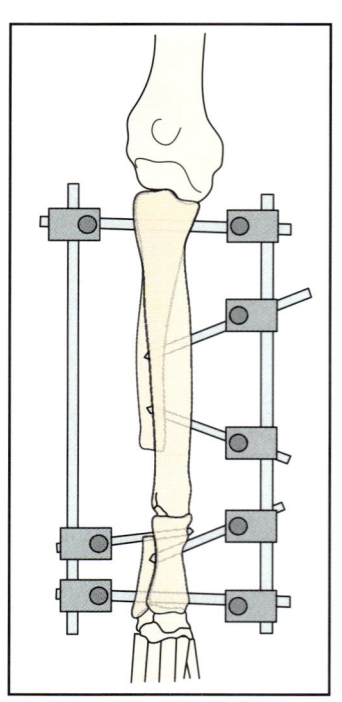

6.34 A bilateral (type II) ESF has been used to stabilize the antebrachium after a corrective closing wedge ostectomy.

Chapter 6 Disturbances of growth and bone development

OPERATIVE TECHNIQUE 6.3 continued
Radial and ulnar osteotomy

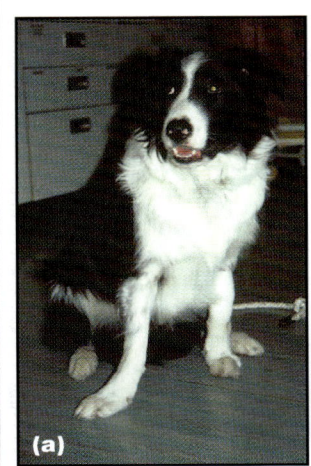

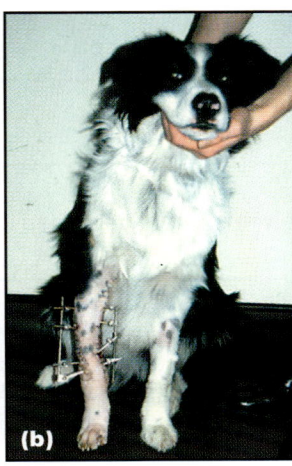

6.35 **(a)** Border Collie with carpal valgus subsequent to a distal radial fracture and a Salter–Harris type V closure of the distal ulnar growth plate. **(b)** A bilateral ESF has been applied after a closing wedge ostectomy to correct the carpal valgus. The ostectomy was performed more proximally than the true point of maximal deformity, to give a large enough distal piece of bone to stabilize. This has resulted in a slight bow to the antebrachium; however, the foot and humerus are in line and the elbow and carpal joints are parallel, so the antebrachial deformity should not cause a problem.

Closure
Bone grafting is not necessary but in the mature animal it is worth using a pair of rongeurs and removing the cancellous bone from the wedge ostectomy and placing this at the ostectomy site. Routine skin closure is carried out after flushing with sterile saline.

Postoperative care
A firm padded support bandage is applied under the ESF for 3 days. Radiographs are taken every 4 weeks to monitor healing.

Chapter 6 Disturbances of growth and bone development

OPERATIVE TECHNIQUE 6.4
Dynamic proximal ulnar osteotomy/segmental ostectomy

Positioning
Dorsal recumbency with the affected leg retracted cranially.

Assistant
Essential.

Tray extras
Two Hohmann retractors; periosteal elevator; Gigli wire; wire passer/fine curved forceps; Steinmann pin, drill bits and drill if intramedullary pin to be used.

Surgical approach
A caudal skin incision is made extending from the olecranon to mid antebrachium. Dissection is performed through the caudal subcutaneous tissue and the periosteum on the caudal ulna is incised using a scalpel blade. The muscles are elevated off the medial and lateral aspects of the ulna distal to the elbow joint.

Surgical technique
The lateral epicondyle and radial head are palpated. The ulnar osteotomy should be performed at least 1 cm distal to the level of the radial head. The Gigli wire is pulled between the radius and ulna using a curved haemostat.

> **PRACTICAL TIP**
> **Passing the Gigli wire between the radius and ulna can be difficult. Dissection of the muscles a reasonable extent distal and proximal to the osteotomy level (the extent of the skin incision) will make muscle retraction and hence passage of the wire easier.**

Two Hohmann retractors are placed laterally and medially to protect and retract musculature. A 'three-handed' assistant is useful during this part of the procedure to hold both Hohmann retractors and the antebrachium whilst the surgeon cuts the bone with the Gigli wire. The ulna can be cut perpendicular to the long axis or in a distocranial to proximocaudal direction to limit caudal rotation of the proximal fragment (Figure 6.36).

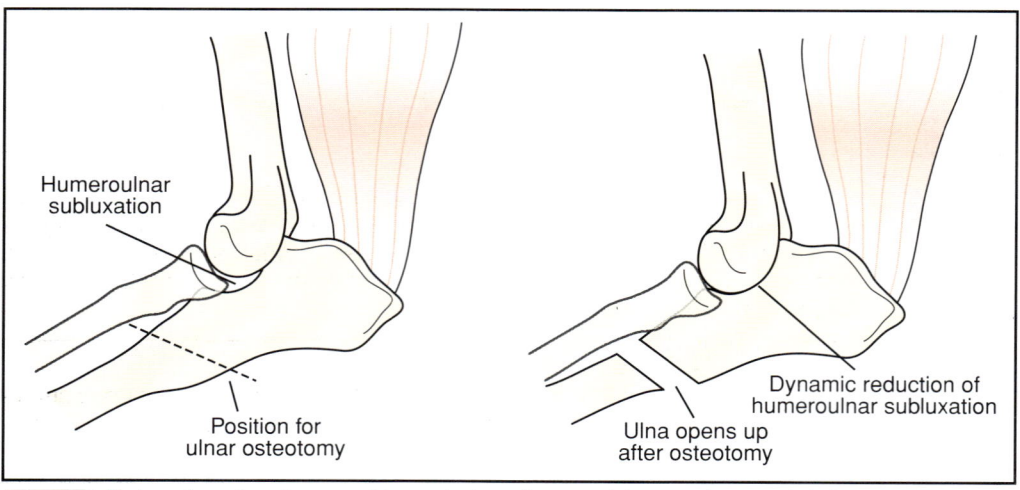

6.36 To lengthen the ulna, a cut is made in a distocranial to proximocaudal direction. The triceps muscle should pull the bone proximally.

Chapter 6 Disturbances of growth and bone development

OPERATIVE TECHNIQUE 6.4 continued
Dynamic proximal ulnar osteotomy/segmental ostectomy

If an ulnar ostectomy is being performed then the second cut can be started prior to completing the first cut whilst the leg is more stable (Figures 6.37 and 6.38).

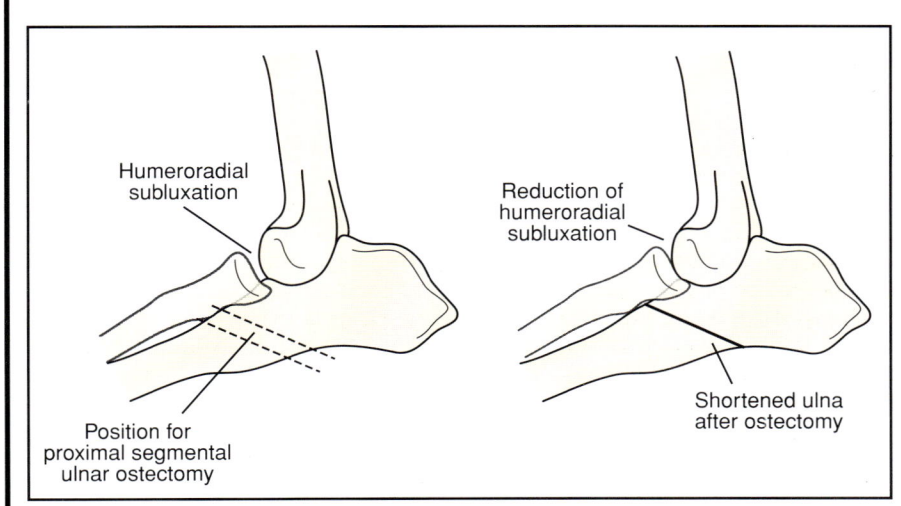

6.37 To shorten the ulna, a segmental ulnar ostectomy is performed equivalent to or slightly greater in size than the humeroradial gap.

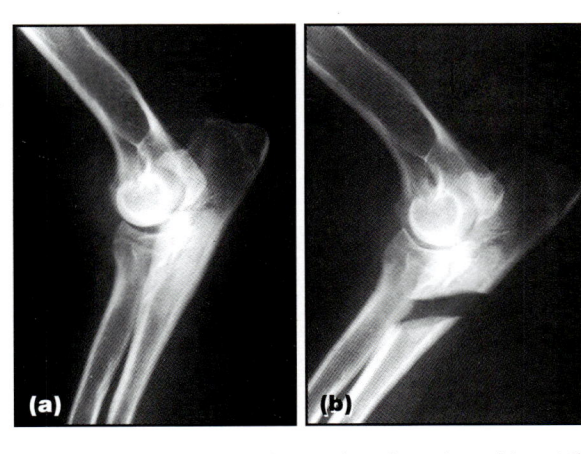

6.38 (a) Preoperative mediolateral radiograph of the elbow of a German Shepherd Dog with a humeroradial subluxation (and panosteitis). (b) Postoperative mediolateral radiograph showing reduction of the joint subluxation after a proximal segmental ulnar ostectomy.

An intramedullary pin can be placed to aid stability of the osteotomy. It is passed in a normograde fashion from the proximocaudal aspect of the olecranon. Predrilling with a slightly smaller drill bit can aid passage of the trocar-tipped pin through the dense olecranon bone. The pin will decrease motion and hence pain and morbidity associated with the osteotomy/ostectomy but it will also restrict dynamic motion of the ulna and therefore may adversely alter the end result.

Closure
The surgical incision site is flushed with sterile saline. The fascia is apposed with a simple continuous suture of slowly absorbable monofilament material, such as polydioxanone. Routine closure of subcutaneous tissue and skin is performed.

Postoperative care
A firm padded support bandage is applied for 10 days postoperatively. Radiographs are taken every 4 weeks to monitor healing. Dogs will often remain lame until the osteotomy site is stable, which can take up to 12 weeks. The osteotomy site will often heal with a large palpable and visible callus, which the owners should be warned about. This will remodel and lessen with time.

Chapter 6 Disturbances of growth and bone development

OPERATIVE TECHNIQUE 6.5
Resection of a partially closed distal radial physis

Positioning
Dorsal recumbency with affected leg retracted caudally.

Assistant
Useful but not essential.

Tray extras
Gelpi retractors; periosteal elevator; rongeurs; hypodermic needles.

Surgical approach and technique
A craniolateral approach to the distal radius is used, and an incision is made in the fascia over the epiphysis. A small-gauge hypodermic needle is used to locate the physis probing from medial to lateral (Figure 6.39). The needle should easily penetrate the normal physis. A curette, rongeurs or an oscillating saw is used to remove the bony bridge completely until there is a visible physis remaining in the point of the V (Vandewater and Olmstead, 1983). A small piece of fat from the abdominal wall or flank area is packed into the defect left after removal of the bony bridge. A partial distal ulnar ostectomy is usually also indicated as there is often additional distal ulnar physeal closure (Operative Technique 6.1).

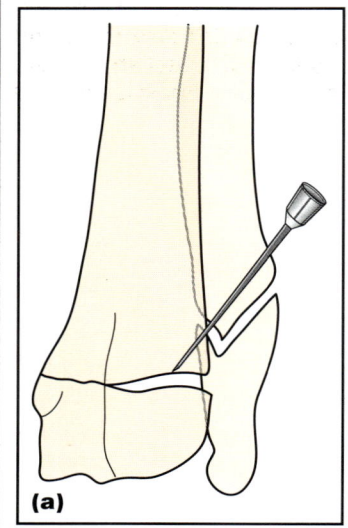

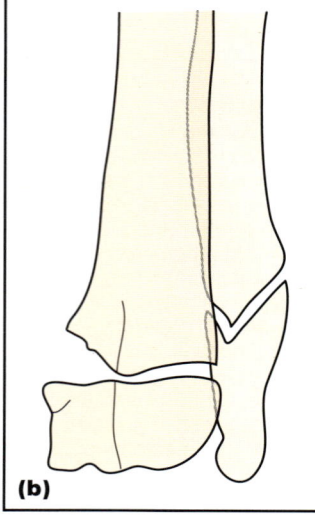

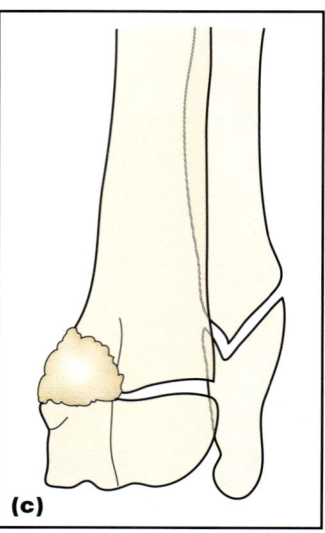

6.39 (a) A hypodermic needle is used to locate the open part of the physis and thus determine the limits of the bony bridge (shown on the medial aspect of the radius). (b) The bony bridge is resected and a distal ulnar ostectomy is often also performed. (c) The defect is then packed with a fat graft.

Closure
The surgical incision site is flushed with sterile saline. The fascia is apposed with a simple continuous suture of slowly absorbable monofilament material, such as polydioxanone. Closure of subcutaneous tissue and skin for both incisions over the radius and flank incision is routine.

Postoperative care
A firm padded support bandage is applied for 10 days postoperatively. Radiographs are taken every 4 weeks to monitor whether growth returns.

Chapter 6 Disturbances of growth and bone development

OPERATIVE TECHNIQUE 6.6
Dynamic lengthening of the radius

Planning
Orthogonal radiographs of both antebrachia and additional radiographs centred on the elbow joint are taken. The size of humeroradial gap is calculated. The need for angular and/or rotational correction is assessed from clinical examination of the dog and from the radiographs.

Positioning
Dorsal recumbency with leg pulled caudally.

Assistant
Useful.

Tray extras
Oscillating saw (or mallet and osteotome or Gigli wire); two Hohmann retractors (or Gelpi retractors); periosteal elevator; battery drill and drill bits; linear ESF distractor, ESF pins and sliding clamps.

Surgical approach and technique
A centrally threaded ESF pin is placed in the proximal radius. A second pin is placed in the distal radius.
 A small medial skin incision is made centred on the proximal third of the radius and dissection is performed down to the radius. A longitudinal incision is made through the periosteum and it is elevated proximally and distally. Two Hohmann retractors or Gelpi retractors are placed, cranially and caudally, to reflect and protect the antebrachial flexor and extensor muscles (Figure 6.40). The radius is cut at the predetermined level using an oscillating saw, osteotome and mallet, or a Gigli wire.

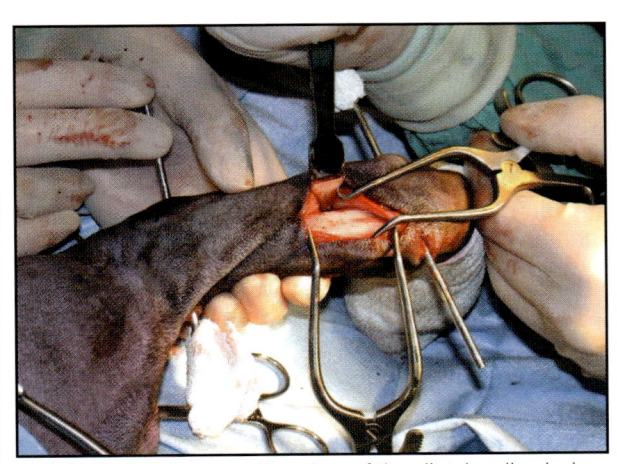

6.40 An intraoperative view of the distal radius being exposed prior to osteotomy.

PRACTICAL TIP
If an osteotome and mallet are used small holes should be drilled along the osteotomy line first.

→

Chapter 6 Disturbances of growth and bone development

> **OPERATIVE TECHNIQUE 6.6** *continued*
> **Dynamic lengthening of the radius**

The sliding clamps are preplaced on threaded bars, with nuts and knurled nuts. Additional half pins are added through the spare clamps on the sliding clamps (Figure 6.41). All pins on clamps are tightened.

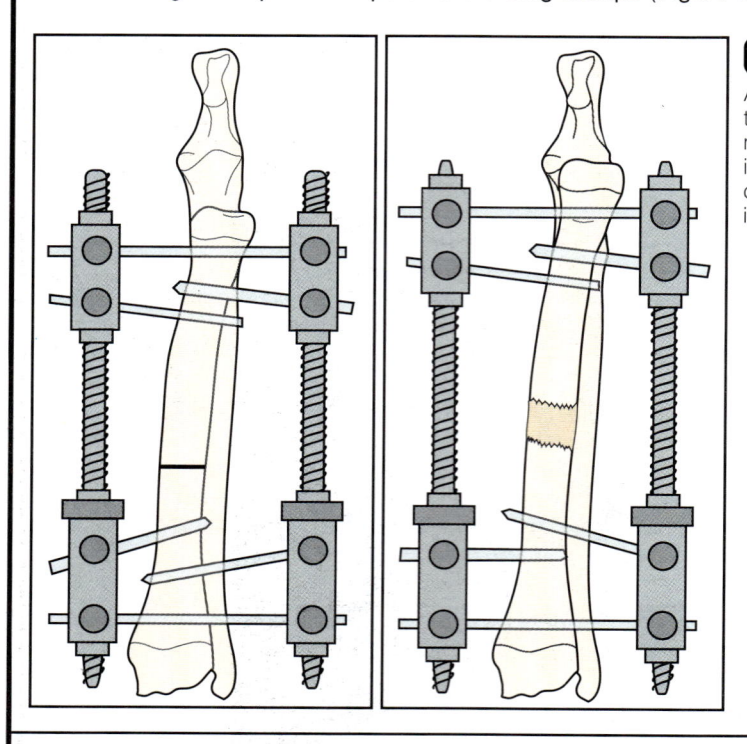

6.41 A bilateral ESF with threaded bars, knurled nuts and sliding clamps is applied in order to distract the bones and increase radial length.

Closure
The periosteum and fascia over the osteotomy site are sutured using a slowly absorbable synthetic suture material, such as polydioxanone. Subcutaneous tissue and skin are closed in a routine fashion.

Postoperative care
The dog is left for 2–5 days after the osteotomy before distraction is started. Distraction of 0.5 mm twice daily is carried out for an average-sized dog. The limb is radiographed regularly to assess the humeroradial joint space and regeneration of bone. Once elbow subluxation is reduced, the ESF can be left in place with the clamps tightened until sufficient bone healing occurs for weightbearing.

A second osteotomy may be needed in immature dogs. Alternatively, both the radius and ulna can be cut. Lengthening can then be continued until the affected leg is longer than the unaffected, making an allowance for continued growth. However, if the ulna continues to grow after radial healing there is still a risk of recurrence of luxation. Removal of the distal ulnar growth plate or removal of the periosteum from around the ulna can prevent this.

Chapter 6 Disturbances of growth and bone development

OPERATIVE TECHNIQUE 6.7
Tibial osteotomy for tarsal varus or valgus

Planning
Orthogonal radiographs of the tibia are taken, including the hock and stifle. The radiographs are traced. The point of maximal deformity and the size and orientation of the wedge is determined using the bisection technique or by drawing lines parallel to the articular surfaces (Figure 6.42, 6.43). The position, number and type of ESF pins that will be needed to stabilize the bone after osteotomy are established.

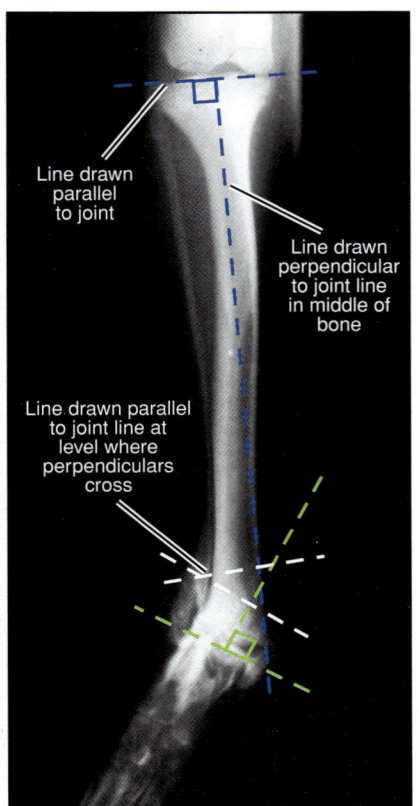

6.42 Application of the lining method for determining the point of maximal deformity and size of wedge required in order to straighten the tibia.

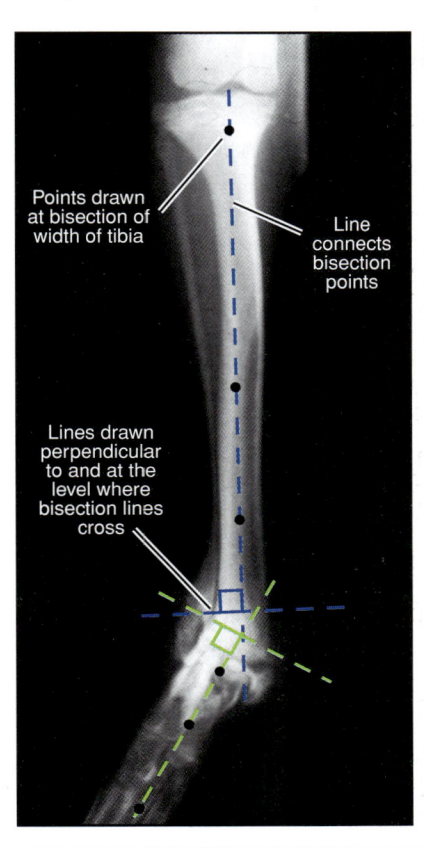

6.43 Application of the bisection technique for determining the point of maximal deformity and size of wedge required in order to straighten the tibia.

Positioning
Dorsal recumbency.

Assistant
Useful.

Tray extras
Periosteal elevator; oscillating saw; two Hohmann retractors; external skeletal fixation set.

Surgical approach and technique
For tibial valgus, two appropriately sized, centrally threaded, positive profile ESF pins are placed parallel to the proximal and distal articular surfaces of the tibia. A small skin incision is made over the medial aspect of the tibia and a predetermined wedge of bone is removed using an oscillating saw, protecting the soft tissues with Hohmann retractors. ESF bars and the predetermined number of clamps are placed (Figure 6.44). The distal tibia is orientated in line with the proximal tibia so that angulation and rotation are corrected. The clamps are tightened. The alignment is reassessed and additional half pins are placed as necessary.

Chapter 6 Disturbances of growth and bone development

OPERATIVE TECHNIQUE 6.7 *continued*
Tibial osteotomy for tarsal varus or valgus

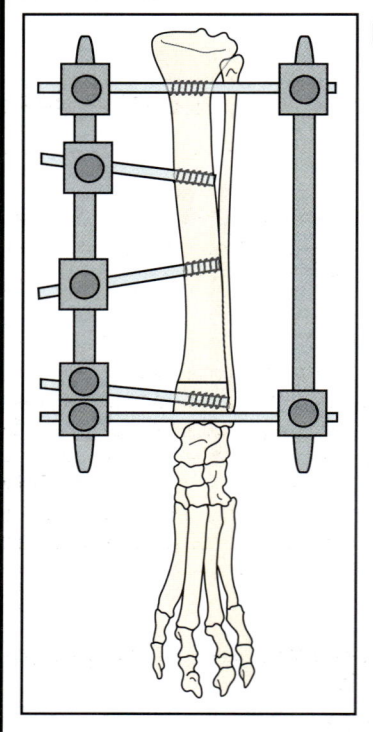

6.44
A bilateral ESF has been applied with three half pins medially after closing wedge ostectomy for tarsal valgus correction.

For tibial varus in Dachshunds, an opening wedge osteotomy has been described (Figure 6.45). Planning is done in a similar fashion but to avoid shortening the tibia further an opening wedge osteotomy is performed rather than a closing wedge ostectomy.

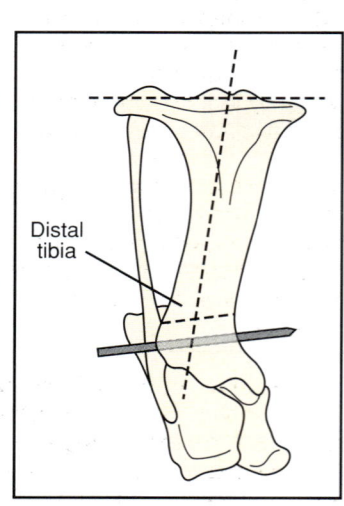

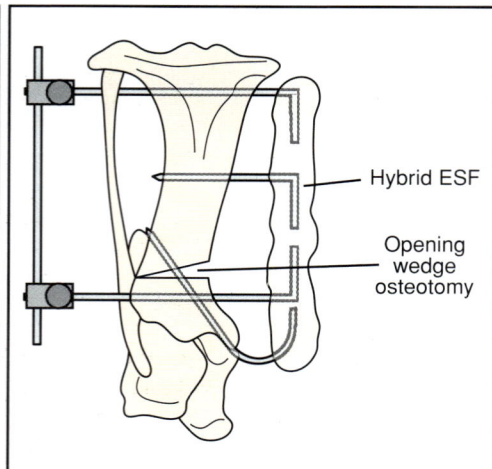

6.45
Opening wedge osteotomy for pes varus in a Dachshund. (Modified from Johnson *et al.*, 1989, with permission.)

Distal tibia

Hybrid ESF

Opening wedge osteotomy

Closure
The skin incision is closed routinely.

Postoperative care
A bandage is placed under and around the ESF for 3 days postoperatively. The tibia is radiographed every 4 weeks to evaluate healing of the osteotomy.

7

Arthritis

Ralph Abercromby, John Innes and Chris May

Introduction

Arthritis is a broad and loose term used to describe any condition affecting the synovial joint. Any abnormality of the synovial joint will cause inflammation to a greater or lesser extent and hence can be said to cause 'arthritis'. Thus, there are many causes of arthritis and many of these initiating factors (e.g. ligament rupture, osteochondrosis) are dealt with elsewhere in this Manual. For the purposes of this chapter, the term 'arthritis' is used to bring together the diagnosis and management of the disease processes involved in three main categories of joint disease: osteoarthritis; immune-mediated polyarthritis; and infective arthritis.

Arthritis can be subdivided into 'inflammatory' and 'non-inflammatory' (or 'degenerative') subtypes (Figure 7.1); however, this subdivision reflects the *relative* degree of inflammation in these disease processes, as all forms of arthritis involve inflammation to some extent. While classification systems are helpful to structure a diagnostic and therapeutic approach, many pathogenic processes are common to all forms of joint disease, although the relative importance of these different processes and the rate at which they progress may differ.

Non-inflammatory
Osteoarthritis: idiopathic (primary); secondary Traumatic Coagulopathic
Inflammatory
Immune-mediated (see Figure 7.5) Infective: viral; bacterial; ehrlichial; mycoplasmal; fungal; protozoal Crystal-induced: hydroxyapatite; calcium pyrophosphate (pseudogout); sodium urate (gout)

7.1 Classification of canine and feline arthritis (adapted from Bennett, 1990). Crystal-induced arthropathies are very rare in dogs and cats.

General diagnostic approach to arthritis

The diagnosis of arthritis lends itself to a problem-oriented approach, with a minimum database of history and physical examination leading to the formation of a problem list and hence the development of a diagnostic plan for further investigation. This logical approach is covered in detail in Chapter 1. However, there are particular observations and findings that are pertinent to lameness associated with arthritis.

History

Signalment and background information
In dogs (more than cats), many arthritides show predilections for a particular age, breed or type, and the signalment is therefore the first essential piece of information in the investigation of joint disease. This is especially true of the primary diseases that lead to secondary osteoarthritis in dogs, notably hip dysplasia, elbow dysplasia and cruciate disease.

Specific history
Specific details that are often pertinent to the investigation of arthritis include:

- Duration of lameness
- The nature of the onset of lameness (peracute, acute, subacute, gradual)
- Progression of lameness over time since onset (constant, deteriorating, improving, variable)
- The nature of any associations with the severity of the lameness (e.g. worse after rest, worse after activity, worse during activity, variation in association with climatic conditions, variation without obvious reason)
- Evidence of unusual swellings, deformities or muscle wastage noted by the owner
- Any evidence that might suggest systemic illness noted by the owner (e.g. changes in appetite or thirst, lethargy, mental depression, excessive panting, respiratory changes).

A history of stiffness after rest is highly likely to indicate joint disease. General stiffness after rest in the pelvic limbs, or difficulty rising from a sit position, may also be associated with caudal lumbar or lumbosacral spinal problems.

It is often useful to establish whether there are any activities the dog or cat used to be able to perform that can no longer be performed, especially with respect to the extent of exercise, running, jumping (e.g. into the back of the car for dogs) or climbing (e.g. stairs). If there are such activities, then it can be useful to establish whether the owner thinks the cessation of the activity is because the animal 'won't' or 'can't' perform the activity any longer.

Chapter 7   Arthritis

Physical examination

- Signs of systemic illness in the general physical examination are especially relevant to the problems that may be associated with inflammatory arthritides.
- The patient should be observed both standing and in one or more gaits. Particular attention should be paid to: which limb or limbs show lameness; conformation; posture; body contours; evidence of deformities; and muscle wastage.
- The joints should be palpated for evidence of heat, pain or swelling (inflammation). Joint swelling that cannot be seen is often detected by careful palpation and in this respect it can be helpful to palpate left and right limbs simultaneously. Palpation also adds information about the texture of any swelling (e.g. differentiating bony, soft tissue and fluid swellings).
- The joints should be manipulated first through their expected normal range of movement, detecting any loss of normal range of movement, any resentment associated with normal range of movement and any evidence of crepitus. Manipulation for abnormal movements (e.g. draw test, tibial compression test, Ortolani sign) can also be helpful in detecting structural failures, especially with respect to joint congruity and ligament failures. It is often rewarding to repeat these manipulations with the patient anaesthetized or sedated, and this can often be combined with further investigations.

Further investigations

If systemic disease is a possibility, further investigations might include haematology, serum biochemistry and serology.

Imaging

Radiography is the index imaging technique for any suspected joint in all suspected arthritis cases. Plain radiography of a joint will allow the joint to be classified as showing no radiographic abnormality, showing evidence of soft tissue swelling only, showing evidence of new bone proliferation (usually with soft tissue swelling) or showing evidence of joint erosion (usually with soft tissue swelling and new bone proliferation). Features characteristic of a primary disease, such as osteochondritis dissecans (OCD), hip dysplasia or elbow dysplasia, may also be apparent in osteoarthritis cases and in some cases there will be extra-articular radiographic features, such as dystrophic mineralization.

> **Radiographic features may be characteristic of a given joint disease, but they are rarely pathognomonic for a cause of lameness. They should always be interpreted in the context of other findings, notably those of the physical examination and joint fluid analysis.**

Additional imaging techniques for joint disease include contrast arthrography (see Chapter 2), ultrasonography, computed tomography and magnetic resonance imaging (see Chapter 4) and arthroscopy (see Chapter 15). Perhaps with the exception of arthroscopy, these imaging modalities are not often used in veterinary medicine as part of the primary clinical investigation of arthritis, but are more often used in investigating primary joint diseases, some of which may lead to osteoarthritis.

Joint fluid analysis

Synoviocentesis and joint fluid analysis (see Chapter 3) is one of the most accessible and powerful aids to diagnosis of arthritis. Joint fluid analysis should be a part of the diagnostic investigation of any joint suspected as having an arthritic problem. The minimum analysis should consist of gross observation and cytological evaluation. Culture and antibiotic sensitivity testing is indicated in selected cases (see Infective arthritis).

Joint inspection and synovial biopsy

Synovial biopsy (see Chapter 3) is especially indicated when a diagnosis of inflammatory arthritis has been confirmed (by history, physical examination, imaging and synovial fluid analysis), but the definitive diagnosis remains occult. Synovial biopsy may be performed using open arthrotomy or arthroscopy, both of which allow for a visual inspection of the joint during sampling. Biopsy samples are commonly submitted for routine histopathology and for bacterial culture and antibiotic sensitivity testing, but may also be submitted for immunohistochemical studies in selected cases. In some osteoarthritis cases with an underlying primary surgical disease (e.g. cruciate ligament disease) the synovium may appear more inflamed than expected at the time of arthrotomy for treatment of the primary disease. Synovial membrane biopsy is a useful adjunct to surgery in these cases to rule out other underlying pathology.

Osteoarthritis

Osteoarthritis (OA) (also termed degenerative joint disease or osteoarthrosis), the most common form of arthritis in dogs and cats, should be thought of as a disease process rather than a disease entity. Importantly, in the dog OA is almost always a secondary phenomenon to an initiating abnormality (e.g. joint laxity or instability, osteochondrosis, trauma).

> **Articular cartilage is considered the key tissue in OA, but it must be remembered that the synovial joint is an organ with interactions ('crosstalk') between the various tissues (cartilage, synovium, bone, ligament, synovial fluid, fat).**

The relative importance of interactions between different joint tissues (e.g. between synovium and cartilage) is still unknown (Figure 7.2). There is no doubt that a morphological marker of progression of OA is the gradual loss of articular cartilage. An understanding of OA requires some information on the metabolism of the tissues of the joint (see Chapter 11).

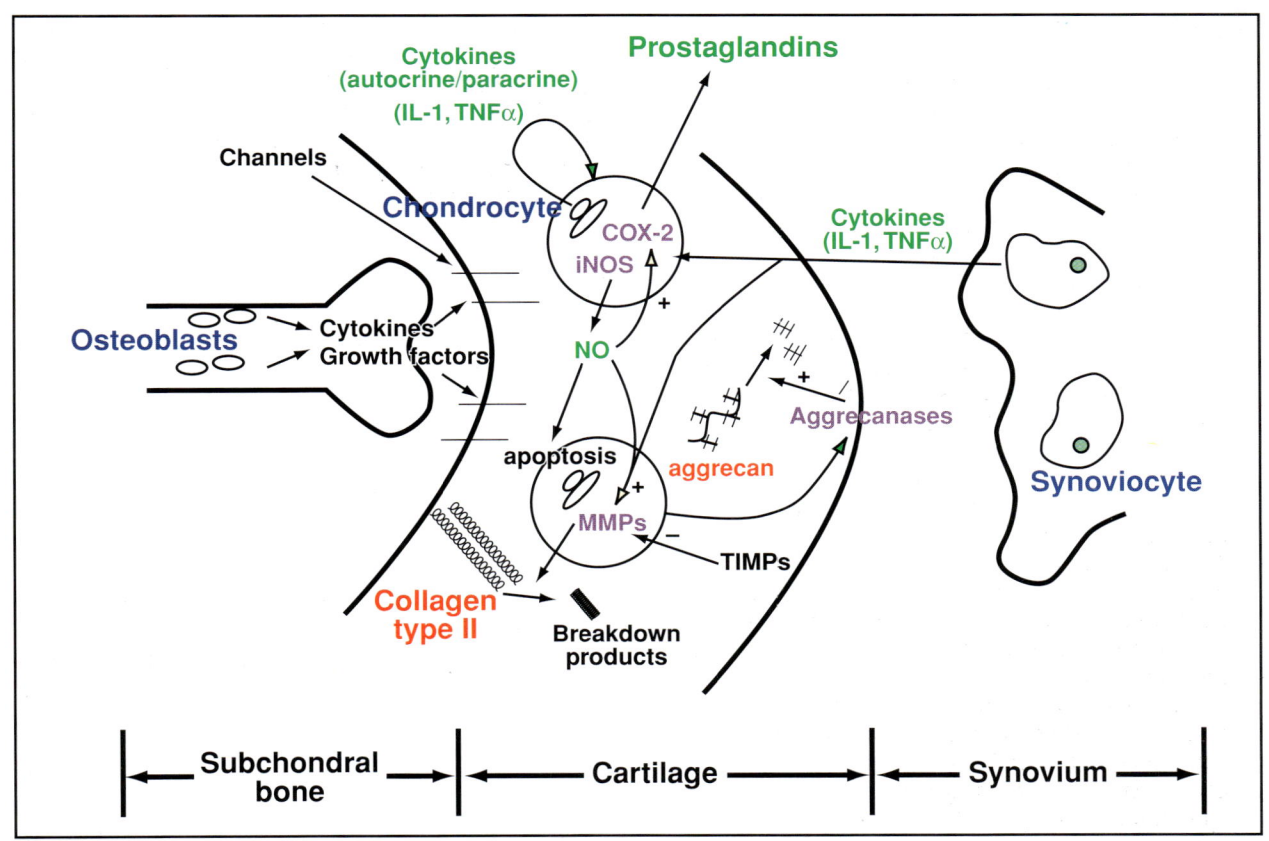

7.2 Cellular 'cross-talk' in osteoarthritis. (COX, cyclo-oxygenase; IL, interleukin; iNOS, inducible nitric oxide synthase; MMP, matrix metalloproteinase; NO, nitric oxide; TIMP, tissue inhibitor of metalloproteinase; TNF-α, tumour necrosis factor α).

Cartilage metabolism

It appears that there are major alterations in cellular activity in OA. Although there is a tendency to think of OA as merely a degenerative disease, there are repair mechanisms within cartilage. It is likely that this capacity for repair decreases with age and this may partly explain the association between OA and ageing. By way of an example, when a dog ruptures a cranial cruciate ligament, there is a marked anabolic response from the cartilage such that tissue DNA is increased and there is increased production of matrix components. In the first year following cranial cruciate ligament rupture, the cartilage actually increases in thickness (Adams and Brandt, 1991; Innes et al., 2002). This is due to a combination of increased hydration of the tissue caused by the disrupted collagen network, and increased matrix production.

Degradative mechanisms are also activated in OA and the tendency is for the balance between synthesis and degradation to swing towards degradation. Experimentally, it takes 3–5 years for full thickness cartilage lesions to appear following cruciate transection in the dog (Brandt et al., 1991). However, the sequence and timeframe of events in the cruciate-deficient stifle joint may differ from those in other joints with other primary diseases (e.g. elbow dysplasia, hip dysplasia). For example, it would appear that the progression to full-thickness cartilage lesions is more rapid in the medial compartment of the elbow with elbow dysplasia.

Diagnosis

OA is generally not a diagnosis of sufficient accuracy in canine orthopaedics because the disease is usually the result of some other primary joint abnormality (e.g. instability, laxity, fracture).

Other chapters in this Manual deal with methods to reach diagnoses of primary joint abnormalities and there is often a seamless transition between the primary joint disease and the process of OA. Management decisions are more often based on the stage of the disease, or perhaps the age of the animal. In cats, it may be difficult to identify a primary joint abnormality (e.g. idiopathic elbow OA in older cats).

Clinical signs

The clinical signs of OA are similar to those of many joint-related conditions:

- Inactivity, stiffness
- Lameness
- Reluctance to exercise
- Muscle atrophy
- Reduced range of motion
- Crepitus
- Altered gait (reduced stride length, altered swing phase)

Chapter 7 Arthritis

- Altered behaviour (aggression, reduced general activity)
- Unkempt appearance (cats).

Radiographic signs
The radiographic signs of OA are non-specific:

- Osteophytosis
- Enthesophytosis
- Intra-articular mineralization
- Subchondral sclerosis
- Subchondral cysts (geodes)
- Soft tissue enlargement.

All joints with OA will show osteophyte formation eventually, but this can occur at different rates. In dogs with complete cranial cruciate ligament rupture, osteophytes are usually visible radiographically within 3–4 weeks. In some dogs with elbow dysplasia, osteophytes may take several months to develop despite significant cartilage loss. In addition, data from the PennHIP scheme indicate that some breeds produce more osteophytes than others, given the same degree of hip laxity (Smith et al., 1995). This highlights the heterogeneity of OA between joints and individuals. The relationship between osteophyte severity and cartilage pathology is poorly defined in dogs and cats but it is likely to change with disease progression. In other words, osteophytes seem to appear early in disease but they may remodel and appear less severe with time, despite the progression of cartilage pathology (Innes et al., 2004).

> Although osteophytes and enthesophytes are used as markers of OA, it should be remembered that these occur with other forms of joint disease.

Intra-articular mineralization seems to occur only in some individuals (Innes et al., 2004). It probably represents deposition of hydroxyapatite crystals within soft tissues such as menisci and ligaments. The significance of this change is unknown.

Subchondral sclerosis is a change traditionally associated with chronic disease. Care must be taken when using plain radiographs to derive information regarding bone density. In a study of boarded radiologists, the reliability of deciding whether sclerosis was present in osteoarthritic canine stifles was unacceptably low (Innes et al., 2004).

Synovial fluid analysis
The characteristics of synovial fluid in OA can change as the disease progresses. Early in disease there may be significant effusion but later on there may be a reduced synovial fluid volume. The viscosity of the fluid is usually near normal and the fluid is a clear white–yellow. The cell count is usually low (1.0–5.0 x 10^9/l) with only 2–5% neutrophils. Hydroxyapatite crystals may be seen under polarized light microscopy.

There have been several studies on the measurement of biomarkers in synovial fluid in the hope that these might be diagnostic or prognostic in OA (Rorvik and Grondahl, 1995; Innes et al., 1998; Johnson et al., 2002; Misumi et al., 2002). These markers are usually macromolecules, or part thereof, derived from articular cartilage, such as keratan sulphate, chondroitin sulphate, degraded collagen and cartilage oligomeric matrix protein (COMP). To date, no such marker has been fully validated in dogs.

Advanced imaging
Arthroscopy can be used to help diagnose and stage OA but this is not usually necessary from a purely clinical standpoint. Arthroscopy can be used to grade the depth and extent of cartilage loss in a semi-quantitative way.

Scintigraphy has been used to image osteoarthritic joints in dogs (Innes et al., 1996; Canapp et al., 1999; Geels et al., 2000). Compared with normal joints, osteoarthritic joints show increased uptake of ^{99m}technetium-labelled diphosphonate. However, the clinical significance of these findings remains uncertain.

Computed tomography can provide detailed information on the bony changes associated with OA, including bone density. However, the direct clinical relevance of such examinations remains unknown at present.

Magnetic resonance imaging (MRI) is now the established gold standard for assessing the loss of cartilage from human joints. There are several methods to acquire and process the magnetic resonance data, including estimating whole cartilage volumes, thickness mapping and delayed gadolinium-enhanced MRI of cartilage (dGEMRIC). In the context of imaging canine cartilage, protocols are not yet standardized and the technique is likely to remain a clinical research tool in the short to medium term (Figure 7.3).

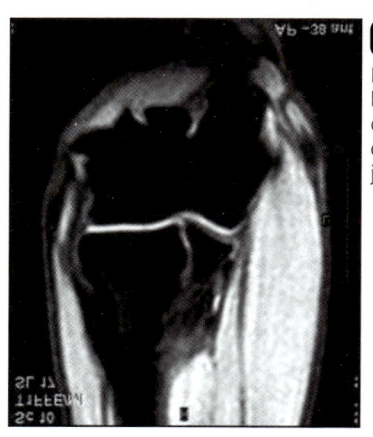

7.3 Coronal fat suppression MRI scan, showing high signal from canine articular cartilage in the elbow joint.

Management
Identification of the primary cause of OA may direct the clinician to surgical treatment of the primary condition (e.g. cranial cruciate ligament rupture, fragmentation of the medial coronoid process, hip laxity) but, because most joint disorders will cause some degree of OA, consideration must be given to this disease process. This chapter will discuss only the medical management of OA. In end-stage disease, surgical treatment may be considered (e.g. total hip replacement) and the reader is referred to the relevant chapter for appropriate discussion of such techniques. Conservative management of OA can be subdivided into the following categories:

- Client education
- Weight control
- Exercise control
- Physiotherapy (including hydrotherapy)
- Medical management: symptom-modifying drugs; structure-modifying drugs
- Nutritional supplementation (nutraceuticals): for pain relief; for structure modification.

Client education and clinical monitoring

Education of the client is very important in managing OA. An understanding of the disease keeps the client motivated and 'onside'. The client needs to know that the disease can only be managed, rather than cured, and that this may have an impact on the patient's (and the owner's) lifestyle. The use of a variety of educational aids (e.g. models, CD-ROMs, websites) and strategies is extremely useful at the start of the management process. Nurse-led arthritis clinics can also aid this process and reinforce management concepts.

Recent studies have evaluated the use of client questionnaires in canine OA and lameness. These tools allow clients to score their dog's clinical problem in a multidimensional way (e.g. effects on different activities, behaviour). The reliability of owners has been assessed in this situation (Innes and Barr, 1998; Hudson et al., 2004) and questionnaires have been statistically tested and refined (Hudson et al., 2004). Use of such questionnaires in clinical practice is likely to become more widespread, as it allows the clinician to track progress and monitor treatments.

Weight control

In human patients there is a strong epidemiological link between OA and obesity, particularly for the knee. There are fewer data for the dog, but previous studies have shown a link between higher body condition score and progression of OA secondary to hip dysplasia (Kealy et al., 1997, 2000). Within the constraints of the current knowledge base, it seems sensible to recommend avoidance of obesity in dogs and cats with joint disease. Body condition scoring is a useful and accessible way to assess the level of obesity in dogs and cats. Proprietory weight-reduction diets are available and participation in veterinary nurse-led weight control clinics is recommended as a means to encourage compliance of owners in this respect. Reduction in bodyweight is also somewhat dependent on activity levels, and other aspects of disease management (e.g. analgesia) are aimed at increasing activity which will, in turn, help to manage obesity.

Exercise control

The aim of exercise control is a balance between avoiding excessive stress on the osteoarthritic joint, and limiting the joint stiffness often noted following prolonged inactivity.

The general recommendation is that exercise should be controlled (lead) and in moderation, with perhaps an increased frequency, but decreased duration. Exercise on flat even ground is likely to be less problematical than on rough uneven ground, and slightly soft surfaces (grass, firm sand) may be preferred to concrete. However, there are few firm data to guide the clinician in this respect and much of this is extrapolated from reports on human patients. On a very practical level, some clients who work may have different expectations of their animal during their leisure time (e.g. weekends) compared to when they are busy working. It may be that exercise may vary with the day of the week and due allowance for this might need to be built into the management protocol (e.g. increasing the dose of analgesics at these times).

Physiotherapy

There is increasing evidence that physiotherapy can help the injured canine joint. Most of this information concerns the postoperative joint (see Chapter 16), but it is also likely that physiotherapy may help the arthritic joint. In human medicine, physiotherapy and exercise protocols have shown functional and pain-relieving benefits for patients with OA (Foley et al., 2003). Swimming and hydrotherapy have become very popular for dogs but to date the effects on dogs with OA have not been widely documented. Swimming does result in a greater range of motion of joints and there does appear to be some benefit for hydrotherapy in human patients with arthritis (Queneau et al., 2001; Eps et al., 2002, Stener-Victorin et al., 2004). Further information is required on the role of swimming and hydrotherapy in dogs with OA.

Medical management

Medications for OA may affect symptoms (clinical signs) and/or modify structure (joint pathology). The Osteoarthritis Research Society International (OARSI) has suggested that the term 'symptom-modifying OA drug' (SYMOAD) be used for agents that relieve pain, including those with a rapid or a slow onset of action (Altman et al., 1996). Agents with the potential for structural modification in OA (STMOADs) have previously been labelled as 'chondroprotective', 'disease-modifying drugs for OA' (DMOADs), 'anatomy-modifying agents', etc., although STMOAD is the current recommended group name (Altman et al., 1996). The demonstration of structure-modification in OA requires randomized controlled clinical trials with appropriate outcome measures. Such measures (e.g. MRI of cartilage) are not yet developed for dogs.

SYMOADs:

Non-steroidal anti-inflammatory drugs: NSAIDs act to inhibit cyclo-oxygenase (COX) and therefore decrease the production of pro-inflammatory prostaglandins, e.g. PGE_2. For some time, COX has been known to exist in two isoforms: the constitutive COX-1 and the inducible COX-2. COX-2 is induced at sites of inflammation and has been an important target for pharmaceutical companies for some years. Effective inhibition of COX-2 appears to reduce pain and inflammation, and sparing of COX-1 appears to reduce the side-effects of NSAID administration (e.g. gastrointestinal irritation, reduced renal blood flow).

Chapter 7 Arthritis

Recently, splice variants of COX-1 have been identified, including COX-3 and partial COX-1 proteins (PCOX-1a and PCOX-1b). COX-3 is expressed in canine cerebral cortex and appears to be somewhat pharmacologically distinct from COX-1 and COX-2. It seems likely that the nomenclature for COX enzymes may change to account for the differences in genetic isoform and enzyme function. (The reader is referred to alternative texts for a full discussion of the pharmacology of NSAIDs.)

The currently available NSAIDs for veterinary species vary somewhat in their selectivity for COX-1 and COX-2. Those licensed for long-term use tend to be either non-selective or have a preference for COX-2. This has advantages in terms of reducing side effects whilst maintaining efficacy. It is probably better to describe these newer agents as COX-1 sparing drugs because of their rapidly reversible blockade of COX-1. Some COX-1 sparing drugs, such as firocoxib, have recently appeared on the canine market.

NSAIDs have been the mainstay of medical management of OA for a considerable time. Aspirin was used for many years in dogs but concerns regarding toxicity with long-term use, and the negative effects of chronic aspirin use on articular cartilage in dogs (Palmoski and Brandt, 1983), have significantly decreased its use. The NSAIDs licensed for use in the dog and cat in Europe and the USA are listed in Figure 7.4.

Because the pain of OA is likely to be chronic and persistent, veterinary surgeons need to think about long-term treatment, not merely short-term treatment for an acute flare in pain. Chronic pain does not seem to serve a useful physiological role: chronic joint pain leads to decreased joint usage, muscle wastage, and increased joint instability, none of which is helpful. Relief of chronic pain can therefore be of benefit to the diseased joint and to quality of life for the patient. Thus long-term use of NSAIDs may be necessary. The licence for some drugs facilitates long-term use (28 days or more) in OA; currently, examples of such drugs include carprofen, deracoxib, etodolac, firocoxib, meloxicam and tepoxalin.

In the UK, paracetamol (acetaminophen) is only licensed for up to 5 days in combination with codeine but it does not appear to inhibit COX peripherally and hence has a very good safety profile if dosed appropriately. There is some evidence that paracetamol may act centrally via COX-3.

Tepoxalin also inhibits lipoxygenase but this effect appears to be short acting (3–5 hours) and the clinical benefits remain unclear.

> **The efficacy of individual agents in individual patients appears somewhat variable and it may be necessary to try different agents to find the most effective one for a particular patient.**

Various studies have compared these agents in terms of efficacy but it is difficult to give a firm opinion as to the preferred agents based on efficacy. Certainly, clinical trials, including those using objective measures such as force platform evaluation, have indicated that this class of drug is effective in reducing synovial joint pain and lameness. However, because safety of NSAIDs can be a concern with long-term use, it can be advisable to reduce the maintenance dose to the lowest effective dose; flare ups of pain and lameness may need to be treated with a return to a higher dose.

The use of NSAIDs in cats can be problematical because of toxicity issues. Currently only ketoprofen is licensed for cats in the UK and that is only for up to 5 days. Anecdotal evidence suggests that meloxicam at 0.05 mg/kg once daily may be a safe and effective longer-term option but this is not currently a licensed use of this product.

By virtue of their action on COX-1, NSAIDs may cause side effects. The pharmacology of individual agents influences the frequency and severity of these,

Drug	Formulation	Licensed dose for dogs in UK	Licensed dose for cats in UK
Carprofen	Tablets	4 mg/kg q24h	No current licence for use in OA in the cat
Deracoxib [a]	Tablets	1–2 mg/kg q24h [b]	Contraindicated [c]
Etodolac [a]	Tablets	10–15 mg/kg q24h [b]	Contraindicated [c]
Firocoxib	Palatable tablets	5 mg/kg q24h	No current licence for use in OA in the cat
Ketoprofen	Tablets	1 mg/kg q24h (for up to 5 days)	1 mg/kg q24h (for up to 5 days)
Meloxicam	Oral suspension	0.2 mg/kg on day 1; thereafter 0.1 mg/kg q24h	No current licence for use in OA in the cat
Paracetamol + codeine	Tablets	33 mg/kg q8h (for up to 5 days)	Contraindicated [c]
Phenylbutazone	Tablets	2–20 mg/kg q24h for 14 days, then review	Contraindicated [c]
Tolfenamic acid	Tablets	4 mg/kg q24h (for up to 3 days); may be repeated every 7 days	No current licence for use in OA in the cat (only licensed for febrile syndromes)
Tepoxalin	Lyophilized tablets	10 mg/kg q24h	No current licence for use in OA in the cat
Vedaprofen	Gel	0.5 mg/kg q24h for 28 days, then review	No current licence for use in OA in the cat

7.4 NSAIDs licensed for dogs and cats in Europe and the USA. [a] not available in Europe; [b] dose in USA; [c] experience indicates this drug is not suitable for long-term use in the cat or no information is available regarding use in cats.

but the common adverse events are vomiting and diarrhoea due to irritation of the gastrointestinal mucosa. COX-1 is also involved in control of renal blood flow and so care should be taken in any patient with renal impairment. This is also true of cardiovascular impairment where renal perfusion may be decreased.

NSAIDs inhibit platelet COX to a variable degree and this should be borne in mind in patients with bleeding disorders or in immunosuppressed patients. NSAIDs may be metabolized in the liver and hepatic disease may also be a contraindication to use of NSAIDs. Furthermore, the displacement of protein-bound agents in animals on concomitant treatment is also sometimes a concern.

The gastrointestinal side-effects of NSAIDs may be ameliorated with gastroprotectants (e.g. sucralfate), H_2 antagonists (e.g. ranitidine, cimetidine) or proton pump inhibitors (e.g. omeprazole). PGE_1 agonists, such as misoprostol, can be used in severe incidents. The reader is referred to the *BSAVA Manual of Canine and Feline Gastroenterology* for further information.

Pentosan polysulphate: PPS is a semi-synthetic sulphated glycosaminoglycan prepared from an extract of beech. It is licensed in several countries around the world, including the UK, Australia, New Zealand and Canada. For a review of the potential effects of this drug the reader is referred elsewhere (Ghosh, 1999). There are three published clinical trials of PPS in dogs.

The first study tested the injectable sodium salt of PPS against placebo in dogs with established OA. It used clinical scores as the primary outcome measure (Read *et al.*, 1996). Results showed positive benefit on clinical signs of OA.

A second study compared the use of PPS against surgical treatment (fragment removal via arthrotomy) in dogs with elbow dysplasia; the results failed to show a difference between the two treatment regimens.

The third study was a 1-year, placebo-controlled study and investigated use of the oral calcium salt of PPS in dogs immediately after surgery for cruciate ligament deficiency; the results failed to show any clinical benefit (Innes *et al.*, 2000). Thus, there is conflict in the literature as to the efficacy of PPS; anecdotally, it may be that the drug is more useful for pain relief in chronic OA.

Potential STMOADs: Many of the candidate STMOAD agents remain in the nutritional supplementation class. A few licensed drugs purport structure-modifying properties but, to date, none has satisfied appropriate criteria, such as those described by the OARSI (Altman *et al.*, 1996).

Polysulphated glycosaminoglycans: Injectable polysulphated glycosaminoglycan is available in the USA but not in the UK. There are several reports that suggest some efficacy as a disease-modifying agent in canine OA. *In vitro* studies suggest effects on chondrocyte viability as well as protecting against extracellular matrix degradation (Sevalla *et al.*, 2000). Studies in puppies susceptible to hip dysplasia given intramuscular gycosaminoglycan polysulphates from 6 weeks to 8 months of age resulted in less subluxation, as determined radiographically. In addition, treated pups had closer coxofemoral congruity when they were 8 months old.

Pentosan polysulphate: Studies in experimental dogs with cruciate ligament transection suggested some structure-modifying potential for PPS (Rogachefsky *et al.*, 1993), although these studies were complicated by the additional use of human recombinant insulin-like growth factor (IGF)-I. The results of these studies indicated that IGF-I showed the more dramatic effects.

Carprofen: There is some evidence that carprofen may have potential for structure-modification in OA. *In vitro* studies suggest some positive effects on glycosaminoglycan synthesis at concentrations up to 10 µg/ml (Benton *et al.*, 1997). Studies in experimental dogs (cruciate transection model) indicated some possible structure modification, mostly on bone turnover (Pelletier *et al.*, 2000).

Future possibilities: There are many avenues for structure modification in OA, from nutritional supplements through to tissue engineering (Hunziker, 2002; Jorgensen *et al.*, 2004) and gene therapy (Evans, 2005). A major goal must be to develop measures of structure modification in dogs, such that clinical trials can proceed in a meaningful manner. The greater understanding of the pathophysiology of OA has identified new therapeutic targets and undoubtedly others will be discovered. The challenge will be to sort the effective drugs from those with mild or minimal effects.

Nutritional supplementation

In recent years the use of nutritional supplementation to support synovial joint health has become very popular. Regulation of these products is confused in that in some countries products are licensed, whereas in many countries products such as glucosamine are available through regular retail outlets. There are many candidate nutritional supplements for OA; the most commonly used products are:

- Glucosamine
- Chondroitin sulphate
- Essential fatty acids (e.g. eicosapentaenoic acid (EPA))
- Extract of turmeric
- Extract of green-lipped mussel
- Methylsulphonylmethane (MSM)
- Combination products.

Glucosamine: Glucosamine is a naturally occurring amino sugar essential for the normal growth and repair of joints and articular cartilage, where it is a normal constituent of glycosaminoglycans, both in the extracellular matrix and in the synovial fluid. Many studies have been conducted on the *in vitro* and *in vivo* effects of glucosamine but its clinical efficacy and mechanism of action are still matters of debate.

A series of experiments conducted since the mid 1980s in rats, dogs and human patients, have shown that up to 90% of oral glucosamine sulphate is absorbed from the gastrointestinal tract, although there is some species variation. Many tissues, including articular cartilage, show uptake of glucosamine from plasma. Thus, it does seem that glucosamine reaches the intended site of action.

The actions of glucosamine are a subject of current debate. Many *in vitro* studies have been conducted to assess anti-inflammatory and cell-stimulatory effects but results are not consistent (Mobasheri et al,. 2002).

Numerous clinical trials of varying quality and duration have been conducted in humans but there have been fewer in veterinary species (McNamara et al., 1996; Hanson et al., 1997; Canapp et al., 1999). Many of the results presented are conflicting and inconclusive. Some of these studies have shown effects on pain, or improvements in arthritis indices, coupled with a good safety profile; others have shown little or no response. A meta-analysis and quality assessment of 15 double-blind randomized placebo-controlled clinical trials of glucosamine compounds have evaluated the efficacy of these agents to treat human OA (McAlindon et al., 2000). All but one of these trials was classified as positive, and the studies collectively demonstrated mild to moderate effects for glucosamine. However, quality scoring showed major deficiencies in study design. A thorough quality assessment detected significant publication bias, poor trial design, including small sample size (Pujalte et al., 1980; Vaz, 1982), lack of long-term follow up (Reichelt et al., 1994) and potential bias resultant from commercial sponsorship of research. In addition, the trials in the meta-analysis only measured symptoms, not disease modification of OA.

There was much excitement in 2001 when Reginster and co-workers published the results of a randomized placebo-controlled study of glucosamine for human knee OA, which indicated a degree of disease-modifying activity (Reginster et al., 2001). A second study showed similar results (Pavelka et al., 2002). At the time of writing, the National Institutes of Health in the USA are funding a large multicentre study on glucosamine (and chondroitin) in OA. The results of this large independent study are awaited eagerly. At the current time, there are not any good quality published, randomized, controlled studies in dogs or cats to demonstrate disease modification from the use of glucosamine.

Chondroitin sulphate: CS is a glycosaminoglycan that is a normal constituent of the major proteoglycan of articular cartilage, aggrecan. Studies in rats and human patients have shown that only a small amount of oral CS is absorbed from the gut. The absolute bioavailability of CS has been calculated as 13.2% of the amount ingested (Conte et al., 1991). Studies in rats using ^{3}H-labelled CS are consistent with extensive depolymerization following oral administration (Ronca et al., 1988, 1998). Interestingly, a study using orally administered ^{14}C-radiolabelled CS in a 3-month-old Beagle failed to show any radioactivity in the articular cartilage, although some did reach physeal cartilage (Bernard et al., 2000), suggesting that intact CS does not reach canine articular cartilage.

Demonstrated *in vitro* and *in vivo* effects of exogenous CS include anti-inflammatory effects (reduced macrophage and neutrophil infiltration in soft tissue) and stimulation of hyaluronan synthesis in rabbit synoviocytes and human synovial fluid (Ronca et al., 1998). Studies on human articular chondrocytes have shown that CS significantly increases ^{35}S incorporation rates into aggrecan (Verbruggen et al., 1999).

There are many studies in human medicine investigating the efficacy of CS in OA. Meta-analyses suggest some effect in relieving symptoms (McAlindon et al., 2000; Richy et al., 2003) but, as with glucosamine, there is likely to be publication bias as well as quality issues (McAlindon et al., 2000). To the author's [JFI] knowledge, there are no good quality veterinary studies addressing the efficacy of CS (in isolation) in canine OA.

Essential fatty acids: The EFAs are a group of polyunsaturated fatty acids (PUFAs). The two principal EFAs are linoleic acid (18:2 *n*-6 LA) and α-linolenic acid (18:3 *n*-3 ALA). The *n* annotation denotes the position of the first double bond in the carbon chain, counting from the methyl end. Arachidonic acid (eicosatetraenoic acid), an *n*-6 fatty acid, and eicosapentaenoic acid (EPA) and docosahexaenoic acid (DHA), *n*-3 fatty acids, may be derived from dietary LA and ALA, respectively, via desaturation and elongation. The EFAs are normal constituents of cell membranes and are involved in lipid transport. Critically, they are also precursors to the eicosanoid family that regulate inflammatory processes. The *n*-3 and *n*-6 fatty acids compete for incorporation into phospholipids and as substrates for cyclo-oxygenases (COX) 1 and 2 and 5-lipoxygenase. While the metabolism of both types of fatty acid leads to eicosanoid production, a higher proportion of *n*-6 fatty acids within cell membranes is believed to promote the production of the inflammatory prostaglandins, leucotrienes and thromboxanes. There has been recent interest in the use of *n*-3 fatty acids in OA.

In vitro studies of human and bovine cartilage have provided direct evidence that *n*-3 EFA supplementation can abrogate the inflammatory and matrix degradative response elicited by chondrocytes (Curtis et al., 2000, 2002), specifically downregulating aggrecanase activity. Clinical trials are currently underway in human knee OA. Current information in dogs suggest that only EPA is efficiently incorporated into canine chondrocyte membranes and that, in vitro, only EPA is able to abrogate the aggrecanase-mediated aggrecan catabolism induced by catabolic cytokines. Recent randomized placebo-controlled clinical studies in dogs suggested clinical benefits from a diet containing high levels of EPA.

Extract of turmeric: Curcumins within turmeric have been proposed as phytochemicals that might be useful in OA. There is evidence that curcumins may act to block the transcription factor, nuclear factor kappa-B. *In vitro* studies suggest an ability to abrogate the cytokine-mediated degradation of cartilage. However, to date, the efficacy in the clinic remains debatable. One randomized placebo-controlled study of an extract of turmeric (P54FP) in clinically affected dogs failed to show a positive treatment effect using peak vertical force of the index limb as the primary outcome measure (Innes *et al.*, 2003).

Combination products: The majority of nutritional supplements marketed for veterinary species are combination products consisting of glucosamine and chondroitin sulphate, often with other ingredients (e.g. methylsulphonylmethane, turmeric, manganese ascorbate). In addition, the majority of clinical studies have used combination products, although there are a very limited number of peer-reviewed studies in the veterinary literature. One recent double-blind comparator study involved 71 osteoarthritic dogs and compared the efficacy, tolerance and ease of administration of two routinely prescribed NSAIDs (carprofen and meloxicam) and a combination glucosamine–CS nutraceutical (Moreau *et al.*, 2003). The authors found significantly improved ground reaction forces for the index limbs following NSAID treatment, but not following nutraceutical therapy. It was concluded that both NSAIDs had a beneficial functional effect, whilst the glucosamine–CS nutraceutical did not.

Summary of management

1. Stage disease and educate client.
2. Weight-reduction strategy if obese.
3. Redesign exercise regimen.
4. Consider physiotherapy/hydrotherapy.
5. Consider prescription diet or nutritional supplementation.
6. Provide analgesia (usually NSAIDs).
7. Monitor response and adapt to change.
8. Consider surgery if medical management fails.

Immune-mediated arthritis

The classification of immune-mediated polyarthritis (IMPA) is summarized in Figure 7.5. Classification primarily hinges on the presence or absence of: erosive changes in the affected joints; extra-articular disease in addition to polyarthritis; and any identifiable primary aetiopathogenic event. Assignment of individual cases to a specific diagnosis within the classification can be difficult (see below) and it is helpful always to bear in mind the classification when IMPA is a differential diagnosis.

Aetiopathogenesis

Perhaps the earliest recognizable phase of all immune-mediated arthritides is damage to the microvascular endothelium within the synovial membrane. This has led to the commonly held hypothesis that the inciting cause is carried to the joint via the circulation in all cases. The early changes within the synovial membrane are consistent with a normal immune response to an antigen, and the production and phagocytosis of immune complexes in response to a chronic antigenic stimulus is thought to be central to the development of chronic disease in IMPA. Persistence of the antigenic stimulus may stem from recurrence or persistence of the inciting antigen(s) or from a derangement of normal

---

Erosive IMPA

Rheumatoid arthritis
Criteria for diagnosis:
1. Stiffness after rest persistent for at least 6 weeks
2. Pain or tenderness on motion of at least one joint persistent for at least 6 weeks
3. Swelling of at least one joint persistent for at least 6 weeks
4. Swelling of one other joint within 3 months
5. Symmetrical joint swelling persistent for at least 6 weeks
6. Subcutaneous nodules
7. Erosive changes on joint radiographs
8. Serological positive test for rheumatoid factor
9. Synovial fluid cytology consistent with IMPA
10. Synovial membrane histopathology typical of rheumatoid arthritis
11. Subcutaneous nodule histopathology typical of rheumatoid arthritis

Seven criteria must be fulfilled, including two of criteria 7, 8 and 10. Subcutaneous nodules are rare in dogs

Erosive polyarthritis of Greyhounds

Erosive feline chronic progressive polyarthritis (cats only)

Non-erosive IMPA without multi-system involvement

Idiopathic syndromes

Non-erosive feline chronic progressive polyarthritis (cats only)

Uncomplicated idiopathic IMPA (Type 1 IMPA)

Syndromes with known antigenic associations

IMPA associated with infection remote from the joint (Type II IMPA)

IMPA associated with gastrointestinal disease (Type III IMPA)

IMPA associated with neoplasia remote from the joint (Type IV IMPA)

Drug-induced IMPA

Vaccine-associated IMPA

Non-erosive IMPA with multi-system involvement

Systemic lupus erythematosus
Criteria for diagnosis:
1. Multi-system disease (see text)
2. Circulating ANA at elevated levels
3. Immunopathological features consistent with the body system involved.

Criteria 1 and 2 must always be satisfied and all three criteria must be satisfied to establish a definitive diagnosis of SLE

Polyarthritis/polymyositis syndrome

Polyarthritis/meningitis syndrome

Polyarteritis nodosa

Breed-associated non-erosive IMPA syndromes

Familial amyloidosis of the Chinese Shar Pei ('Shar Pei Fever')

Juvenile-onset polyarthritis in the Japanese Akita

7.5 Classification of immune-mediated arthritides. Criteria for diagnosis are included for those with specific criteria. Synovial fluid changes consistent with IMPA should be demonstrated in all cases.

---

down-regulation of the immune system following successful elimination of the inciting antigen(s). Many theories have been proposed for a mechanism of failure of normal immunoregulation that might lead to immune-mediated disease. The actual mechanism(s) of failure remains unclear, but possibilities include:

- Molecular mimicry, in which normally tolerated host antigens are mimicked by similar antigens on an invading organism and the resulting cross-reactivity of the immune system leads to a breach in tolerance
- Apoptosis (programmed cell death) may result in enzymatic or oxidative modification of cellular macromolecules. The modified autologous macromolecules may form neoantigens to which autologous T-cells are not tolerant.

In humans, advances in genetics have shown significant genetic predispositions to IMPA syndromes, most notably in HLA-B27-related disease (see below). Associations have also been shown between allelic polymorphisms of the major histocompatibility complex (MHC) in the HLA-DR region and the occurrence of human rheumatoid arthritis (RA). It is estimated that MHC genes confer 30–50% of the genetic component of susceptibility to human RA. Furthermore, there are additional correlations between the presence of allelic polymorphisms and the severity of disease, including the tendency to show seropositivity for rheumatoid factor (RF), joint erosions and extra-articular disease. It is probable that the role of genetics in the occurrence and severity of IMPA will be further elucidated in humans in the near future; as the canine and feline genomes are unravelled, it is likely that similar associations will be identified.

In some forms of IMPA the inciting antigen can be identified. Good examples of this are seen in cases where the IMPA is associated with infection distant from the joints (van der Wel and Meyer, 1995) or in drug-induced IMPA (Giger *et al.*, 1985). Most cases of IMPA remain idiopathic, but it is widely considered that the antigenic source in many of such cases is likely to be an infective agent(s).

In erosive forms of IMPA there is proliferation of granulation tissue, which invades the articular cartilage and subchondral bone. Granulation tissue that behaves in this way is called 'pannus' and both the pannus and the inflamed synovial membrane can be a source of enzymes that are directly responsible for destruction of the affected joints. Immune complex deposition in the damaged cartilage may also be a contributing factor to continued cartilage destruction.

Extra-articular manifestations of disease are important in many IMPA cases and are often a consequence of either immune complex disease (e.g. immune complex glomerulopathy giving rise to proteinuria) or autoantibody formation (e.g. anti-platelet antibodies giving rise to immune-mediated thrombocytopenia). Such changes are epitomised in systemic lupus erythematosus (SLE), which is characterized by the presence of idiopathic immune-mediated multi-system disease that includes antinuclear antibodies and the presence of IMPA in the majority of cases.

Diagnosis

IMPA should be considered as a differential diagnosis for any dog or cat with signs of generalized stiffness and pyrexia, whether or not there are also signs of extra-articular disease. The complex nature of the classification of IMPA can be daunting at the outset of an investigation of a suspected case, but the diagnosis can be simplified if the investigation is broken down into two distinct stages:

1. Establishment of a diagnosis of IMPA and radiographic evaluation of multiple joints to allow an initial classification of the case as either 'erosive' or 'non-erosive'.
2. Classification of the IMPA. Additional steps to classify the condition further should be taken only after the diagnosis of IMPA is established. Classification provides a definitive diagnosis that improves the accuracy of the prognosis and allows an appropriate therapeutic plan to be made.

Establishing the diagnosis

IMPA can present in any age, breed or sex of dog and cat, and with an onset that can be acute or chronic. Clinical severity is very variable, with presentations ranging from complete inability to stand, with multiple and obvious joint effusions, to only vague stiffness or lameness in a single limb. Most cases show the following characteristics:

- *Pyrexia.* IMPA is the most common diagnosis in dogs presenting with pyrexia of unknown origin (PUO). In one study, IMPA accounted for 22% of all PUO cases and it was suggested that IMPA should always be excluded before less common causes of PUO are considered (Dunn and Dunn, 1998)
- *Stiffness after rest.* This is typically more severe and persistent than that seen in osteoarthritis
- *Multiple and symmetrical joint involvement.* Symmetrical involvement of multiple joints is rarely seen in any condition other than IMPA, particularly in combination with pyrexia. In cases with erosive disease there may be multiple joint deformities, instability (subluxation or luxation) and crepitus (Figure 7.6). It is important to note that obvious joint swelling and pain are not always palpable in IMPA cases and cytological evaluation of multiple joint fluid samples is mandatory to demonstrate

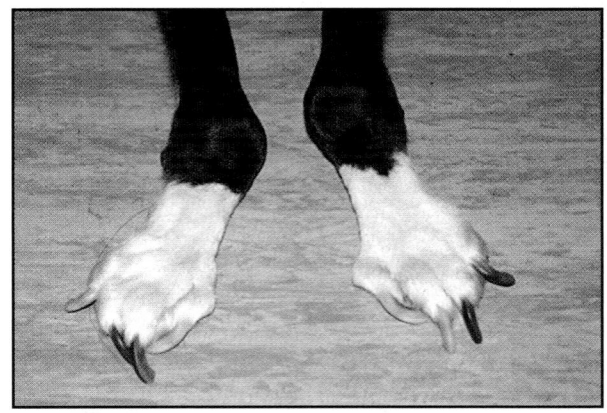

7.6 The forefeet of a dog with canine rheumatoid arthritis. There are multiple joint swellings and deformities involving the carpi and joints of the feet. The changes are symmetrical.

multiple and symmetrical joint inflammation if IMPA is suspected. In some cases, especially early in disease, inflammation may be present only in a limited number of joints, or may be monoarticular; more joints may then become involved with the passage of time. This phenomenon is known as 'recruitment'.

A diagnosis of IMPA can often be established on the basis of the cytological analysis of multiple symmetrical joint fluid samples. Synovial fluid bacterial culture and antibiotic sensitivity testing can sometimes help to exclude bacterial synovitis from the differential diagnosis list. Additional investigations that are relevant in the investigation of suspected IMPA cases include:

- *Radiography.* Any suspected joint should be radiographed early in the course of the clinical investigation to assess for the presence of intra-articular soft tissue swelling consistent with effusion or joint capsule thickening, and to evaluate for the presence of erosions. Erosions are seen when there is destruction of subchondral bone. Osteophytes are uncommon in non-erosive disease, but marked periosteal proliferative bone formation may be seen in some specific forms of erosive IMPA. Radiological features often show bilateral symmetry in all forms of IMPA and in erosive forms it is the large joints distal in the limb that often show the earliest and most obvious changes (Figure 7.7)

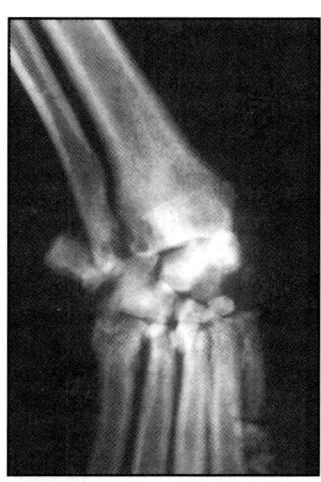

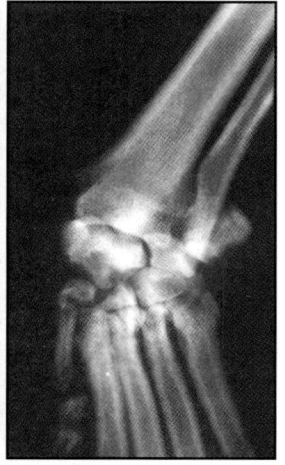

7.7 Dorsopalmar radiographs of the left and right forefeet of a dog with RA. Note the presence of erosions and subluxations and the symmetrical nature of the radiological features.

- *Haematology.* There may be an anaemia (autoimmune or anaemia of chronic disease), leucocytosis or leucopenia, neutrophilia with a left shift, and thrombocytopenia. Thrombocytopenia and leucopenia are especially seen in cases with SLE
- *Serum biochemistry.* Serum urea, creatinine, alkaline phosphatase, alanine transferase and aspartate transferase levels may all be elevated. Raised serum creatine kinase and aldolase levels may be seen in cases complicated by myositis. Globulins may be increased as a consequence of antibody production, and albumin may be reduced as a result of protein loss consequential to immune complex glomerulopathy or immune-mediated damage to nephrons or the bowel leading to protein-losing nephropathy or enteropathy
- *Urinalysis.* Proteinuria may be detected as a result of glomerulopathy or nephropathy
- *Synovial membrane biopsy.* Synovial membrane histopathology is not always essential to establish a diagnosis of IMPA, but it can help to classify the disease more accurately
- *Others.* As some cases of IMPA are complicated by extra-articular disease, there may be an indication for additional investigations, such as: CSF analysis, when aseptic meningitis is suspected because of concurrent spinal pain (Webb *et al.,* 2002); electromyography, if immune-mediated myositis is suspected; or biopsy of other tissues (muscle, skin, liver, kidney) to confirm the presence of immunopathology, including amyloidosis, in some chronic cases.

Classifying the IMPA

Once a diagnosis of IMPA has been made by multiple joint fluid analyses, further evidence can be gathered to classify the condition in more detail. Criteria have been established to standardize the diagnosis of the immune-mediated arthritides. These are derived from similar criteria for the diagnosis of comparable conditions in humans, but have been adapted for use in dogs and cats. A definitive diagnosis is made when the criteria for a given condition are satisfied and other causes of IMPA have been excluded. This can sometimes be difficult because there is a great deal of overlap between the different syndromes, reflecting common pathways in the pathogenesis. Some cases will satisfy the criteria for more than one syndrome simultaneously and it may be impossible to ascribe a definitive diagnosis reliably in such cases. In classifying IMPA, the division into those showing erosive and those showing non-erosive disease is fundamental.

Erosive IMPA

Rheumatoid arthritis: RA in humans can be defined as a chronic systemic inflammatory disorder, characterized by deforming symmetrical polyarthritis associated with synovitis of joint and tendon sheaths, articular cartilage loss, erosion of juxta-articular bone and, in most patients, the presence of IgM RF in the blood. Syndromes similar to RA in humans have been recognized in both cats and dogs but are perhaps best characterized in dogs. A symmetrical destructive arthropathy simultaneously affecting several joints in a dog is highly likely to be RA, but the diagnosis must be confirmed by reference to the published criteria (see Figure 7.5). Although erosive joint disease is typical of RA, erosions are not always present in the early stages and the criteria allow for the diagnosis to be made in the absence of subchondral bone destruction. In some cases erosions are initially only seen in a small number of joints, even though inflammation is present in many joints. Chronic cases often show joint collapse, subluxation or luxation and, in some cases, there is periarticular bone proliferation and mineralization of peri-articular soft tissues.

The role of RF in RA is often misunderstood. 'Rheumatoid factor' is a collective term for antibodies (most commonly IgM) with specificity for the Fc receptor of IgG. These antibodies play a normal role in immunoregulation, influencing both cellular and humoral immunity. An important physiological role of RF is to facilitate opsonization and the elimination of immune complexes. As a result, circulating RF levels may be elevated in many disease processes involving antigenic stimuli and can often return to normal with recovery from disease. An elevated RF level does not, therefore, equate to a diagnosis of RA. Furthermore, it is important to note that approximately 25% of dogs with RA do not have significant circulating levels of RF, so the absence of RF does not exclude the diagnosis (Bennett and Kirkham, 1987). The presence or absence of circulating RF is only one of the criteria applied in the diagnosis of RA and it is important only to make a diagnosis of RA on the basis of a *full application* of the criteria.

A further confounding factor in diagnosis can be the presence of other antibodies in the circulation as a result of the polyclonal activation of lymphocytes. This derangement of immunoregulation is associated with chronic immunopathology, including IMPA, and is especially prevalent in RA and SLE. Polyclonal activation is the non-specific re-activation of memory B lymphocytes, with a consequential non-specific production of antibodies, often in large quantities. As a result, affected patients may show increased circulating levels of many antibodies, including some that are important in the diagnosis of other IMPA syndromes, such as: antinuclear antibodies; antibodies against infective agents such as viruses and bacteria that have been associated with IMPA (e.g. *Borrelia burgdorferi*, see below); and antibodies against routine vaccine components (e.g. canine distemper virus). This can confuse attempts at definitive diagnosis and at unravelling aetiopathogenesis. It is therefore important to be aware of the possibility of polyclonal activation in any IMPA case and to interpret antibody tests in the context of all the other criteria for classification of the IMPA syndromes.

Extra-articular manifestations of disease are also important. Although these are most commonly associated with SLE, they can also be significant in patients with RA and in patients with multiple bacterial arthritis, especially when this is associated with bacterial endocarditis. SLE is invariably a non-erosive disease, but multiple bacterial arthritis and RA may both show joint erosions and differentiating these two conditions can be extremely difficult in some cases.

Other erosive joint diseases: Other syndromes of erosive IMPA have been described in dogs and cats, but there is often a considerable overlap with RA and it remains unclear whether these are truly separate syndromes or simply variants of RA. The term 'Felty's syndrome' is used to describe a rare variant of RA, but with additional features of splenomegaly and leucopenia.

An erosive polyarthritis has been described with specificity to Greyhounds in Australia and the USA (Barton *et al.*, 1985; Woodard *et al.*, 1991); it has not yet been reported in the UK. The condition primarily affects young dogs aged between 3 months and 3 years. No familial predisposition has been recognized. The condition remains idiopathic, and affected dogs are negative for serological titres to *Ehrlichia*, *Brucella*, *Borrelia*, *Rickettsia* and *Chlamydia* and also for RF and antinuclear antibody (ANA). The pathology in these cases is similar to that seen in other erosive polyarthritides and the prognosis for racing dogs is grave.

Feline chronic progressive polyarthritis (FCPP, also called periosteal proliferative polyarthritis) is an IMPA most commonly seen in young adult male cats. The syndrome has been reported in both erosive and non-erosive forms, though it remains uncertain whether these are truly the same syndrome. The erosive form has many similarities to RA in pathology, progression and prognosis but affected cats are usually seronegative for RF. The non-erosive form is more common (see below).

Non-erosive IMPA

A number of non-erosive IMPA syndromes have been described. The most typical are uncomplicated idiopathic (Type I) IMPA and SLE. The nomenclature for non-erosive polyarthritis of dogs and cats in the literature can be confusing and warrants some discussion. Bennett (1987) initially described four conditions under the classification of canine idiopathic polyarthritis (CIP, Types I to IV). The same syndromes have more recently been referred to as Types I to IV immune-mediated polyarthritis. Type I IMPA is the typical condition in this class and the term is applied to any IMPA for which an underlying antigenic source cannot be identified and which is not complicated by extra-articular disease. This differentiates truly idiopathic and straightforward IMPA from cases of IMPA with known antigenic sources (infection – Type II; gastrointestinal disease – Type III; tumours – Type IV; drug or vaccine reactions) as well as from more complex multi-systemic syndromes (e.g. SLE) and cases with an apparent breed association (e.g. familial renal amyloidosis in Shar Pei dogs). Although there is much overlap in pathogenesis, it is useful to classify IMPA in this way as it assists greatly in formulating a prognosis and treatment plan.

From the above, it is clear that in any case confirmed to have a non-erosive IMPA, further diagnostic steps should include a search for evidence of extra-articular disease and a search for possible antigenic sources. The general investigation has been outlined above; specific investigations relevant to individual syndromes are discussed in more detail below.

Non-erosive IMPA without multi-system disease: This group includes IMPAs that are truly idiopathic and those that have a recognizable potential antigenic source. Included in this group are the non-erosive form of feline chronic progressive polyarthritis and those cases of canine IMPA that have been classified as Types I to IV IMPA.

Non-erosive feline chronic progressive polyarthritis: The non-erosive form of FCPP is characterized radiographically by an absence of erosions and by marked periosteal proliferation of bone adjacent to joints, often with marked mineralizing enthesopathies (Figure 7.8). This latter form is reported to occur only in male cats (Goring and Beale, 1993) and this has led to comparisons with reactive arthritis in humans (see below). A similar syndrome is seen, rarely, in young adult male dogs.

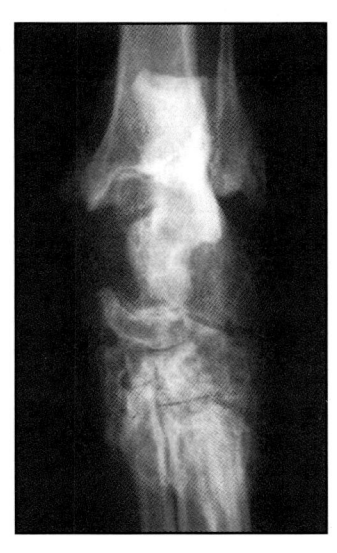

7.8 Dorsoplantar radiograph of the tarsus of a cat with the non-erosive form of FCPP. There is periarticular new bone formation but no evidence of erosion. Symmetrical changes were present in the contralateral limb.

The clinicopathological findings (haematology, serum biochemistry, joint fluid analyses) are similar to those of other IMPA syndromes in both the erosive and non-erosive forms of FCPP. Affected cats are usually negative for RF and ANA, but are often seropositive for both feline syncytium forming virus (FeSV) and feline leukaemia virus (FeLV). The incidence of seropositivity to these viruses was greater in cats with FCPP than in a normal population of cats (Pederson *et al.,* 1980). However, care should be taken in interpreting these results because both viruses are common in the general population and the results may reflect an increased risk of secondary viral infection in immunocompromised animals or could be an artefact due to polyclonal activation rather than truly reflecting a causal role for the viruses in IMPA.

Uncomplicated idiopathic (Type I) IMPA: Uncomplicated idiopathic IMPA is the most common form of IMPA in dogs, accounting for approximately 50% of the cases of non-erosive IMPA without multi-system involvement. The condition is diagnosed when non-erosive IMPA is confirmed and all other forms of non-erosive IMPA have been excluded.

IMPA associated with infection remote from the joint (Type II): This accounts for approximately 25% of the cases of non-erosive IMPA without multi-system involvement in dogs. Sites of infection that have been associated with IMPA include the endocardium, genitourinary tract, respiratory tract and skin. It is thought that the chronic infection acts as a persistent source of antigens which drive the chronic immune complex disease. In some cases it is difficult to determine whether the cause of joint disease is infective as a result of haematogenous spread of bacteria from the primary focus, or a result of secondary immune-mediated phenomena.

Comparisons have been drawn between this group of conditions and reactive arthritis (Reiter's syndrome) in humans. Reactive arthritis is a syndrome of IMPA most commonly occurring in young adult males secondary to an infection. Although multiple infections can trigger the syndrome, it predominantly occurs in response to either genitourinary infections (especially with *Chlamydia trachomatis*) or enteric infections (especially with some strains of *Salmonella* or *Shigella*). A genetic susceptibility is recognized in humans; more than two-thirds of reactive arthritis sufferers have the HLA-B27 genotype. Furthermore, many of the HLA-B27-negative patients with reactive arthritis carry genes for antigens that cross-react with the protein encoded by HLA-27. Although this syndrome has some similarities with Type II IMPA in dogs there are also many dissimilarities. Notably, in the canine syndrome elimination of the primary infection often leads to a resolution of the IMPA, whereas in reactive arthritis IMPA persists for months or even years after resolution of the primary disease. Reactive arthritis has more similarities with the non-erosive form of FCPP (see above).

IMPA associated with gastrointestinal disease (Type III): This accounts for approximately 15% of the cases of non-erosive IMPA without multi-system involvement in dogs. The most common gastrointestinal signs are vomiting and diarrhoea. The gut is potentially a source of bacterial and food antigens that could trigger an immune complex disease. There may be a predilection in young Boxers (see below).

IMPA associated with neoplasia remote from the joints (Type IV): Tumour cells may provide a source of persistent antigens that can trigger a secondary IMPA.

Drug-induced IMPA: Rarely, IMPA is seen as a side effect of drug therapy, notably some antibiotics, especially sulphonamides (probable predisposition in Dobermanns), erythromycin, lincomycin, cephalosporins and penicillin derivatives. Sometimes these cases present with multi-systemic disease. It is thought that immune complex hypersensitivity occurs as a result of drug–antibody interactions. The drug may also combine with host proteins to form neoantigens. There is usually a rapid resolution of signs in response to drug withdrawal.

IMPA associated with vaccination: Occasionally an IMPA is recognized following vaccination, especially during a primary vaccination course in puppies and kittens. In cats, this may be associated with the calicivirus component of the vaccine (Dawson *et al.,* 1993). The problem is normally self-limiting within a few days. A recent study of Type I IMPA in dogs found no association between the time of vaccination and the onset of disease (Clements *et al.,* 2004).

Non-erosive IMPA with multi-system disease

Systemic lupus erythematosus: Even though it is rare in dogs and cats, SLE is often taken as the type syndrome in non-erosive IMPA complicated by multi-system disease because it epitomises the systemic pathogenic events that can occur in association with IMPA. Most dogs and cats with SLE are presented with pyrexia and a symmetrical non-erosive IMPA. Other common manifestations include:

- Skin disease
    - Mucocutaneous ulceration
    - Skin rashes (typical histopathology on biopsy)
- Renal disorders
    - Immune complex glomerulopathy
    - Nephropathy (proteinuria; casts on urinalysis)
- Haematological disorders
    - Haemolytic anaemia (autoagglutination or positive Coombs' antiglobulin test)
    - Leucopenia or lymphopenia (antibodies to white cells)
    - Autoimmune thrombocytopenia (antibodies to thrombocytes demonstrated by the platelet factor 3 test or by immunofluorescence)
- Neurological or muscular disorders
    - Aseptic meningitis (aseptic inflammation demonstrated by CSF cytology)
    - Polymyositis (electromyographic changes; elevated circulating creatine kinase levels; typical histopathology)
- Serositis
    - Pleuritis
    - Pericarditis
- Ocular disorders
    - Keratoconjunctivitis sicca
    - Retinopathy
    - Uveitis.

To confirm the diagnosis, circulating ANA must be present and there must be evidence of multi-systemic disease with an immune-mediated pathogenesis. Polyarthritis, though common, is not invariably present.

For definitive diagnosis in dogs and cats it is generally accepted that circulating levels of ANA must be elevated. In humans there is a recognized syndrome of 'ANA-negative SLE'. Diagnosis in human patients is based on the American Rheumatism Association criteria of 1982 (Tan et al., 1982) and has since been refined further (Gill et al., 2003). It is still accepted that an ANA titre <1:40 usually rules out SLE in humans, but patients with a negative ANA titre and persistent multi-systemic disease can undergo further evaluation for possible ANA-negative SLE. Furthermore, human patients with an ANA titre >1:40 but no evidence of multi-system disease can still be diagnosed with SLE following tests for additional abnormal circulating antibodies, including antibodies to double-stranded DNA and to Sm nuclear antigen. These tests increase the sensitivity and specificity of the diagnosis. This is important because circulating ANA levels may be elevated in normal patients and in patients with diseases other than SLE. Current understanding of the immunopathogenesis of SLE in dogs and cats is not as detailed as that in humans and there are no equivalent clinical tests for antibodies to double-stranded DNA or the Sm antigen. It is therefore appropriate that the criteria should remain simpler in dogs and cats at the present time, even though this is likely to result in a loss of sensitivity and specificity in the diagnosis.

Other multi-systemic IMPA syndromes: All forms of IMPA can occasionally be associated with some manifestations of extra-articular disease. Those cases with multi-system involvement clearly overlap in pathogenesis with SLE, but in the absence of positive circulating ANA levels they should not be diagnosed as such with the current state of understanding in dogs and cats. True (ANA-positive) SLE is worthy of differentiation, because it carries a poorer prognosis.

Though many body systems can be affected by immune complex or autoimmune disease in association with IMPA, specific associations have been made with polymyositis (especially in Spaniels) (Bennett and Kelly, 1987) and with aseptic meningitis. The combination of IMPA and aseptic meningitis shows a predisposition for certain breeds, including the Weimaraner, German Short-haired Pointer, Bernese Mountain Dog and Boxer. In young Boxers an acute syndrome of IMPA with or without aseptic meningitis (presenting as acute spinal pain) is sometimes seen in association with gastrointestinal upset, particularly diarrhoea, acute inappetence or abdominal discomfort, and sometimes with elevated circulating amylase. Cases often respond to dietary management alone and this suggests a possible enteropathic source of inciting antigen.

Polyarteritis nodosa is a rare disease characterized in humans by the presence of a generalized necrotising vasculitis of small and medium-sized arteries. It has a severe morbidity and mortality. Unsurprisingly, this generalized vasculitis is clinically characterized by multi-system disease, predominantly presenting with disorders of the kidneys, muscles and joints, central and peripheral nervous systems, gastrointestinal tract, skin, genitals and cardiovascular system. The diagnosis is assisted by the demonstration of typical arteritis in biopsies from affected tissues. Similar syndromes have rarely been recognized in dogs and are clinically difficult to differentiate from SLE and other IMPA syndromes in the absence of biopsy of affected tissues.

Sjögren's syndrome is a chronic autoimmune syndrome of humans characterized by antibody production against salivary and lacrimal gland tissue, though other secretory tissues can also be involved. It primarily affects middle-aged women. Approximately half of human patients are considered to have the condition as a primary disease with no other associations; the other half have Sjögren's syndrome as a secondary condition in association with other immune-mediated disorders, most commonly RA and SLE. Immune-mediated keratoconjunctivitis sicca has been documented in dogs, both in association with IMPA and in isolation. This has often been compared to Sjögren's syndrome in people, although xerostomia is less well recognized in dogs.

Breed-associated non-erosive IMPA syndromes: Specific forms of IMPA associated with breeds have been recognized in the Chinese Shar Pei (Di Bartola *et al.*, 1990; May *et al.*, 1992) and Japanese Akita (Dougherty *et al.*, 1991). The term 'Shar Pei fever' has been applied to a recurring inflammatory disease of the distal limb joints, especially the hock, in this breed. The disorder is characterized by brief episodes of acute joint swelling, with some evidence of synovitis. In the long term affected individuals are also prone to a familial amyloidosis, which has a high mortality because of renal involvement. Comparisons have been drawn between this condition and familial Mediterranean fever of humans, a genetic disease primarily characterized by recurring serositis but that can also present with immune-mediated arthritis and predisposes patients to amyloidosis. IMPA in the Japanese Akita usually has onset in adolescence and may also be associated with aseptic meningitis.

Treatment

Treatment of all IMPA syndromes is based on: elimination of the inciting cause (if this can be achieved); or immunosuppressive therapy. The inciting cause can be identified and removed, leading to remission of the IMPA, in a limited number of cases (i.e. those IMPA cases associated with a recognizable inciting antigenic source) and this should always be the main goal. However, the majority of cases require some form of immunosuppressive therapy, even sometimes after a recognized inciting antigenic source has been successfully eliminated. In some cases therapy can eventually be withdrawn without relapse (see Figure 7.9 for guidelines). The majority of cases require lifelong therapy, however, and in these the aim should always be to work towards the minimum effective dose of immunosuppressive or anti-inflammatory drugs for long-term control of remission. In this group of patients the aims of treatment may be summarized as follows:

- To relieve symptoms and signs of disease
- To maintain physical function
- To prevent structural damage to the affected joints
- To restore and maintain an optimal quality of life
- To minimize the morbidity and mortality associated with both the disease and the therapies
- To correct abnormal parameters of disease activity.

Drug therapy: In humans, NSAIDs form the cornerstone of drug therapy for most IMPA syndromes. Corticosteroids are used sparingly because of their toxicity in long-term use, which is related to both the dose and the duration of exposure. So-called disease-modifying anti-rheumatoid drugs (DMARDs) or slow-acting anti-rheumatoid drugs (SAARDs) are used as the mainstay of treatment for progressive forms of IMPA (such as RA). Drugs that are usually classified in this group include methotrexate, sulfasalazine, hydroxychloroquine, injectable gold aurothiomalate, azathioprine, ciclosporin, D-penicillamine and leflunomide. Their use in the management of IMPA has occurred either through serendipity or by extension from their use as immunosuppressive agents in association with transplant surgery. Although placebo-controlled clinical trials of these drugs and drug combinations have shown improved efficacy for controlling signs and symptoms, evidence for true modification of the progression of RA remains sparse; hence, the controversy over drug terminology. Few of these drugs have been fully evaluated for use in dogs and cats with IMPA and most have the potential for serious side effects. The drugs in this class that have been documented for use in dogs and cats are listed in Figure 7.9

WARNING
The administration of these drugs is not recommended without a full understanding of their use in clinical practice. Figure 7.9 is intended as a guide only. Specialist advice should be sought if necessary.

Drug	Usage
Prednisolone	Cornerstone of therapy for IMPA in dogs and cats. Initial use at immunosuppressive doses (dogs 2–4 mg/kg daily, divided; cats 4–6 mg/kg daily, divided). Tapering dose over a period of 4–6 months after the first 2–4 weeks if remission achieved. Aim for a minimum effective dose, ideally q48h
Azathioprine	Initially, 2 mg/kg q48h in combination with prednisolone (on alternate days), reducing to 0.5–2 mg q48h once remission achieved. Significant risk of bone marrow suppression, haematology and serum biochemistry; monitor every 7–14 days initially. NOT FOR USE IN CATS
Cyclophosphamide	Initially, 50 mg/m^2 q48h in combination with prednisolone (on alternate days). Used for no more than 12–16 consecutive weeks because of risk of haemorrhagic cystitis (especially in dogs). Significant risk of bone marrow suppression, haematology and serum biochemistry; monitor every 7–14 days initially
Colchicine	Inhibits the synthesis and secretion of serum amyloid A. Has been used as lifelong therapy in cases at risk of amyloidosis ('Shar Pei Fever'). Dose 0.03 mg/kg q12h–48h but no conclusive evidence published for a positive effect. Reported side effects in humans include gastrointestinal disturbance and, rarely, renal damage, bone marrow suppression, myopathy or peripheral neuropathy

7.9 Drugs commonly used in the treatment of immune-mediated arthritis.

In dogs and cats with IMPA syndromes, NSAIDs rarely control signs of disease adequately to maintain physical function. Furthermore, toxicity in cats is problematical for long-term NSAID therapy. Most dogs or cats with IMPA require some form of immunosuppressive therapy, and high doses of prednisolone have traditionally been the mainstay. Many cases can be managed with this drug alone, weaning to the lowest effective dose. Refractory cases, patients with marked corticosteroid-related side effects and those with erosive or multi-system disease usually require more aggressive drug therapy. In these cases an immunosuppressive drug (most commonly cyclophosphamide or azathioprine) is often used in combination with prednisolone. Combination therapy will often result in remission in 1–4 weeks and the drugs are then usually continued for a further 1–3 months before withdrawing gradually and reverting to low-to-moderate doses of prednisolone to maintain remission. In some cases side effects of therapy may be significant; this requires either dose reduction or substitution of a different drug.

The success of drug therapy in achieving remission and the risks of drug-related side effects should not be judged on clinical findings alone. Regular assessment of clinicopathological parameters, including haematology, serum biochemistry, synovial fluid analysis and urinalysis, is necessary.

Recent advances in human medicine have led to the development of agents that antagonize the cytokines which promote inflammation in IMPA. Notable amongst these are agents antagonizing the activity of tumour necrosis factor (TNF) and interleukin 1 (IL-1). Though there is some evidence that these agents provide good relief from signs and symptoms and may also be disease-modifying in humans, there have been no reported trials in dogs and the cost of such treatment is likely to be prohibitive in the near future for veterinary patients.

Non-pharmacological support: The patient's body weight should be optimised. Rest is usually indicated in acute phases of disease but moderate activity, within the abilities of the patient, should be encouraged during remission. Swimming is excellent activity for maintaining joint mobility in a relatively non-weightbearing environment.

Diets rich in fish oils and omega fatty acids appear to be of some benefit in humans, as does a vegetarian diet. None of these has been fully evaluated in dogs and cats, and a balanced vegetarian diet is difficult to achieve in carnivores.

Routine vaccination should be avoided in animals on immunosuppressive therapy. The advantages and disadvantages should be weighed carefully, even in patients that are in remission, as some vaccine components may contribute to joint inflammation.

Surgical management: Surgery is rarely indicated in dogs and cats with IMPA. Surgical correction may be indicated for luxations and subluxations resulting from ligament injuries. Arthrodesis, excision arthroplasty or joint replacement arthroplasty may all be considered as potential salvage procedures. Synovectomy has been used as a procedure to reduce pain and possibly slow the progression of disease in people, but it has not been widely reported in the veterinary literature.

Surgical failure rates are high in these patients and the potential benefit of any surgery must be weighed against the surgical risk for patients that have a seriously deranged immune system and may be on drugs that cause further immunosuppression or adversely affect tissue healing.

Prognosis

The classification of IMPA patients into specific syndromes allows a more accurate prognosis to be given. Prognoses are summarized in Figure 7.10.

Syndrome	Prognosis
Erosive IMPA	
Rheumatoid arthritis	Poor. Inevitably progressive erosion and destruction of joints leads to severe disability. Frequent extra-articular disease. Aggressive therapy may preserve quality of life for some time. Euthanasia often ultimately necessary
Erosive polyarthritis of Greyhounds	Extremely poor. Hopeless for a return to athletic ability. Often have a poor response to immunosuppressive therapy
Erosive feline chronic progressive polyarthritis	As for RA
Non-erosive IMPA	
Non-erosive feline chronic progressive polyarthritis	Immunosuppressive therapy usually required permanently to preserve quality of life. Euthanasia may ultimately be necessary
Uncomplicated idiopathic IMPA (Type I)	Usually good. Some dogs are cured with therapy over several months. Many are controlled with lifelong therapy at manageable low doses. A small percentage progress to full-blown rheumatoid arthritis and carry a correspondingly poor prognosis
IMPA associated with gastrointestinal disease, infection or neoplasia (Types II–IV)	Often good if the primary condition can be identified or resolved. Some persist with IMPA after resolution of the primary problem, but this often responds to therapy and therapy can often be withdrawn once remission is achieved
Drug-induced IMPA	Excellent. Normally a full recovery within days of withdrawal of the causative drug
Vaccine-associated IMPA	Very good. Generally self-limiting within a few days to weeks
Systemic lupus erythematosus	Guarded. Often requires aggressive combination therapies to control and remission may not be maintained. Euthanasia may ultimately be necessary

7.10 Summary of prognoses for immune-mediated arthritis. (continues) ▶

Syndrome	Prognosis
Non-erosive IMPA (continued)	
Polyarthritis/polymyositis	Guarded. Approximately 30% make a full recovery. Most have permanent stiffness or relapse once therapy is withdrawn
Polyarthritis/meningitis	Good in most cases. Therapy can sometimes be withdrawn after several months without relapse
Polyarteritis nodosa	Rare. Reported to be a good prognosis in dogs, but is a very aggressive disease in people
Familial amyloidosis of the Chinese Shar Pei	Good for response to joint disease in early life, but high rates of mortality associated with amyloidosis. Colchicine therapy may help
Juvenile-onset polyarthritis in the Japanese Akita	Poor. Often responds poorly to therapy. Euthanasia is often necessary

7.10 (continued) Summary of prognoses for immune-mediated arthritis.

Infective arthritis

Infective arthritis is an inflammatory arthropathy from which an infective organism can be identified or cultured. From an empirical position, however, it also includes inflammatory arthritides that are thought highly likely to be the result of an infective organism but from which the specific organism cannot be identified. This failure may be due to the inherent limitations of microorganism culture, or the previous use of antibiotics. In addition, there are cases of inflammatory joint disease in which there is an ongoing immune-mediated inflammation, even though the infective organism has been eradicated from the joint or rendered no longer infectious. Infective arthritis is a potentially devastating joint condition. In a small number of cases, particularly the neonate suffering from polyarthritis with concomitant systemic infection, it can be associated with fatalities.

A wide variety of organisms has been reported to cause infective arthritis in the dog. These include viruses, bacteria, bacterial L forms, mycoplasmas, *Chlamydia,* fungi and protozoans. Bacteria, especially haemolytic streptococci and *Staphylococcus intermedius,* are the most common cause of infective arthritis in the UK. This section will concentrate on such disease; other conditions, which, given changes in climate, alterations in available vectors and the greater ease of pet animal movement into and out of the UK, are likely to increase in prevalence, will be mentioned briefly.

Infective arthritis affects the cat but the veterinary literature has paid considerably less attention to this species. Typically, the condition results from a cat bite wound close to or actually penetrating a joint (Wilkinson, 1984) and therefore the infective organism is usually part of the normal bacterial flora of the feline oropharynx, i.e. *Pasteurella multocida, Bacteroides* spp., streptococci and spirochaetes.

Bacterial arthritis

Route of infection
Bacteria can be introduced into the joint directly – during surgery, at the time of an open wound, or by a penetrating foreign body. In addition, infection can reach the joint as an extension of a contiguous soft tissue or bone infection, or following haematogenous spread. Penetrating wounds, traumatically exposed joint surfaces, foreign bodies, infected surgery and contaminated injections are relatively common causes of infection in dogs and cats, though less so than in large animal practice. It is a credit to the immune system, and to some extent veterinary attention, that the majority of small animal patients with open wounds secondary to accidents do not result in clinically evident severe infective joint disease. Of greater concern, however, is the observation that the majority of the cases of infective arthritis referred (admittedly a small number) are subsequent to surgery (Clements *et al.*, 2005). Cruciate/stifle surgery appears over-represented, possibly because it is one of the most frequently performed joint surgeries in small animal practice. There may be considerable tissue damage and many 'corrective' procedures rely on foreign material in or close to the joint (Marchevsky and Read, 1999).

Haematogenous spread in the dog (Fearnside and Preston, 2002) and cat is uncommon and is usually limited to neonates and debilitated animals, or to immunosuppressed patients. An ageing cat appears to have been affected by *Streptococcus pneumoniae* septicaemia and septic arthritis secondary to transmission from a child (Stallings *et al.*, 1987). Systemic spread of infection can localise in the synovium due to the loop configuration of the blood supply in the synovial villi. The skin, bladder, prostate, kidneys, digestive tract, lungs, gingivae and anal glands have all been implicated as possible primary foci of infection. There is the potential for a bacterial endocarditis lesion to shed organisms that may localise and become established in the synovium (of particular note if steroid medication is being considered for a culture-negative inflammatory joint condition). In many cases, however, the distant infective nidus for the haematogenous seeding of bacteria is not identified. Bacterial arthritis secondary to systemic spread is more likely when corticosteroid therapy, immunosuppressive drugs, debilitating illness, OA or joint trauma coexist. This may be due to host defence mechanisms being rendered ineffective and/or an increase in the local blood supply, thereby increasing the number of organisms reaching the joint. It should therefore be noted that the potential exists for a sterile inflamed joint, as might occur in a severe sprain or subsequent to surgery, to become secondarily infected via the haematogenous route.

Chapter 7   Arthritis

Infections tend to affect single joints only. However, in the relatively immunoincompetent puppy or kitten, or in the immunsuppressed patient, systemically borne infective organisms may affect several joints. Typically, this infective polyarthritis is generally secondary to omphalophlebitis, mammary or uterine infections of the bitch/queen, or streptococcal pharyngitis. *Staphylococcus canis* is most commonly incriminated in bacterial arthritis resulting from congenital or neonatal exposure. In the adult, polyarthritis may be encountered secondary to septicaemia, such as that which accompanies bacterial endocarditis. Bacterial polyarthritis is, however, considerably less common than infective monoarticular disease.

Infective arthritis secondary to extension from an adjacent soft tissue infection or osteomyelitis is uncommon. In one survey (Bennett and Taylor, 1988) only 2 of 58 cases were as a result of extension of osteomyelitis.

Pathogenesis

The synovium is a highly vascular, areolar connective tissue that *does not have a lining to act as a limiting basement membrane*. Intra-articular bacteria are engulfed by the synovial phagocytes and migrating polymorphonuclear neutrophils. A complex interaction of host defence, enzymes, exotoxins and endotoxins results.

The degree of articular cartilage damage is variable and depends on the number, type and virulence of the organism, the extent to which organisms multiply, and the local and general resistance of the patient. Initially, infection causes inflammation of the synovium. This is reflected in the synovial fluid, which becomes hypercellular with a preponderance of polymorphonuclear leucocytes (see Chapter 3). Bacteria may or may not be seen in the synovial fluid or in synovial membrane. The hypercellular joint fluid is a potent source of lysosomal enzymes. Proteolytic enzymes are also released from the lysosomal granules of synovial cells, which results in synovial, cartilage and bone necrosis. Within synovial fluid of infective arthritis patients, inflammatory mediators such as tumour necrosis factor and interleukins are found in high concentrations. The local supply of proteinase inhibitors is rapidly depleted, resulting in rapid cartilage destruction.

In experimental bacterial arthritis, chondroitin sulphate is lost before collagen. The breakdown of the supporting cartilage matrix leaves the collagen fibrils without support. Once the matrix is broken down, the collagen fibrils suffer mechanical damage by the pressure and grinding of joint motion. If the cartilage is to be preserved, aggressive measures must be taken before matrix breakdown occurs. Experimentally, antibiotic therapy begun within 24 hours of infection decreases collagen loss but does not prevent proteoglycan loss from the cartilage matrix (Smith *et al.,* 1987).

Granulation tissue and synovial abscesses can eventually result in articular cartilage and bone erosion, in a fashion similar to the pannus of rheumatoid patients. The inflammatory processes occurring within the joint not only affect synovial fluid and articular cartilage, but also weaken the subchondral bone. Direct pressure necrosis of the cartilage may also result from joint effusions.

There is convincing evidence that inflammatory synovitis and cartilage destruction can continue even when there are few or no viable bacteria remaining. It can result from ongoing inflammatory processes once the organisms have been eliminated. Alternatively, immune complexes resulting from distant infections can spread systemically, localize in joint tissues, and result in immune complex-mediated injury. The use of antibiotics can result in cell wall-free bacteria (bacterial L-forms) which can be difficult to detect but can cause continued inflammation.

Synovial fluid is usually free of all the factors of the blood clotting system but in septic arthritis fibrin deposits form. The deposition of fibrin on the cartilage surface limits the normal exchange of cartilage metabolites and nutrients with the synovial fluid. This further contributes to maintaining the vicious cycle of inflammation, causing permanent joint damage.

Clinical features

Medium and large breed dogs (Figure 7.11) are affected more frequently than small and toy breeds (Clements et al, 2005), possibly because the joints have a larger surface area. The carpus, hock, stifle and hip are reported as being most commonly affected. The smaller joints of the foot are infrequently infected, in contrast to immune-based primary inflammatory disease. In these joints, where infection does occur, penetrating wounds or spread from contiguous infection are the likely source. This pattern is also noted in human patients, where the knee and the hip are most affected (approximately 50% and 15%, respectively, dependent on the age of the patient) (Goldenberg, 1993).

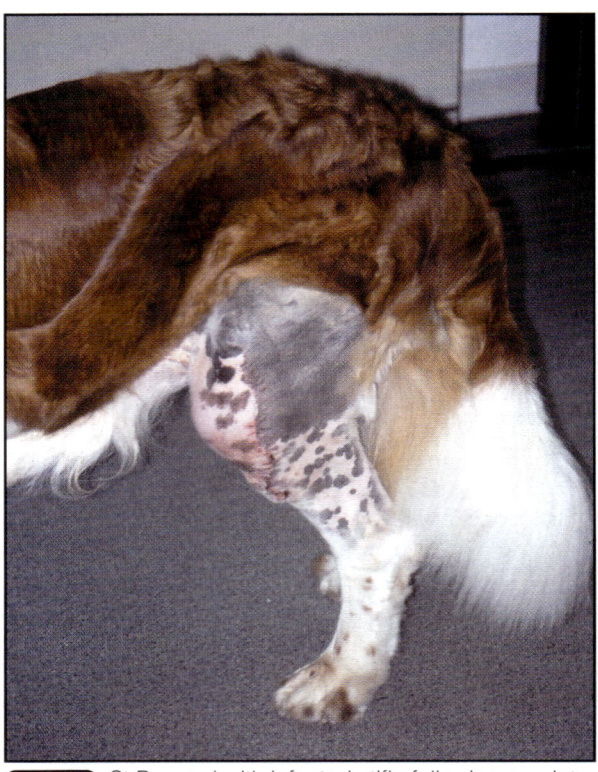

7.11 St Bernard with infected stifle following cruciate repair.

Monoarthropathy: Acute-onset severe lameness in one limb is typical. In 30–40% of cases, however, it may be more gradual in onset if the pathological changes are less severe. The majority of cases will affect one of the larger joints of the appendicular skeleton of a medium or large breed dog. Males are affected nearly twice as frequently as females (Bennett and Taylor, 1988). Patients can be affected at any age.

Periarticular swelling is generally, though not always, noted. Tenderness, pain and perhaps crepitus are evident on manipulation of the affected joint. The joint may be warmer to the touch than unaffected joints and there may be erythema of the overlying skin. Muscle atrophy is often quite marked, even relatively early in the disease process. Regional lymphadenitis and distal limb oedema are also noted in some cases.

The presence of a penetrating wound, bite or surgical incision may be evident. Signs of systemic disease, such as pyrexia, anorexia, weight loss and lethargy, are uncommon or variable.

Polyarthropathies: Severity of lameness and degree of joint swelling range from mild to severe and are often variable. Where significant pain or discomfort is present in a number of joints, the patient may be reluctant to rise or to walk. A number of such cases will be presented as possible neurological patients. Signs of systemic disease may be present in addition to the articular changes.

The degree of lameness will deteriorate significantly if joint instability occurs secondarily to the infection. Severe inflammatory disease may result in weakening and rupture of intra-articular structures, such as the cranial cruciate ligament, or may result in luxation of joints such as the hip. Care should be taken to avoid misdiagnosing a potentially severe infective arthritis as a joint sprain or hip dysplasia (Schrader, 1982), although either could become secondarily infected.

Diagnosis
Early and correct diagnosis is essential to limit irreversible intra-articular changes, to allow correct drug management, and to prevent inappropriate medication with immunosuppressive drugs. Diagnosis and differentiation from other arthritides is based on a combination of history, physical findings, radiographic interpretation and laboratory analysis, including synovial fluid analysis, synovial membrane biopsy, haematology and bacteriology. Whilst clinical signs may provide a presumptive diagnosis of infective arthritis, a definitive diagnosis can only be reached with identification or culture of the organism.

Radiography: Radiographic signs depend on the stage of the disease and the organism involved. Radiographic evidence alone is insufficient to make a diagnosis of infection. Plain radiographs should be obtained to provide a baseline assessment of the infected joint and to assess the presence/absence of contiguous osteomyelitis. In the immature patient, epiphyseal growth plates should be carefully assessed. Serial radiography over a period allows assessment of the progression of the disease, at least as far as bone involvement is concerned.

Whilst radiographs may indicate the degree of osseous involvement, they rarely permit assessment of the articular cartilage. Weightbearing radiography is rarely performed in small animal practice, making assessment of the joint space an unreliable index. Thus, in some cases radiographic changes may be absent or subtle, even though synovial fluid analysis indicates infection.

Radiographic signs (Figure 7.12) are divided into those seen early in the disease process and those seen later during the persistent or chronic phase. Changes are likely to be more marked with time, with

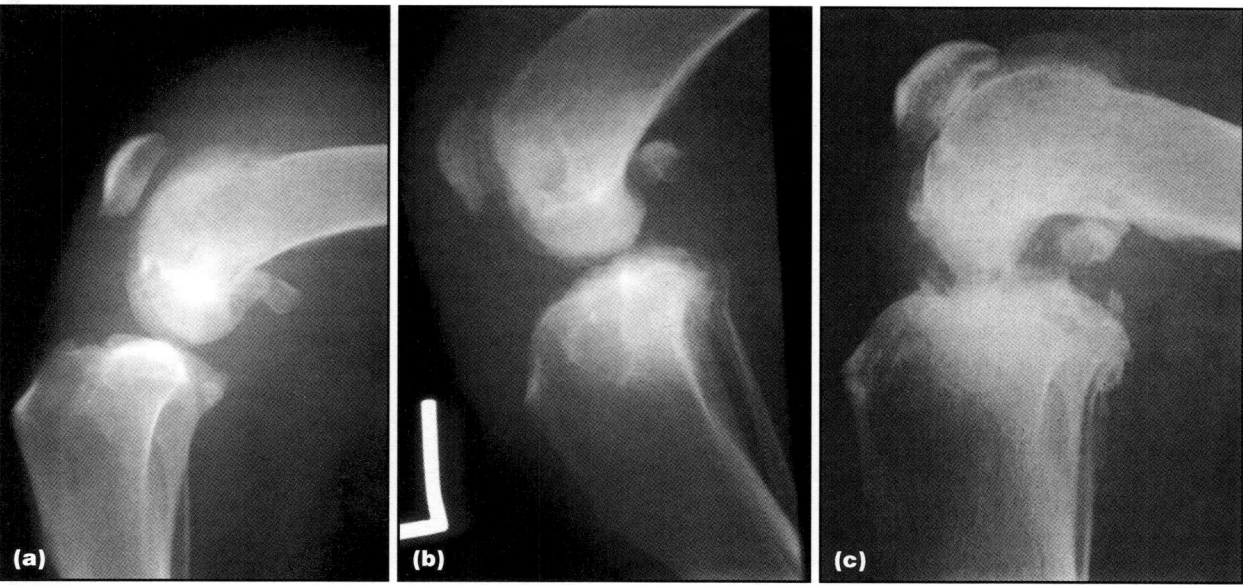

7.12 **(a)** Radiograph of infected stifle, demonstrating marked effusion, limited bone lysis and displacement of the patella. **(b)** Radiograph showing moderate bone destruction, widened tunnels within the femur and tibia (from previous surgery), and new bone formation. **(c)** Radiograph of infected stifle, showing advanced changes. Note the widespread osteolysis, osteoproduction, soft tissue swelling and collapse of the joint space. (c, Courtesy of John Houlton)

Chapter 7 Arthritis

many taking several weeks to become apparent. Some organisms, such as *Staphylococcus* spp., are more destructive than others, i.e. *Erysipelothrix* and *Streptococcus* spp. (Pederson *et al.*, 1989). Soft tissue changes (swelling, effusion) will precede osseous changes. Changes seen in the latter phase can be useful in providing a prognosis. Early changes are on the whole non-specific but, together with clinical and laboratory evidence, may help confirm the diagnosis.

Early changes: These are restricted to the soft tissues. The earliest sign is joint effusion with displacement of fat pads and fascial planes. The joint capsule becomes thickened and there may be a subjective widening of the joint space secondary to effusion. Periarticular swelling or oedema may be present. A degree of periarticular osteopenia may become evident.

Early changes may be subtle and easily overlooked. Familiarity with the normal radiographic appearance of joints and periarticular structures/fascial planes is required and high-quality radiographs are essential to allow their observation and interpretation (see Chapter 2). Dependent on the joint and patient size, the use of mammography film/screens may be of help.

In the early stages of infective arthritis, osseous changes are only likely to be observed in the uncommon event of osteomyelitis extending into the joint. Radiographs may also demonstrate the presence of a radiopaque intra-articular foreign body.

Gas shadows within the joint are rare. If present, they may indicate a recent penetrating joint wound, or infection with a gas-forming organism such as *Escherichia coli* or anaerobes (Meredith and Rittenberg, 1978).

Later changes: Bone changes are more likely to be observed in the later stages of infection. Once again, they are non-specific and can be confused with severe chronic OA, erosive immune-mediated arthritis and, perhaps, neoplasia. Changes observed include destruction of subchondral bone, and an irregular joint space secondary to the effects of pannus, synovial hypertrophy or enzymatic attack. Dystrophic calcification of intra-articular or periarticular structures may occur.

As articular cartilage is destroyed, the joint collapses and the joint space becomes narrowed. Discrete bone loss, generalized osteopenia, especially after an extended period of disuse, and subchondral osteosclerosis may be evident. Inflammation and oedema of the periosteum can produce faintly identifiable periosteal proliferative bone adjacent to the affected joint. Osteophyte production becomes more evident as the disease progresses and may be severe in advanced cases.

Fibrous or bony ankylosis may occur following cartilage destruction and exposure of the subchondral bone. Evidence of osteomyelitis may become more obvious. Spontaneous bony fusion (arthrodesis) is unlikely; it is more likely for bone bridges to develop between adjacent bones and around a radiolucent abscess that forms within the exudate. A reduction in range of motion of a joint may be inferred from the joint position observed on the radiographs. Evidence of ligamentous injury, i.e. cruciate or plantar ligaments, may also be inferred from radiographs.

Advanced imaging

Scintigraphy: Abnormalities may be noted within hours or days of onset of signs. Technetium scans are, however, not specific for infection; gallium scans may demonstrate joint infection when technetium does not. Indium-labelled leucocyte scintigraphy is less sensitive than technetium but is more specific for joint sepsis, relying on chemotaxis of labelled leucocytes to the area of infection (Lisbona and Rosenthall, 1977; Norris *et al.*, 1979).

Magnetic resonance imaging: MRI may provide earlier diagnosis than plain radiography. It can detect fluid earlier and provides better definition of soft tissue extension and involvement (Beltran *et al.*, 1987; Mitchell *et al.*, 1988).

Computed tomography: CT provides good detail of osseous changes, perhaps identifying bone erosions earlier than plain radiography (Resnick *et al.*, 1987).

Synovial fluid analysis: Definitive diagnosis of bacterial arthritis can only be achieved by recovering the organism from synovial fluid or synovium, or by visualizing it in a smear. Whenever there is a suspicion of bacterial infection, arthrocentesis should be performed (see Chapter 3) and synovial fluid examined.

The synovial fluid is inflammatory, increased in volume and with reduced viscosity. It may be turbid and frequently clots on exposure to air due to the presence of fibrinogen. The mucin clot will be poor. The fluid is often haemorrhagic (Figure 7.13) but this does not differentiate it from the haemarthrosis of trauma or coagulopathies.

White cell counts are elevated, in some cases as high as 200×10^9 cells/l, with the predominant cell being the polymorphonuclear leucocyte. In low-grade disease it may be as low as 4×10^9 cells/l. Both relative and

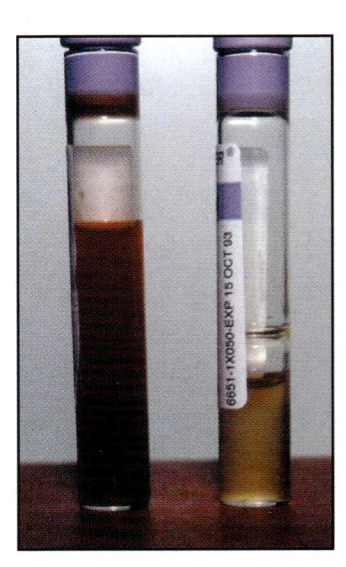

7.13 Two samples of synovial fluid. The sample on the left is haemorrhagic; that on the right is from an infected joint.

absolute neutrophil counts overlap ranges found in non-infective inflamed joints; therefore, a neutrophilia does not necessarily indicate infection. Neutrophils often show degenerative and toxic changes, such as pyknotic nuclei, degranulation and cell rupture. Similar changes can be present in non-erosive arthritis and RA, but are less likely.

Where synovial fluid volumes permit, protein and glucose levels may be measured. Protein will be elevated (4–5 mg/dl) and the synovial fluid to blood glucose ratio may be very low (<0.5) as the provision of glucose in the joint is reduced and the uptake by bacteria, white blood cells and synovium is increased. Blood and synovial fluid samples must be taken at the same time if a glucose ratio is to be determined. These tests may be of interest but are unlikely to provide additional useful diagnostic information beyond that provided by the leucocyte total and differential counts when differentiating between infected and sterile synovial fluid.

Haematology and biochemistry: The results of haematology and biochemical tests are neither diagnostic nor consistent. Neutrophilia, low-grade anaemia, mild thrombocytopenia, increased erythrocyte sedimentation rate, elevated liver enzymes, hyperglobulinaemia, hypoglycaemia and low titres for antinuclear antibody and rheumatoid factor may all be present (Bennett and Taylor, 1988).

Bacteriology: Although confirmation of infective arthritis requires culture or identification of the responsible organism, a speculative diagnosis may be made on the basis of history and synovial fluid cytology (Clements et al., 2005). Arthrocentesis should be performed in a sterile fashion, much as one would perform blood cultures. The area of sampling (see Chapter 3) should be clipped and prepared as for surgery. If fluid is to be inoculated into growth medium, the needle used for sampling should be replaced with a fresh sterile needle. Cytology and Gram staining should be performed on a synovial fluid smear (Figure 7.14).

An attempt should be made to culture the organism in both aerobic and anaerobic media. The bacteria most commonly isolated are *Staphylococcus intermedius*, *S. aureus* and β-haemolytic *Streptococcus* of Lancefield Group G (Bennett and Taylor, 1988; Marchevsky and Read, 1999). Less commonly, coliforms or anaerobes are responsible; only occasionally are *Pasteurella multocida*, *Pseudomonas aeruginosa*, *Proteus* spp. and *Nocardia asteroides* cultured. The significance of any diphtheroid-like organisms is uncertain. *Brucella abortus* (Clegg and Rorrison, 1968) and *Erysipelothrix rhusiopathiae* (Houlton and Jefferies, 1989) have been identified in the UK from joints with infective arthritis. Arthritis can be a feature of canine tuberculosis (Olsson, 1957) but this is now extremely rare; this could alter with the current increase in the incidence of human tuberculosis in the UK.

Some investigators have claimed that, with correct technique, a positive culture can be obtained from the synovial fluid of most infected joints (Pederson and Pool, 1978). Similarly, in human patients nearly 100% positive culture is achieved in non-gonococcal bacterial arthritis. This degree of success is, however, not enjoyed by other veterinary investigators (Marvel and Marsh, 1977; Montgomery et al., 1989; Clements et al., 2005). Even in an experimental model, direct culture of synovial fluid yielded a positive result in only approximately 50% of cases (Montgomery et al., 1989). Culture of the synovial membrane has been claimed to be more successful (Sledge, 1978; Wolski, 1978) but this too is inconsistent. Montgomery et al. (1989) found direct culture of synovial fluid and of synovial membrane to be disappointing but culture of synovial fluid following a 24-hour period of incubation in blood culture medium at 37°C was 100% reliable. Previous medication with antibiotics may prevent a successful culture, though Clements et al. (2005) reported no association between positive/negative culture of synovial fluid samples and either previous administration of antimicrobials or identifying bacteria on a synovial fluid smear.

Both aerobic and anaerobic culture should be performed, as anaerobic bacterial osteomyelitis/arthritis (*Peptostreptococcus* sp., *Propionibacterium* sp.) has been reported (Hodgin et al., 1992).

Culture of blood or urine is not generally rewarding but a positive culture from either in the absence of a positive joint fluid culture may give an indication of the organism responsible.

Histology: The severity of changes differs with the course and time of the infection and may differ between joints within an individual patient.

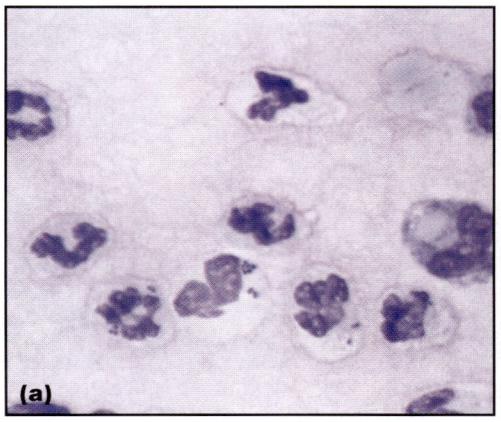

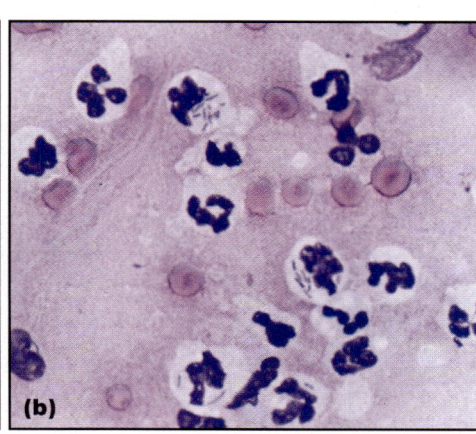

7.14 Intracellular cocci **(a)** and rods **(b)** in synovial fluid. Original magnification x1000. (Courtesy of Chris Belford, Cytopath)

Chapter 7   Arthritis

- **Synovium:** non-specific inflammatory changes. In some cases the infiltrate is predominantly polymorphonuclear leucocytes (PMNs), in others lymphocytes and plasma cells. The primary lesion is a synovitis. The synovium is thickened and discoloured, perhaps with obvious haemorrhages or fibrin deposits. In low-grade infections the lining cells are hypertrophied and hyperplastic with a mononuclear infiltration of the supporting layer. PMNs are present in relatively small numbers and haemosiderin deposits may be present. In more severe cases PMNs are present in larger numbers and may form micro-abscesses; haemorrhages will be seen in the synovium. Frequently bacteria are not evident.
- **Cartilage:** degeneration secondary to the effects of enzymatic destruction of the matrix, or to the inflamed granulation tissue (pannus) which adheres to and gradually replaces/under-runs the cartilage.
- **Bone:** evidence of subchondral bone destruction and inflammatory infiltrate into the periosteum or periosteal new bone associated with a periostitis.

Treatment
Early aggressive therapy is indicated. The aims of treatment are to eradicate the infective organism, preserve the articular cartilage and preserve joint function. Analgesics and attention to general nursing care will improve the quality of life of the affected animal.

Drug therapy: Effective treatment depends on early and correct identification of the causative organism, the acquisition of an antibiotic sensitivity profile and the removal of purulent material from the joint. Until culture and sensitivity results are obtained, a broad-spectrum β-lactamase-resistant agent such as amoxicillin/clavulanate should be administered (Kornegay and Anson, 1990). Antibiotic therapy may be altered on receipt of laboratory results.

Systemic administration (intramuscular or intravenous) of antimicrobials gives adequate levels of drug within the synovial membrane and fluid (Nelson, 1971). It should be maintained for 48–96 hours before being replaced by oral administration. There appears to be no need for intra-articular administration; indeed, such administration increases the risk of introducing further infection or, perhaps, a chemical arthritis (Argen et al., 1966; Rvedy, 1973).

Bactericidal agents are preferred to bacteriostatic drugs and should be administered for at least 2 weeks following clinical resolution, negative culture results from repeat synovial fluid samples and a return of normal or near-normal synovial fluid cytology. Treatment is often required for at least 6–8 weeks.

In some instances the antibacterial of choice (based on culture sensitivity) will have a toxicity profile that precludes long-term systemic use. Should the use of such drugs prove necessary, local slow-release preparations may be useful (Figure 7.15). The temporary intra-articular use of gentamicin-impregnated polymethylmethacrylate (PMMA) beads (Brown and Bennett, 1988) has been shown to maintain good intra-articular levels of the drug with very low systemic levels (Walenkamp et al., 1986). This avoids nephrotoxic and ototoxic effects. Originally intended for the treatment of osteomyelitis, the limited intra-articular use of these beads does not appear to result in a clinically significant chemical synovitis. More recently, gentamicin-impregnated collagen sponges (GICSs) have been reported for the successful management of septic arthritis (Hirsbrunner and Steiner, 1998; Steiner et al., 1999; Owen et al., 2005). In contrast to PMMA beads, GICSs are absorbed (in 9 days to 3 months in humans; Stemberger et al., 1989), which precludes the need for a second surgery for removal. These sponges, however, do not currently have a licence in the UK, unlike in some European countries, for treatment of infection.

Immune-mediated arthritis associated with infection: In a number of cases, even after eradication of all viable bacteria, a sterile synovitis and lameness persist. This may be an immune complex-mediated disease. As long as there is *no* evidence of remaining infection, corticosteroid therapy may be indicated (Bennett and Taylor, 1988).

Drainage: Although antibiotics alone may suffice for early low-grade infections, in more severe cases it may be preferable to drain and lavage the joint (Figure 7.16).

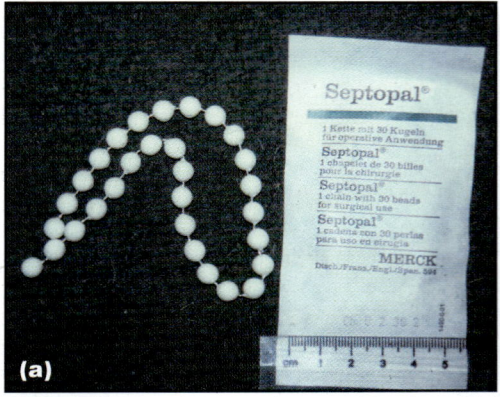

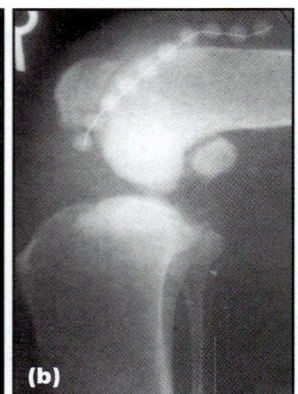

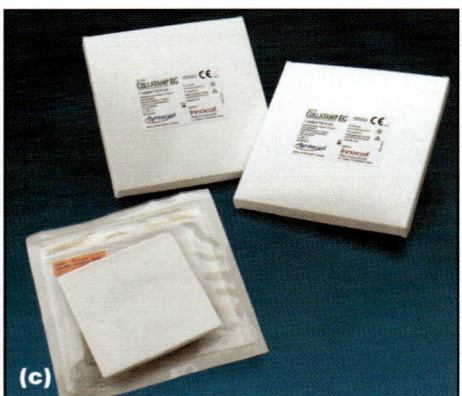

7.15   Examples of antibacterial implants. **(a)** Septopal beads. **(b)** Radiograph of an infected stifle with implanted Septopal beads. **(c)** Collatamp sponges. (c, Courtesy of David Prior, Innocoll)

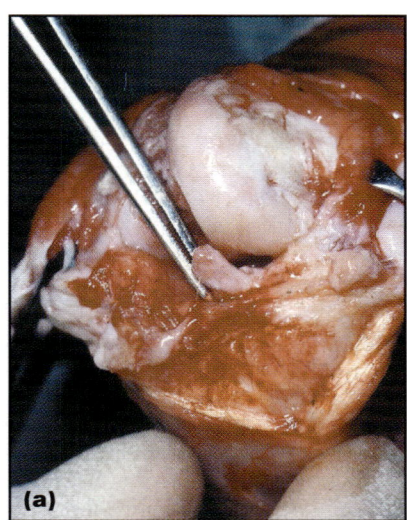

7.16
(a) Debridement of an infected stifle in a Cavalier King Charles Spaniel.
(b) Lavage and placement of wide bore drains following open debridement.

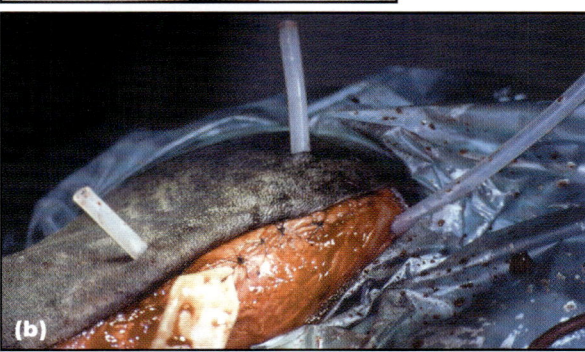

Arthrotomy or arthroscopy (Fearnside and Preston, 2002) assists removal of purulent exudate, reduces the bacterial load, and removes chondrodestructive enzymes and fibrin deposits, although Clements *et al.* (2005) found no difference between those cases managed surgically and those treated conservatively. Decompression in the immature patient may avoid further vascular embarrassment of the epiphysis.

Needle or catheter aspiration may prove satisfactory but where fibrin deposits have formed they are unlikely to be adequate. In such cases arthrotomy is required. Whichever is performed, an aseptic protocol should be followed and the joint flushed with large volumes – several litres – of sterile isotonic fluid such as lactated Ringer's.

Where arthrotomy is performed, fibrin deposits and necrotic tissue can be carefully removed. Articular cartilage should be assessed critically for prognostic purposes but iatrogenic damage studiously avoided. Drains should be placed as far apart as possible to limit local flow between them and ensure lavage of the whole joint. Thereafter, the joint should be flushed twice daily until the fluid contains no or little inflammatory exudate. Practically, this is often for 3–4 days. Whilst flushing the joint it is useful to occlude the egress drain temporarily. This ensures distension of the joint, assists in breaking down adhesions, and helps prevent the formation of localized pockets of pus. Depending on circumstances, the arthrotomy wound can be closed surgically or allowed to heal by second intention (Brown, 1978). At all times the wounds and drains must be kept scrupulously clean. They should be protected with sterile dressings to prevent further infection or self-inflicted injury; such management is time- and staff-intensive.

Indications for arthrotomy rather than needle aspiration are: infections of more than 3 days duration; penetrating wounds; infection following surgery; and infection in skeletally immature animals (Brown, 1978). Arthrotomy is not generally appropriate for polyarthritic patients.

Physiotherapy: The cartilage should be protected from excessive wear and weightbearing activity, but passive manipulation will assist with the expression of exudate from the joint. Gentle controlled exercise will assist with provision of nutrients to, and removal of metabolites from, the joint. In addition, it will assist in limiting the reduction in range of joint motion that typically occurs following joint disease and immobilization. Whilst on antibiotics, exercise should be restricted to walking on the lead. Hydrotherapy may be of assistance once the wounds have healed completely (see Chapter 16).

Prognosis

Final clinical outcome depends on: the degree of damage present at the time of initial diagnosis; the organism responsible; and the effectiveness of treatment. Chronic infections, severely chondrodestructive organisms or extensive joint destruction do not augur well for a successful outcome. Multiple joints are more difficult to treat than a single one, and haematogenous infection, such as that accompanying bacterial endocarditis, may be difficult or impossible to eradicate.

Early treatment with systemic antibiotics will result in satisfactory outcome in most circumstances. In one study (Bennett and Taylor, 1988) 56% of 57 cases made a full clinical recovery and 32% remained only slightly lame. Only 12% of cases responded poorly to treatment, with persistent lameness. Where considerable joint damage occurs prior to eradication of infection, the outcome will be considerably worse.

MRSA

Methicillin-resistant *Staphylococcus aureus* (MRSA) infection is uncommonly diagnosed in veterinary medicine but, as in human medicine, it is increasing in frequency and is causing mounting concern (Tomlin *et al.*, 1999; Duquette and Nuttall, 2005). Animal infection can be associated with chronically colonized (infected) but clinically unaffected owners, hospital staff or other patients. Because infection appears able to be transmitted from owner to pet (Scott *et al.*, 1988; Cefai *et al.*, 1994) there is cause for concern in the reverse direction. Animals most at risk include acutely ill hospitalized patients, especially those who are immunosuppressed or those with implants or indwelling catheters.

Where there is an increased index of suspicion for the presence of MRSA, such as a chronic non-healing wound, patients should be screened for its presence. If possible, swabs (nasal, throat, any skin lesions, intravenous catheter sites, urine if there is an indwelling catheter or urinary tract infection, faeces if diarrhoea is present) should be taken, sent to a laboratory capable of identifying MRSA, and results obtained before the patient is admitted to the hospital. This is clearly more practical for the referral case than in the 'first opinion' situation.

Chapter 7 Arthritis

Patients admitted with MRSA, or a high suspicion of infection, must be managed with strict barrier nursing techniques/protocol. Contact with other patients should be prevented and numbers of staff in contact must be limited; their contact with other patients must also be controlled. Hand washing between patients using hot water and soap followed by 70% alcohol rub, 4% chlorhexidine wash or 7.5% povidone–iodine, and the wearing of gloves and suitable disposable protective clothing for contact with wounds and body fluids should be practised. Face and eye protection should be worn if aerosols are likely.

The floor and the environment should be cleaned with a chlorinated phenol disinfectant. Disposable bedding is preferred and the patient can be bathed with chlorhexidine on alternate days.

Staff must pay particular attention to personal hygiene and take all possible precautions to prevent contaminating/infecting other patients, areas of the hospital, veterinary personnel or contacts. Screening staff for MRSA may become necessary if multiple infections suggest that the problem has become endemic in the clinic. Routine surveillance might also include any resident or visiting animals belonging to staff. It is important to differentiate transient carriage from true colonization and persistent carrier status. Transient carriage is far more common and is most effectively controlled by hand washing. Colonized staff should be encouraged to seek medical advice from their doctor.

MRSA is a major nosocomial pathogen and is being isolated from animal specimens with increasing frequency. There are a number of web-based sources of information. The reader is referred to the Health Protection Agency website (www.hpa.org.uk) for advice and (www.hpa.org.uk/infections/topics_az/staphylo/guidelines.htm) for guidelines. The Centers for Disease Control and Prevention in the USA have a similar website (www.cdc.gov/ncidod/hip/aresist/mrsafaq.htm).

Treatment depends on the extent of the infection, clinical signs present and microbiological results. Owen et al. (2005) report successful management of MRSA septic arthritis of a stifle with intra-articular GICSs, systemic gentamicin and oral clindamcyin.

Infected joint prostheses

Total hip replacement is performed in an increasing number of veterinary practices and elbow replacement is now commercially available. Infection of joint prostheses is rare but potentially catastrophic. Radiographically, it may be difficult to differentiate between aseptic loosening, loosening secondary to infection, and early neoplastic changes. Indium-linked leucocyte scintigraphy, where available, may be useful for diagnosis (Magnuson et al., 1988). Confirmation of infection is likely to require aspiration or biopsy. Where infection is suspected, it is usual to remove the implants and, if used, all cement (Dyce and Olmstead, 2002). The commercial availability of cementless prostheses may allow subsequent implantation of a replacement once all infection is cleared, though there is a risk of subclinical infection persisting and therefore the vast majority of infected hip replacement cases are currently converted into femoral neck excision arthroplasties.

Borrelial arthritis

The tick-borne spirochaete *Borrelia burgdorferi* can cause a multi-systemic inflammatory disorder in humans as well as other animals. It has been called Lyme disease following its isolation from a group of Americans with an inflammatory arthropathy who lived in Lyme, Connecticut. Small mammals serve as a reservoir for the spirochaete, with the sheep tick *Ixodes ricinus* probably the most important vector in the UK. Once in the body *B. burgdorferi* may act as a persistent pathogen. The disease has been diagnosed with increasing frequency but it is only relatively recently that Koch's postulates have been satisfied (Appel, 1992). The organism is rarely cultured from, or seen in, blood, synovial fluid or synovial membrane samples. The presence of *Borrelia burgdorferi* may also be an incidental finding. Borrelial arthritis may be associated with immune-mediated disease; in such cases it may be considered as a form of Type II idiopathic polyarthritis.

Clinical features: An expanding erythematous skin lesion (erythema chronicum migrans) and other organ involvement is recognized in human patients, but in the dog the most frequently reported clinical sign is an inflammatory non-erosive arthropathy with shifting lameness and swollen joints. Clinical signs in experimentally infected animals occur about 2–5 months after exposure to ticks (Appel et al., 1993).

Diagnosis: Diagnosis usually relies on the presence of lameness due to mono- or pauci-arthritis and perhaps pyrexia and lymphadenopathy in association with a positive antibody titre. Serological evidence of disease is, however, unreliable. A large number of asymptomatic dogs from an endemic region will be seropositive and there is considerable overlap between those animals considered to be clinically affected and those that are asymptomatic. Titres in clinically affected animals range from 1/512 to 1/16,384 with a mean of 1/2700; asymptomatic animals may have a titre as high as 1/8192, and 42% have a titre of 1/512 or greater (Kornblatt et al., 1985). False positive reactions have been found in human patients with autoimmune disorders, rheumatoid arthritis and certain viral, rickettsial and other bacterial infections (Blank et al., 1991) and from dogs with periodontal disease (Schillhorn van Veen, et al., 1993). There is cross-reaction with other spirochaetes. PCR testing shows promise, but currently is not totally reliable.

Dogs in many parts of Britain have serum antibodies to *B. burgdorferi* (May et al., 1991). A putative diagnosis of canine Lyme disease in this country has been made on the basis of clinical signs, serology and response to antibiotic therapy (May et al., 1990) but no attempt was made to culture the organism and none was observed in samples.

Serum levels of antibodies to *Borrelia burgdorferi* have been measured in the cat (Magnarelli et al., 1990). As in the dog, there was a seasonal effect on antibody levels and an uncertain relationship between seropositivity and clinical signs.

Radiographs show only soft tissue changes.

Examination of synovial fluid reveals an increase in leucocytes, typically in the region of 46.3 x 10^9 cells/l, 85% being polymorphonuclear leucocytes (Kornblatt et al., 1985).

Treatment: Treatment with tetracycline is reported to result in rapid clinical improvement. Doxycycline is probably the drug of choice for early treatment of arthritis in the mature patient, and amoxicillin in immature ones. Other drugs recommended for use in humans include ampicillin, ceftriaxone and minocycline. Clinical response is often seen within 24–48 hours. Treatment is instituted for a minimum of 30 days but it is questionable whether there is clearance of the organism after this period. Chronic non-erosive polyarthritis may, however, persist despite therapy.

Rickettsial arthritis

Infection with a granulocytic strain of canine ehrlichiosis can cause non-erosive polyarthritis (Stockham et al., 1986). It is a tick-transmitted rickettsial disease not native to the UK.

Clinical signs are often non-specific, including pyrexia, but can involve an acute lameness of several joints. Haematological and biochemical findings may be non-specific; they include non-regenerative anaemia, thrombocytopenia, leucopenia, pancytopenia, hyperglobulinaemia and hypoalbuminaemia. Cytology of affected synovial fluid confirms inflammation (cell count typically 30–50 x 10^9 cells/l: 80% non-degenerative PMNs, 20% mononuclear cells). Radiographic signs are restricted to soft tissue changes. Diagnosis depends on clinical signs, haematology/biochemistry results, serology and observing *Ehrlichia* morulae. These are seen in 1–2% of the synovial fluid polymorphonuclear leucocytes of affected animals (Cowell et al., 1988).

The polyarthritis responds well to doxycycline and minocycline but patients may remain asymptomatic carriers.

Bacterial L-forms

Bacterial L-forms are cell wall-deficient bacteria that morphologically resemble *Mycoplasma*. They can, with time, revert to their parental cell-walled state in culture. Their formation is aided by the use of cell wall damaging antimicrobials and by host immune responses. L-forms are difficult to culture or to identify with a light microscope but they can be identified with electron microscopy. Their presence in both diseased and healthy animals makes their significance uncertain. It is often not possible to fulfil Koch's postulates.

A progressive disease syndrome that is non-responsive to most antibiotics was reported in cats (Carro et al., 1989). Fistulating subcutaneous wounds develop and spread haematogenously or by direct extension to the joints. It is thought that the source of infection is from infected cat bites or infected ointment (Keane, 1983). Affected animals have swollen painful crepitant joints, which eventually drain purulent material. A non-specific systemic illness with pyrexia, anorexia, depression, marked leucocytosis (up to 54 x 10^9 WBC/l), mature neutrophilia, lymphocytosis and mild anaemia may be present. Radiographs demonstrate periarticular swelling and periosteal proliferation, which can progress to severe articular cartilage and subchondral bone destruction. Confirmation by routine means is difficult, and a speculative diagnosis is based on clinical signs and an inability to demonstrate aerobic/anaerobic bacteria, mycobacteria, mycoplasmas or fungi. Case details of a large series are lacking.

An L-form of *Nocardia asteroides* was retrieved from a dog with progressive polyarthritis that was non-responsive to steroids and antibiotics (Buchanan et al., 1983).

The disease appears to be responsive to tetracyclines but not to most other antimicrobials. Response should be seen within 2 days and therapy continued for at least 7 days after cessation of discharge. Erythromycin and chloramphenicol have been used in canine infections.

Mycoplasmal arthritis

Mycoplasma spp. are normal inhabitants of the conjunctival membranes, respiratory passages and urogenital tract of the dog and cat. Only rarely, in these species, do they spread systemically to cause a polyarthritis. Affected animals are usually old, debilitated, immune-deficient (Hooper et al., 1985) or immunosuppressed patients, such as those undergoing treatment for cancer (Pederson et al., 1989). An inflammatory non-erosive polyarthritis with swollen painful joints is present. *Mycoplasma gateae* arthritis and tenosynovitis have been described and reproduced in the cat (Moise et al., 1983) and *M. spumans* was isolated from a polyarthritis in a Greyhound (Barton et al., 1985).

Radiographs show only soft tissue changes. Examination of the watery turbid synovial fluid reveals an increase in polymorphonuclear white cells with non-degenerate nuclei. The organisms can be seen using Giemsa, Wright's or Leishman stains.

Mycoplasmas are sensitive to fluoroquinolones, macrolides (tylosin, erythromycin, tiamulin), tetracycline, spiramycin, chloramphenicol, lincomycin, clindamycin and aminoglycosides. As none of these is bactericidal, treatment for an extended period is necessary.

Chlamydial arthritis

Although rare, a systemic disease associated with pyrexia, lymphadenopathy and arthropathy of several joints in which *Chlamydia* spp. was considered to be implicated has been described (Lambrechts et al., 1999).

Fungal arthritis

Fungal arthritis is uncommon in the dog and cat (Codner, 1992). Apart from discospondylitis associated with *Aspergillus* (Butterworth et al., 1995), fungal arthritis has not been reported in the UK. A case of fungal osteomyelitis has been reported (Brearley and Jeffery, 1993).

Haematogenous spread following inhalation is thought to be the major cause of joint infection, though direct contamination or spread from a contiguous soft tissue or bone infection can occur. Changes in synovial fluid and synovial membrane are inflammatory and the organism may be seen on histology. Radiographically, the joint and periarticular tissues are swollen, and there is likely to be cartilage and bone erosions and osteopenia. The signs may be confused with those of rheumatoid arthritis. Confirmation is based on fungal culture or on serological examination. A variety of fungi have been cultured as causes of infective arthritis, including *Coccidioides immitis* (Maddy, 1958), *Cryptococcus neoformans* (Kavit, 1958), *Blastomyces dermatitidis* (Maskic, 1968), *Sporothrix schenkii* (Goad and Pecquet-Goad, 1986) and *Aspergillus fumigatus* (Oxenford and Middleton, 1986). The organism responsible depends largely on the geographical location of the host. Treatment with antifungal drugs such as amphotericin B, ketoconazole, itraconazole and fluconazole has been variably successful.

Viral arthritis

Post-viral arthropathies are quite common in humans, especially in the post-convalescent period following mumps, coxsackie or adenovirus infection. This may be due to immune complex hypersensitivity rather than to a direct pathogenic effect of the virus. A transient polyarthritis is sometimes seen in the dog 5–7 days after vaccination. It is usually associated with a multivalent live vaccine but can also be seen with killed vaccines. Corticosteroid therapy may be used if the lameness is severe and persistent but is usually unnecessary and may interfere with the effectiveness of vaccination.

Natural calicivirus infection has been demonstrated to produce a transient (24–48 hours' duration) pyrexia, lameness and stiffness in 8–14-week-old kittens (Pederson *et al.*, 1983). Although pain could be demonstrated on joint manipulation, and joint fluid contained an increased number of macrophages, some containing phagocytosed polymorphonuclear leucocytes, synovial membrane histology and synovial fluid analysis did not demonstrate the organism or inflammation. This, however, could reflect the timing of examination (Bennett *et al.*, 1989). Long-term effects on the joint are unknown. Acute arthritis has been induced experimentally with both field-strain and vaccine-strain calicivirus (Dawson *et al.*, 1994) and calicivirus has been isolated from the joint of a kitten with arthritis (Levy and Marsh, 1992).

Cats with effusive feline infectious peritonitis may have inflammation of the synovium and yellow cloudy synovial fluid containing an increase in polymorphonuclear cells. Although lameness may be evident, many animals with synovial inflammation do not show evidence of lameness or stiffness.

A chronic progressive polyarthritis that was not caused by identifiable bacteria or mycoplasmas but was aetiologically linked to feline leukaemia virus and feline syncytium-forming virus (FeSFV) infections has been reported by Pederson *et al.* (1980). The condition is not caused by inoculation of FeSFV alone. Serology or virus isolation can be used to identify infection. Two forms were determined on radiographic examination. The first, and most prevalent, was characterized by osteopenia and periosteal new bone in the region of the affected joints. The other had severe subchondral marginal erosions, joint instability and deformity. The condition may be partially controlled by corticosteroid therapy alone (prednisolone 10–15mg/cat/day) or in combination with cyclophosphamide, but in most cases it is relentlessly progressive.

Protozoal arthritis

Infection with the protozoan *Leishmania donovani* can cause a proliferative systemic disease of the reticuloendothelial system, of which the synovial membrane is a component (Slappendel and Greene, 1990). The natural cycle of infection is through bloodsucking sandflies serving as vectors, transmitting the disease among wild or domestic animals and people (zoonosis). Wild and domestic dogs serve as the main reservoir for *Leishmania*.

Clinical signs include weight loss, lethargy, skin lesions, lymphadenopathy, hepatosplenomegaly, pyrexia and lameness. In the UK, affected animals are likely to have been imported from the Mediterranean region, Africa, Asia, South America or the southern and central states of the USA. Diagnosis is based on the identification of the organism within macrophages, especially those in aspirates of lymph nodes or bone marrow. When joints are affected, leishmania bodies will be observed within the large number of macrophages that infiltrate the synovium. Serological tests may verify the presence of antibodies but do not prove or disprove the presence of active infection; however, a seropositive patient with compatible clinical signs is likely to be suffering from leishmaniasis. Radiographs may appear normal.

Leishmania has been implicated in an immune-based polyarthritis (Bennett, 1990).

Meglumine antimonate and sodium stilbogluconate appear to be the most effective treatments, but leishmaniasis in dogs is resistant to therapy and relapses are to be expected (Codner, 1992). This protozoan can infect humans and therefore public health implications must be considered.

References and further reading

Adams ME and Brandt KD (1991) Hypertrophic repair of canine articular cartilage in osteoarthritis after anterior cruciate ligament transection. *Journal of Rheumatology* **18**, 428–435

Altman R, Brandt K, Hochberg M *et al.* (1996) Design and conduct of clinical trials in patients with osteoarthritis: recommendations from a task force of the Osteoarthritis Research Society – Results from a workshop. *Osteoarthritis and Cartilage* **4**, 217–243

Angevine DM and Rothband S (1940) The significance of the synovial villus and the ciliary process as factors in the localisation of bacteria in the joints and eyes of rabbits. *Journal of Experimental Medicine* **71**, 129

Appel MJG (1992) Canine Lyme disease: towards satisfying Koch's postulates. In: *Current Veterinary Therapy: Small Animal Practice, XI*, ed. RW Kirk, pp. 256–259. WB Saunders, Philadelphia

Appel MJ, Allan S, Jacobson RH *et al.* (1993) Experimental Lyme disease in dogs produces arthritis and persistent infection. *Journal of Infectious Diseases* **167**, 651–664

Argen RJ, Wilson CH and Wood P (1966) Suppurative arthritis: clinical features of 42 cases. *Archives of Internal Medicine* **117**, 661–666

Barth WF and Segal K (1999) Reactive arthritis (Reiter's syndrome). *American Family Physician* **60**, 499–507

Barton MD, Ireland L, Kirschner JL and Forbes C (1985) Isolation of *Mycoplasma spumans* from polyarthritis in a Greyhound. *Australian Veterinary Journal* **62**, 206–210

Beltran J, Noto AM, McGee RB, Freedy RN and McCalla MS (1987) Infections of the musculoskeletal system: high-field-strength MR imaging. *Radiology* **164**, 449–454

Bennett D (1987) Immune based non-erosive inflammatory joint disease of the dog. Canine idiopathic polyarthritis. *Journal of Small Animal Practice* **28**, 909–920

Bennett D (1990) Joints and joint diseases. In: *Canine Orthopedics*, 2nd edn, ed. W Whittick, pp. 776–778. Lea and Febiger, Philadelphia

Bennett D, Gaskell RM, Mills A *et al.* (1989) Detection of feline calicivirus antigens in the joints of infected cats. *Veterinary Record*, **124**, 329–332

Bennett D and Kelly DF (1987) Immune based non-erosive inflammatory joint disease of the dog. 2. Polyarthritis/polymyositis syndrome. *Journal of Small Animal Practice* **28**, 891–901

Bennett D and Kirkham D (1987) The laboratory identification of serum rheumatoid factor in the dog. *Journal of Comparative Pathology* **97**, 542–550

Bennett D and Taylor DJ (1988) Bacterial infective arthritis in the dog. *Journal of Small Animal Practice* **29**, 207–230

Benton HP, Vasseur PB, BroderickVilla GA and Koolpe M (1997) Effect of carprofen on sulfated glycosaminoglycan metabolism, protein synthesis, and prostaglandin release by cultured osteoarthritic canine chondrocytes. *American Journal of Veterinary Research* **58**, 286–292

Bernard P, Germain C, Bousquet E and Segal O (2000) Radioactivity distribution in a young dog dosed orally with (acetyl-1-14C) chondroitin sulphate. *Proceedings, BSAVA Congress, Birmingham* p.85

Blank EC, Quan TJ, Mayer LW *et al.* (1991) In: *Proceedings of the First National Conference on Lyme Disease Testing* p.79. American Society for State Public Health Laboratory Directors, Washington

Brandt KD, Myers SL, Burr D and Albrecht M (1991) Osteoarthritic changes in canine articular cartilage, subchondral bone, and synovium fifty-four months after transection of the anterior cruciate ligament. *Arthritis and Rheumatism* **34**, 1560–1570

Brearley MJ and Jeffery N (1992) Cryptococcal osteomyelitis in a dog. *Journal of Small Animal Practice* **33**, 601

Brown A and Bennett D (1988) Gentamicin-impregnated polymethyl methacrylate beads for the treatment of septic arthritis. *Veterinary Record* **123**, 625–626

Brown SG (1978) Infectious arthritis and wounds of joints. *Veterinary Clinics of North America* **8**, 501–510

Buchanan AM, Beaman BL and Pederson NC (1983) *Nocardia asteroides* recovery from a dog with steroid and antibiotic unresponsive idiopathic arthritis. *Journal of Clinical Microbiology* **18**, 702–709

Butterworth SJ, Barr FJ, Pearson GR and Day MJ (1995) Multiple discospondylitis associated with *Aspergillus* species infection in a dog. *Veterinary Record* **136**, 38–41

Canapp SO, McLaughlin RM, Hoskinson JJ, Roush JK and Butine MD (1999) Scintigraphic evaluation of dogs with acute synovitis after treatment with glucosamine hydrochloride and chondroitin sulfate. *American Journal of Veterinary Research* **60**, 1552–1557

Carro T, Pederson NC, Beaman BL and Munn R (1989) Subcutaneous abscesses and arthritis caused by a probable bacterial L-form in cats. *Journal of the American Veterinary Medical Association* **194**, 1583–1588

Cefai C, Ashurst S and Owens C (1994) Human carriage of methicillin-resistant *Staphylococcus aureus* linked with a pet dog. *Lancet* **344**, 539–540

Clegg FG and Rorrison JM (1968) *Brucella abortus* infection in the dog: a case of polyarthritis. *Research in Veterinary Science* **9**, 183–185

Clements DN, Gear RN, Tattersall J, Carmichael S and Bennett D (2004) Type I immune-mediated polyarthritis in dogs: 39 cases (1999–2002). *Journal of the American Veterinary Medical Association* **224**, 1323–1327

Clements DN, Owen MR, Mosley JR *et al.* (2005) Retrospective study of bacterial infective arthritis in 31 dogs. *Journal of Small Animal Practice* **46**, 171–176

Codner EC (1992) Infectious polyarthritis in the dog and cat. In: *Current Veterinary Therapy: Small Animal Practice, XI*, ed. RW Kirk, pp. 246–252. WB Saunders, Philadelphia

Conte A, Debernard M, Palmieri L *et al.* (1991) Metabolic fate of exogenous chondroitin sulfate in man. *Arzneimittel-Forschung/Drug Research* **41**, 768–772

Cowell RL, Tyler RD, Clinkenbeard KD and Meinkoth JH (1988) Ehrlichiosis and polyarthritis in three dogs. *Journal of the American Veterinary Medical Association* **192**, 1093–1095

Curtis CL, Hughes CE *et al.* (2000) n-3 fatty acids specifically modulate catabolic factors involved in articular cartilage degradation. *Journal of Biological Chemistry* **275**, 721–724

Curtis CL, Rees SG *et al.* (2002) Pathologic indicators of degradation and inflammation in human osteoarthritic cartilage are abrogated by exposure to n-3 fatty acids. *Arthritis and Rheumatism* **46**, 1544–1553

Dawson S, Bennett D, Carter SD *et al.* (1994) Acute arthritis of cats associated with feline calicivirus infection. *Research in Veterinary Science* **56**, 133–143

Dawson S, McCardle F, Bennett D *et al.* (1993) Investigation of vaccine reactions and breakdowns after feline calicivirus vaccination. *Veterinary Record* **132**, 418–419

DiBartola SP, Tarr MJ, Webb DM and Giger U (1990) Familial renal amyloidosis in Chinese Shar Pei dogs. *Journal of the American Veterinary Medical Association* **197**, 483–487

Dougherty SA, Center SA, Shaw EE and Erb HA (1991) Juvenile-onset polyarthritis syndrome in Akitas. *Journal of the American Veterinary Medical Association* **198**, 849–856

Dunn KJ and Dunn JK (1998) Diagnostic Investigations in 101 dogs with pyrexia of unknown origin. *Journal of Small Animal Practice* **39**, 574–580

Duquette RA and Nuttall TJ (2005) Methicillin-resistant *Staphylococcus aureus* in dogs and cats: an emerging problem? *Journal of Small Animal Practice* **45**, 591–597

Dyce J and Olmstead ML (2002) Removal of infected canine cemented total hip prostheses using a femoral window technique. *Veterinary Surgery* **31**, 552–560

Eps HA, Utley M, Southwood T *et al.* (2002) A multi-centred randomised controlled trial investigating the effectiveness of hydrotherapy in children with juvenile idiopathic arthritis. *Arthritis and Rheumatism* **46**, S608–S608

Evans CH (2005) Gene therapy: what have we accomplished and where do we go from here? *Journal of Rheumatology* **32**, 17–20

Fearnside SM and Preston CA (2002) Arthroscopic management of septic polyarthritis in a dog. *Australian Veterinary Journal* **80**, 681–683

Foley A, Halbert J, Hewitt T and Crotty M (2003) Does hydrotherapy improve strength and physical function in patients with osteoarthritis? A randomised controlled trial comparing a gym based and a hydrotherapy based strengthening programme. *Annals of the Rheumatic Diseases* **62**, 1162–1167

Geels JJ, Roush JK, Hoskinson JJ and McLaughlin RM (2000) Evaluation of an intracapsular technique for the treatment of cranial cruciate ligament rupture. Clinical, radiographic, scintigraphic and force plate analysis findings in 20 dogs. *Veterinary and Comparative Orthopaedics and Traumatology* **13**, 197–203

Ghosh P (1999) The pathobiology of osteoarthritis and the rationale for the use of pentosan polysulfate for its treatment. *Seminars in Arthritis and Rheumatism* **28**, 211–267

Giger U, Werrer LL, Millichamp NJ and Gorman NT (1985) Sulfadizine-induced allergy in six Doberman pinschers. *Journal of the American Veterinary Medical Association* **186**, 479–484

Gill JM, Quisel AM, Rocca PV and Walters DT (2003) Diagnosis of systemic lupus erythematosus. *American Family Physician* **68**, 2179–2186

Goad DL and Pecquet Goad ME (1986) Osteoarticular sporotrichosis in a dog. *Journal of the American Veterinary Medical Association* **189**, 1326–1328

Goldenberg DL (1993) Infectious arthritis. In: *Textbook of Rheumatology*, ed. WN Kelly *et al.*, pp.1449–1466. WB Saunders, Philadelphia

Goring RL and Beale BS (1993) Immune-mediated arthropathies. In: *Disease Mechanisms in Small Animal Surgery, 2nd edition*, ed. Bojrab MJ, pp. 743–757 Lea and Febiger, Philadelphia

Hanson RR, Smalley LR *et al.* (1997) Oral treatment with a glucosamine-chondroitin sulfate compound for degenerative joint disease in horses: 25 cases. *Equine Practice* **19**(9), 16–30

Hirsbrunner G and Steiner A (1998) Treatment of infectious arthritis of the radiocarpal joint cattle with gentamicin-impregnated collagen sponges. *Veterinary Record* **142**, 399–402

Hodgin EC, Michaelson F, Howerth EW, Austin F, Davis F and Haase AS (1992) Anaerobic bacterial infections causing osteomyelitis/arthritis in a dog. *Journal of the American Veterinary Medicine Association* **201**, 886–888

Hooper PT, Ireland LA and Carter A (1985) Mycoplasma polyarthritis in a cat with probable severe immune deficiency. *Australian Veterinary Journal* **62**, 352

Houlton JEF and Jefferies AR (1989) Infective polyarthritis and multiple discospondylitis in a dog due to *Erysipelothrix rhusiopathiae*. *Journal of Small Animal Practice* **30**, 35–38

Hudson JT, Slater MR, Taylor L, Scott HM and Kerwin SC (2004) Assessing repeatability and validity of a visual analogue scale questionnaire for use in assessing pain and lameness in dogs. *American Journal of Veterinary Research* **65**, 1634–1643

Hunziker EB (2002) Articular cartilage repair: basic science and clinical progress. A review of the current status and prospects. *Osteoarthritis and Cartilage* **10**, 432–463

Innes J and Barr A (1998) Can owners assess outcome following surgical treatment of canine cranial cruciate ligament deficiency? *Journal of Small Animal Practice* **39**, 373–378

Innes JF, Barr ARS, Patteson MW and Dieppe PA (1996) Scintigraphy in the evaluation of osteoarthritis of the canine stifle joint – relationship with clinical, radiographic and surgical observations. *Veterinary and Comparative Orthopaedics and Traumatology* **9**, 53–59

Innes JF, Barr ARS and Sharif M (2000) Efficacy of oral calcium pentosan polysulphate for the treatment of osteoarthritis of the canine stifle joint secondary to cranial cruciate ligament deficiency. *Veterinary Record* **146**, 433–437

Innes JF, Costello M, Barr FJ, Rudorf H and Barr ARS (2004) Radiographic progression of osteoarthritis of the canine stifle

Chapter 7 Arthritis

joint: a prospective study. *Veterinary Radiology and Ultrasound* **45**, 143–148

Innes JF, Fuller CJ, Grover ER, Kelly AL and Burn JF (2003) Randomised, double-blind, placebo-controlled parallel group study of P54FP for the treatment of dogs with osteoarthritis. *Veterinary Record* **152**, 457–460

Innes JF, Sharif M and Barr ARS (1998) Relations between biochemical markers of osteoarthritis and other disease parameters in a population of dogs with naturally acquired osteoarthritis of the genual joint. *American Journal of Veterinary Research* **59**, 1530–1536

Innes JF, Shepstone L, Holder J, Barr ARS and Dieppe PA (2002) Changes in the canine femoropatellar joint space in the postsurgical, cruciate-deficient stifle joint. *Veterinary Radiology and Ultrasound* **43**, 241–248

Johnson KA, Hay CW, Chu QL, Roe SC and Caterson B (2002) Cartilage-derived biomarkers of osteoarthritis in synovial fluid of dogs with naturally acquired rupture of the cranial cruciate ligament. *American Journal of Veterinary Research* **63**, 775–781

Jorgensen C, Gordeladze J and Noel D (2004) Tissue engineering through autologous mesenchymal stem cells. *Current Opinion In Biotechnology* **15**, 406–410

Kavit AY (1958) Cryptococcic arthritis in a Cocker Spaniel. *Journal of the American Veterinary Medical Association* **133**, 386–388

Kealy RD, Lawler DF, Ballam JM et al. (1997) Five-year longitudinal study on limited food consumption and development of osteoarthritis in coxofemoral joints of dogs. *Journal of the American Veterinary Medical Association* **210**, 222

Kealy RD, Lawler DF, Ballam JM et al. (2000) Evaluation of the effect of limited food consumption on radiographic evidence of osteoarthritis in dogs. *Journal of the American Veterinary Medical Association* **217**, 1678–1680

Keane DP (1983) Chronic abscesses in cats associated with an organism resembling mycoplasma. *Canadian Veterinary Journal* **24**, 289–291

Kornblatt AN, Urband PH and Steere AC (1985) Arthritis caused by *Borrelia burgdorferi* in dogs. *Journal of the American Veterinary Medical Association* **186**, 960–964

Kornegay JN and Anson LW (1990) Joint infections. In: *Infectious Diseases of the Dog and Cat*, 2nd edn, ed. CE Greene, pp. 94–96. WB Saunders, Philadelphia

Lambrechts N, Picard J and Tustin RC (1999) *Chlamydia*-induced septic arthritis in a dog. *Journal of the South African Veterinary Association* **70**, 40–42

Layton CT (1999) *Pasteurella multocida* meningitis and septic arthritis secondary to a cat bite. *Journal of Emergency Medicine* **17**, 445–448

Levy JK and Marsh A (1992) Isolation of calicivirus from the joint of a kitten with arthritis. *Journal of the American Veterinary Medical Association* **201**, 753–755

Lisbona R and Rosenthal L (1977) Observations on the sequential use of 99m Tc-phosphate complex and 67Ga imaging in osteomyelitis, cellulites and septic arthritis. *Radiology* **123**, 123

Maddy KT (1958) Disseminated coccidioidomycosis of the dog. *Journal of the American Veterinary Medical Association* **137**, 483–489

Magnarelli LA, Anderson JF, Levine HR and Levy SA (1990) Tick parasitism and antibodies to *Borrelia burgdorferi* in cats. *Journal of the American Veterinary Medical Association* **197**, 63–66

Magnuson JE, Brown ML, Hauser ME et al. (1988) In-III-labelled leukocyte scintigraphy in suspected orthopaedic prosthesis infection: comparison with other imaging modalities. *Radiology* **168**, 235–239

Marchevsky AM and Read RA (1999) Bacterial septic arthritis in 19 dogs. *Australian Veterinary Journal* **77**, 233–237

Marvel JE and Marsh HQ (1977) Management of penetrating injuries of the knee. *Clinical Orthopaedics* **122**, 268–272

Maskic D (1968) North American blastomycosis. In: *Current Veterinary Therapy: Small Animal Practice, III*, ed. RW Kirk, pp. 621–622. WB Saunders, Philadelphia

May C, Bennett D and Carter SD (1990) Lyme disease in the dog. *Veterinary Record* **126**, 293

May C, Carter SD, Barnes A, Bell S and Bennett D (1991) Serodiagnosis of Lyme disease in UK dogs. *Journal of Small Animal Practice* **32**, 170–174

May C, Hammill J and Bennett D (1992) Chinese Shar-Pei fever syndrome: a preliminary report. *Veterinary Record* **131**, 586–587

McAlindon TE, LaValley MP, Gulin JP and Felson DT (2000) Glucosamine and chondroitin for treatment of osteoarthritis – a systematic quality assessment and meta-analysis. *Journal of the American Medical Association* **283**, 1469–1475

McNamara PS, Spencer DVM et al. (1997) Slow-acting, disease-modifying osteoarthritis agents. *Veterinary Clinics Of North America: Small Animal Practice* **27**(4), 863

Meredith HC and Rittenberg GM (1978) Pneumoarthrography: an unusual radiographic sign of gram-negative septic arthritis. *Radiology* **128**, 642

Misumi K, Vilim V, Carter SD et al. (2002) Concentrations of cartilage oligomeric matrix protein in dogs with naturally developing and experimentally induced arthropathy. *American Journal of Veterinary Research* **63**, 598–603

Mitchell M, Howard B, Haller J, Sartoris DJ and Resnick D (1988) Septic arthritis. *Radiology Clinics of North America* **26**, 1295–1313

Mobasheri A, Vannucci SJ, Bondy CA et al. (2002) Glucose transport and metabolism in chondrocytes: a key to understanding chondrogenesis, skeletal development and cartilage degradation in osteoarthritis. *Histology and Histopathology* **17**, 1239–1267

Moise NS, Crisman JW, Fairbrother JF and Baldwin C (1983) *Mycoplasma gateae* arthritis and tenosynovitis in cats: case report and experimental reproduction of the disease. *American Journal of Veterinary Research* **44**, 16–21

Montgomery RD, Long IR, Milton JL, DiPinto MN and Hunt J (1989) Comparison of aerobic culturette synovial membrane biopsy and blood culture medium in detection of canine bacterial arthritis. *Veterinary Surgery* **18**, 300–303

Moreau M, Dupuis J et al. (2003) Clinical evaluation of a nutraceutical, carprofen and meloxicam for the treatment of dogs with osteoarthritis. *Veterinary Record* **152**, 323

Nelson JD (1971) Antibiotic concentration in septic joint effusions. *New England Journal of Medicine* **284**, 349–353

Norris R, Ehrlich MG and McKusick K (1979) Early diagnosis in disc space infection with 67 Ga in an experimental model. *Clinical Orthopaedics Related Research* **144**, 293–298

Olsson S-E (1957) On tuberculosis in the dog. A study with special reference to X-ray diagnosis. *Cornell Veterinarian* **47**, 193–219

Owen MR, Moores AP and Coe RJ (2005) Management of MRSA septic arthritis in a dog using a gentamicin-impregnated collagen sponge. *Journal of Small Animal Practice* **45**, 609–612

Oxenford CJ and Middletone DJ (1986) Osteomyelitis and arthritis associated with *Aspergillus fumigatus* in a dog. *Australian Veterinary Journal* **63**, 59–60

Palmoski M and Brandt K (1983) In vivo effects of aspirin on canine osteoarthritic cartilage. *Arthritis and Rheumatism* **26**, 994–1001

Pavelka K, Gatterova J, Olejarova M et al. (2002) Glucosamine sulfate use and delay of progression of knee osteoarthritis. A 3-year, randomized, placebo-controlled, double-blind study. *Archives of Internal Medicine* **162**, 2113–2123

Pederson NC, Laliberte L and Elman S (1983) A transient febrile 'limping' syndrome of kittens caused by two different strains of Feline Calicivirus. *Feline Practice* **13**, 26–35

Pederson NC and Pool RR (1978) Canine joint disease. *Veterinary Clinics of North America* **8**, 465–493

Pederson NC, Pool RR and O'Brien T (1980) Feline chronic progressive polyarthritis. *American Journal of Veterinary Research* **41**, 522–535

Pederson NC, Wind A, Morgan JP and Pool RR (1989) Joint diseases of the dog and cat. In: *Textbook of Veterinary Medicine*, 3rd edn, ed. SJ Ettinger, pp.2329–2377. WB Saunders, Philadelphia

Pelletier JP, Lajeunesse D, Jovanovic DV et al. (2000) Carprofen simultaneously reduces progression of morphological changes in cartilage and subchondral bone in experimental dog osteoarthritis. *Journal of Rheumatology* **27**, 2893–2902

Pujalte JM, Llavore EP et al. (1980) Double-blind clinical evaluation of oral glucosamine sulfate in the basic treatment of osteoarthrosis. *Current Medical Research and Opinion* **7**, 110–114

Queneau P, Francon A and Graber-Duvernay B (2001) Methodological reflections on 20 randomized clinical hydrotherapy trials in rheumatology. *Therapie* **56**, 675–684

Read RA, Cullishill D and Jones MP (1996) Systemic use of pentosan polysulfate in the treatment of osteoarthritis. *Journal of Small Animal Practice* **37**, 108–114

Reginster JY, Deroisy R, Rovati LC et al. (2001) Long-term effects of glucosamine sulphate on osteoarthritis progression: a randomised, placebo-controlled clinical trial. *Lancet* **357**, 251–256

Reichelt A, Forster KK et al. (1994) Efficacy and safety of intramuscular glucosamine sulfate in osteoarthritis of the knee - a randomized, placebo-controlled, double-blind-study. *Arzneimittel-Forschung* **44**, 75–80

Resnick CS, Ammann AM and Walsh JW (1987) Chronic septic arthritis of the adult hip: computed tomographic features. *Skeletal Radiology* **16**, 513–516

Richy F, Bruyere O, Ethgen O et al. (2003) Structural and symptomatic efficacy of glucosamine and chondroitin in knee osteoarthritis: a comprehensive meta-analysis. *Archives of Internal Medicine* **163**, 1514–1522

Rogachefsky RA, Dean DD et al. (1993) Treatment of canine osteoarthritis with IGF-1 and sodium pentosan polysulphate. *Osteoarthritis and Cartilage* **1**, 105–114

Ronca F, Palmieri L, Panicucci P and Ronca G (1998) Anti-inflammatory activity of chondroitin sulfate. *Osteoarthritis and Cartilage* **6**, 14–21

Ronca G, Roncatestoni S and Lualdi P (1988) Pharmacokinetics of H-3 chondroitin sulfate Following oral administration in animals. *Zeitschrift für Rheumatologie* **47**, 325–326

Rorvik AM and Grondahl AM (1995) Markers of osteoarthritis: a review of the literature. *Veterinary Surgery* **24**, 255–262

Rvedy J (1973) Treatment of septic arthritis. *Clinical Orthopaedics and Related Research* **96**, 150–151

Schillhorn van Veen TW, Murphy AJ and Colmery B (1993) False positive *Borrelia burgdorferi* antibody titres associated with periodontal disease in dogs. *Veterinary Record* **132**, 512

Schrader SC (1982) Septic arthritis and osteomyelitis of the hip in six mature dogs. *Journal of the American Veterinary Medical Association* **181**, 894–898

Scott GM, Thomson R, Malonelee J and Ridgway GI (1988) Cross-infection between animals and man: possible feline transmission of *Staphylococcus aureus* infection in humans. *Journal of Hospital Infection* **12**, 29–34

Sevalla K, Todhunter RJ, Vernier-Singer M and Budsberg SC (2000) Effect of polysulfated glycosaminoglycan on DNA content and proteoglycan metabolism in normal and osteoarthritic canine articular cartilage explants. *Veterinary Surgery* **29**, 407–414

Slappendel RJ and Greene CE (1990) Leishmaniasis. In: *Infectious Diseases of the Dog and Cat*, ed. CE Greene, pp. 769–777. WB Saunders, Philadelphia

Sledge CB (1978) Surgery in infectious arthritis. *Clinics in Rheumatic Diseases* **4**, 149

Smith GK, Popovitch CA, Gregor TP and Shofer FS (1995) Evaluation of risk factors for degenerative joint disease associated with hip dysplasia in dogs. *Journal of the American Veterinary Medical Association* **206**, 642–647

Smith RL, Schurman DJ, Kajiyama G, Mell M and Gilkerson E (1987) The effects of antibiotics on the destruction of cartilage in experimental infectious arthritis. *Journal of Bone and Joint Surgery* **69A**, 1063–1068

Stallings B, Ling GV, Lagenaur LA, Jang SS and Johnson DL (1987) Septicaemia and septic arthritis caused by *Streptococcus pneumoniae* in a cat: possible transmission from a child. *Journal of the American Veterinary Medical Association* **191**, 703–704

Steiner A, Hirsbrunner G, Miserez R and Tschudi P (1999) Arthroscopic lavage and implantation of gentamicin-impregnated collagen sponges for treatment of septic arthritis in cattle: 14 cases (1995–1997). *Veterinary and Comparative Orthopaedics and Traumatology* **12**, 64–69

Stemberger A, Sorg KH, Machka K and Blumel G (1989) Technologische und biochemische aspekte von kollagen-implanaten. In: *Kollagen als Wirkstofftrager*, ed. A. Stemberger *et al.*, pp.17–29. Schattauer, Stuttgart

Stener-Victorin E, Kruse-Smidje C and Jung K (2004) Comparison between electro-acupuncture and hydrotherapy, both in combination with patient education and patient education alone, on the symptomatic treatment of osteoarthritis of the hip. *Clinical Journal of Pain* **20**, 179–185

Stockham SL, Schmidt DA and Tyler JW (1986) Polyarthritis associated with canine granulocytic ehrlichiosis. *Veterinary Clinical Pathology* **15**, 8

Sundberg SB, Savage JP and Foster BK (1989) Technetium phosphate bone scan in the diagnosis of septic arthritis in childhood. *Journal of Paediatric Orthopaedics* **9**, 579–585

Tan EM, Cohen AS, Fries JF *et al.* (1982) The 1982 revised criteria for the classification of systemic lupus erythematosus. *Arthritis and Rheumatism* **25**, 1271–1277

Tomlin J, Pead MJ, Lloyd DH *et al.* (1999) Methicillin resistant *Staphylococcus aureus* infections in 11 dogs. *Veterinary Record* **144**, 60–64

van der Wel TJ and Meyer HP (1995) Discospondylitis and immune-mediated polyarthritis in a Bernese mountain dog. *Tigdschrift voor Diergeneeskunde* **120**, 75–77

Vaz AL (1982) Double-blind clinical evaluation of the relative efficacy of ibuprofen and glucosamine sulfate in the management of osteoarthrosis of the knee in out-patients. *Current Medical Research and Opinion* **8**, 145–149

Verbruggen G, Cornelissen M, Elewaut D *et al.* (1999) Influence of polysulfated polysaccharides on aggrecans synthesized by differentiated human articular chondrocytes. *Journal of Rheumatology* **26**, 1663–1671

Walenkamp GHIM, Vree TB and Van Rens TJG (1986) Gentamicin-PMMA beads: pharmacokinetic and nephrotoxicological study. *Clinical Orthopaedics and Related Research* **205**, 171–183

Webb AA, Taylor SM and Muir GD (2002) Steroid-responsive meningitis-arteritis in dogs with noninfectious, nonerosive, idiopathic, immune-mediated polyarthritis. *Journal of Veterinary Internal Medicine* **16**, 269–273

Wilkinson GT (1984) Arthritis associated with infection in the cat. *Veterinary Annual* **24**, 292–296

Wolski KP (1978) Staphylococcal and other Gram-positive coccal arthritides. *Clinics in Rheumatic Diseases* **4**, 181

Woodard JC, Riser WH, Bloomberg MS, Gaskin JM and Goring RL (1991) Erosive polyarthritis in two greyhounds. *Journal of the American Veterinary Medical Association* **198**, 873–876

8a

Muscle and tendon injuries

Angus Anderson

Anatomy and physiology

Skeletal muscle constitutes the single largest tissue mass in the body and makes up 40–50% of the total body weight. The basic structural element of muscle is the muscle fibre, which is a syncytium of many cells fused together, with multiple nuclei. Muscle fibres are organized by the surrounding connective tissue that serves to bind them together to ensure integrated movement among fibres. This connective tissue also provides a scaffold for regenerating muscle fibres following injury (Figure 8.1). Skeletal muscle is innervated by axons that terminate at the motor end plate. The axon and all the muscle fibres that it contacts are referred to as a motor unit. The number of muscle fibres per motor unit varies enormously. Where fine control is required, the number of muscle fibres per unit may be small (e.g. extraocular muscles), whereas the number may be very large in large muscles, such as the triceps.

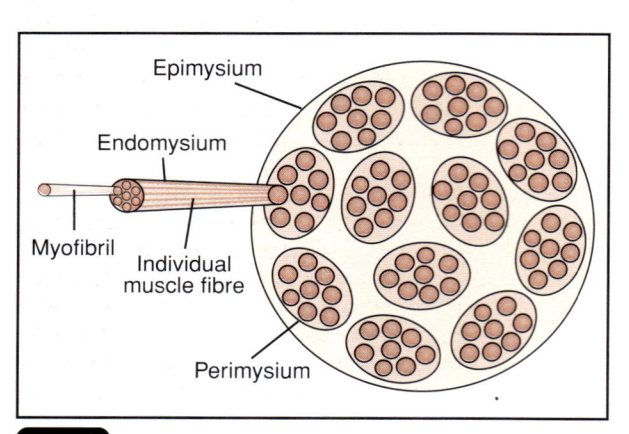

Skeletal muscles are attached to bone or cartilage by cord-like tendons or flat aponeuroses. Some muscles attach directly to bone by fleshy attachments. Tendon is a composite material consisting of collagen fibrils embedded in a matrix of proteoglycans. There is a relative paucity of cells, the majority of which are fibroblasts arranged in parallel rows between collagen bundles (Figure 8.2). The major constituent of tendon is type I collagen (~85% of dry weight), which is organized in a highly structured way (with elastin and proteoglycans) resulting in a tissue with one of the highest tensile strengths in the body. The tensile properties of tendon vary with its anatomical location, amount of activity and age (Woo *et al.*, 1994).

Tendons that bend sharply, such as the flexor tendons of the digits, are enclosed by a sheath that allows the tendon to move smoothly and helps to direct the path of the tendon. A mesotenon originating on the side of the bend opposite the friction surface joins the epitenon covering the tendon. Sliding of the tendon is assisted by the presence of synovial fluid that also provides some nutrition to the tendon by diffusion. In regions where tendons wrap around an articular surface (e.g. biceps brachii tendon) large compressive stresses are generated, and in these areas tendon can take on a cartilage-like appearance (Woo *et al.*, 1994). Tendons not enclosed in a sheath move in a straight line and are surrounded by a loose areolar connective tissue called the paratenon. There are significant differences in the blood supply to sheathed tendons compared with non-sheathed tendons and this has a profound influence on the healing responses following injury.

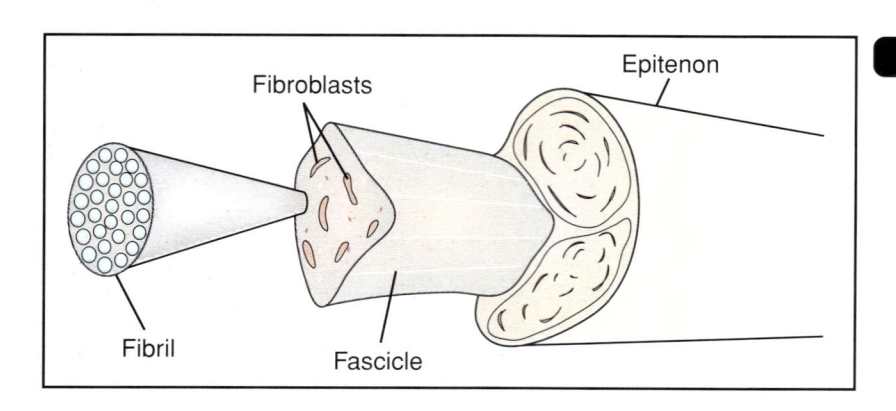

8.1 Schematic drawing of the structure of muscle.

8.2 Schematic drawing of the structure of tendon.

Chapter 8a   Muscle and tendon injuries

Response of muscle to injury

Muscle injury can occur by a variety of mechanisms, ranging from ischaemia to direct injury by crushing or laceration. Muscle cells are capable of regeneration if their sarcolemmal nuclei are not destroyed. Where the endomysium is intact, fibre regeneration can replace degenerate fibres. Where the endomysium has been damaged, the process of regeneration is less organized and its success depends upon the absence of any obstruction from haematoma or fibrous scar tissue. New muscle cells can also originate from a population of relatively undifferentiated satellite cells that exist in a quiescent state beside the original muscle syncytium. The process of regeneration occurs simultaneously with proliferation of fibrous connective tissue. The latter may interfere with the ability of the muscle fibres to function normally, particularly where there are excessive amounts of fibrous connective tissue. The blood supply from adjacent tissues is important in the recovery of muscle following injury. Large devascularized areas of muscle heal by fibrous scar tissue formation. Functional regeneration also requires intact motor and sensory nerves. Damaged motor nerves that are left intact can regenerate and form new neuromuscular junctions but sensory nerves cannot regenerate their specialized sensory receptors (Fitch *et al.*, 1997).

Classification of muscle injuries

Injuries can be classified (in increasing order of severity) as contusions, strains, lacerations and ruptures. The clinical signs of muscle injury will vary with the severity of the injury, the function of the individual muscle that is affected, and its chronicity.

Muscle contusion

Contusions result from non-penetrating blunt injuries that cause an initial inflammatory reaction and haematoma. Later, scar tissue with variable amounts of muscle regeneration may be seen. These inflammatory responses tend to resolve more quickly, and there is a faster recovery of tensile strength, in mobilized muscle. Severe blunt injury may result in the formation of bone within muscle (myositis ossificans). Contusions do not usually require any specific treatment unless they are very large. Initial treatment in acute injuries consists of cold compresses and immobilization. After 24 hours warm compresses or baths may be used with compression bandaging, or immobilization, depending on severity.

Indirect muscle strain injuries

Injuries involving the muscle–tendon unit are referred to as *strains* (in contrast to injuries of ligaments that are referred to as *sprains*). Strain injuries result from overstretching or overuse of the muscle–tendon unit and can be classified qualitatively as mild, moderate or severe, depending on the severity of the clinical signs (Farrow, 1978). Strain injuries are particularly important and more common in athletic dogs such as Greyhounds. Muscles that cross more than one joint are particularly at risk. Injuries generally occur at the myotendinous junction and are characterized initially by haematoma formation and then by the development of scar tissue.

Muscle laceration

Muscle lacerations usually result from direct trauma from sharp objects but may also result from surgical exposures. For normal function to return, muscle must regenerate across the repair site and denervated tissue must be re-innervated. Functional recovery following laceration is rarely complete but partial recovery is usually possible. Where muscles are lacerated and sutured, healing occurs primarily by the formation of a dense connective tissue scar. Small numbers of myotubes may penetrate the scar but good regeneration of muscle tissue across the laceration is not usually seen. This results in a reduced ability of the muscle to produce tension, which may affect function.

Muscle rupture

Muscle ruptures may be partial or complete and are most frequently seen in athletic dogs such as Greyhounds. Muscle ruptures are caused by the active contraction of a muscle unit occuring simultaneously with forced passive extension of this unit. Examples of specific injuries include rupture of the triceps, gracilis and gastrocnemius muscles.

Clinical signs of muscle rupture include lameness, pain and swelling. Lameness and muscle atrophy may be present in chronic injuries. Muscle ruptures occur more commonly through the musculotendinous junction than the muscle belly. Differentiating partial from complete tears may be difficult on clinical examination and may require surgical exploration to be certain. Delaying surgical treatment may result in the formation of excessive surgical scar tissue with a reduced range of movement and consequent deterioration in function.

Muscle contracture

Muscle contracture is a state of shortening of a muscle not caused by active contraction (Vaughan, 1979). It usually results from fibrous connective tissue replacement of muscle; this occurs secondary to degenerative changes that may be induced by trauma or damage to the nerve or blood supply. It can also be a congenital abnormality or may be secondary to an infection or immune-mediated disease.

Surgical repair of muscle injuries

The need for surgery corresponds with the severity of the injury. Treatment of muscle lacerations depends on whether the injury is acute or chronic, and on the likely effect of any loss of function on limb use. Severed muscles should be sutured with minimal delay.

Because muscles have an inherently poor ability to hold sutures these should be placed through the muscle sheath using a horizontal mattress pattern (Figure 8.3a). A tension-relieving suture pattern such as near–far, far–near can be useful where retraction of the muscle edges makes apposition difficult (Figure 8.3b). Monofilament non-absorbable or slowly absorbable

Chapter 8a Muscle and tendon injuries

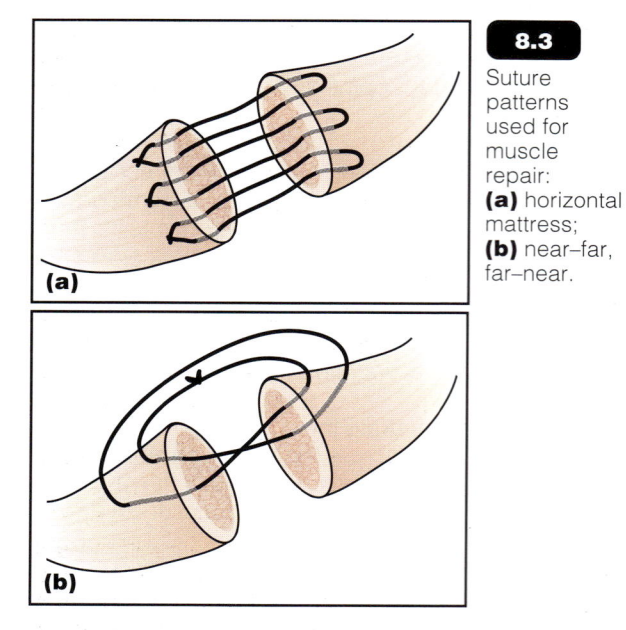

8.3 Suture patterns used for muscle repair: **(a)** horizontal mattress; **(b)** near–far, far–near.

suture material (PDS or polyglyconate) should be used. The latter should retain its tensile strength for long enough to allow healing to occur.

Immobilization is very important in the postoperative period to minimize the risk of breakdown of the repair. Affected muscles should be kept immobilized for 3 weeks followed by a very gradual return to activity over the following 4–6 weeks (restraint by cage confinement, bandaging, lead activity). Physical therapy may be of considerable value during this rehabilitation period. Prolonged immobilization can lead to reduced tensile strength and excessive scar tissue contraction.

Tendon injury and healing

Tendon injury can result from direct trauma, laceration or contusion and from indirect trauma as a result of acute or chronic tensile overload. Indirect injury is often multifactorial since most tendons can withstand tensile forces greater than can be exerted by muscles or sustained by bone. For this reason avulsion fractures and ruptures at the musculotendinous junction are commoner than mid-substance tears. The presence of other pathological processes, such as inflammation, may also influence the tendency for tendons to become injured. Tendon injuries frequently occur with injury to adjacent soft tissues and consequently their healing does not occur in isolation. This frequently results in the formation of adhesions that can limit gliding function. Restoration of gliding function is less critical in veterinary species compared with certain situations in humans (e.g. hand surgery), and restoration of adequate tensile strength is usually more important. The healing process varies, depending upon whether the tendon is surrounded by paratenon or a tendon sheath.

Healing in paratenon-covered tendons

Following laceration of the tendon and paratenon the wound fills with blood clot and inflammatory products. Proliferating capillary buds and fibroblasts rapidly invade this area from the paratenon and form granulation tissue between the tendon ends. Collagen synthesis can be detected within a few days and a fibrous bridge forms between the tendon ends over a period of several weeks. After 3–4 weeks the collagen fibres and fibroblasts orientate themselves along the long axis of the tendon as a result of stress. This is the process of secondary remodelling and results in increased biomechanical strength and a reduction in scar tissue. This process continues for several months until there are minimal differences between the scar and the original tendon.

Healing in sheathed tendons

Healing responses in sheathed tendons are much more limited compared with those of paratenon-covered tendons. The severed ends of the tendon will tend to distract within the sheath creating a gap. Following surgical repair and immobilization, healing occurs predominantly through the ingrowth of connective tissue from the sheath and the cellular response from the endotenon (Woo *et al.*, 1994). The formation of adhesions between the tendon and its sheath may restrict gliding function but this can be minimized by appropriate surgical technique and postoperative care.

General principles of tendon repair

Certain general principles must be adhered to in order to optimize the healing process. These include gentle tissue handling and adequate haemostasis. The goals of surgery are to minimize adhesion formation and, when required, to restore gliding function. There should be a minimal delay in the timing of the repair unless there is severe contamination. When contamination is present the area should be debrided and lavaged, and, if there is adequate healthy soft tissue with an adequate blood supply, primary tenorrhaphy can be performed. If contamination is severe, repair can be delayed, but the limb should be immobilized to reduce the likelihood of the tendon ends distracting; coloured suture can be placed in the tendon ends to aid identification when definitive repair is performed. In this situation adhesions are more likely to develop, however, and the repair will be more prone to breakdown.

The choice of suture material is to some extent determined by the preference of the surgeon but it should have the following qualities:

- Easy to pass through tissue
- Non-irritant
- Good knot security
- Adequate strength that is maintained during the healing process.

The materials that fulfil these properties most effectively are monofilament nylon and polypropylene (non-absorbable); in some situations, polydioxanone (absorbable) can be used (where loading on tendon during healing is not great and blood supply is good). There is often a tendency to select a suture with a large diameter but this may distort tissues and not tie or loop properly.

Suture patterns

A number of suture patterns have been described for tendon repair. No one suture technique is satisfactory in all cases. The three commonest suture patterns for use in round tendons are shown in Figure 8.4. The locking-loop (modified Kessler) is superior to the Bunnell–Mayer because it is less constrictive to the intrinsic blood supply and provides greater tensile strength (Berg and Egger, 1986). The three-loop pulley suture provides greater tensile strength and resistance to gap formation than the locking-loop patterns (Berg and Egger, 1986; Moores et al., 2004). Short, flat or aponeurotic tendons are most easily repaired with interrupted horizontal mattress sutures or a baseball suture (Figure 8.5).

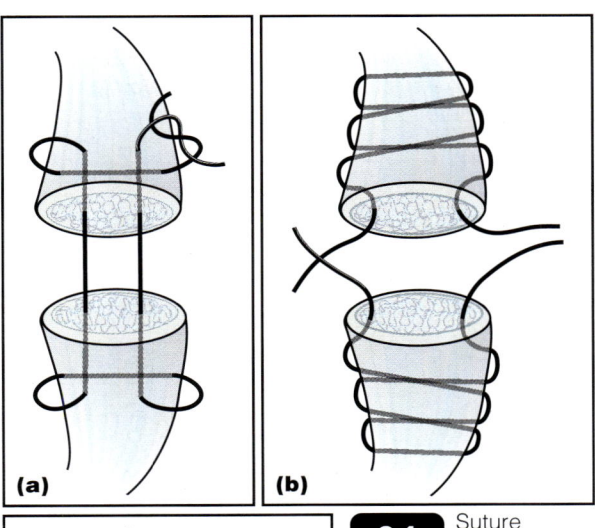

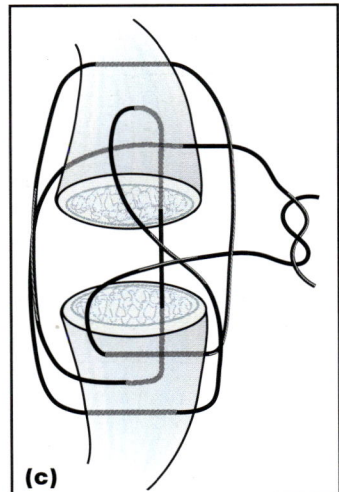

8.4 Suture patterns for repair of round tendons: **(a)** locking loop; **(b)** Bunnell–Mayer; **(c)** three-loop pulley.

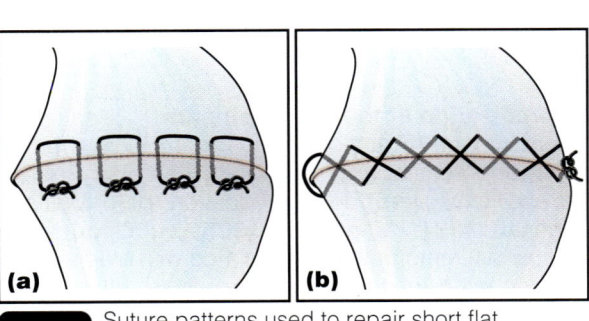

8.5 Suture patterns used to repair short flat tendons: **(a)** horizontal mattress; **(b)** baseball.

Whatever suture pattern is chosen, for the first 2 weeks the strength of the anastomosis relies entirely on the suture. A strong anastomosis may allow early mobilization, which may help to maximize final tensile strength. By 6 weeks after surgery tensile strength is approximately 50% of normal and by 1 year this rises to about 80% (Woo et al., 1994).

Specific muscle disorders: thoracic limb

Rupture of the serratus ventralis muscle

This is an uncommon injury, occurring more frequently in cats than dogs, which results in a very characteristic upward displacement of the scapula on weightbearing (Bloomberg, 1993). Treatment consists of suturing the dorsal border of the scapula to the torn soft tissues. Holes are drilled in the dorsal border of the scapula to facilitate suture placement. An alternative is to place a wire suture from the caudal border of the scapula around rib 6 or 7. Postoperatively, either the limb should be supported in a Velpeau sling for 10–14 days or the animal should be cage-confined for 3–4 weeks.

Rupture of the long head of the triceps

This injury occurs most commonly in the racing Greyhound and results from the avulsion of a small part of the triceps origin (Eaton-Wells, 1998). Treatment options include surgical re-attachment of the muscle or conservative management with ice packs in the acute stage to reduce swelling and oedema. Prognosis for return to racing is good.

Disorders of the supra- and infraspinatus muscles

Contracture of the supra/infraspinatus

Contracture of the infraspinatus, and less commonly the supraspinatus muscle, is an uncommon cause of lameness that has been reported mainly in working dogs (Vaughan, 1979; Bennett, 1986). Usually, medium to larger breeds of dog are affected and, although the lameness is usually unilateral, bilateral lameness has been reported. Typically, lameness is acute in onset at exercise and over a period of several weeks a characteristic gait abnormality develops. At rest the affected limb is held with the elbow joint adducted and the foot and carpus abducted (Figure 8.6). Shoulder

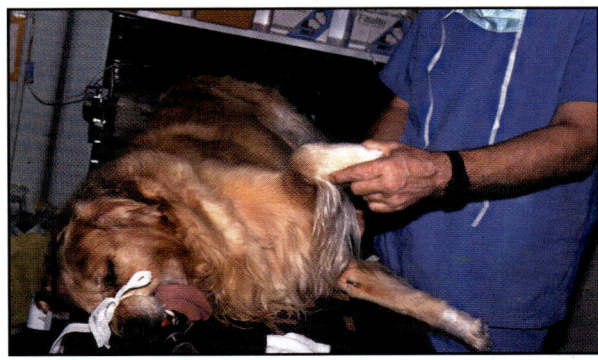

8.6 Infraspinatus contracture in a Golden Retriever, showing lateral deviation of the carpus when the limb is flexed.

Chapter 8a Muscle and tendon injuries

flexion is reduced but non-painful and during flexion of the limb the foot and carpus swing outwards instead of in a straight line. Supra- and infraspinatus are usually atrophied on examination. During locomotion the lower limb is circumducted in a characteristic fashion.

Radiographs of the shoulder joint do not show any specific abnormalities, although if the contracture is severe there may be a reduction in joint space width on lateral and craniocaudal radiographs of the joint (Figure 8.7). Ultrasonography has been used to identify changes to the affected muscles (Siems *et al.*, 1998) and electromyography will sometimes show abnormalities consistent with a myopathic origin (Pettit *et al.*, 1978). Treatment is by tenotomy of the affected tendon and breaking down adhesions between the tendon and joint capsule.

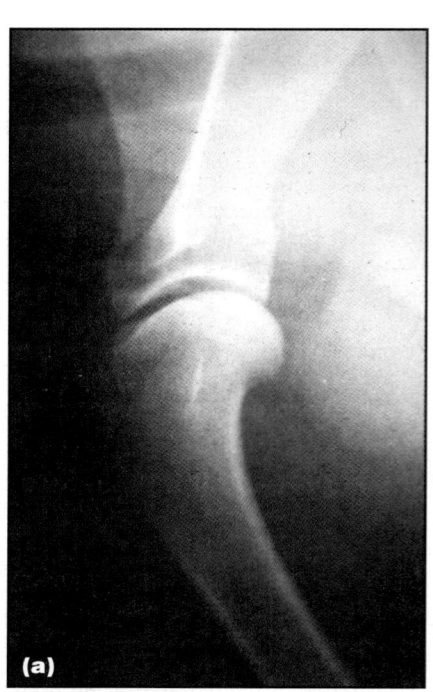

8.7 Infraspinatus contracture: shoulder joint radiographs. **(a)** Lateral view showing narrowing of caudal joint space. **(b)** Craniocaudal view showing reduced space between the acromion and the greater tubercle.

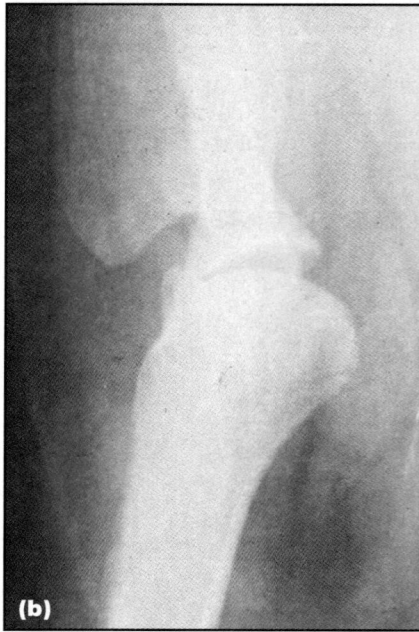

Infraspinatus bursal ossification

Infraspinatus bursal ossification (IBO) has been recognized in a number of medium-sized to larger breeds of dog, particularly the Labrador Retriever (McKee *et al.*, 2002). Muscle atrophy in the shoulder region is usually present and focal pain may be detected on direct pressure over the point of insertion of the infraspinatus on the greater tubercle of the humerus. Radiographic abnormalities are most obvious on craniocaudal views of the shoulder and consist of discrete areas of calcification between the acromion and the greater tubercle of the humerus (Figure 8.8). Sclerosis of the humerus at the attachment site of the infraspinatus may be visible on lateral radiographs. It should be remembered that other abnormalities of the shoulder joint may also be present that are not obvious on plain or contrast radiography of the joint (McKee *et al.*, 2002). Full evaluation of the joint requires arthroscopy to rule out the presence of other abnormalities.

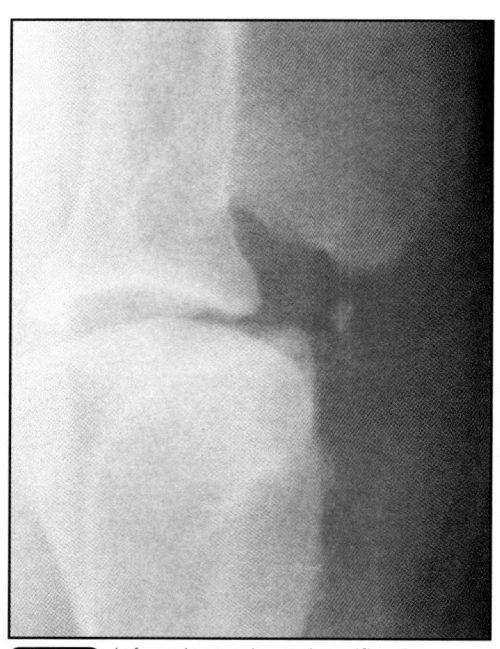

8.8 Infraspinatus bursal ossification: craniocaudal radiograph of the shoulder joint.

Treatment initially should be conservative and consist of rest and either non-steroidal anti-inflammatory drugs (NSAIDs) or an intra-articular injection of a long-acting corticosteroid (methylprednisolone). If this fails to resolve the lameness, surgical excision of the mineralized bodies may result in improvement (McKee *et al.*, 2002).

Mineralization of the supraspinatus

Supraspinatus mineralization has been reported mainly in larger breeds of dog, particularly Labrador Retrievers and Rottweilers (Flo and Middleton, 1990; Muir and Johnson, 1994; Krieglender, 1995), but its presence may be asymptomatic or associated with other abnormalities of the shoulder joint. The precise aetiology and pathogenesis of supraspinatus mineralization are not fully understood but indirect trauma to the tendon may

Chapter 8a Muscle and tendon injuries

disrupt the blood supply leading to hypoxia. This may result in collagen transforming into fibrocartilage that undergoes dystrophic calcification (Uhthoff *et al.*, 1976).

Muscle atrophy may be present over the affected shoulder and pain may be elicited on manipulation of the joint. Direct palpation of the greater tubercle or supraspinatus tendon may elicit pain in some dogs. Diagnosis is made on radiography of the shoulder and mineralization is seen adjacent to the greater tubercle. It is usually present as well circumscribed foci (Figure 8.9a). Arthrography to delineate the biceps tendon and skyline views of the intertubercular groove (Figure 8.9b) may assist in the localization of calcified deposits. It has been proposed that mineralization adjacent to the biceps tendon may cause a mechanical tenosynovitis that is responsible for lameness (Krieglender, 1995). Accordingly, more superficial mineralization may not be of clinical significance. Supraspinatus mineralization as a cause of lameness can only be made after excluding other causes of shoulder and forelimb lameness.

Conservative treatment should be attempted initially (restricted activity for 6–8 weeks and NSAIDs or intra-articular injection of a long-acting corticosteroid) but if this fails surgery should be considered. The muscle can be exposed by a standard craniomedial approach to the shoulder and calcified deposits removed. If they are difficult to identify, longitudinal incisions can be made in the tendon. Lameness has also been reported to resolve following extracorporeal shock wave therapy (Danova and Muir, 2003).

Disorders of the biceps tendon

A number of disorders are commonly recognized affecting the origin of the biceps tendon and the intra-articular tendon body as it courses through the intertubercular groove over the craniomedial aspect of the shoulder. These conditions are listed and their treatment options summarized in Figure 8.10. Disorders of the biceps tendon are covered in detail in Chapter 17.

Avulsion of the origin or insertion of extensor carpi radialis

Avulsion of the origin of the extensor carpi radialis is reported to be common in Greyhound puppies and has been observed in pet dogs (Anderson *et al.*, 1993; Eaton-Wells, 1998). The injury occurs at exercise and

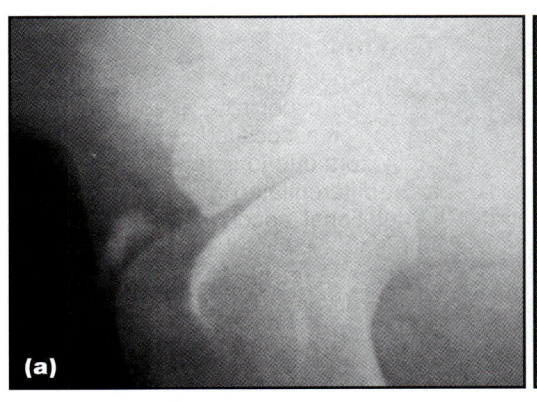

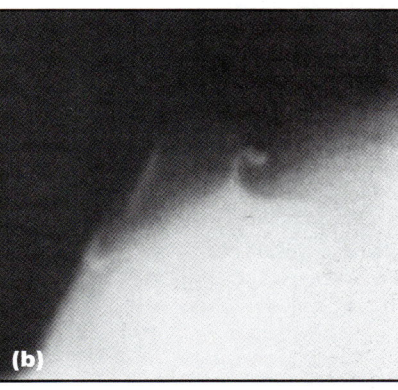

8.9 Mineralization of the supraspinatus muscle. **(a)** Lateral radiograph of the shoulder joint. **(b)** Skyline radiograph of the intertubercular groove.

Disorder	Management options	References
Avulsion from supraglenoid tubercle	• Re-attach tendon if shoulder joint unstable • Conservative if shoulder joint is stable	Denny and Butterworth (2000)
Rupture or partial rupture of tendon	• Conservative if shoulder joint is stable • Total and partial ruptures can be sutured if the shoulder joint is unstable • Partial ruptures can be tenotomized via arthroscopy or tenodesed to bicipital groove with screw and washer or staple (if shoulder joint stable)	Denny and Butterworth (2000)
Medial instability of tendon	• Repair transverse humeral ligament • Screws placed in greater and lesser tubercles connected by sutures to restrain tendon in groove	Bennett and Campbell (1979); Boemo and Eaton-Wells (1995)
Tenosynovitis	• Conservative (rest and NSAIDs) • Intra-articular methylprednisolone (20–40 mg depending on size of dog) and rest for 4–6 wk • Arthroscopic tenotomy • Tenodesis to bicipital groove with staple or screw and washer	Stobie *et al.* (1995); Denny and Butterworth (2000); Beale *et al.* (2003)
Rupture of biceps tendon sheath	• Tenotomy • Tenodesis	Innes and Brown (2004)

8.10 Treatment options for dogs with biceps brachii tendon disorders.

Chapter 8a Muscle and tendon injuries

often results from collisions. Avulsions of the origin of this muscle are associated with pain and swelling at this site. Radiographs may reveal the presence of periosteal new bone at the origin of the muscle in more chronic cases (Figure 8.11) (Anderson *et al.*, 1993). Surgical repair can be performed but most cases are likely to go sound if treated conservatively. Avulsions of the insertion of this muscle will cause lameness but these injuries are managed conservatively because the incidence of failure of surgical repair is high, and fibrosis results in good return of function (Eaton-Wells, 1998).

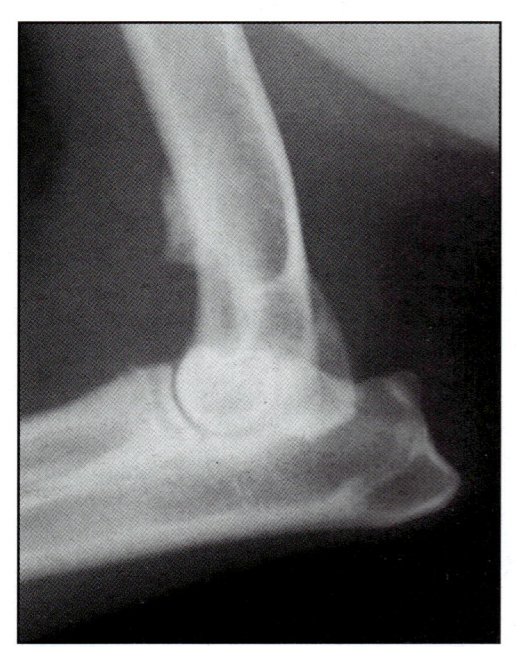

8.11 Radiograph of humerus, showing calcification of the origin of extensor carpi radialis.

Injury to the insertion of flexor carpi ulnaris
Flexor carpi ulnaris (FCU) is comprised of two heads. These originate from the olecranon and medial epicondyle of the humerus and insert on the accessory carpal bone. A strain injury of the tendons of insertion can cause lameness in racing dogs and pets (Roe, 1998). Avulsions of these tendons can occur with acute overextension of the carpus with lateral stress. Pain and swelling are present immediately proximal to the accessory carpal bone. Mild strain injuries are treated by rest whereas avulsion of the insertion should be repaired surgically. Lacerations of the tendon of insertion will result in mild to moderate carpal hyperextension and should be repaired.

Flexor carpi ulnaris tendon contracture
In young dogs, typically 6–12 weeks of age, carpal hyperflexion can develop associated with excessive tautness in the FCU tendons (Vaughan, 1992). Dobermann and Shar Pei breeds appear to be most commonly affected. The condition can develop uni- or bilaterally and is usually acute in onset. Affected puppies will show carpal hyperflexion and a lateral bowing of the carpus (Figure 8.12). Treatment consists of restricting activity (avoid stairs and jumping) for several

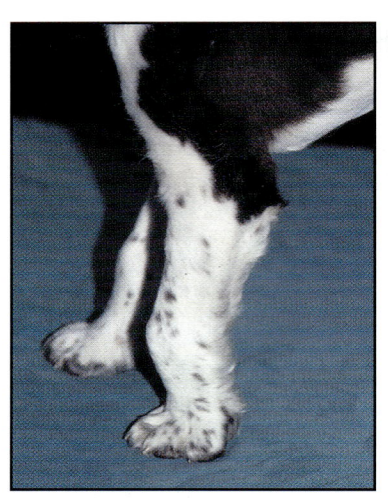

8.12 Flexural deformity of the carpus in a puppy caused by flexor carpi ulnaris tendon contracture.

weeks and improvement is usually rapid and complete within about 4 weeks. Occasionally severely affected pups will not improve over this period and in these cases one or both of the FCU tendons can be sectioned just proximal to the accessory carpal bone. The condition is likely to be due to an unequal rate of bone growth relative to that of the soft tissues.

Carpal hyperextension
Spontaneous carpal hyperextension can occur in puppies of 2–3 months of age, especially German Shepherd Dogs. This appears to be associated with poor muscle tone of the carpal flexors due to inadequate exercise. The condition can be differentiated from hyperextension associated with nutritional secondary hyperparathyroidism by radiographic examination. Treatment is by encouraging controlled exercise to improve muscle tone (Shires *et al.*, 1985). External support is contraindicated as this will exacerbate the problem.

Specific muscle disorders: pelvic limb

Injury to the tensor fasciae latae muscle
This injury has been reported primarily in racing Greyhounds. The range of injuries include:

- Rupture of the origin
- Vertical splits along the muscle fibres
- Avulsion of the attachment to the fascia lata (Eaton-Wells, 1998).

On examination, pain can be elicited on extension of the hip. Either pain and swelling are present over the muscle, or a deficit can be palpated. Complete or partial avulsions can be managed by surgical repair or laser therapy. Surgical repair involves reattaching the muscle to the fascia. Care should be taken not to place sutures in the vastus lateralis because this will cause pain when the dog is exercised (Eaton-Wells, 1998). Dogs should be kept confined to lead exercise for 10 days and then allowed increasing amounts of exercise over the following 6 weeks. The prognosis for these injuries is good.

Chapter 8a Muscle and tendon injuries

Injury of the iliopsoas muscle
Traumatic injury of the iliopsoas muscle is an unusual injury causing pelvic limb lameness with pain on extension and internal rotation of the hip (Breur and Blevins, 1997). Pain can be detected on palpation of the muscle cranial to its attachment to the lesser trochanter and in small dogs rectal examination may allow evaluation of the muscle. Injury to the muscle can be identified by ultrasonography. Conservative treatment of a small number of dogs has been reported to be successful. If this fails, tenomyectomy may be performed.

Quadriceps contracture
Quadriceps contracture is a condition characterized by stifle hyperextension and atrophy of the quadriceps muscle (Figure 8.13). The condition is most commonly a sequel to fractures of the femur, particularly where complications such as osteomyelitis and non-union have occurred, or where these fractures have been managed in young animals by application of external support that has maintained the stifle in extension (Bardet, 1987). The condition can also be a congenital disorder (Stead *et al.*, 1977) or a complication of *Toxoplasma* or *Neospora* infection.

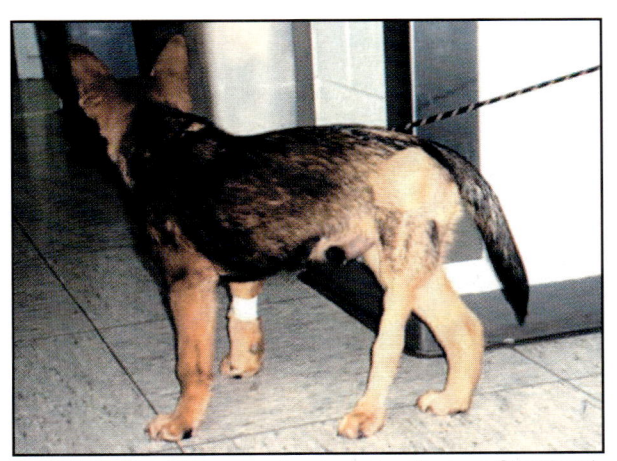

8.13 Quadriceps contracture in a German Shepherd Dog. (Courtesy S. Langley-Hobbs.)

Quadriceps contracture results in a severe lameness where the limb is not used when walking or when the dorsum of the paw becomes excoriated from being dragged on the floor. The patella is drawn proximally in its groove or may be luxated medially. In young dogs the condition can result in secondary hip subluxation with associated degenerative changes. In the congenital form the rigidity can be very profound and result in the stifle bending caudally (genu recurvatum). The growth and development of the distal femur and proximal tibia may be affected.

In cases secondary to femoral fracture, the initiating factor is fibrous adhesion formation between the vastus intermedius muscle and the femur. Muscle trauma appears to have little role in the aetiology; immobilization with concurrent muscle trauma was not found to cause joint stiffness in young dogs (Shires *et al.*, 1982). Severe restriction of stifle movement causes progressive degenerative changes in the articular and periarticular tissues that can result in a fibrous ankylosis. Many of these changes to articular tissues, and the generalized muscle atrophy that develops in the limb, reach a stage where they become irreversible.

Treatment of quadriceps contracture can be very difficult and prognosis must be only guarded to poor. The surgical options include excision of the vastus intermedius, stifle arthrodesis and amputation (Bardet, 1987). Excision of the vastus intermedius can be performed by a craniomedial approach to the femur and dissecting between the cranial and caudal bellies of the sartorius muscle. Any excess callus associated with the fracture healing should be removed. This procedure should allow restoration of a reasonable degree of flexion to the stifle provided the condition has not become too advanced. Following surgery, the challenge is preventing the disorder from recurring by maintaining stifle movement. This can be achieved by application of an Ehmer sling for a short period and then application of aggressive physiotherapy, which may require heavy sedation and prolonged pain relief. A dynamic stifle flexion apparatus has been described where external fixator pins are placed in the proximal femur and distal tibia and connected by rubber bands (De Haan *et al.*, 1995; Liptak and Simpson, 2000). This allows stifle movement and physiotherapy but prevents the joint from fully extending.

Stifle arthrodesis may be performed if the above surgery fails, but where there is concurrent significant limb shortening and other abnormalities, such as hip subluxation, amputation is recommended.

Gracilis muscle injury
Rupture of the gracilis muscle is the commonest major muscle injury in the racing Greyhound. Injury to the muscle can occur at the muscular origin and/or the tendinous insertion in one or both pelvic limbs (Eaton-Wells, 1992). Avulsions may be partial (usually the caudal margin) or complete. Diagnosis is based on clinical observation and palpation of the medial thigh (Figure 8.14). Acute injuries will show signs of haemorrhage extending down the inner thigh, and a swelling with ventral displacement of the muscle where the origin of the muscle has ruptured, or dorsal displacement of the muscle if the insertion has ruptured. Swelling and subcutaneous haemorrhage become more obvious 12–24 hours following injury.

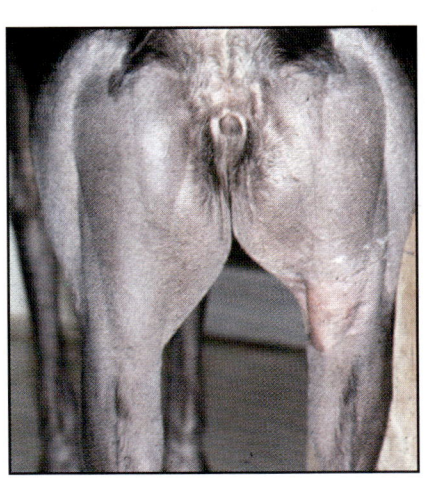

8.14 Greyhound with avulsion of its gracilis origin. (Courtesy of R. Eaton-Wells.)

Chapter 8a Muscle and tendon injuries

Surgical repair is the treatment of choice if a full return to racing is desired. For injuries to the origin of the muscle, a horizontal skin incision is made directly over this region. The muscular origin is friable and is best sutured by pre-placing a series of near–far, far–near pulley sutures of PDS or polyglyconate from the muscle to the subpubic tendon. Injuries of the insertion of the muscle can be approached by a longitudinal incision placed in a similar fashion to the origin from the muscle to its fascial attachment to the tibia. Particular attention should be paid to attaching the caudal thick tendinous portion to the tibia. Following surgery, dogs should be kennel confined for 1 week and then their exercise gradually increased over the next 6 weeks. Dogs may return to racing 10–12 weeks after surgery.

Gracilis or semitendinosus contracture

Contracture of the gracilis or semitendinosus (less commonly) muscles results in a very characteristic gait abnormality that has been reported most frequently in middle-aged German Shepherd Dogs (Vaughan, 1979; Lewis *et al.*, 1997). Lameness in affected dogs may be acute or gradual in onset and may be uni- or bilateral. Affected muscles are palpable as distinct firm bands extending from their origin to the caudomedial aspect of the stifle. Weightbearing in affected limbs is normal and dogs will exercise normally. Gait abnormality is most obvious when dogs are trotting. When the limb is raised the hock will hyperflex and be rotated rapidly outwards while the foot is turned inwards.

Although lameness can be resolved immediately by surgery (tenotomy, tendinectomy or myectomy), lameness always recurs within 3–5 months. All forms of adjunctive medical treatment have been reported to be ineffective.

Avulsion of the origin of the lateral or medial head of the gastrocnemius

Avulsions of the lateral or medial head of the gastrocnemius are uncommon injuries that result in hyperflexion of the hock and a semi-plantigrade stance (Muir and Tass Dueland, 1994; Prior, 1994; Robinson, 1999). Pain can be elicited by pressure over the origin of the affected muscle and on extension of the stifle. Radiographs of the stifle show distal displacement of the fabella of the affected muscle belly (Figure 8.15). Surgical reattachment of the tendon is necessary to restore function. The fabella can be used as an anchor for nylon leader line or wire that is attached to the caudal aspect of the femur through a bone tunnel or to a screw. The hock should be maintained in extension for 6 weeks after surgery to reduce tension on the repair.

Avulsion of the popliteus muscle

This is a very rare injury that has been reported in several skeletally immature dogs and a single adult dog (Eaton-Wells and Plummer, 1978; Tanno *et al.*, 1996). Radiographs show distal displacement of the popliteal sesamoid and an avulsed fragment of bone adjacent to the lateral aspect of the lateral condyle of the femur (Figure 8.16). If the bony fragment is sufficiently large it can be re-attached with a screw but, if not, the tendon can be sutured to adjacent soft tissues.

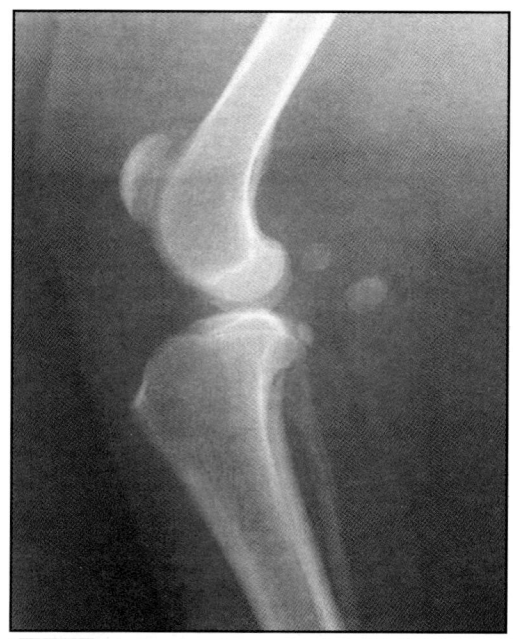

8.15 Lateral radiograph of a stifle joint, showing avulsion of the origin of the lateral head of the gastrocnemius muscle.

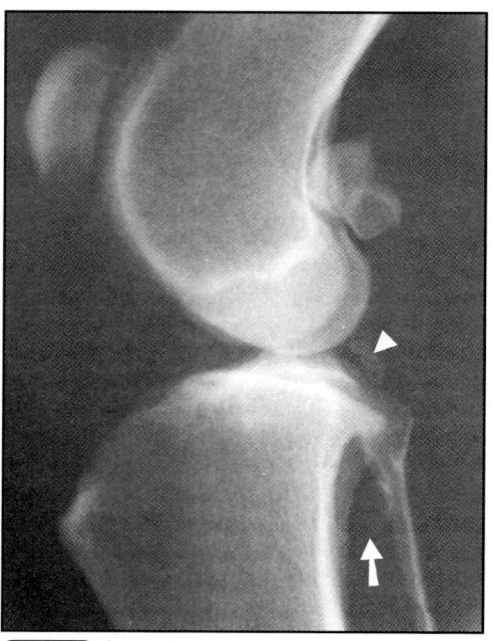

8.16 Lateral radiograph of a stifle joint, showing avulsion of the popliteus muscle. The popliteal sesamoid bone is displaced distally (arrow) and a small avulsion fragment is visible more proximally (arrowhead). (Courtesy S. Langley-Hobbs.)

References and further reading

Alexander JW and Early TD (1984) A carpal laxity syndrome in young dogs. *Journal of Veterinary Orthopaedics* **3**, 22–26
Anderson A, Stead AC and Coughlan AR (1993) Unusual muscle and tendon disorders of the forelimb in the dog. *Journal of Small Animal Practice* **34**, 313–318
Bardet JF (1987) Quadriceps contracture and fracture disease. *Veterinary Clinics of North America* **17**, 957–973
Beale BS, Hulse DA, Schulz KS and Whitney WO (2003) Arthroscopically assisted surgery of the shoulder joint. In: *Small*

Chapter 8a Muscle and tendon injuries

Animal Arthroscopy, ed. BS Beale, pp. 23–49. WB Saunders, Philadelphia

Bennett RA (1986) Contracture of the infraspinatus muscle in dogs: a review of 12 cases. *Journal of the American Animal Hospital Association* **22**, 481–487

Bennett D and Campbell JR (1979) Unusual soft tissue orthopaedic problems in the dog. *Journal of Small Animal Practice* **20**, 27–39

Berg RJ and Egger EL (1986) In vitro comparison of the three loop pulley and locking loop suture patterns for repair of canine weight-bearing tendons. *Veterinary Surgery* **15**, 107–110

Bloomberg M (1993) Muscles and tendons. In: *Textbook of Small Animal Surgery, 2nd edn*, ed. D Slatter, pp. 1996–2020. WB Saunders, Philadelphia

Boemo CM and Eaton-Wells RD (1995) Medial displacement of the tendon of origin of the biceps brachii muscle in 10 greyhounds. *Journal of Small Animal Practice* **36**, 69–73

Breur GJ and Blevins WE (1997) Traumatic injury of the iliopsoas muscle in three dogs. *Journal of the American Veterinary Medical Association* **210**, 1631–1634

Danova NA and Muir P (2003) Extracorporeal shock wave therapy for supraspinatus calcifying tendinopathy in two dogs. *Veterinary Record* **152**, 208–209

De Haan JJ, Goring RL, Renberg C and Bertrand S (1995) Modified transarticular external skeletal fixation for support of Achilles tenorrhaphy in four dogs. *Veterinary Comparative Orthopaedics and Traumatology* **8**, 32–35

Denny HR and Butterworth SJ (2000) The shoulder joint. In: *A Guide to Canine and Feline Orthopaedics, 4th edn*, pp. 303–340. Blackwell, Oxford

Eaton-Wells RD (1992) Surgical repair of acute gracilis muscle rupture in the racing Greyhound. *Veterinary Comparative Orthopaedics and Traumatology* **5**, 18–21

Eaton-Wells RD (1998) Muscle injuries in the racing Greyhound. In: *Canine Sports Medicine and Surgery*, ed. MS Bloomberg, JF Dee and RA Taylor, pp. 84–91. WB Saunders, Philadelphia

Eaton-Wells RD and Plummer GV (1978) Avulsion of the popliteal muscle in an Afghan Hound. *Journal of Small Animal Practice* **19**, 743–747

Farrow CS (1978) Sprain, strain and contusion. *Veterinary Clinics of North America* **8(2)**, 169–182

Fitch RB, Montgomery RD and Jaffe MH (1997) Muscle injuries in dogs. *Compendium on Continuing Education for the Practicing Veterinarian* **19**, 947–957

Flo GL and Middleton D (1990) Mineralisation of the supraspinatus tendon in dogs. *Journal of the American Veterinary Medical Association* **197**, 95–97

Innes JF and Brown G (2004) Rupture of the biceps brachii tendon sheath in two dogs. *Journal of Small Animal Practice* **45**, 25–28

Kriegleder H (1995) Mineralisation of the supraspinatus tendon: clinical observations in seven dogs. *Veterinary Comparative Orthopaedics and Traumatology* **8**, 91–97

Lewis DD, Shelton GD, Piras A et al. (1997) Gracilis or semitendinosus myopathy in 18 dogs. *Journal of the American Animal Hospital Association* **33**, 177–188

Liptak JM and Simpson DJ (2000) Successful management of quadriceps contracture in a cat using a dynamic flexion apparatus. *Veterinary Comparative Orthopaedics and Traumatology* **13**, 44–48

McKee WM, May C and Macias C (2002) Infraspinatus bursal ossification in eight dogs. *Proceedings of the 1st World Orthopaedic Veterinary Congress, Munich*, 141

Moores AP, Owen MR and Tarlton JF (2004) The three-loop pulley suture versus two locking-loop sutures for the repair of canine Achilles tendons. *Veterinary Surgery* **33**, 131–137

Muir P and Johnson KA (1994) Supraspinatus and biceps brachii tendinopathy in dogs. *Journal of Small Animal Practice* **35**, 239–243

Muir P and Tass Dueland R (1994) Avulsion of the origin of the medial head of the gastrocnemius in a dog. *Veterinary Record* **135**, 359–360

Pettit GD, Chatburn CC, Hegreberg A and Meyers KM (1978) Studies on the pathophysiology of infraspinatus muscle contracture in the dog. *Veterinary Surgery* **7**, 8–11

Prior JE (1994) Avulsion of the lateral head of the gastrocnemius muscle in a working dog. *Veterinary Record* **134**, 382–383

Robinson A (1999) Atraumatic bilateral avulsion of the origins of the gastrocnemius muscle. *Journal of Small Animal Practice* **40**, 498–500

Roe S (1998) Injuries and diseases of tendons. *Canine Sports Medicine and Surgery*, ed. MS Bloomberg, JF Dee and RA Taylor, pp. 92–99. WB Saunders, Philadelphia

Shires PK, Braund KG and Milton JL (1982) Effect of localised trauma and temporary splinting in immature skeletal muscle and mobility of the femoro-tibial joint in the dog. *American Journal of Veterinary Research* **43**, 454–460

Shires PK, Hulse DA and Kearney MK (1985) Carpal hyperextension in two-month-old pups. *Journal of the American Veterinary Medical Association* **186**, 49–52

Siems JJ, Breur GJ, Blevins WE and Cornell KK (1998) Use of two dimensional ultrasonography for diagnosing contracture and strain of the infraspinatus muscle in a dog. *Journal of the American Veterinary Medical Association* **212**, 77–80

Stead AC, Camburn MA and Gunn HM (1977) Congenital hindlimb rigidity in a dog. *Journal of Small Animal Practice* **18**, 39–46

Stobie D, Wallace L and Lipowitz A (1995) Chronic bicipital tenosynovitis in dogs: 29 cases. *Journal of the American Veterinary Medical Association* **207**, 201–207

Tanno F, Weber U, Lang J and Simpson D (1996) Avulsion of the popliteus muscle in a malinois dog. *Journal of Small Animal Practice* **37**, 448–451

Uhthoff HK, Sarkar K and Maynard JA (1976) Calcifying tendonitis: a new concept of its pathogenesis. *Clinical Orthopaedics and Related Research* **118**, 164–168

Vaughan LC (1979) Muscle and tendon injuries in dogs. *Journal of Small Animal Practice* **20**, 711–736

Vaughan LC (1992) Flexural deformity of the carpus in puppies. *Journal of Small Animal Practice* **33**, 381–384

Woo SL-Y, An K-N, Arnoczky SP et al. (1994) Anatomy, biology and biomechanics of tendon, ligament and meniscus. In: *Orthopaedic Basic Science*, ed. SS Simon, pp. 45–88. American Academy of Orthopaedic Surgeons, Philadelphia

8b
Diseases of muscle and the neuromuscular junction

G. Diane Shelton

Introduction

Diseases affecting muscle and the neuromuscular junction are commonly overlooked when evaluating a dog with lameness. Orthopaedic disorders occur more frequently than neuromuscular diseases; however, when a diagnosis cannot be reached following a careful orthopaedic evaluation, disorders of muscle and the neuromuscular junction should be considered. Joint diseases such as polyarthritis can appear very similar clinically to polymyositis or myasthenia gravis. This chapter will focus on the most commonly encountered neuromuscular disorders, with particular reference to those that can present as lameness.

Clinical signs

Affected individuals with muscle or neuromuscular junction disease may present with lameness, limb contractures or more generalized locomotor abnormalities, such as a crouched stance and stiff, short-strided gait. Muscle tone and peripheral reflexes are normal or reduced and there may be significant muscle atrophy in chronic myopathies. In some individuals, weakness of the pharyngeal, laryngeal and oesophageal muscles may result in dysphagia, dysphonia or regurgitation. Pyrexia may be present in inflammatory myopathies or be associated with aspiration pneumonia as a result of megaoesophagus.

Diagnostic procedures

A thorough physical, neurological and orthopaedic examination should be performed including gait evaluation. Routine laboratory analysis of blood should include serum creatine kinase (CK), electrolytes, and lactate and pyruvate concentrations. Further special testing would include thyroid evaluation and measurement of serum acetylcholine receptor antibodies (see the *BSAVA Manual of Canine and Feline Clinical Pathology*). If available, electromyography and measurement of nerve conduction velocities can be very useful. Assessment of a muscle biopsy specimen is the single most important diagnostic test for evaluation of muscle diseases.

Myopathies

Myopathies may be classified as inflammatory or non-inflammatory. Inflammatory myopathies (IMs) include generalized diseases, such as polymyositis and dermatomyositis, and focal IMs, such as extraocular and masticatory muscle myositis. Non-inflammatory myopathies include muscular dystrophies, steroid myopathy, endocrine myopathies associated with hypothyroidism and Cushing's syndrome, metabolic myopathies associated with disorders of energy production (including glycogen, lipid and mitochondrial metabolism) and myotonic myopathies.

Inflammatory myopathies

IMs are a result of infiltration of inflammatory cells into striated muscle (Figure 8.17). This discussion will include only the generalized IMs; reviews of canine IMs have recently been published (Podell, 2002; Evans *et al.*, 2004). The prognosis for most of these disorders is favourable if they are diagnosed early in the course of the disease and treated appropriately. If there is a delay in reaching a diagnosis, or if therapy is inappropriate, severe loss of muscle mass (Figure 8.18) and irreversible fibrosis may result in limb deformities or contractures.

Clinical signs highly suggestive of generalized IMs include a stiff, stilted gait or an unexplained lameness in the absence of detectable orthopaedic abnormalities. CK levels are persistently elevated, mildly to moderately (10–20 times normal values); *persistently elevated serum CK concentrations must not be ignored*. Muscle pain may not be a prominent clinical sign (Evans *et al.*, 2004) although the presence of inflammation in muscle biopsy specimens suggests that this should be the case. Affected animals will have progressive muscle atrophy.

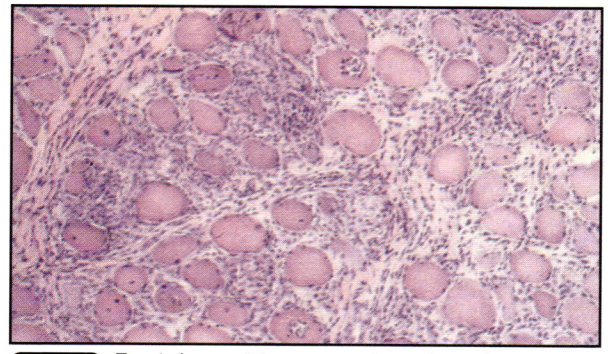

8.17 Fresh frozen biopsy specimen from the vastus lateralis muscle of a dog with chronic inflammatory myopathy. There is myofibre loss and atrophy, endomysial fibrosis, and diffuse mononuclear cell infiltration with a perimysial and endomysial distribution (invasion of non-necrotic fibres). (H&E stain; original magnification X100)

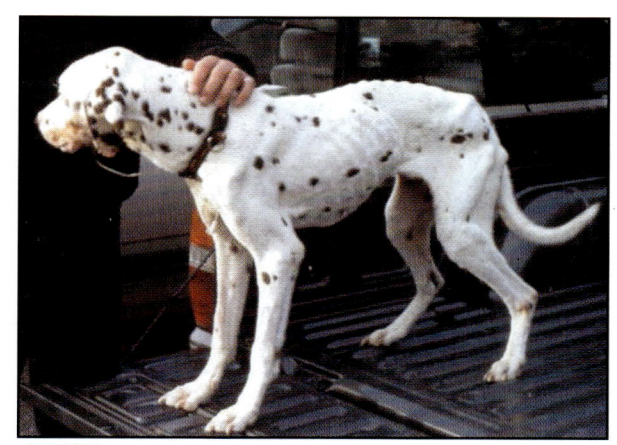

Chapter 8b Diseases of muscle and the neuromuscular junction

8.18 Severe loss of muscle mass in a Dalmatian with chronic inflammatory myopathy.

The single most important diagnostic procedure is muscle biopsy (Dickinson and LeCouteur, 2002). As cellular infiltrates may have a patchy multifocal distribution, biopsy specimens should be taken from at least two different muscles. Muscle biopsy is relatively innocuous and well tolerated. For suspected myopathies, specimens should be taken, using an open biopsy procedure, from large proximal limb muscles such as the triceps brachii from the thoracic limb and the vastus lateralis or biceps femoris muscles from the pelvic limb. Following a histological diagnosis of inflammatory myopathy further investigations and therapies can be undertaken (Figure 8.19).

- Serum antibody titres against infections (e.g. *Toxoplasma gondii*, *Neospora caninum*, tick-related disorders) are assessed. An infectious aetiology for IMs may be more common than previously thought (Evans *et al.*, 2004).
- Screening thoracic and abdominal radiographs are taken for evidence of oesophageal dilatation, aspiration pneumonia and neoplasia.
- Specific therapy is administered for an infectious agent or neoplasia if identified.
- If there is no evidence of an infectious agent or neoplasia, immunosuppressive therapy with prednisolone is initiated at 2 mg/kg q12h orally. Serum CK concentration is monitored until within the normal range. When clinical signs are controlled, the prednisolone is gradually decreased to the lowest alternate day dosage that will keep the dog free of clinical signs. Long-term therapy may be required.
- A fentanyl patch (25–50 μg/hour) is recommended for pain relief during the first few days of treatment.
- If aspiration pneumonia is present, appropriate systemic bactericidal antibiotics are given for 24 hours before the onset of corticosteroid therapy.

8.19 Further investigations and possible therapeutic options for inflammatory myopathies.

Non-inflammatory myopathies

Muscular dystrophies

Muscular dystrophies are a heterogenous group of inherited degenerative mostly non-inflammatory disorders, characterized by progressive muscle weakness and wasting (Shelton and Engvall, 2002). A dystrophic myopathy should be considered in any young dog or cat (male or female, mixed breed or purebred) with persistent muscle weakness, muscle atrophy or hypertrophy, gait abnormality or contractures beginning in the first few months of life. For most disorders that have been identified, neither a cure nor a specific therapy is yet available. It is important to obtain a correct diagnosis because most dystrophic myopathies occur in purebred animals and knowledge of inheritance patterns is of utmost importance to animal breeders.

Clinical signs of muscular dystrophy include weakness and muscle atrophy or hypertrophy beginning in the first few months of life (Figure 8.20). Affected animals may have dramatically and persistently elevated serum CK concentrations (10–100 times normal values). The muscle biopsy is critical for confirmation of the diagnosis and shows a typical dystrophic phenotype, which includes myofibre degeneration, regeneration and fibrosis (Figure 8.21). Calcific deposits are found in tissues (Figures 8.21 and 8.22). Immunohistochemical evaluation of the expression of relevant muscle proteins, including dystrophin, dystrophin-associated proteins, laminins and other proteins (Figure 8.23), may

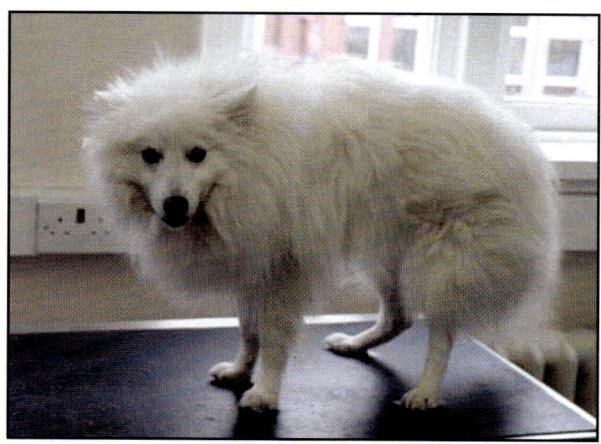

8.20 Young Japanese Spitz diagnosed with muscular dystrophy associated with a truncated form of dystrophin. Note the hunched posture with pelvic limbs tucked under the body. (Courtesy of Dr Boyd Jones)

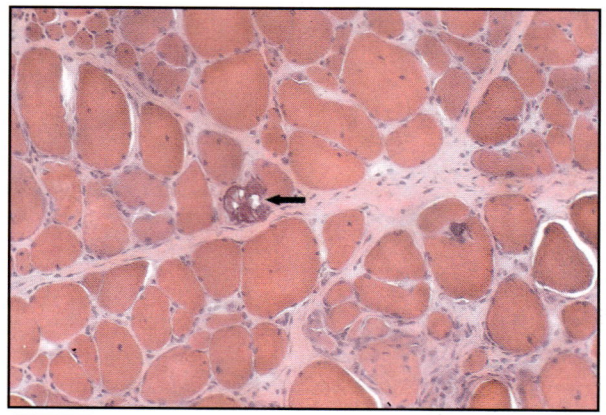

8.21 Fresh frozen biopsy specimen from the biceps femoris muscle of a 10-month-old DSH cat with clinical signs of muscle weakness and hypertrophy from an early age. There is variation in myofibre size, endomysial fibrosis and degenerating fibres; a calcific deposit is arrowed. (H&E stain; original magnification X100)

121

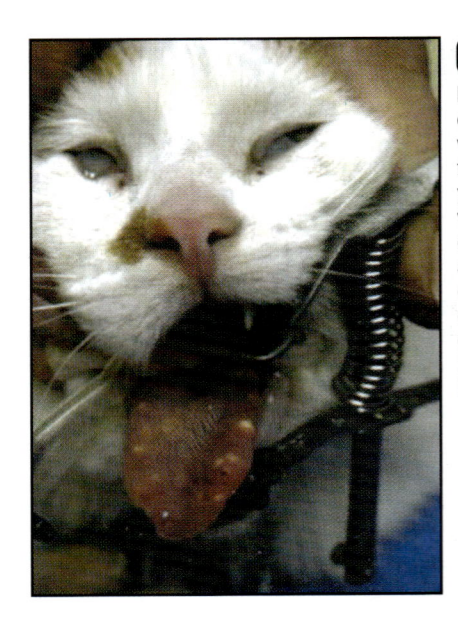

Chapter 8b Diseases of muscle and the neuromuscular junction

8.22 Numerous calcific deposits were found on the tongue of a young DSH cat with muscular dystrophy associated with dystrophin deficiency. (Courtesy of Dr Randy Longshore)

determine the type of muscular dystrophy and direct specific mutational analyses. This is a cost-effective and sensitive method, which can be performed directly on freshly frozen muscle biopsy specimens.

The most common form of muscular dystrophy described in humans is Duchenne muscular dystrophy, caused by a lack of the muscle protein dystrophin. A major reason why Duchenne muscular dystrophy is the most common is the extremely large size of the dystrophin gene, making it the target of more frequent mutations than a smaller gene. This may also be the case for dystrophies affecting dogs and cats, although few have been described and precise classifications are only in the early stages. Recently, congenital muscular dystrophies have been identified in dogs and cats associated with deficiency of merosin (laminin α-2) (O'Brien *et al.*, 2001; Poncelet *et al.*, 2003), and in dogs associated with deficiency of sarcoglycans (Schatzberg and Shelton, 2004). Muscular dystrophies described to date in dogs and cats are listed in Figure 8.24.

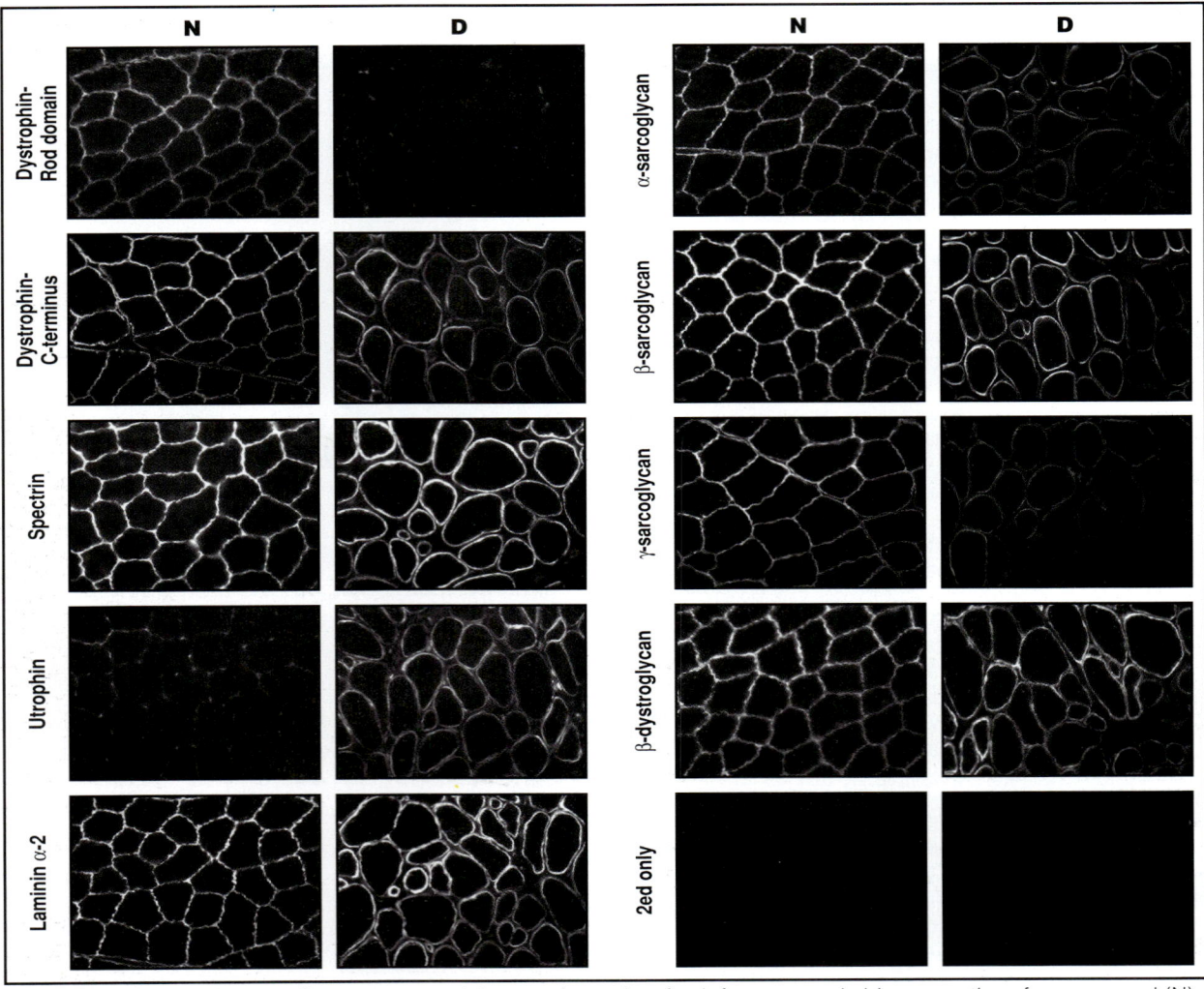

8.23 Example of immunofluorescence stainings performed on fresh frozen muscle biopsy sections from a normal (N) and a dystrophic (D) dog for the clinical diagnosis of different forms of muscular dystrophy. Samples from the dystrophic dog show an absence of staining for the rod domain of dystrophin with near normal staining for the carboxy terminus. Staining for α and γ sarcoglycans is decreased. Staining for utrophin is more intense than for the normal dog, suggesting overexpression. Normal staining for spectrin is present confirming the presence of membrane integrity (Jones *et al.*, 2004).

Chapter 8b Diseases of muscle and the neuromuscular junction

Muscular dystrophy	Pathogenesis	Animals affected	Clinical signs	Clinical pathology	Treatment	Heritability?
Dystrophin-deficient muscular dystrophy in dogs (see Figure 8.20) and cats (see Figure 8.22)	Dystrophin links myofibre cytoskeleton to extracellular matrix and is crucial in stabilization of muscle fibre membranes during contraction	Several breeds of dog Mixed-breed dogs Cats (Shelton and Engvall, 2002; Schatzberg and Shelton, 2004)	Dysphagia, regurgitation and dyspnoea may occur as a result of hypertrophy of the lingual, pharyngeal and oesophageal musculature and the diaphragm. Cardiomyopathy may result in heart failure	Serum CK is dramatically elevated (may be 100X normal values). Diagnosis is confirmed by demonstration of the dystrophic phenotype on muscle biopsy and lack of membrane dystrophin on immunohistochemical staining	No specific therapy available. Prognosis poor	X-linked disorder that typically affects males. Females can be affected if a carrier female is bred to an affected male. Affected animals should not be used in a breeding programme
Merosin (laminin α-2) deficiency in dogs and cats (Figure 8.25)	Laminin α-2 is the major component of the basal lamina that surrounds each muscle fibre	Brittany and Springer Spaniels Flame point Siamese cat DSH cat (O'Brien et al., 2001; Poncelet et al., 2003)	Muscle weakness and atrophy, or stiffness and rigidity	Serum CK is moderately elevated (10–20X normal values). Dystrophic phenotype is confirmed by muscle biopsy and exact classification determined by immunohistochemical staining showing an absence of laminin α-2	No specific therapy available. Prognosis poor	Unknown, but likely autosomal recessive
Sarcoglycan deficiency in dogs	The sarcoglycan (SG) complex spans the sarcolemmal membrane, bridging dystrophin and the dystroglycan complex in muscle. Mutations in the SG complex result in limb girdle muscular dystrophies in humans	Boston Terrier Cocker Spaniel Chihuahua (Schatzberg and Shelton, 2004)	Presenting clinical signs are similar to those of dystrophin-deficient muscular dystrophy	Serum CK is dramatically elevated (100X normal values). Diagnosis is confirmed by muscle biopsy and demonstration of reduced or absent SG complex on immunohistochemical staining	No specific treatment available. Prognosis poor	Unknown, but likely autosomal recessive

8.24 Muscular dystrophies in dogs and cats.

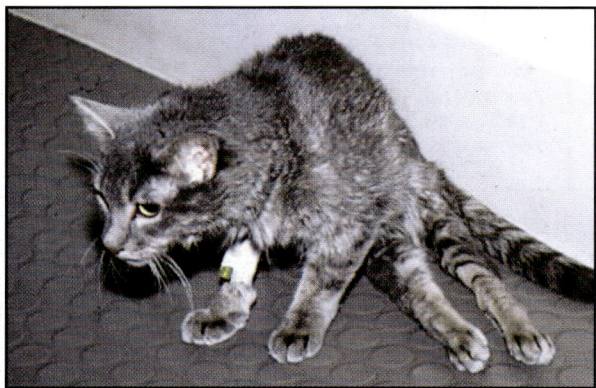

8.25 Muscle contracture resulted in pelvic limb stiffness and rigidity in a young cat with congenital muscular dystrophy resulting from a deficiency of laminin α-2 (merosin). (Courtesy of Dr Dennis O'Brien)

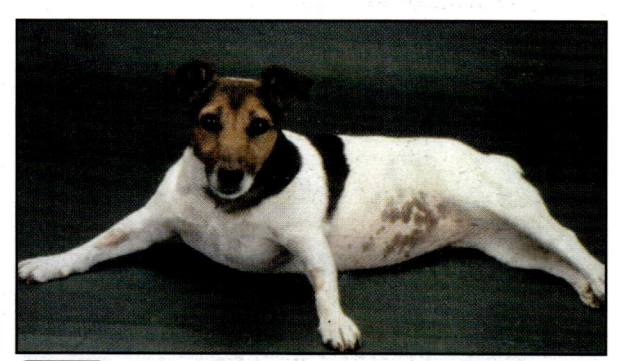

8.26 A 10-year-old female spayed Jack Russell Terrier with pelvic limb spasticity and proximal muscle hypertrophy associated with Cushing's syndrome. Electrophysiology was consistent with a myotonia associated with this endocrine disorder. (Courtesy of Dr Mark Jackson)

Endocrine disorders

Weakness, stiffness, myalgia and lameness occur relatively commonly in endocrine disorders (Figure 8.26), particularly in geriatric animals (Platt, 2002). In some affected dogs and cats, muscle involvement may be an incidental finding or may be subclinical. In other cases, muscle weakness or stiffness may be the first clinical sign of an underlying endocrine disorder and may lead to a diagnosis. It is important to remember that the most common clinical presentations of endocrine disorders, such as the overweight, heat-seeking dog in hypothyroidism, do not have to be present. The most common endocrine disorders that can result in myopathic clinical signs are summarized in Figure 8.27.

123

Chapter 8b Diseases of muscle and the neuromuscular junction

Endocrinopathy	Clinical signs	Results of investigations	Treatment and prognosis	Comments
Glucocorticoid excess: exogenous corticosteroid therapy (iatrogenic steroid myopathy) or endogenous Cushing's syndrome	**Steroid myopathy:** weakness and muscle atrophy may be profound **Cushing's syndrome:** muscle atrophy and weakness. Severe pelvic limb rigidity and clinical myotonia have been found (see Figure 8.26.) Unilateral limb stiffness that can progress to involvement of all limbs may be an initial clinical sign	Type 2 fibre atrophy is a consistent finding in muscle biopsy specimens from dogs with steroid myopathy or spontaneous Cushing's syndrome	**Steroid myopathy:** The treatment of choice is dose reduction if the underlying condition is controlled. Exercise may partially prevent the development of weakness **Cushing's syndrome:** Muscle weakness and atrophy improve with specific therapy for Cushing's syndrome. The prognosis for resolution of clinical myotonia has not been as favourable	Muscle atrophy resulting from exogenous corticosteroid therapy should be reversible once treatment is discontinued
Hypothyroidism	Classical clinical signs (e.g. lethargy, weight gain, seborrhoea, alopecia) may or may not be obvious. Weakness, stiffness and myalgia may be the initial presenting clinical signs. A neuropathy has also been described	Serum CK may be mildly elevated if muscle necrosis is present	Prognosis for recovery of muscle strength in hypothyroid myopathy is excellent once a euthyroid state is restored	Although there are no long-term studies of the response of neuropathy to thyroid replacement, it is this author's opinion that the prognosis for recovery is not as favourable
Hyperthyroidism in cats	Clinical signs of muscle weakness in hyperthyroid cats include neck ventroflexion, tremors, fatigue, gait disturbances, decreased ability to jump and breathlessness after exertion	Serum CK may be markedly elevated with normal muscle biopsy. Hypokalaemia may be a complicating factor	Prognosis is good for resolution of muscle weakness following treatment to achieve a euthyroid state	Reversible myasthenia gravis with autoantibodies to acetylcholine receptors (AChRs) may occur in a small percentage of cats treated with methimazole. Weakness should resolve and the anti-AChR antibody titres return to the normal range following discontinuation of the drug
Hypoadrenocorticism (Addison's disease)	Muscle weakness occurs frequently in association with hypoadrenocorticism in dogs and cats. The weakness is usually generalized but may selectively involve the pharyngeal or oesophageal musculature	Hyperkalaemia and hyponatraemia. Minimal or no response to stimulation with ACTH	Correction of the electrolyte imbalance and glucocorticoid deficiency usually results in resolution of clinical weakness	Although hypoadrenocorticism classically includes mineralocorticoid and glucocorticoid deficiency, an atypical form with a deficiency of glucocorticoids alone and normal concentrations of sodium and/or potassium has been described. Because reversible megaoesophagus has been associated with this atypical form, all dogs with an unexplained megaoesophagus should be tested for glucocorticoid deficiency
Hyperinsulinism secondary to pancreatic islet cell tumours	Weakness and collapse may be a result of profound hypoglycaemia, although the most prominent clinical signs are related to the central nervous system. In rare cases insulinoma produces clinical signs of peripheral neuropathy	Hypoglycaemia	In general, prognosis for complete remission and recovery from an accompanying peripheral neuropathy, even with surgical intervention, is poor	Pancreatic islet cell carcinoma is a relatively common neoplasm in middle-aged to older dogs

8.27 Common endocrine disorders that can result in myopathic clinical signs.

Metabolic disorders

Metabolic myopathies make up a diverse group of disorders caused by biochemical defects of the skeletal muscle energy-generating systems (Platt, 2002). These disorders can result in poor exercise tolerance, myalgia, atrophy, cramping and myoglobinuria. The biochemical defects primarily affect ATP production. Relatively few of these disorders have been characterized in veterinary medicine. In the dog, the presence of predominantly oxidative muscle fibre types, in the absence of classical type 2B fibres (purely glycolytic), may make clinical presentations associated with aberrant glycogen metabolism difficult to recognize. Clinical signs may be referable to abnormalities in other body systems that can overshadow muscle-associated weakness. A good example of this is phosphofructokinase deficiency in Springer Spaniels, in which the primary clinical signs are associated with haemolytic anaemia. Elevated CK concentrations and glycogen deposits in muscle biopsy specimens from affected dogs support a concurrent myopathy. The following defects of glycogen metabolism have been confirmed:

- Glycogenosis type II in Lapland dogs
- Glycogenosis type III in German Shepherd Dogs and Akitas
- Glycogenosis type IV in Norwegian Forest cats
- Glycogenosis type VII (phosphofructokinase deficiency) in English Springer Spaniels and American Cocker Spaniels.

Chapter 8b Diseases of muscle and the neuromuscular junction

The highly oxidative nature of canine muscle may predispose dogs to disorders of oxidative metabolism, including mitochondrial myopathies and disorders of fatty acid oxidation, or of carnitine metabolism. Although confirming a diagnosis of a defect in oxidative metabolism may be difficult, evaluation of plasma lactic and pyruvic acid concentrations (Platt and Garosi, 2004) and muscle biopsy specimens should be helpful diagnostic procedures. To date, the following disorders have been confirmed or suspected in dogs:

- Pyruvate dehydrogenase (PDH) deficiency
- Mitochondrial myopathy
- Lipid storage myopathy.

PDH deficiency has been confirmed in Clumber and Sussex Spaniels (Platt, 2002; Abramson *et al.*, 2004). Clinical presentation is one of exercise intolerance. A presumptive diagnosis can be made by demonstration of marked elevations in plasma lactate and pyruvate concentrations with a lactate:pyruvate ratio <10. Confirmation of PDH deficiency is made through measuring enzyme activity in cultured fibroblasts. Although no specific therapy is available, dietary modifications, including feeding a high-fat, low-carbohydrate diet and addition of thiamine, may be of some benefit (Abramson *et al.*, 2004).

Mitochondrial myopathy associated with altered cytochrome C oxidase activity and reduced mitochondrial DNA was documented in Old English Sheepdog littermates with exercise intolerance.

Lipid storage myopathy has been described in dogs but the precise biochemical defect(s) have not yet been characterized. The clinical presentation is variable and includes muscle atrophy, weakness, and, in some cases, dramatic myalgia. Lactic acidaemia is found in most dogs with lipid storage myopathy. Diagnosis is confirmed by identification of numerous, large lipid droplets within muscle fibres. Therapy includes supplementation of L-carnitine (50 mg/kg q12h), coenzyme Q_{10} (100 mg q24h) and B vitamins.

Diseases resulting in myotonia

Myotonia is a myogenic condition defined as prolonged contraction or delayed relaxation of a muscle after voluntary movement or after mechanical or electrical stimulation. Myotonia is characterized by muscle stiffness without cramping (action myotonia), muscle dimpling after being struck by a reflex hammer (percussion myotonia) and characteristic EMG changes (myotonic discharges). Diseases resulting in myotonia may be associated with diminished sarcolemmal chloride conductance, altered sodium channel inactivation, from unknown mechanisms associated with myotonic dystrophy, and with various metabolic conditions and intoxications. Vite (2002) provides an in-depth review of myotonia and disorders of muscle cell membrane excitability.

Myotonia congenita: This condition has been reported in dogs and cats:

- Chow-Chows affected with myotonia congenita present with evident muscle stiffness soon after pups become ambulatory. The clinical signs of muscle stiffness diminish with exercise
- In the Miniature Schnauzer myotonia congenita is inherited as an autosomal recessive trait (Figure 8.28). The mutation has been identified and has been shown to be a result of a mis-sense mutation in both alleles of the gene encoding the skeletal muscle voltage-dependent chloride channel C1C-1. A DNA-based test capable of detecting the mutant allele in affected and carrier Miniature Schnauzers has been developed and is available at the Josephine Deubler Genetic Testing Laboratory of the University of Pennsylvania (www.vet.upenn.edu/penngen)
- Myotonia congenita has also been described in domestic cats, although the mode of inheritance and molecular defect have not been determined.

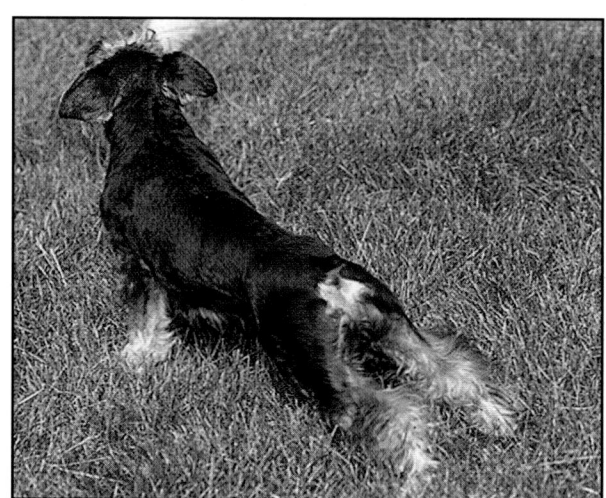

8.28 Muscle stiffness observed in a young Miniature Schnauzer with myotonia congenita. This condition is inherited as an autosomal recessive trait in this breed.

Treatment for myotonia congenita is directed at decreasing repetitive activity in muscle by using antagonists to voltage-gated sodium channels. These drugs include procainamide, quinidine, phenytoin and mexiletine. Certain drugs have been reported to worsen myotonia congenita and should be avoided. These include dantrolene, beta-blocking adrenergic agents, fenoterol, diuretics, monocarboxylic aromatic acids, cholesterol-lowering drugs, depolarizing muscle relaxants and anaesthetics acting on the sarcolemma or end plate, including decamethonium, succinylcholine, neostigmine and physostigmine. Bromide may also be contraindicated (Vite, 2002).

Miscellaneous non-inflammatory disorders

Scattered reports of breed-associated, non-dystrophic myopathies affecting young dogs are to be found in the literature (Shelton and Engvall, 2002). Hereditary myopathy of Labrador Retrievers (HMLR) (Figure 8.29) has recently been shown to be associated with the same genetic mutation as centronuclear-like myopathy (CLM) described in the French Labrador Retriever pedigree (Tiret *et al.*, 2003). A genetic test is

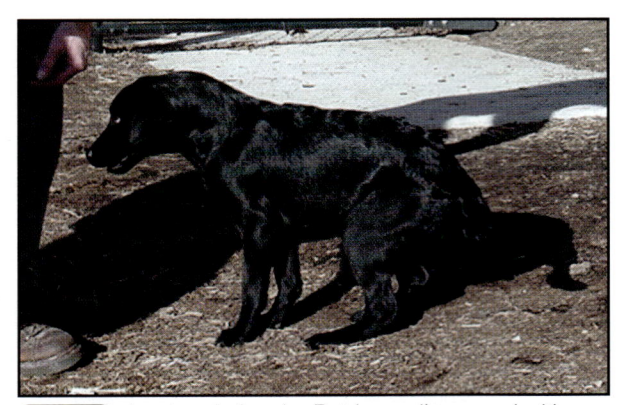

Chapter 8b Diseases of muscle and the neuromuscular junction

8.29 A young Labrador Retriever diagnosed with hereditary myopathy. The puppy is looking up with its eyes as its neck muscles are too weak to lift its head. (Courtesy of Drs Joan Coates and Dennis O'Brien)

now available for this myopathy and to detect carriers (www.labradorcnm.com). These disorders can be readily distinguished from dystrophin-deficient muscular dystrophy, which also occurs in this breed, by the serum CK concentration (markedly elevated in dystrophin deficiency and only mildly elevated in HMLR and CLM) and by immunohistochemical staining of muscle biopsy specimens for dystrophin (normal staining in HMLR and CLM).

For comparative purposes, the previously described 'central-core' like myopathy (Targett *et al.*, 1994) occurring in the Great Dane has been reclassified as 'inherited myopathy of the Great Dane' (IMGD) with distinct histological features (Lujan Feliu-Pascual, in press). The clinical presentation of muscle weakness and atrophy in this breed with age of onset less than 1 year, combined with typical pathological changes on muscle biopsy specimens, should make this diagnosis relatively straightforward.

Disorders of neuromuscular transmission

Myasthenia gravis
Myasthenia gravis is caused by an autoimmune attack against nicotinic acetylcholine receptors, which results in depletion of post-synaptic receptors. It is the most completely characterized autoimmune disease affecting the neuromuscular system, and probably the most completely characterized autoimmune disease in general. For a general review of this topic see Shelton (2002). In the author's opinion, acquired myasthenia gravis is the most common neuromuscular disease that can be diagnosed and treated in dogs. Clinicians should become familiar with the spectrum of clinical signs, as dogs with myasthenia gravis have been initially misdiagnosed with disc disease or acute abdominal crisis, and undergone anaesthesia and surgical procedures that could potentially exacerbate the myasthenic condition. Although less common in cats, myasthenia gravis should also be considered in any cat that is presented with a recent onset of muscular weakness.

Clinical forms of acquired myasthenia gravis include:

- Focal myasthenia gravis, including oesophageal dilation and pharyngeal weakness without clinically detectable limb muscle weakness. This is seen in 43% of cases (Shelton *et al.*, 1997). Laryngeal paralysis alone, in the absence of oesophageal or pharyngeal weakness, has not been identified in myasthenia gravis
- Generalized weakness, present in 57% of cases with or without oesophageal or pharyngeal dysfunction (Shelton *et al.*, 1997). The absence of a megaoesophagus cannot eliminate the diagnosis of acquired myasthenia gravis; these dogs are sometimes misdiagnosed with disc disease
- Acute fulminating generalized myasthenia gravis can occur in a small number of cases and these require intensive care, including ventilatory support

Similar clinical forms occur in cats. Cranial mediastinal masses are more common in cats (25%) (Shelton *et al.*, 2000) than in dogs (3%). Diagnosis of acquired myasthenia gravis is described in Figure 8.30.

Demonstration of circulating serum anti-acetylcholine receptor antibodies

Immunoprecipitation radioimmunoassay continues to be the gold standard for the diagnosis of acquired myasthenia gravis in both dogs and cats. This test is sensitive, specific and documents an autoimmune response

Edrophonium chloride challenge test

A dramatic response would give a presumptive diagnosis of myasthenia gravis, and therapy can be initiated. False-positive and false-negative results can occur. A negative test should not rule out a diagnosis of myasthenia gravis

Compound muscle action potential (CMAP)

A decrease in the amplitude of the CMAP in response to repetitive nerve stimulation can also provide a presumptive diagnosis of myasthenia gravis; however, there is a lack of sensitivity and specificity, in addition to the requirement for general anaesthesia in a possibly critical patient

Single-fibre EMG

This is a sensitive method for detecting delayed or failed neuromuscular transmission, and a methodology has been established for the dog. Specificity is lacking, with positive findings in other disorders of the nerve, muscle and neuromuscular junction. This procedure is also technically difficult and not performed routinely even in speciality neurology practices

8.30 Diagnosis of acquired myasthenia gravis.

An early and accurate diagnosis of acquired myasthenia gravis, followed by appropriate therapy, is the most important factor in obtaining a good clinical outcome. If megaoesophagus is present, altered feeding procedures (elevation of food and water or placement of a gastrostomy tube) are critical for nutritional support, hydration and drug delivery. Anticholinesterase drugs are the cornerstone of therapy. Available drugs include pyridostigmine (1–3 mg/kg orally q8–12h) and neostigmine (2 mg/kg/day orally in divided doses to effect). Pyridostigmine has fewer cholinergic side effects than neostigmine. If an optimal response to therapy is not obtained with supportive care and anticholinesterase drugs alone, low-dose prednisolone therapy is suggested. Immunosuppressive dosages of prednisolone should be avoided early in the course of treatment as increased weakness often occurs, requiring hospitalization and sometimes intensive medical care with respiratory support (Shelton, 2002).

In the absence of immunosuppression, determination of serial anti-acetylcholine receptor antibody titres is a good indicator of disease status and helps to determine duration of therapy. Treatment should be continued while anti-acetylcholine receptor antibody titres are positive. In dogs, in the absence of immunosuppression, there is an excellent correlation between resolution of clinical signs, including megaoesophagus, and return of anti-acetylcholine receptor antibody titres to the normal range (Shelton and Lindstrom, 2001). Spontaneous remissions frequently occur in canine myasthenia gravis (Shelton *et al.*, 2000), but whether this is also the natural course of the disease in feline myasthenia gravis is yet to be evaluated.

Miscellaneous disorders of neuromuscular transmission

Other disorders of neuromuscular transmission encountered in practice include tick paralysis and botulism, organophosphate intoxication in the cat and drug-induced neuromuscular blockade (Shelton, 2002). These disorders should result in a fairly rapid onset of lower motor neuron tetraparesis and would probably not be a consideration for the lame dog or cat.

References and further reading

Abramson CJ, Platt SR and Shelton GD (2004) Pyruvate dehydrogenase deficiency in a Sussex spaniel. *Journal of Small Animal Practice* **45**, 162–165

Dickinson PJ and LeCouteur RA (2002) Muscle and nerve biopsy. *Veterinary Clinics of North America: Small Animal Practice* **32**, 63–102

Evans J, Levesque D and Shelton GD (2004) Canine inflammatory myopathies: a clinicopathologic review of 200 cases. *Journal of Veterinary Internal Medicine* **18(5)**, 679–691

Jones BR, Brennan S, Mooney CT *et al.* (2004) Muscular dystrophy with truncated dystrophin in a family of Japanese Spitz dogs. *Journal of the Neurological Sciences* **217**, 143–149

Lujan Feliu-Pascal A, Shelton GD, Targett MP *et al.* (in press) Inherited myopathy of Great Dane (IMGD) dogs with distinct histological features. *Journal of Small Animal Practice*

O'Brien, Johnson GC, Liu LA *et al.* (2001) Laminin α2 (merosin)-deficient muscular dystrophy and demyelinating neuropathy in two cats. *Journal of the Neurological Sciences* **189**, 37–43

Olby NJ (2005) Laboratory evaluation of muscle disorders. In: *BSAVA Manual of Canine and Feline Clinical Pathology, 2nd edn,* ed. E Villiers and L Blackwood, pp. 364–72. BSAVA Publications, Gloucester

Platt SR (2002) Neuromuscular complications in endocrine and metabolic disorders. *Veterinary Clinics of North America: Small Animal Practice* **32**, 125–146

Platt SR and Olby NJ (eds) (2004) *BSAVA Manual of Canine and Feline Neurology, 3rd edn.* BSAVA Publications, Gloucester

Platt SR and Garosi LS (2004) Neuromuscular weakness and collapse. *Veterinary Clinics of North America: Small Animal Practice* **34(6)**, 1281–1306

Podell M (2002) Inflammatory myopathies. *Veterinary Clinics of North America: Small Animal Practice* **32**, 147–167

Poncelet L, Resibois A, Engvall E and Shelton GD (2003) Laminin α2 deficiency-associated muscular dystrophy in a Maine coon cat. *Journal of Small Animal Practice* **44**, 550–552

Schatzberg SJ and Shelton GD (2004) Newly identified neuromuscular disorders. *Veterinary Clinics of North America: Small Animal Practice* **34(6)**, 1497–1524

Shelton GD (2002) Myasthenia gravis and disorders of neuromuscular transmission. *Veterinary Clinics of North America: Small Animal Practice* **32**, 189–206

Shelton GD and Engvall E (2002) Muscular dystrophies and other inherited myopathies. *Veterinary Clinics of North America: Small Animal Practice* **32**, 103–124

Shelton GD, Ho M and Kass PH (2000) Risk factors for acquired myasthenia gravis in cats: 105 cases (1986–1998). *Journal of the American Veterinary Medical Association* **216**, 55–57

Shelton GD and Lindstrom JM (2001) Spontaneous remission in canine myasthenia gravis: implications for assessing human myasthenia gravis therapies. *Neurology* **57**, 2139–2141

Shelton GD, Schule A and Kass PH (1997) Risk factors for acquired myasthenia gravis in dogs: 1,154 cases (1991–1995). *Journal of the American Veterinary Medical Association* **211**, 1428–1431

Targett MP, Franklin RJM, Olby NJ and Houlton JEF (1994) Central core myopathy in a Great Dane. *Journal of Small Animal Practice* **35**, 100–103

Tiret L, Blot S, Kessler JL *et al.* (2003) The cnm locus, a canine homologue of human autosomal forms of centronuclear myopathy, maps to chromosome 2. *Human Genetics* **113**, 297–306

Vite CH (2002) Myotonia and disorders of altered muscle cell membrane excitability. *Veterinary Clinics of North America: Small Animal Practice* **32**, 169–187

9

Tumours of the musculoskeletal system

B. Duncan X. Lascelles

Introduction

The musculoskeletal system comprises the bones, joints, muscles, nerves and associated structures that are concerned with locomotion. As such, there are many different tumour types that can result in lameness. The most common tumours of the musculoskeletal system presenting as lameness cases are primary bone tumours of the appendicular system, followed by joint tumours of the appendicular system. This chapter covers these tumours. As a summary, Figures 9.1 and 9.2 outline the tumour types of the musculoskeletal system, their clinical features, biological behaviour and broad treatment options in dogs and cats. Readers are referred to the *BSAVA Manual of Canine and Feline Oncology* for information regarding primary muscle tumours (Kirpensteijn and Rutteman, 2003) and axial skeletal tumours and less common appendicular skeletal tumours (Dernell, 2003). Readers are also referred to the *BSAVA Manual of Canine and Feline Oncology* for information regarding the control of pain associated with tumours of the musculoskeletal system (Lascelles, 2003). Tumours of the peripheral nerves that result in locomotor interference are covered in Chapter 10 and in the *BSAVA Manual of Canine and Feline Oncology* (Jeffery, 2003).

Tumour type	Clinical features	Biological behaviour	Treatment options
Primary muscle tumours			
Rhabdomyosarcoma	Striated muscle	Locally aggressive; early metastasis	Surgical resection
Haemangiosarcoma	Any muscle can be affected	Locally invasive; presumed highly metastatic	Surgical resection with adjuvant chemotherapy
Joint tumours			
Synovial cell sarcoma	Mainly stifle, tarsus, elbow and carpus	Locally aggressive; variable (low) metastasis	Amputation; chemotherapy
Histiocytic sarcoma	Mainly stifle and tarsus	Locally aggressive; highly metastatic	Amputation; chemotherapy
Synovial myxomas	Mainly stifle, carpus, tarsus	Locally invasive; low to no metastatic potential	Amputation
Other sarcomas of the synovium (malignant fibrous histiocytoma, fibrosarcoma, chondrosarcoma, undifferentiated sarcoma)	Mainly stifle and tarsus	Locally aggressive; variable metastasis	Amputation; chemotherapy
Primary bone tumours			
Endosteal osteosarcoma	Appendicular skeleton, metaphyseal locations	90% have micrometastases at presentation	Surgery with adjuvant chemotherapy; radiation
Periosteal osteosarcoma	Appendicular or axial skeleton	Locally invasive; highly metastatic	Surgery with adjuvant chemotherapy; radiation
Parosteal or juxtacortical osteosarcoma	Appendicular or axial skeleton	Minimally invasive, variable (low) metastasis	Surgical resection
Chondrosarcoma	Mainly axial skeleton	Locally invasive, moderate metastasis	Surgical resection; adjuvant chemotherapy

9.1 Tumour type, clinical features, biological behaviour and treatment options for the most common tumours of the musculoskeletal system (muscles, joints, bones) of the dog. (continues) ▶

Chapter 9 Tumours of the musculoskeletal system

Tumour type	Clinical features	Biological behaviour	Treatment options
Primary bone tumours (continued)			
Haemangiosarcoma	Appendicular skeleton, variable locations	90% have micrometastases at presentation	Surgery with adjuvant chemotherapy
Fibrosarcoma	Appendicular	Locally invasive, low to moderate metastasis	Surgical resection; chemotherapy; radiation therapy
Multilobular osteochondrosarcoma	Axial skeleton, primarily skull	Low to moderate invasion, low metastasis	Surgical resection
Bone cysts	Metaphyseal locations, long bones	Non-invasive, benign	Surgical curettage with stabilization
Multiple cartilaginous exostoses	Any skeletal site	Benign; rare transformation to malignant type	None or surgical cytoreduction
Osteoma	Axial skeleton	Non-invasive	None or surgical cytoreduction

9.1 (continued) Tumour type, clinical features, biological behaviour and treatment options for the most common tumours of the musculoskeletal system (muscles, joints, bones) of the dog.

Tumour type	Clinical features	Biological behaviour	Treatment options
Osteosarcoma	Appendicular or axial skeleton, variable sites	Locally invasive, low metastasis	Surgical resection, adjuvant chemotherapy for axial lesions
Multiple cartilaginous exostoses (osteochondromas)	Any skeletal site, especially vertebrae; feline leukaemia virus positive	Local invasion, malignant transformation	None or surgical removal for palliation

9.2 Tumour type, clinical features, biological behaviour and treatment options for the most common tumours of the musculoskeletal system (muscles, joints, bones) of the cat.

Canine primary bone osteosarcoma

Osteosarcoma (OSA) accounts for up to 85% of malignancies originating in the skeleton, and primary OSA accounts for approximately 5% of all canine tumours. The most common sites for primary OSA are the long bones of the thoracic and pelvic limbs. The metaphyseal region of long bones is the most common primary site, with thoracic limbs being affected twice as often as pelvic limbs. The distal radius and proximal humerus are the two most common locations. In the pelvic limbs, the incidence of tumours is fairly evenly distributed between the distal femur, distal tibia and proximal tibia, with the proximal femur a slightly less common site.

OSA is an aggressive tumour, with over 90% of cases having micrometastatic disease at the time of diagnosis.

OSA is largely a disease of middle-aged to older dogs, with a median age of 7 years. There is a large range in age of onset with a small peak in incidence in the 18–24 months age range, although for certain breeds this may not hold true. Increasing weight and, more specifically, height appear to be the most predictive factors for the disease in the dog. The breeds most at risk for OSA are St Bernard, Great Dane, Irish Wolfhound, Scottish Deerhound, Irish Setter, Dobermann, German Shepherd Dog and Golden Retriever. The overall male:female ratio of OSA appears to be fairly equal, with a reported slightly increased incidence in males, although this may not be true for all breeds.

Diagnosis

Very often, a presumptive diagnosis of OSA can be made based on signalment, history, physical examination and radiographic findings. Dogs with OSA usually present with lameness and/or swelling at the primary site. Pain on direct palpation over the site is a very common finding. Onset and, initially, degree of lameness are variable; some will present acutely lame following pathological fracture whilst lameness is mild in others. An associated history of mild recent trauma is not uncommon. Lateral and craniocaudal radiographs should be obtained. The overall radiographic appearance of the bone varies from almost entirely osteoblastic or osteogenic changes (Figure 9.3) to mostly bone lysis. There is often soft tissue extension with an obvious soft tissue swelling. New bone (tumour bone) may form in these areas in a palisading pattern perpendicular to, or radiating from, the axis of the cortex ('sun-burst' effect). As the tumour invades the cortex, the periosteum is elevated and new bone is laid down by the cambium layer. This results in an apparently triangular deposition of dense new bone on the cortex at the periphery of the lesion (Codman's triangle). OSAs do not generally cross articular cartilage, but the tumours may extend into periarticular soft tissues, and adjacent bones are at risk by extension.

OSA can occasionally occur at previous fracture sites and in association with chronic osteomyelitis or other chronic inflammatory processes.

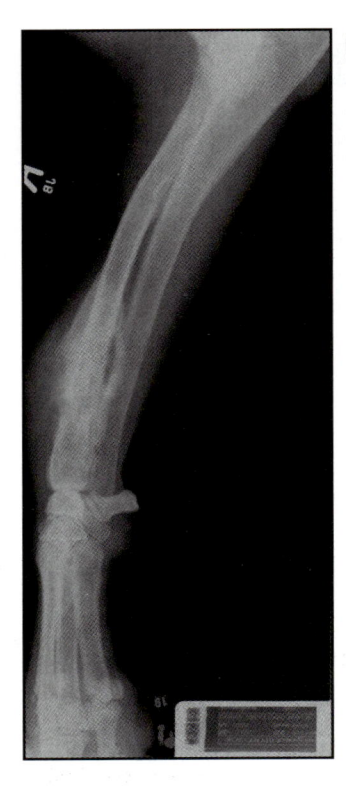

Chapter 9 Tumours of the musculoskeletal system

9.3 Radiographic appearance of a predominantly osteoblastic OSA in a Great Dane.

Biopsy method	Equipment needed	Comments	Accuracy of the technique
Fine needle aspiration	18 or 20 gauge needles	Technique is as for any fine needle aspirate; less likely to get a diagnostic sample in very osteoblastic tumours; minimally invasive; only requires sedation	Approx. 65% conclusive for OSA when OSA present (65% specific); approx. 20% suggestive
Needle core biopsy	Jamshidi needles; trephine needles	More likely to need general anaesthesia; longer processing time; reduced risk of complications seen with open biopsy	Approx. 92% for detecting tumour; approx. 82% (specific) for diagnosing specific tumour type (Powers *et al.*, 1988)
Incisional biopsy	Surgical kit and scalpel, trephine or curette	Large sample can be obtained, increasing sensitivity; disadvantages of an operative procedure; risk of postsurgical complications including pathological fracture	

9.4 Overview of biopsy methods for the diagnosis of appendicular OSA.

Differential diagnoses of lytic, proliferative or mixed pattern aggressive bone lesions identified on radiographs include:

- Other primary bone tumours
- Metastatic bone cancer (e.g. prostate, thyroid)
- Multiple myeloma or lymphoma of bone
- Systemic mycosis with bony localization
- Bacterial osteomyelitis.

If the client is willing to allow treatment based on the presumptive diagnosis, histological confirmation of the presumptive diagnosis following surgical treatment of local disease (amputation or limb sparing) can be considered. Otherwise, a tissue biopsy is indicated (Figure 9.4). When performing a biopsy of bone, the *centre* of the radiographic lesion is chosen for biopsy, as well as more peripheral sites. During the biopsy process, imaging should be used to ensure accurate placement (Figure 9.5). Biopsy at the lesion periphery alone will often result in sampling the reactive bone surrounding the tumour growth. If there is a possibility of limb sparing, the biopsy site should be chosen so as not to interfere with the subsequent approach (during surgical removal, biopsy tracts should be removed and treated as tumour tissue). Material for culture and cytology may be taken from the samples prior to fixation.

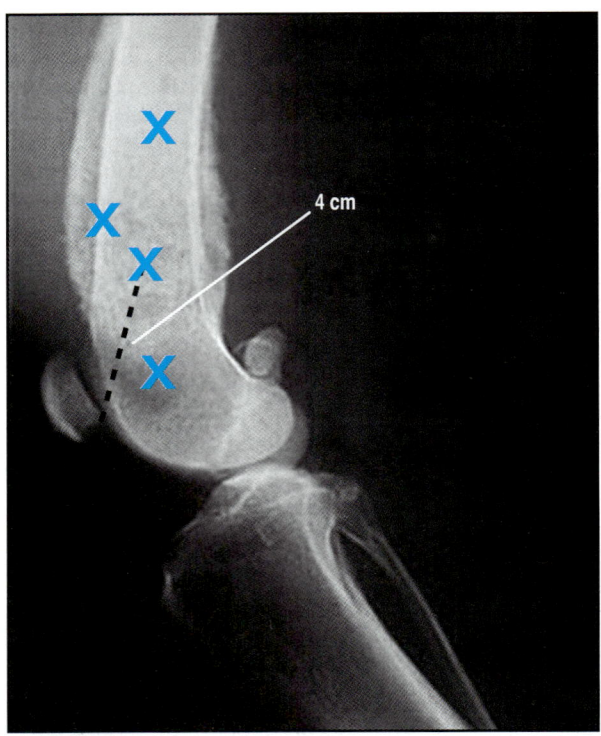

Staging and patient assessment

The presence of detectable metastases is the single most important prognostic indicator, and as such, appropriate 'staging' should be performed. Regional lymph nodes should be palpated and fine needle cytology performed on any enlarged node. Although it is relatively rare to detect pulmonary metastatic disease at the time of diagnosis (<10% of dogs), three

9.5 During the biopsy process, imaging should be used to ensure accurate placement. A measurement is made from an easily palpable landmark (the distal patella in this case) to the centre of the lesion. The dog's leg is placed in the same position as it is on the radiograph, and this measurement is used to locate accurately the centre of the lesion in the dog. A biopsy (or two) is performed at this site. Other sites chosen for biopsy (marked by blue crosses) can be accurately identified in the same manner. For less easily identified locations, a needle can be placed, then a radiograph taken to ensure accurate location of the biopsy instrument. In some centres, fluoroscopy allows accurate placement of biopsy instruments.

Chapter 9 Tumours of the musculoskeletal system

radiographic views of the thorax, including both right and left lateral views, should be taken. Pulmonary metastases cannot be detected radiographically until the nodules are 6–8 mm in diameter. Computed tomography (CT) of the lung may increase detection levels at presentation (Waters *et al.*, 1998) but the sensitivity of CT may result in a number of false-positive results. Not all microscopically detectable lesions are detected by CT; in one study only 44% of metastases ≤5 mm in diameter were detected compared with 91% metastases >5 mm in diameter (Waters *et al.*, 1998). Sites of bone metastasis may be detected by careful orthopaedic examination, bone survey radiography or nuclear scintigraphy (Lamb, 1987). Scintigraphy can also be used to evaluate the degree of bone involvement from a primary bone tumour. It has been demonstrated that scintigraphy overestimates the length of OSA disease by 30%, allowing its use to guide resection safely (Lamb *et al.*, 1990; Leibman *et al.*, 2001).

The patient's overall health status requires careful assessment. Advancing years do not preclude treatment; however, prolonged anaesthesia and chemotherapy may not be tolerated in dogs with compromised organs.

Treatment and prognosis

Dogs presented with stage III disease (measurable metastases) have a very poor prognosis. Although the actual survival times in such dogs have not been well defined, it is generally accepted to be only weeks. Occult metastatic disease is present in approximately 90% of dogs at presentation and the median survival is only 2–4 months if amputation or some other form of treatment of the local disease is the only therapy used. Some form of systemic therapy is necessary if survival is to be significantly improved. With no treatment at all, dogs experience severe pain because of extensive destruction of bone and surrounding tissue by the primary tumours, and most owners elect for euthanasia. Because of progressive pain in untreated dogs, dogs that have limbs amputated are likely to live longer than dogs that do not undergo amputation, even without systemic therapy. Whether this is statistically significant is unknown, but amputation dramatically improves the quality of life of affected dogs, even though longevity is minimally affected.

There is some evidence that dogs younger than 5 years survived less well than older dogs (Spodnick *et al.*, 1992). Additional studies have related large tumour size (Misdorp and Hart 1979; Kuntz *et al.*, 1998) and location in the humerus (Bergman *et al.*, 1996) to poor outcome. The degree of tumour necrosis has also been correlated with poor prognosis (Kirpensteijn *et al.*, 2002). Preoperative elevation of either total (serum) or the bone isoenzyme of alkaline phosphatase is associated with a shorter disease-free interval and survival (Ehrhart *et al.*, 1998; Garzotto *et al.*, 2000; Kirpensteijn *et al.*, 2002). In one of these studies (Ehrhart *et al.*, 1998) dogs that had elevated preoperative values that did not return to normal within 40 days following surgical removal of the primary lesion also failed earlier from disease. Recent work has shown a potential relationship between histological grade, based on microscopic features, and systemic behaviour (metastasis) (Kirpensteijn *et al.*, 2002).

Figure 9.6 (after Dernell, 2003) gives approximate survival times with various treatments.

Treatment	Methods	Median survival
Pain management	Non-steroidal anti-inflammatory drugs (NSAIDs), Narcotics, N-methyl-D-aspartate (NMDA) antagonists (Lascelles, 2003)	2–3 months (the advent of more specific inhibitors of osteoclast activity and of more selective cyclo-oxygenase-2 (COX-2) inhibitors may extend this)
Palliative radiation	Megavoltage	2 months of pain relief; further doses of palliative radiation may be effective and allow for longer survival (2–6 months) (Bateman *et al.*, 1994; Ramirez *et al.*, 1999)
Surgery	Amputation or limb sparing alone	3–6 months
Radiation and chemotherapy	Fractionated megavoltage with platinum chemotherapy	6–12 months (estimate – little research in this area)
Amputation and chemotherapy	Cisplatin, carboplatin, doxorubicin or combinations	10–14 months (generally improved survival after dual agent chemotherapy (Chun *et al.*, 2000) compared with single agent (Shapiro *et al.*, 1988; Berg *et al.*, 1992; Bergman *et al.*, 1996))
Surgical limb sparing (Figures 9.7 and 9.8) and chemotherapy	Cisplatin, carboplatin, doxorubicin or combinations	12–16 months (infection following limb salvage appears to improve survival (Lascelles *et al.*, in press))

9.6 Survival times with various treatments for OSA in dogs.

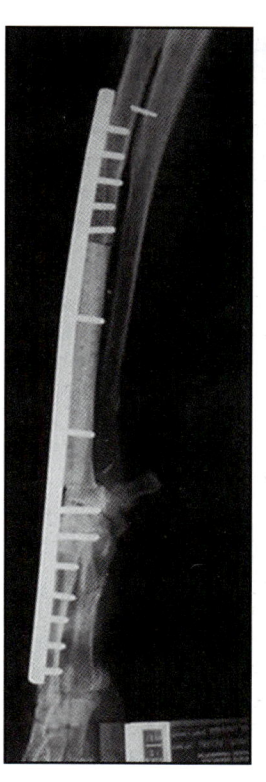

9.7 The distal radius is the site associated with the best outcome following limb salvage surgery. A fresh frozen allograft, filled with bone cement replacing the resected cancerous bone, is shown being held in place by a bone plate.

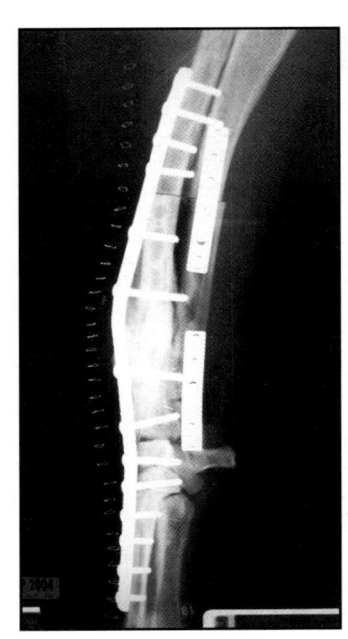

Chapter 9 Tumours of the musculoskeletal system

9.8 This Great Dane had an OSA. The tumour was resected together with the radius and the ulna, and irradiated with 70 Gy. The soft tissues were then resected and the remaining bony tissue placed back into the dog, after filling the cavity with bone cement. The irradiated bones filled with bone cement are held in place with bone plates. The outcome of such *ex vivo* irradiation has not been well defined (Liptak *et al.*, 2004).

Other primary bone tumours in dogs

It can be difficult to distinguish chondroblastic OSA from chondrosarcoma, fibroblastic OSA from fibrosarcoma and telangiectatic OSA from haemangiosarcoma when only small amounts of biopsy tissue are evaluated. This makes interpretation of older reports difficult in terms of trying to establish the true incidence of the different types of primary bone tumours. This also underscores the importance of evaluating the entire excised specimen to validate the preoperative biopsy specimen evaluation. This is also true in cases where initial biopsy might indicate low-grade disease. Primary bone tumours other than OSA make up somewhere between 5% and 10% of bone malignancies in dogs. These tumours are chondrosarcomas, haemangiosarcomas, fibrosarcomas, lymphomas and myelomas.

Canine joint tumours

Synovial cell sarcomas have been described as the most common tumours affecting joints in dogs, although overall they are uncommon tumours (Madewell and Pool, 1978; Lipowitz *et al.*, 1979; McGlennon *et al.*, 1988). They occur most commonly in the large joints of the extremities (especially the stifle) in middle-aged large-breed dogs. The clinical course can be protracted, with clinical signs being evident for months to years (Vail *et al.*, 1994). They are believed to arise from primitive mesenchymal precursor cells outside the synovial membrane of joints and bursae. Histologically, they have been characterized as having two intermingled cellular elements – an epithelioid and a fibroblastic component. The proportions of these can vary tremendously, and in human medicine, synovial cell sarcomas have been classified into two types: biphasic (both cellular elements are present) and monophasic (only one cellular element present). Other joint tumours reported in dogs include fibrosarcoma, rhabdomyosarcoma, OSA, malignant fibrous histiocytoma (MFH), liposarcoma, haemangiosarcoma, myxoma, malignant giant cell tumour of soft tissue and undifferentiated sarcoma (Whitelock *et al.*, 1997). Recently, histiocytic sarcomas have been reported in the periarticular tissue of large appendicular joints.

In one study, most dogs with diagnosed synovial sarcoma that underwent amputation had disease-free intervals and survival times of over 36 months; a high mitotic rate, marked nuclear pleomorphism and a greater percentage of necrotic tumour were associated with a significantly poorer prognosis (Vail *et al.*, 1994). Local excision seems to be associated with a very high recurrence rate (Vail *et al.*, 1994). However, there has been recent discussion regarding the diagnosis of synovial sarcomas (Craig *et al.*, 2002). In one retrospective immunocytochemical evaluation of previously diagnosed synovial cell sarcomas, only 14% were confirmed as synovial cell sarcomas, with 51% being histiocytic sarcomas, 17% synovial myxomas and the remaining 18% being sarcomas of various types (undifferentiated, fibrosarcoma, chondrosarcoma, MFH). This percentage of synovial sarcomas was similar to that of a previous recent review of radiographically similar joint tumours where only 8 of 30 (27%) were identified as synovial cell sarcomas histologically (Whitelock *et al.*, 1997). The importance of this recent information is that knowing the precise tumour type seems to affect prognosis, but at the moment the specific details of this are difficult to define. In the study by Vail and colleagues (1994) overall median disease-free interval was 30 months for dogs that were rendered tumour-free (by amputation); positive cytokeratin staining had a negative influence on survival. However, in the study by Craig *et al.* (2002), the average survival was 32 months for dogs with positive cytokeratin-staining tumours, significantly better than that for dogs with histiocytic sarcoma or undifferentiated sarcoma.

Local invasion of underlying bone by joint tumours is common in later stages of the disease and is easily recognizable on routine radiographs by punched-out bone lesions. The tumour invades the bone at the attachment of the joint capsule or tendons to the bone. Amputation is the treatment of choice for local disease, with wide resection margins. However, joint myxomas may be amenable to complete local resection if they have not invaded local tissues (Craig *et al.*, 2002). Metastasis rates appear to vary depending on tumour type, and, therefore, the need for chemotherapy should be based on precise evaluation of what tumour type is present, as defined by immunohistochemical staining. Overall for all joint tumours, an eventual metastasis rate of between 40% and 55% can be expected (Vail *et al.*, 1994). When metastasis occurs, it is seen in the lymph nodes, lungs, spleen and liver. Given that metastasis rates appear to vary greatly between histological types of synovial tumours, immunohistochemical staining is recommended, and should include cytokeratin, CD18 and smooth muscle actin (Craig *et al.*, 2002).

Chapter 9 Tumours of the musculoskeletal system

Feline primary bone tumours

Bone tumours in cats are rare (Dorn et al., 1968). The majority (up to 90%) of bone tumours in cats are histologically malignant (Bitetto et al., 1987). Appendicular and axial sites for primary bone tumours are equally frequent (Heldmann et al., 2000). OSA accounts for the majority (70–80%) of all primary malignant bone cancer of cats. The pelvic limbs are more frequently affected, and the disease is less metastatic than in dogs.

Up to one third of feline OSA may be extraskeletal in origin, with the most common location being interscapular. At this site, local vaccination was considered a predisposing factor (Heldmann et al., 2000).

A histological feature of some feline OSA cases is the presence of multinucleate giant cells, with some people classifying these separately as 'giant cell tumours of bone'. OSA is invasive into surrounding tissue; however, some surrounding soft tissue may be compressed rather than infiltrated. Often, there is variation of the histological appearance within the tumour, with some portions having a more fibrosarcomatous appearance and others being more cartilaginous. A subtype of OSA in cats, termed parosteal osteosarcoma, has been described (14 cases in the literature). This has also been called juxtacortical osteosarcoma. Cortical destruction does not usually occur. Otherwise, the behaviour is very similar to OSA.

Osteochondromatosis or multiple cartilaginous exostosis (MCE) is a disease that occurs in cats, and can have an aggressive natural behaviour. Although differing terms have been used (osteochondromatosis, osteochondroma, multiple osteochondromas, multiple cartilaginous exostosis), there are essentially two 'cancer' syndromes – solitary lesions in older feline leukaemia virus- (FeLV-) negative cats, and multiple lesions in younger FeLV-positive cats. Both solitary and multiple lesions can affect both the axial and appendicular skeleton, but tend to affect the axial skeleton more often. MCE is a disease that occurs after skeletal maturity in cats. This is in contrast to dogs where exostoses develop before closure of growth plates. Also, in contrast to dogs, the lesions seldom affect long bones, are rarely symmetrical and are probably of viral rather than familial origin. Affected cats range in age from 1.3–8 years (mean 3.2 years) (Carpenter et al., 1987). Virtually all cats with MCE will test positive for FeLV.

Diagnosis

Lameness or an obvious mass, or local effects due to the presence of a mass, are the most common clinical signs (Figures 9.9 and 9.10). The lesions may appear radiographically similar to OSA in dogs or can arise from the periosteal surface (juxtacortical OSA) (Bitetto et al., 1987). It is rare for cats to have metastatic OSA, but metastasis can occur.

Cats with virus-associated MCE have rapidly progressing, conspicuous, hard swellings over affected sites, causing pain and loss of function. Common sites for lesion development are the scapula, vertebrae and mandible. However, any bone can become affected. Radiographically the lesions are either sessile or pedunculated protuberances from bone surfaces, with indistinct borders. There may be a loss of smooth contour with evidence of lysis, particularly if there is malignant transformation.

Both OSA and MCE may be suspected by the radiographic appearance of the lesions and MCE by the FeLV status of the cat. Definitive diagnosis is confirmed by histopathological evaluation.

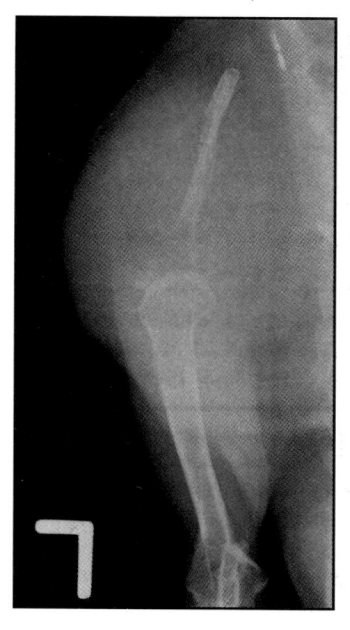

9.9 Radiograph of an OSA of the distal scapula in a 4-year-old cat, showing destruction of the affected bone. The cat had a history of 2.5 years of lameness with a progressively enlarging mass. Metastasis did not occur.

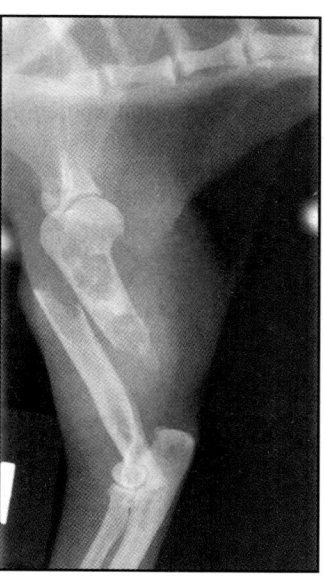

9.10 This radiograph shows the typical appearance of OSA in the cat – a predominance of osteolysis. In this case, there was minimal extension into the surrounding tissues, but the osteolytic nature of the lesion resulted in fracture of the humerus.

Treatment and prognosis

Amputation for appendicular OSA can result in prolonged survival times, or even cure (if there is no detectable metastasis). In two studies of 15 cats, the median survival after amputation alone was 24 and 44 months (Turrel and Pool, 1982; Bitetto et al., 1987). The metastatic potential is much less than for the same disease in dogs or humans. Due to the difficulty of local control, axial sites carry a poorer prognosis. Axial sites are best treated with combination therapy, and chemotherapy has shown a survival advantage in these cases (Heldmann et al., 2000).

Cats with MCE have a guarded prognosis. Lesions may be removed surgically for palliation. However, local recurrences are common, and new, painful, debilitating lesions may occur. No reliably effective treatment is known for this condition in cats, although radiation has been suggested.

Other tumours of the musculoskeletal system in cats

Fibrosarcomas can occur in bones, but the majority are probably extension into bone from surrounding tumours. They appear to occur most often on the maxilla and mandible, but primary fibrosarcomas of long bones have been reported. The biological behaviour for fibrosarcomas of bone is not truly known, and they should probably be treated as for other fibrosarcomas in cats (surgery, radiation and chemotherapy).

Primary bone chondrosarcomas appear to occur more frequently on the appendicular skeleton, but limited numbers are reported in the literature. The presentation and clinical signs are similar to OSA. Small biopsy specimens of masses may be misleading, as many OSAs have predominating cartilaginous areas. The treatment for chondrosarcomas is essentially the same as for OSAs, but the prognosis may be better as the metastatic rate is probably lower.

Haemangiosarcoma of bone is a rare primary bone tumour of cats. Metastasis appears to be common. Surgical resection should be considered palliative, and chemotherapy may be administered to attempt systemic control.

Very few synovial cell sarcomas have been reported in the cat, and it is unclear if these were actually fibrosarcomas.

Osteomas occur rarely, in places similar to OSAs. Clinical signs are related to the physical presence of the tumour. The approach should be as for OSAs, with a biopsy performed to differentiate them. Treatment is surgical resection, and possibly radiation for incomplete resections.

References

Bateman KE, Catton PA, Pennock PW and Kruth SA (1994) 0-7-21 radiation therapy for the palliation of advanced cancer in dogs. *Journal of Veterinary Internal Medicine* **8**, 394–399

Berg J, Weinstein MJ, Schelling SH and Rand WM (1992) Treatment of dogs with osteosarcoma by administration of cisplatin after amputation or limb-sparing surgery: 22 cases (1987–1990). *Journal of the American Veterinary Medical Association* **200**, 2005–2008

Bergman PJ, MacEwen EG, Kurzman ID *et al.* (1996) Amputation and carboplatin for treatment of dogs with osteosarcoma: 48 cases (1991–1993). *Journal of Veterinary Internal Medicine* **10**, 76–81

Bitetto WV, Patnaik AK, Schrader SC and Mooney SC (1987) Osteosarcoma in cats: 22 cases (1974–1984). *Journal of the American Veterinary Medical Association* **190**, 91–93

Carpenter JL, Andrews LK and Holzworth J (1987) Tumors and tumor-like lesions. In: *Diseases of the Cat: Medicine and Surgery*, ed. J Holzworth, pp. 406–596. WB Saunders, Philadelphia

Chun R, Kurzman ID, Couto CG *et al.* (2000) Cisplatin and doxorubicin combination chemotherapy for the treatment of canine osteosarcoma: a pilot study. *Journal of Veterinary Internal Medicine* **14**, 495–498

Craig LE, Julian ME and Ferracone JD (2002) The diagnosis and prognosis of synovial tumors in dogs: 35 cases. *Veterinary Pathology* **39**, 66–73

Dernell W (2003) Tumours of the skeletal system. In: *BSAVA Manual of Canine and Feline Oncology*, 2nd edn, ed. JM Dobson and BDX Lascelles, pp. 179–195. BSAVA Publications, Gloucester

Dorn, CR, Taylor DO, Schneider R, Hibbard HH and Klauber MR (1968) Survey of animal neoplasms in Alameda and Contra Costa Counties, California. II. Cancer morbidity in dogs and cats from Alameda County. *Journal of the National Cancer Institute* **40**, 307–318

Ehrhart N, Dernell WS, Hoffmann WE *et al.* (1998) Prognostic importance of alkaline phosphatase activity in serum from dogs with appendicular osteosarcoma: 75 cases (1990–1996). *Journal of the American Veterinary Medical Association* **213**, 1002–1006

Garzotto CK, Berg J, Hoffmann WE and Rand WM (2000) Prognostic significance of serum alkaline phosphatase activity in canine appendicular osteosarcoma. *Journal of Veterinary Internal Medicine* **14**, 587–592

Heldmann E, Anderson MA and Wagner-Mann C (2000) Feline osteosarcoma: 145 cases (1990–1995). *Journal of the American Animal Hospital Association* **36**, 518–521

Jeffery N (2003) Tumours affecting the nervous system. In: *BSAVA Manual of Canine and Feline Oncology*, 2nd edn, ed. JM Dobson and BDX Lascelles, pp. 317–328. BSAVA Publications, Gloucester

Kirpensteijn J and Rutteman GR (2003) Sarcomas of soft tissues. In: *BSAVA Manual of Canine and Feline Oncology*, 2nd edn, ed. JM Dobson and BDX Lascelles, pp. 196–205. BSAVA Publications, Gloucester

Kirpensteijn J, Teske E, Kik M, Klenner T and Rutteman GR (2002) Lobaplatin as an adjuvant chemotherapy to surgery in canine appendicular osteosarcoma: a phase II evaluation. *Anticancer Research* **22**, 2765–2770

Kuntz CA, Asselin TL, Dernell WS *et al.* (1998) Limb salvage surgery for osteosarcoma of the proximal humerus: outcome in 17 dogs. *Veterinary Surgery* **27**, 417–422

Lamb CR (1987) Bone scintigraphy in small animals. *Journal of the American Veterinary Medical Association* **191**, 1616–1622

Lamb CR, Berg J and Bengtson AE (1990) Preoperative measurement of canine primary bone tumors, using radiography and bone scintigraphy. *Journal of the American Veterinary Medical Association* **196**, 1474–1478

Lascelles BDX (2003) Relief of chronic cancer pain. In ed. JM Dobson and BDX Lascelles: *BSAVA Manual of Canine and Feline Oncology*, 2nd edn, pp. 137–151. BSAVA Publications, Gloucester

Lascelles BDX, Dernell W, Correa MT *et al.* (in press) Improved survival associated with postoperative wound infection in dogs treated with limb-salvage surgery for osteosarcoma. *Annals of Surgical Oncology*

Leibman NF, Kuntz CA, Steyn PF *et al.* (2001) Accuracy of radiography, nuclear scintigraphy, and histopathology for determining the proximal extent of distal radius osteosarcoma in dogs. *Veterinary Surgery* **30**, 240–245

Lipowitz AJ, Fetter AW and Walker MA (1979) Synovial sarcoma of the dog. *Journal of the American Veterinary Medical Association* **174**, 76–81

Liptak JM, Dernell WS, Lascelles BD *et al.* (2004) Intraoperative extracorporeal irradiation for limb sparing in 13 dogs. *Veterinary Surgery* **33**, 446–456

Madewell BR and Pool R (1978) Neoplasms of joints and related structures. *Veterinary Clinics of North America* **8**, 511–521

McGlennon NJ, Houlton JEF and Gorman NT (1988) Synovial sarcoma in the dog – a review. *Journal of Small Animal Practice* **29**, 139–152

Misdorp W and Hart AA (1979) Some prognostic and epidemiologic factors in canine osteosarcoma. *Journal of the National Cancer Institute* **62**, 537–545

Powers BE, LaRue SM, Withrow SJ, Straw RC and Richter SL (1988) Jamshidi needle biopsy for diagnosis of bone lesions in small animals. *Journal of the American Veterinary Medical Association* **193**, 205–210

Ramirez O III, Dodge RK, Page RL *et al.* (1999) Palliative radiotherapy of appendicular osteosarcoma in 95 dogs. *Veterinary Radiology and Ultrasound* **40**, 517–522

Shapiro W, Fossum T, Kitchell B, Couto C and Theilen (1988) Use of cisplatin for treatment of appendicular osteosarcoma in dogs. *Journal of the American Veterinary Medical Association* **192**, 507–511

Spodnick G, Berg J and Rand W *et al.* (1992) Prognosis for dogs with appendicular osteosarcoma treated by amputation alone: 162 cases (1978–1988). *Journal of the American Veterinary Medical Association* **200**, 995–999

Turrel JM and Pool RR (1982) Primary bone tumors in the cat: a retrospective study of 15 cats and a literature review. *Veterinary Radiology* **23**, 152–166

Vail DM, Powers BE, Getzy DM *et al.* (1994) Evaluation of prognostic factors for dogs with synovial sarcoma: 36 cases (1986–1991). *Journal of the American Veterinary Medical Association* **205**, 1300–1307

Waters DJ, Coakley FV, Cohen MD *et al.* (1998) The detection of pulmonary metastases by helical CT: a clinicopathologic study in dogs. *Journal of Computer Assisted Tomography* **22**, 235–240

Whitelock RG, Dyce J, Houlton JEF and Jefferies AR (1997) A review of 30 tumours affecting joints. *Veterinary Comparative Orthopaedics and Traumatology* **10**, 146–152

10

Neurological causes of lameness

T. James Anderson

Introduction

Lameness is generally a consequence of discomfort or physical restriction of a limb or limbs due to pathology of the musculoskeletal structures of that limb. Lameness is, therefore, generally due to pathology involving bones, joints, muscles, tendons and other soft tissue structures. However, the coordinated control of limb movement requires the appropriate influence of the peripheral, and thus the central, nervous system on all these structures, and it is axiomatic that pathology of the nervous system will affect limb function. Traditionally, as limb musculature and reflexes are usually unaffected by abnormalities in limb movement related to brain and spinal cord dysfunction (e.g. proprioceptive deficits, ataxia and tremor) related clinical signs have not been considered as lameness but rather as gait abnormalities. However, disease of the peripheral nerves, particularly focal disease resulting in single limb dysfunction, and characterized by pain and/or weakness, is often considered by the owner and clinician as lameness.

Clinical signs of neurological lameness

Pain and lower motor neuron (LMN) deficits are the cardinal clinical signs of neurological disease causing lameness.

Lower motor neuron deficits

The LMN (neuronal cell body in the grey matter of the spinal cord and axon in the peripheral nerve) connects directly to muscles and is important in reflex activity, muscle tone and in maintaining muscle bulk (Figure 10.1). Upper motor neurons (UMNs) initiate LMN activity and dysfunction is often reflected by ataxia and incoordination. For a fuller discussion of lesion localization see the *BSAVA Manual of Canine and Feline Neurology*. Frank LMN deficits are often a late feature of the disease and may not be evident at first presentation.

Pain

The degree of pain observed is variable. It usually progresses from low grade and intermittent to severe and persistent as the condition becomes more advanced. The discomfort observed is often not associated with limb movement or weight bearing. The degree of pain in advanced disease may be extreme and challenging to control. Examination of the limb may not localize the discomfort to any particular structure. Indeed, the discomfort may be erroneously attributed to an adjacent structure more often associated with lameness. For example, the shoulder joint may be thought to be painful when the true source of the pain is a brachial plexus tumour. Generalized pain associated with a limb or during its manipulation may indicate nerve root signature, a manifestation of compression of an associated peripheral nerve(s) (Figure 10.2) (Sharp and Wheeler, 2005).

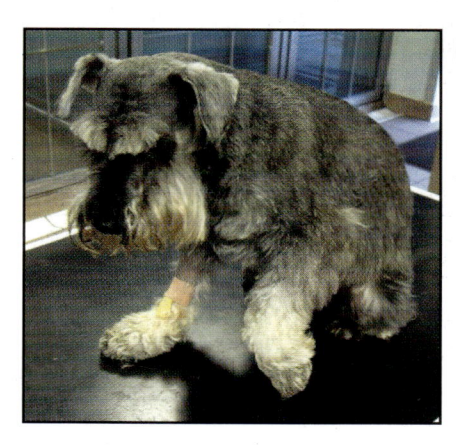

10.2 Left thoracic limb discomfort due to nerve root signature in a Miniature Schnauzer with a cervical disc extrusion. (Courtesy of Simon Platt)

Evidence of discomfort may also be seen in related structures, particularly the axial skeleton. Palpation of the axilla may be painful in patients with brachial plexus tumours, although the mass itself may not be palpable. Deep palpation of the axilla may be required and care must be taken to differentiate discomfort associated with pathology from that related to the technique.

A change in behaviour may be evidence of discomfort, e.g. not jumping up, difficulty with steps or a reluctance to sit or stand.

Feature	LMN disease	UMN disease
Proprioception	Reduced	Reduced
Local reflexes	Reduced	Unaffected or increased
Muscle tone	Reduced	Unaffected or increased
Muscle bulk	Rapid atrophy	Minimal or slow atrophy

10.1 Clinical signs of lower and upper motor neuron disease.

Chapter 10 Neurological causes of lameness

Aids to diagnosis

Examination of the patient, selection of appropriate imaging techniques and other pertinent investigations are covered in Chapters 1–5. Magnetic resonance imaging (MRI) has much to offer in the investigation of a patient with a suspected neurological lameness as the nervous system tissues are imaged directly. In contrast, the more traditional techniques of myelography and epidurography rely on inference rather than direct visualization of the tissues and negative or equivocal findings leave the clinician in an uncertain position. For example, they cannot be relied upon to exclude an event such as an intraforaminal disc extrusion, particularly if the disc material is non-calcified. Electrophysiological studies may be of value when assessing the neuromuscular system of a patient with a suspected neurological lameness (see below). Occasionally, other tests may also be required in the assessment of specific problems (Figure 10.3).

Situation	Test
Suspected endocrine involvement	Assessment of thyroid and adrenal function Assessment of glucose metabolism
Suspected muscle involvement	Serum creatine kinase Muscle biopsy
Suspected electrolyte involvement	Serum electrolytes (Na$^+$, K$^+$, Cl$^-$, Ca^{2+})
Suspected protozoal infection	Serology or polymerase chain reaction (PCR) on cerebrospinal fluid (CSF) for *Neospora* (dogs) and *Toxoplasma* (cats)

10.3 Other tests of potential value in assessing patients with suspected neurological causes of lameness.

Electrophysiology

Electrophysiology techniques provide specific information about muscle and nerve function and thus document their involvement in a disease process. They require specialist equipment.

Electromyography

In many muscle diseases, and also as a consequence of denervation, spontaneous electrical activity develops in affected muscles. Electromyography (EMG) is a sensitive method of detecting this activity. The spontaneous activity reflects instability in the muscle membrane and is detected by recording directly from the muscle. The presence of spontaneous electrical activity in muscle is indicated by a number of EMG findings (Figures 10.4 and 10.5). Although muscle may exhibit spontaneous electrical activity, such an observation in isolation does not differentiate between primary muscle and nerve disease (Niederhauser and Holliday, 1989).

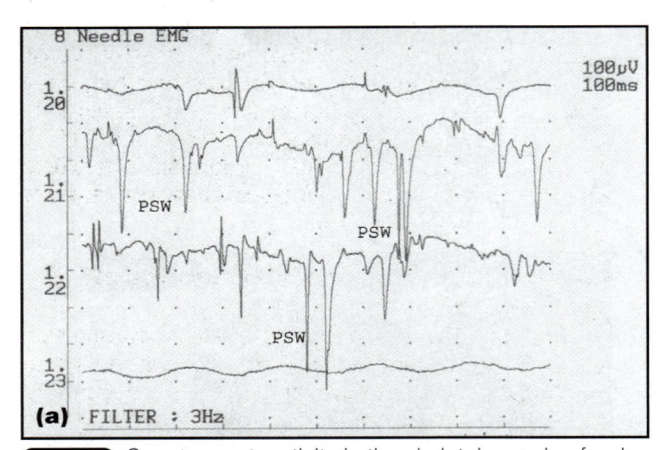

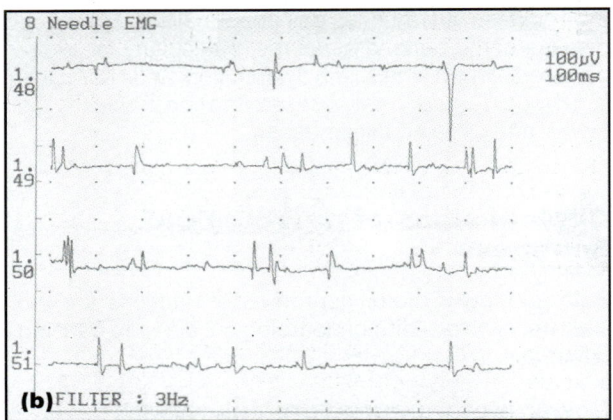

10.4 Spontaneous activity in the skeletal muscle of a dog affected by a peripheral neuropathy. In the normal muscle of an anaesthetized patient an EMG trace should be electrically silent, which is seen as a flat trace.
(a) Predominantly positive sharp waves (PSW). **(b)** Predominantly fibrillation potentials. These findings represent the same electrical event, with the traces reflecting differences in detection by the needle. (Courtesy of Jacques Penderis)

EMG finding	Represents	Significance
Increased insertional activity (a sharply defined period of electrical activity is normally associated with needle insertion and movement)	Prolonged activity following mechanical irritation due to needle insertion	Muscle irritability
Positive sharp waves and fibrillation potentials (represent the same electrical event, their different appearance reflecting how they are detected by the recording electrode)	Spontaneous action potential in a myofibre	Denervation Inflammation Some myopathies
Complex repetitive discharges	Group of myofibres firing in synchrony	Chronic denervation and some myopathies
Myotonic discharges (see also Chapter 8)	Repetitive discharges in myofibres	Potential myopathy

10.5 Summary of the significance of abnormal EMG findings.

Chapter 10 Neurological causes of lameness

Nerve conduction studies

Following nerve stimulation, the recording of the appropriate response depends on whether the nerve fibre type under study is a motor or sensory nerve. Recording should document axon recruitment and conduction velocity. The interpretation of motor nerve conduction studies is summarized in Figure 10.6. The function of nerve roots has to be studied indirectly, as an extension of nerve conduction studies, due to their anatomical inaccessibility. The major techniques are summarized in Figure 10.7.

Nerve conduction abnormality	Interpretation
Decrease in compound muscle action potential (CMAP) without temporal dispersion	• Axonal disease • Decreased neuromuscular transmission (botulism) • Myopathy (reduced number of myofibres from which to develop CMAP)
Decrease in proximal vs distal CMAP of >50%	Conduction block
Prolonged latency or slowed conduction velocity without a decrease in CMAP amplitude	Demyelination ± axonopathy

10.6 Summary of the significance of nerve conduction studies.

Nerve root	Function	Characteristic tested
Ventral (motor) nerve root	F waves	CMAPs generated by stimulation of the ventral horn cells by antidromic conduction from the stimulus point
Dorsal (sensory) nerve root	Cord dorsum potentials	Spinal cord field potential

10.7 Summary of electrophysiology techniques to test nerve root function. (After Poncelet, 2004).

In general, axonal loss is reflected by a reduction in the action potential generated. In contrast, demyelination is indicated by temporal dispersion of the action potential. Motor nerve studies record compound muscle action potential (CMAP) from the associated muscle. The CMAP can be affected by changes at the neuromuscular junction and in the muscle. Sensory conduction is derived directly from recording the nerve action potential.

It is important to remember that peripheral neuropathies do not always exhibit a decrease in conduction velocity, as the fastest conducting fibres may not be involved.

Biopsy

Mass lesions may represent abnormal nervous tissue or changes in other structures with the potential for nerve compression. When identified, either by examination or imaging (Figure 10.8), biopsy is necessary to achieve a specific diagnosis. Abnormalities in nerve conduction and EMG studies are an indication for nerve and possibly muscle biopsy (see Chapter 8b and Long and Anderson, 2004).

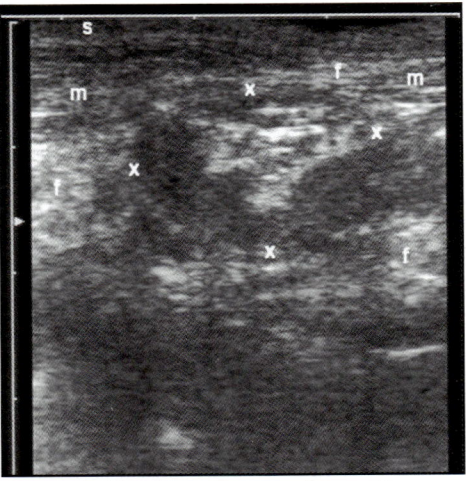

10.8 Ultrasound image of an axillary mass (delineated by x) in a dog with ipsilateral LMN signs in the limb. The mass is of mixed echogenicity and has well defined borders. An ultrasound-guided biopsy confirmed the presence of neoplasia. (f, fat; m, muscle; s, skin). (Courtesy of Alison King)

Specific conditions

Syringomyelia

Cavitation of the spinal cord parenchyma, secondary to obstruction of cerebrospinal fluid (CSF) flow, disrupts cord function and is associated with a wide spectrum of clinical signs. This is an inherited condition in the Cavalier King Charles Spaniel and has been associated with both thoracic limb and pelvic limb neurological deficits and limb pain (Rusbridge *et al.*, 2000). Diagnosis requires MRI. Prognosis is guarded, with the options including medical management and surgery (Rusbridge, 2005).

Peripheral neuropathies as causes of lameness

Several diseases affect the peripheral nervous system leading to generalized LMN signs affecting all four limbs and thus producing a flaccid tetraparesis. These are reviewed by Cuddon (2002) and summarized in Figure 10.9. Some of these diseases have a rapid, if not fulminating, course and consequently, the appearance of significant weakness, areflexia and hypotonia in all limbs means that such problems are unlikely to be considered a lameness. However, the early stages of the acute problems and the early course of the chronic conditions are often characterized by apparent pelvic limb stiffness, which may be considered lameness. Evidence of LMN disease and the appropriate investigation should establish the aetiology. *Neospora canis* infection will be considered as a specific entity (see below).

Paraneoplastic neuropathy

This is a rare cause of peripheral neuropathy in small animals. The clinical picture is ultimately one of generalized LMN signs (see Figure 10.1). However, in common with other chronic polyneuropathies, the signs are

Chapter 10 Neurological causes of lameness

Peripheral neuropathy	Clinical features	Aetiology	Comments
Acute canine polyradiculoneuritis (Coonhound paralysis)	Acute disease. Initially may affect pelvic limbs giving a stiff gait with short strides. Progressing to tetraparesis over 5–10 days	Unknown. Immune-mediated and thought to be canine equivalent of Guillain–Barré syndrome in man. Thought to be related to exposure to raccoon saliva with other precipitating environmental factors	Common in North America; ocasionally described on other continents
Endocrine-related neuropathies	Insidious tetraparesis usually involving the pelvic limbs initially	Associated with diabetes mellitus, hypothyroidism	Rare in diabetes. Uncommon in hypothyroidism
Paraneoplastic neuropathy	Insidious tetraparesis usually involving the pelvic limbs initially	Probably immune-mediated	Not associated with any particular tumour type
Distal denervating disease	Progressive tetraparesis with variable rate of progression	Unknown	Only reported in the UK

10.9 Peripheral neuropathies. (After Cuddon, 2002)

often first noticed in the pelvic limbs and, in the initial stages, may mimic lameness. The syndrome has been reported in association with a range of neoplasms.

Nerve entrapment

Pressure on nerve roots within the spinal column or as they exit the bony foramina causes pain. This can be due to mass lesions compressing the nerve root (e.g. disc herniation or tumour) or changes in the diameter of the exit foramina. Compression of peripheral nerves outside the spinal column may also induce pain. Although one might expect to see LMN signs, these may only occur late in a disease or not at all. Consequently, the specific involvement of nerve roots or peripheral nerves may not be immediately apparent from the physical examination of the patient.

Clinical signs

Clinical signs depend upon the nerve(s) affected; to produce lameness it is likely that affected nerves will be contributors to the brachial plexus (C5–T2) or the lumbosacral plexus (L4–S1) (DeLahunta, 1983). In the cervical region, nerve root entrapment usually produces thoracic limb lameness with little in the way of other clinical signs, though occasionally an ipsilateral hemiparesis may be present due to spinal cord compression. In the lumbosacral region, the commonest region to be affected is the lumbosacral junction. Though intermittent or shifting pelvic limb lameness and a stiff gait are common reasons for presentation, other manifestations are seen. These include changes in behaviour, such as not jumping into vehicles or difficulty in sitting/rising, focal discomfort of the lumbosacral joint, urinary and faecal incontinence, and tail weakness.

Compression of a peripheral nerve away from the exit foramina is rare, other than from involvement in tumours (see below). However, peripheral nerves may be compromised as a consequence of fracture fixation (see *BSAVA Manual of Small Animal Fracture Repair and Management*), for example due to impingement from external fixator pins, or, rarely, by becoming included in callus formation. The commonest neurological complication associated with fracture repair is sciatic compression. Damage may be due either to the postoperative retrograde movement of an intramedullary femoral pin (Figure 10.10) or to poor pin insertion during fracture repair. Retrograde pin migration generally occurs within a few weeks of surgery and results in severe pain, marked lameness and severe muscle atrophy. Lameness is generally resolved following pin removal. An alternative stabilization technique may be required, depending on the degree of fracture healing at the time of pin removal.

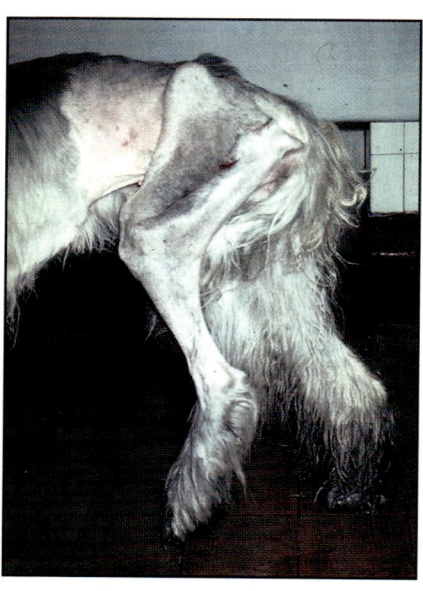

10.10 Dog with impingement of the sciatic nerve caused by an intramedullary pin. (Courtesy of JEF Houlton)

Diagnosis

Diagnosis requires an imaging technique that can be confidently expected to identify the presence of such a lesion. Radiography and myelography/epidurography have been the traditional techniques for assessing patients with lesions affecting the spinal cord and nerve roots, but MRI has proved to be advantageous, particularly for lateralized disc lesions which may not be evident on a myelogram/epidurogram (Figure 10.11) (Chambers *et al.*, 1997). MRI is the technique of choice for assessing the degree of impingement on nerve roots by bony and soft tissue changes altering the bony exit foramen as the nerve root can be specifically imaged.

Chapter 10   Neurological causes of lameness

associated with significant disruption of tissues, poor visualization and excessive cord manipulation (Seim, 2002). There is, therefore, potential for significant postoperative morbidity. An alternative approach in the cervical region is to distract the adjacent vertebrae, thus enlarging the associated foramina (Fitch et al., 2000) (Figure 10.12). In the lumbar region, the foramen may be enlarged by the traditional hemilaminectomy approach, in which the articular facets and surrounding bone are resected. For lumbosacral lateralized disc extrusions, the L7/S1 nerve root can be decompressed via a dorsal approach using either a foraminotomy (preserving the articulation) or a facetectomy. Facetectomy does not appear to compromise stability if it is unilateral (de Riso et al., 2000).

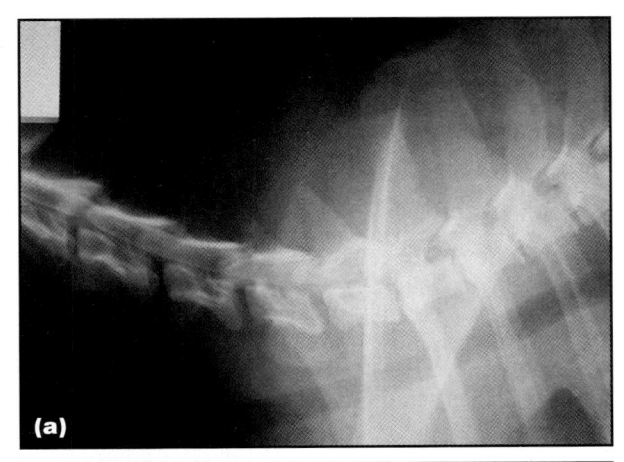

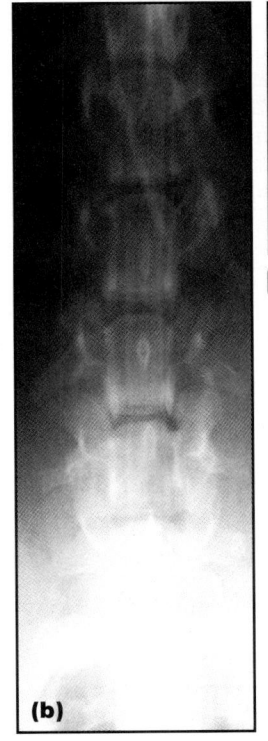

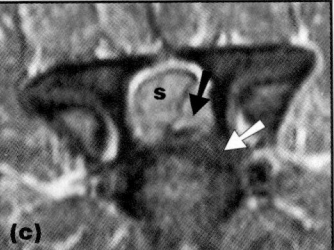

10.11 Imaging the cervical region of a dog with intermittent neck pain and left thoracic limb lameness. The myelograms **(a,b)** of the lower cervical region do not readily identify the lateralized non-calcified disc extrusion. The transverse T2-weighted MRI image of the C5/6 intervertebral space **(c)** shows a lateralized non-calcified disc extrusion (closed arrow). The open arrow points to the nerve root. s, spinal cord.

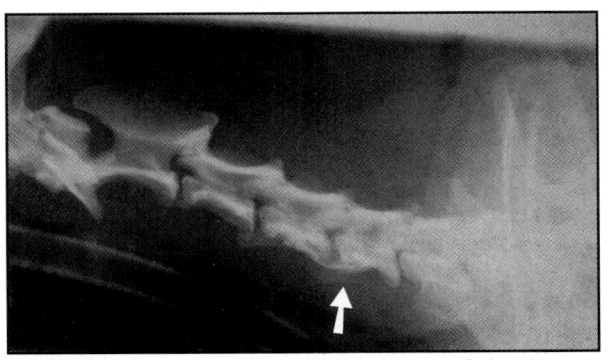

10.12 Lateral postoperative radiograph of a patient showing distraction/fusion with a PMMA plug (arrowed) to decompress a lateralized disc extrusion.

Treatment and prognosis

Analgesia: Control of pain may be challenging. Non-steroidal anti-inflammatory drugs may be effective for some patients, but steroids at an anti-inflammatory dose (e.g. prednisolone 0.5–1.0 mg/kg q24h) are often more effective in the severely affected patient. It is important that patients are adequately confined, a requirement that many owners find difficult in the home environment. Some patients require opioid analgesics to manage the discomfort. Ultimately, in patients where pain is persistent and poorly ameliorated by conservative management, pain control is best effected by decompressing the affected nervous structure(s).

Lateralized/intraforaminal disc extrusion: In the cervical region these present a surgical challenge, as a ventral slot provides poor surgical access. A dorsal hemilaminectomy is a recognized approach to lateralized cervical disc extrusions but it may be associated with significant disruption of tissues, poor visualization and excessive cord manipulation (Seim, 2002). There is, therefore, potential for significant postoperative morbidity. An alternative approach in the cervical region is to distract the adjacent vertebrae, thus enlarging the associated foramina (Fitch et al., 2000) (Figure 10.12). In the lumbar region, the foramen may be enlarged by the traditional hemilaminectomy approach, in which the articular facets and surrounding bone are resected. For lumbosacral lateralized disc extrusions, the L7/S1 nerve root can be decompressed via a dorsal approach using either a foraminotomy (preserving the articulation) or a facetectomy. Facetectomy does not appear to compromise stability if it is unilateral (de Riso et al., 2000).

Benign productive changes in the bony margins of the foramina: Compression of nerve roots is a potential sequel to benign hypertrophy of joint components, for example as in spondylosis (Jeffery, 1995). Spondylosis is a common finding in older animals and is frequently an incidental finding. Thus further investigation is required to confirm whether the changes observed are associated with nerve root compromise. A foraminotomy or facetectomy can be undertaken to relieve any compression. Large-breed dogs with changes in their facet joints as a consequence of cervical spondylopathy may have nerve root compression as part of the syndrome. This will be addressed by techniques employing distraction/fusion but not by procedures such as continuous dorsal laminectomy.

Intraspinal cysts: Thoracic (Dickinson et al., 2001) and shifting pelvic limb lameness (Webb et al., 2001) have been reported as a consequence of extradural cysts compressing nerve roots. These cysts are derived from the periarticular soft tissues of the facet joints. Although the histological nature of the cysts is variable, surgical resection of the mass carries a favourable prognosis.

Fractures and luxations: Narrowing of the exit foramen due to spinal column instability may compress nerve roots (Okin, 1983). Surgical intervention may be required to distract and stabilize the components of the foramen, maintaining appropriate dimensions.

Chapter 10 Neurological causes of lameness

Discospondylitis: This has been reported as a cause of L7 nerve root compression (Lipscombe and Muir, 2000). MRI was essential to confirm the diagnosis as more traditional techniques of imaging had been unremarkable. Appropriate medical therapy effected a cure.

Vertebral tumours: Tumours of the vertebral bodies may compress or invade nerve roots. Such tumours are challenging to manage and have a generally poor prognosis (Dernell *et al.*, 2000).

Compromise of peripheral nerve trunks by abnormal soft tissues: Compromise of peripheral nerves by altered soft tissues is common in humans (e.g. carpal tunnel syndrome). In small animals such problems are rare. Occasionally, peripheral nerves can become compromised by fracture callus formation.

Tumours

Tumours of peripheral nerves are relatively common in dogs (27% of all nervous system tumours (Hayes *et al.*, 1975)) but rare in cats. Controversy exists over their nomenclature and the determination of their cellular origin (Summers *et al.*, 1995). The majority are characterized by their malignant histopathological characteristics and aggressive biological behaviour and there is a recommendation to consider these tumours as a broad group titled 'malignant peripheral nerve sheath tumours' (MPNSTs). Tumours of neuronal origin affecting peripheral nerves are extremely rare.

MPNSTs most commonly affect the ventral roots, although they can develop in the dorsal roots or along the length of a peripheral nerve. As they develop they can spread both distally and proximally. The tumour is initially within a single nerve, but if it invades a plexus it may spread to other nerve trunks. Affected nerves become thickened, enabling them to be identified with appropriate imaging (Figure 10.13).

Compression or invasion of peripheral nerves by tumours developing along their anatomical course will lead to pain and dysfunction. In the thoracic limb extension of extradural lymphoma (Spodnick *et al.*, 1992) and a lung tumour (Ferreira *et al.*, 2005) have been described compromising the brachial plexus, whilst in the pelvic limb tumours of the pelvis (e.g. a primary bone tumour) commonly compromise sciatic function (Figure 10.14).

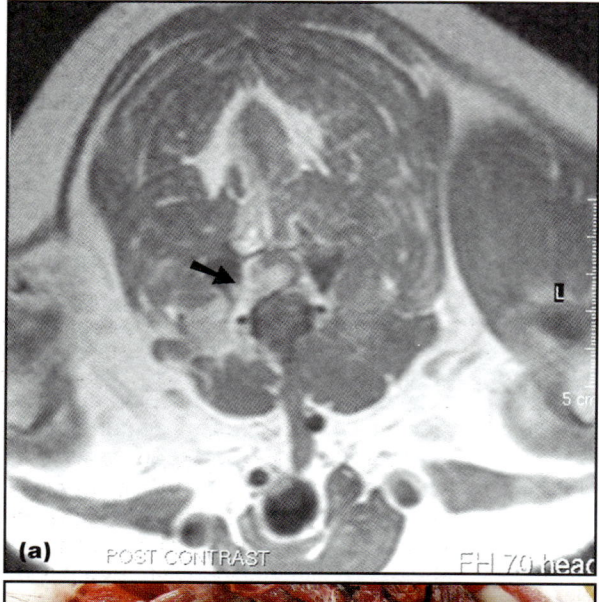

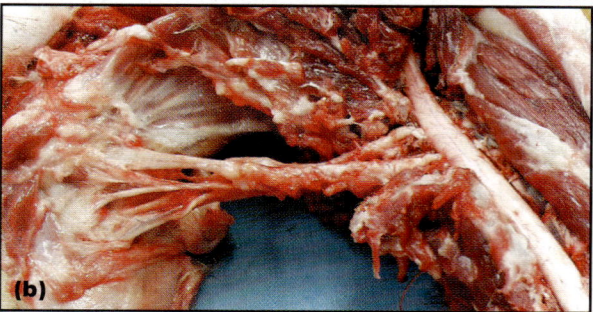

10.13 MPNST of the brachial plexus. **(a)** T1-weighted MRI image with contrast medium, showing enhancement of a nerve root (arrowed) and involvement of the spinal cord. **(b)** Post-mortem appearance of the brachial plexus, showing gross thickening of the peripheral nerves extending into the spinal canal.

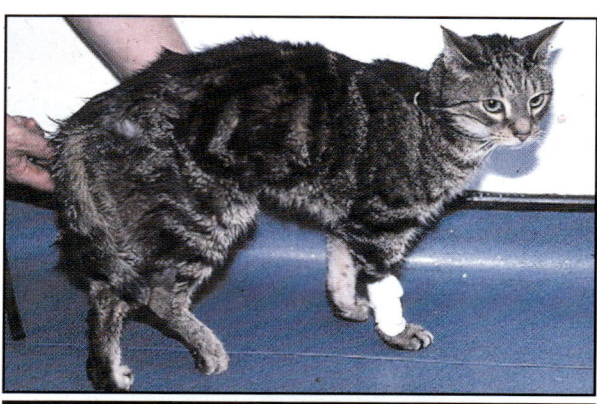

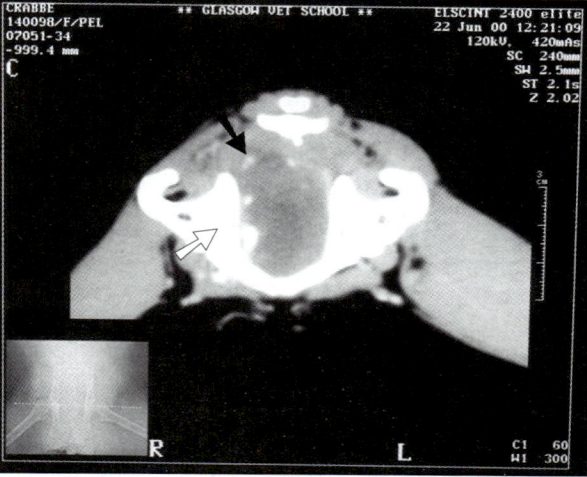

10.14 Cat with a primary bone tumour extending to affect the right sciatic nerve, resulting in right pelvic limb lameness and muscle atrophy. The CT scan of the pelvis shows a destructive lesion of the right ischium (white arrow) and extensive intrapelvic soft tissue swelling extending dorsally to the region of the sciatic nerve (black arrow).

Brachial plexus disease

Avulsion

Brachial plexus avulsion is a common traumatic polyneuropathy in the dog. The nerve roots are stretched or torn from the spinal cord during forced abduction of the limb, resulting in their intradural avulsion. Although both dorsal and ventral roots are involved, the major clinical signs are related to the ventral roots of C6–T2. Signs include hypotonia, an absence of myotatic reflexes, proprioceptive deficits and loss of superficial and deep sensation; the pattern depends on the nerve roots involved (Bailey, 1984). Neurogenic atrophy can develop rapidly and Horner's syndrome may be seen in caudal avulsions. This results from damage to the sympathetic innervation of the pupils and eyelids. In a series of 18 dogs, Griffiths *et al.* (1983) noted 55% of dogs with an avulsion of the brachial plexus had a partial Horner's syndrome with miosis. Loss of the ipsilateral cutaneous trunci reflex may also occur with caudal lesions.

The prognosis for this injury varies with the extent of avulsion. Caudal and complete lesions are the most common and severe as they involve the radial nerve. Thus the ability of the patient to bear weight is diminished as triceps function is impaired. The prognosis depends on whether there is physical division of the nerve or a temporary functional block in conduction (neuropraxia) from which recovery is possible. This can be difficult to establish. Clinically, the strongest predictor of a good outcome is the preservation of sensation following the injury, whilst decreased or absent radial nerve conduction velocity was a negative prognostic indicator (Faissler *et al.*, 2002). Caudal and complete avulsions have a guarded to poor prognosis (Faissler *et al.*, 2002).

Patients with preserved sensation may be managed conservatively for up to 2 months to assess potential recovery of the motor deficit. Patients may develop significant complications, including excoriation of the dorsal surface of the manus, self-mutilation injuries and muscle contractures, and should be managed accordingly. Amputation is indicated for persistent severe dysfunction or significant complications.

Patients with function in the elbow flexors/extensors may be candidates for muscle tendon transposition procedures (Bennett and Vaughan, 1976; Steinberg, 1988). For such techniques to be effective it is imperative that the transplanted muscle has some function. Though electrophysiology (e.g. EMG) may be of value in further investigation, it should not be the only parameter in decision making.

Tumours

MPNSTs are more common in the thoracic limb of dogs (Wright, 1985) than in the pelvic limb. The more peripherally located MPNSTs of the brachial plexus are characterized by progressive thoracic limb lameness with persistent non-localizable pain, the eventual development of LMN deficits (see Figure 10.1) and often a palpable axillary mass. In contrast, tumours originating from the nerve roots are likely to also exhibit signs associated with spinal cord compression (Targett *et al.*, 1993). Ipsilateral Horner's syndrome and ipsilateral loss of the panniculus reflex may be observed with tumours affecting the caudal brachial plexus. Diagnosis is challenging in the early stages before the LMN deficits become evident or a mass becomes palpable (Carmichael and Griffiths, 1981). The success of tumour resection reflects location and spread. Tumours that have invaded the spinal cord have a poor prognosis due to the inability to resect them fully and the high likelihood of recurrence. The more peripherally located tumours have the potential for successful resection, although this may necessitate limb amputation. This may be curative for some patients (Targett *et al.*, 1993).

Inflammatory disease

Brachial plexus neuritis: This is a rare bilaterally symmetrical condition of the thoracic limbs, characterized by a flaccid paralysis and the classic clinical findings of LMN dysfunction (see Figure 10.1) affecting both motor and sensory functions (Cummings *et al.*, 1973). Reported myelographic studies and CSF analyses have been unremarkable. The proposed mechanism is an immune-mediated inflammation and the condition has been reported following rabies vaccination with a modified live vaccine (Steinberg, 1988). The reported cases of the more severe form of brachial plexus neuritis have exhibited little in the way of recovery.

A milder manifestation associated with shifting thoracic limb lameness has been described. Similarly, an underlying immune-mediated mechanism is suspected, with some cases responding to steroids, whilst others have responded to dietary manipulation (Steinberg, 1988).

There is only one feline case described in the literature, which was temporally associated with a modified live rabies vaccine. The patient recovered spontaneously over a 3-week period (Bright *et al.*, 1978).

An equivalent syndrome affecting the lumbosacral plexus causing lameness has yet to be described in small animals. A rare syndrome of cauda equina neuritis has been reported in the dog, characterized by marked LMN deficits (Griffiths *et al.*, 1983).

Inflammation of isolated nerve roots: Inflammatory disease of single nerve roots has been confirmed in dogs and in at least one cat and is currently considered a rare phenomenon. Clinical descriptions are limited but the cardinal sign is persistent pain associated with the affected limb, resulting in a non-specific lameness. Cases affecting both thoracic and pelvic limbs have been observed. LMN effects might be expected to be a differentiating feature, but these appear to be mild initially thus reducing the confidence of localizing the lesion to the peripheral nervous system early in the disease (similar to MPNSTs, see above).

An MRI scan is the imaging modality of choice to identify the affected nerve root (Figure 10.15), although confirmation of the inflammatory nature of the pathology requires histopathology. The clinical signs, gross pathological appearance and imaging share many similarities with MPNSTs, and the two conditions can only be distinguished by histopathology. However, MPNSTs are commoner and have a different prognosis (see above).

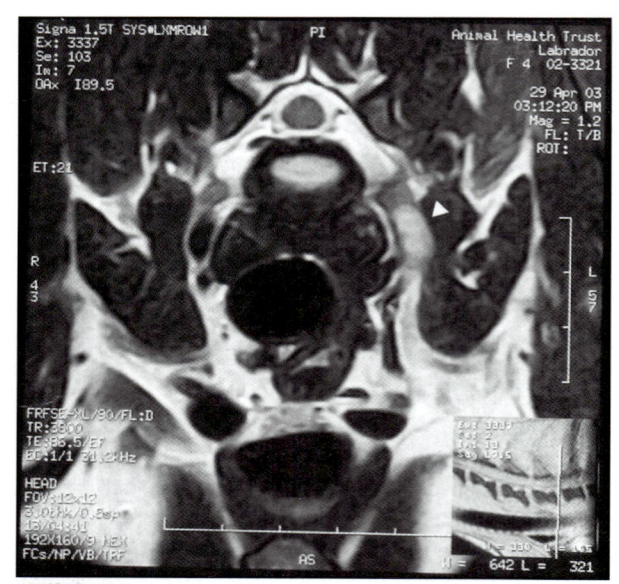

Chapter 10 Neurological causes of lameness

10.15 Transverse T2-weighted MRI scan of C7/T1 spinal cord showing an enlarged nerve root in a 5-year-old Labrador Retriever. The changes in the left nerve root (arrow head) have a similar appearance to a MPNST, but an inflammatory process was confirmed by histopathology. (Courtesy of Simon Platt)

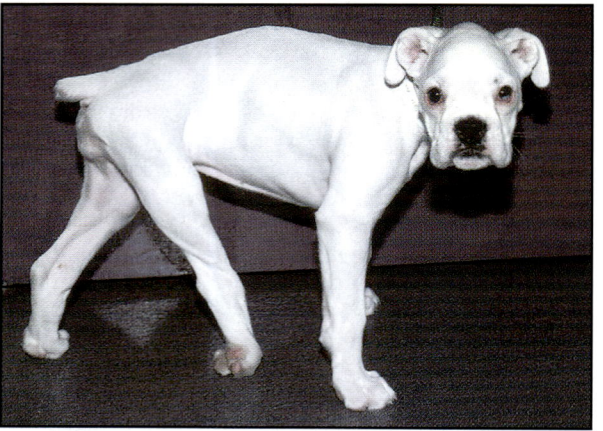

10.16 A 4-month-old Boxer puppy with *Neospora caninum* myositis–neuritis. The stifle is fixed in extension and there is generalized muscle atrophy of the right pelvic limb.

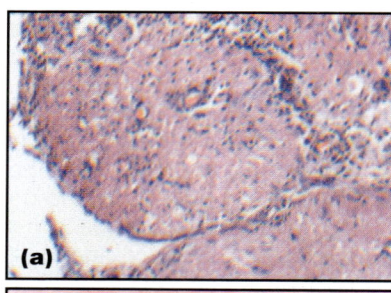

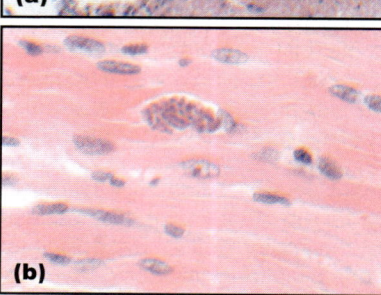

10.17 Photomicrographs of *Neospora caninum* infection. **(a)** Nerve root, showing massive cellular infiltration and radiculoneuritis (H&E; original magnification X100). **(b)** Skeletal muscle showing presence of tissue cyst (H&E; original magnification X400). (Courtesy of Adrian Philbey)

Information on management is limited. Resection of the affected nerve root may relieve pain but there is the potential for persistent neurological deficits. The value of medical therapy has not been established, although anti-inflammatory doses of steroids have been observed to have a beneficial effect.

Neosporosis

Neospora caninum is a protozoan parasite for which the dog is the definitive host (Lindsay *et al.*, 1999). The commonest manifestation of disease is a congenital infection of puppies, which tends to cause outbreaks in kennels. As puppies are usually homed by the time the clinical signs become apparent the identification of an outbreak depends on the accumulation of clinical information at a central point, and with the dispersion of litters at weaning this may not happen.

Clinical signs are first observed at 3–8 weeks of age, with progressive LMN disease (see Figure 10.1) affecting the pelvic limbs. Often one limb is more affected than the other. The patellar reflex is characteristically reduced or absent. The affected limb(s) become atrophied and stiff (Figure 10.16).

Diagnosis is by serology or polymerase chain reaction (PCR) of CSF and biopsy of affected nerves and muscle. CSF analysis may reveal pleocytosis. Histopathology confirms an inflammatory peripheral neuropathy and myopathy (Figure 10.17). Positive identification of the organism is achieved by immunocytochemistry.

Treatment has been reviewed by Vite (2005). A number of regimens have been described, including clindamycin (10–40 mg/kg orally, divided q8–12h) or trimethoprim/sulphonamide (15–20 mg/kg combined dose orally q12h) with pyrimethamine (at 1 mg/kg orally q24h) for a prolonged period (4–8 weeks). To be effective, therapy must be instituted promptly.

Once the patient has developed pelvic limb muscle contracture, therapy is ineffective. Prognosis for a return of limb function is generally poor, as the disease is usually identified in the chronic form, and amputation may be required.

There is no equivalent syndrome in kittens associated with *Toxoplasma gondii* infection.

References and further reading

Adams WH, Daniel GB, Pardo AD and Selcer R (1995) Magnetic resonance imaging of the caudal lumbar and lumbosacral spine in 13 dogs. *Veterinary Radiology and Ultrasound* **36**, 1–13

Bailey CS (1984) Patterns of cutaneous anaesthesia associated with brachial plexus avulsion in the dog. *Journal of the American Veterinary Medical Association* **185**, 889–899

Bennett D and Vaughan LC (1976) The use of muscle relocation techniques in the treatment of peripheral nerve injuries in dogs and cats. *Journal of Small Animal Practice* **17**, 99–108

Bright RM, Crabtree BJ and Knecht CD (1978) Brachial plexus neuropathy in the cat: a case report. *Journal of the American Animal Hospital Association* **14**, 612–615

Carmichael S and Griffiths IR (1981) Tumours involving the brachial plexus in seven dogs. *Veterinary Record* **108**, 435–437

Chambers JN, Selcer BA, Sullivan SA and Coates JR (1997) Diagnosis of lateralised lumbosacral disk herniation with magnetic resonance imaging. *Journal of the American Animal Hospital Association* **33**, 296–297

Cuddon PA (2002) Acquired canine peripheral neuropathies. *Veterinary Clinics of North America: Small Animal Practice* **32**, 207–249

Cummings JF, Lorenz MD, DeLahunta A and Washington LD (1973) Canine brachial plexus neuritis: a syndrome resembling serum neuritis in man. *Cornell Veterinarian* **63**, 589–617

DeLahunta A (1983) Lower motor neuron – general somatic efferent system. In: *Veterinary Neuroanatomy and Clinical Neurology, 2nd edn*, ed. A DeLahunta, pp. 53–94. WB Saunders, Philadelphia

de Riso L, Thomas WB and Sharp NJH (2000) Degenerative lumbosacral stenosis. *Veterinary Clinics of North America: Small Animal Practice* **20**, 111–132

Dernell WS, Van Vechten BJ, Straw RC *et al.* (2000) Outcome following treatment of vertebral tumours in 20 dogs (1986–1995). *Journal of the American Animal Hospital Association* **36**, 245–251

Dickinson PJ, Sturges BK, Berry WL *et al.* (2001) Extradural spinal synovial cysts in nine dogs. *Journal of Small Animal Practice* **42**, 502–509

Faissler D, Cizinauskas S and Jaggy A (2002) Prognostic factors for functional recovery in dogs with suspected brachial plexus avulsion. *Journal of Veterinary Internal Medicine* **16**, 370

Ferreira AJA, Peleteiro MC, Correia JHD, Jesus SO and Goulão A (2005) Small-cell carcinoma of the lung resembling a brachial plexus tumour. *Journal of Small Animal Practice* **46**, 286–290

Fitch RB, Kerwin SC and Hosgood G (2000) Caudal cervical intervertebral disk disease in the small dog: role of distraction and stabilization in ventral slot decompression. *Journal of the American Animal Hospital Association* **36**, 69–74

Garosi L (2004) Lesion localization and differential diagnosis. In: *BSAVA Manual of Canine and Feline Neurology, 3rd edn*, ed. SR Platt and NJ Olby, pp. 24–34. BSAVA Publications, Gloucester

Griffiths IR, Carmichael S, Mayer SJ and Sharp NJ (1983) Polyradiculoneuritis in two dogs presenting as neuritis of the cauda equina. *Veterinary Record* **112**, 360–361

Griffiths IR, Duncan ID and Lawson DD (1974) Avulsion of the brachial plexus. 2. Clinical aspects. *Journal of Small Animal Practice* **15**, 177–183

Hayes HM, Priester WA and Pendergrass TW (1975) Occurrence of nervous-tissue tumours in cattle, horses, cats and dogs. *International Journal of Cancer* **15**, 39–47

Jeffery ND (1995) Degenerative conditions. In: *Handbook of Small Animal Spinal Surgery*, ed. ND Jeffery, pp. 85–110. WB Saunders, London

Lindsay DS, Dubey JP and Duncan RB (1999) Confirmation that the dog is a definitive host for *Neospora caninum*. *Veterinary Parasitology* **82**, 327–333

Lipscombe VJ and Muir P (2000) Magnetic resonance imaging of a dog with sciatic nerve root signature. *Veterinary Record* **147**, 393–395

Long SN and Anderson TJ (2004) Tissue biopsy. In: *BSAVA Manual of Canine and Feline Neurology, 3rd edn*, ed. SR Platt and NJ Olby, pp. 84–96. BSAVA Publications, Gloucester

Niederhauser UB and Holliday TA (1989) Electrodiagnostic studies in diseases of muscle and neuromuscular junctions. *Seminars in Veterinary Medicine and Surgery (Small Animal)* **4**, 116–125

Okin R (1983) Vertebral fracture with L6 nerve root entrapment. *Canine Practice* **10**, 30–34

Poncelet L (2004) Electrophysiology. In: *BSAVA Manual of Canine and Feline Neurology, 3rd edn*, ed. SR Platt and NJ Olby, pp. 54–69. BSAVA Publications, Gloucester

Rusbridge C, MacSweeny JE, Davies JV *et al.* (2000) Syringomyelia in Cavalier King Charles spaniels. *Journal of the American Animal Hospital Association* **36**, 34–41

Rusbridge C (2005) Neurological diseases in the Cavalier King Charles spaniel. *Journal of Small Animal Practice* **46**, 265–272

Seim III HB (2002) Surgery of the cervical spine. In: *Small Animal Surgery, 2nd edn*, ed. WT Fossum, pp. 1213–1268. Mosby, St Louis

Sharp NJH and Wheeler SJ (2005) Cervical disc disease. In: *Small Animal Spinal Disorders: Diagnosis and Surgery, 2nd edn*, ed. NJH Sharp and SJ Wheeler, pp. 93–120. Elsevier Mosby, Edinburgh

Spodnick GJ, Berg J, Moore FM and Cotter SM (1992) Spinal lymphoma in cats: 21 cases (1976–1989). *Journal of the American Veterinary Medical Association* **200**, 373–376

Steinberg HS (1988) Brachial plexus injuries and dysfunctions. *Veterinary Clinics of North America: Small Animal Practice* **18**, 565–580

Summers B, Cummings J and de Lahunta A (1995) Diseases of the peripheral nervous system. In: *Veterinary Neuropathology*, ed. B Summers *et al.*, pp. 402–501. Mosby, St Louis

Targett MP, Dyce J and Houlton JEF (1993) Tumours involving the nerve sheaths of the forelimb in dogs. *Journal of Small Animal Practice* **34**, 221–225

Vite CH (2005) Inflammatory diseases of the central nervous system. In: *Braund's Clinical Neurology in Small Animals: Localization, Diagnosis and Treatment*, ed. CH Vite. International Veterinary Information Service, Ithaca (www.ivis.org) A3228.0205

Webb AA, Pharr JW, Lew LJ and Tryon KA (2001) MR imaging findings in a dog with lumbar ganglion cysts. *Veterinary Radiology and Ultrasound* **42**, 9–13

Wright JA (1985) The pathological features associated with spinal tumours in 29 dogs. *Journal of Comparative Pathology* **95**, 549–557

11

Surgical biology of joints

Rory Todhunter

Introduction

The goals of surgical intervention in joint disease are: to prevent or ameliorate the progression of osteoarthritis; to reduce or eliminate pain; and to improve joint function for a prolonged period. This chapter offers a solid foundation to enable the surgeon to make the critical decision to operate on a joint and to know what to do during and after the operation that may benefit the patient. A more in-depth review can be found in Todhunter and Johnston (2003).

Anatomy and physiology

Synovial joints facilitate predictable, energy-efficient and pain-free movement. Translational movement in normal joints is restricted by the joint capsule, ligaments, articular contour and the periarticular tendons and muscles. Muscles acting across the joint contribute to mechanical stability and control movement. Load is transmitted and distributed across the joint surface while maintaining the contact stresses across the joint surfaces at acceptably low levels and over a wide range of loads and oscillating speeds. More than 1–3-fold body weight during walking, and 5–10-fold body weight during running must be transmitted through the loadbearing joints (Simon and Radin, 1997).

Ligaments and tendons

Ligaments and tendons consist of collagen, mostly type I, which forms the fibrils and fibres of the tissue. The ligaments connect bone to bone. Collateral ligaments prevent excessive valgus and varus distortion of the joint. The cruciate ligaments in the stifle prevent translation of the joint surfaces, contribute to proprioceptive function, and the cranial cruciate ligament resists internal rotation of the tibia relative to the femur. The cranial cruciate ligament consists of a craniomedial and caudolateral band. Partial tears most commonly affect the craniomedial band. Partial tears of this band tend to heal poorly. Ligaments are poorly vascularized and heal slowly once injured. They never regain their original architecture and remain mechanically inferior to the strength of the uninjured ligament.

Tendons connect muscle to bone. Injuries tend to occur at the muscle–tendon junction. Severe tendon injuries heal poorly and also remain mechanically inferior due to loss of the original architecture.

Menisci

In the stifle, the menisci contribute to rotational, translational and varus/valgus stability. The menisci also alter the load that is borne by the subjacent articular cartilage. These fibrocartilaginous structures contain approximately 65% water and 70–80% collagen on a dry weight basis in the dog, accompanied by a differential distribution of collagen and proteoglycan. The axial portion has a proportionally higher proteoglycan content and is preferentially compressed, while the peripheral portion has a proportionally higher collagen content and is preferentially loaded in tension. The axial portion is poorly vascularized and heals poorly. In dogs, axial tears of the meniscus are most commonly excised. Peripheral injuries may heal partially, due to better blood supply at the capsular attachments. The meniscus is innervated and can indirectly cause joint pain through impingement and by causing tension on the joint capsule. The medial meniscus is subject to injury in the cruciate-deficient stifle as it cannot move as freely as the lateral meniscus when the tibia translates cranially. The lateral meniscus has a meniscofemoral ligament which allows it to move more freely. Tears in the caudal horn of the medial meniscus are usually excised as they heal poorly and can cause joint pain.

Synovium and fibrous capsule

The joint capsule has a thick fibrous portion, produced by fibroblasts, which is lined by a thin subsynovium or lamina propria and the synovium, an incomplete layer, one to four synoviocytes thick, with no basement membrane. Synoviocytes form a continuum of cells and have secretory (type B) or phagocytic (type A) functions (Henderson and Pettipher, 1985). The synovium is in contact with the synovial fluid (Figure 11.1). The fibrous joint capsule and ligaments are innervated; synovial inflammation and effusion, and stretching aggravate mechano- and chemoreceptors.

Synovial fluid

The synovial fluid is a colourless or pale yellow viscous liquid that occupies the intra-articular space. It is an ultrafiltrate of plasma with the addition of hyaluronan synthesized by type B synoviocytes. In inflamed joints synoviocytes also secrete pro-inflammatory cytokines that can affect chondrocyte metabolism.

Chapter 11 Surgical biology of joints

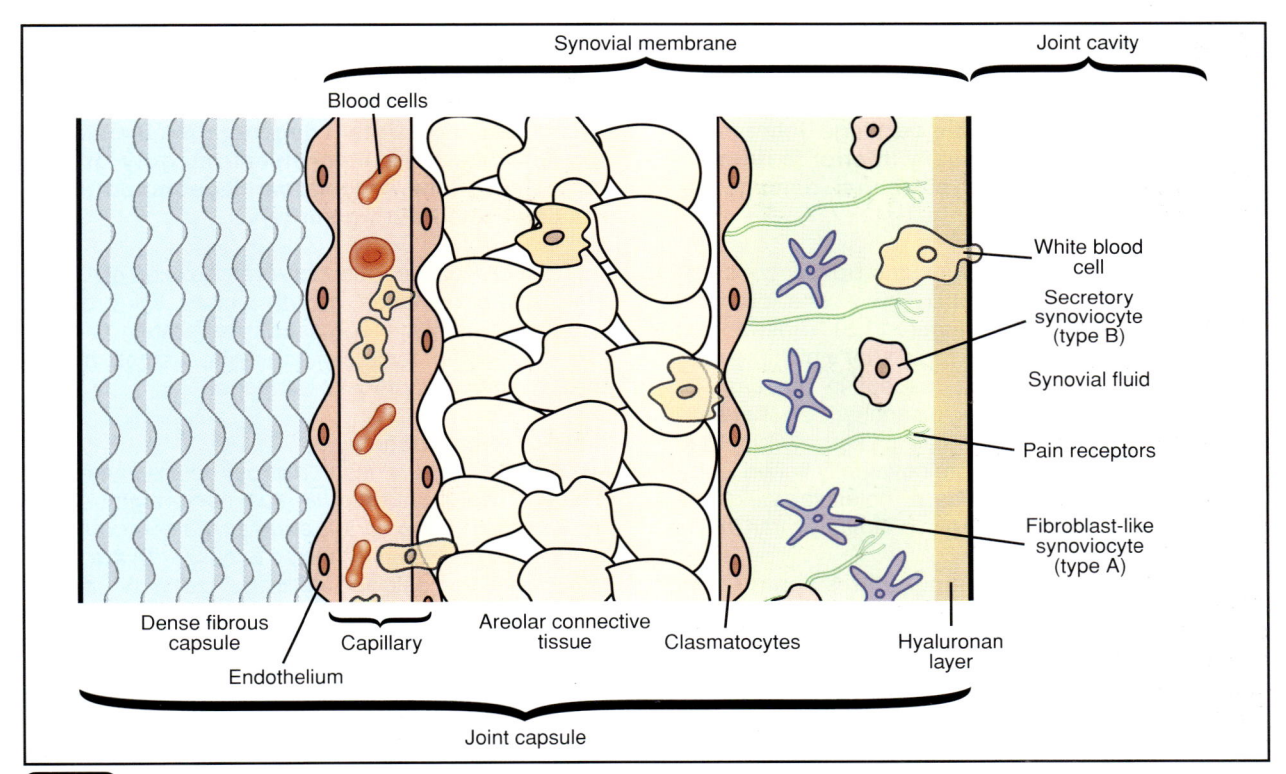

11.1 The joint capsule of a dog.

Synovial fluid from normal canine joints contains <1000 nucleated cells per microlitre. Most of these are mononuclear (synoviocytes, monocytes and lymphocytes make up 95%); the remainder are neutrophils. Fluid exchange between plasma and synovial fluid is governed by hydrostatic and colloid osmotic pressure differences. Lipophilic molecules, oxygen and carbon dioxide diffuse freely into and out of the synovial fluid (Simkin *et al.*, 1990). Synovial fluid nourishes articular cartilage, intra-articular ligaments and menisci. Subatmospheric intra-articular pressure (−2 to −6 cmH$_2$O) assists in stabilizing the normal joint (Lust *et al.*, 1980).

Hyaluronan is a long-chain polysaccharide that is synthesized at the plasma membrane of the fibroblastic synoviocyte and extruded into the extracellular space. Its high concentration in synovial fluid imparts a high viscosity that allows the synovial fluid to support transient shear stresses (Schurz and Ribitsch, 1987). Synovial fluid undergoes shear-thinning behaviour under stress and strain, a feature called thixotropy. Hyaluronan in the extracellular matrix may behave like a molecular sieve. The interstitial space is one of the two main routes (the other is the synovial capillary bed) by which fluid leaves the joint. Maintaining normal concentration and size of hyaluronan molecules is critical for preserving joint health: proliferation of synovial lining cells is inhibited *in vitro* at the molecular weight and concentration of hyaluronan present in normal synovial fluid. Following intra-articular injection, hyaluronan escapes from the joint within 1–2 days, although the majority is cleared within hours. Hyaluronan also has a critical function in the extracellular matrix of articular cartilage by aggregating large numbers of aggrecan monomers along its chain (see below).

Articular cartilage

Composition

Articular cartilage is composed of collagen and proteoglycans.

The translucent, glass-like (hyaline) appearance of articular cartilage is due primarily to its high water content (70% by weight in mature healthy cartilage and 80–90% in neonatal canine cartilage) (Todhunter *et al.*, 1998) and the fine structure of its collagen fibril network. It is a multiphasic material with a major fluid phase of water and electrolytes and a solid phase, which on a dry-weight basis, consists of about 50% collagen, 35% proteoglycan, 10% glycoproteins, 3% mineral, 1% lipid and 1–2% chondrocytes (by volume) (Figure 11.2). Most of the collagen in articular cartilage is of type II (85–90%); small amounts of types VI, IX, X, XI, XII and XIV are present.

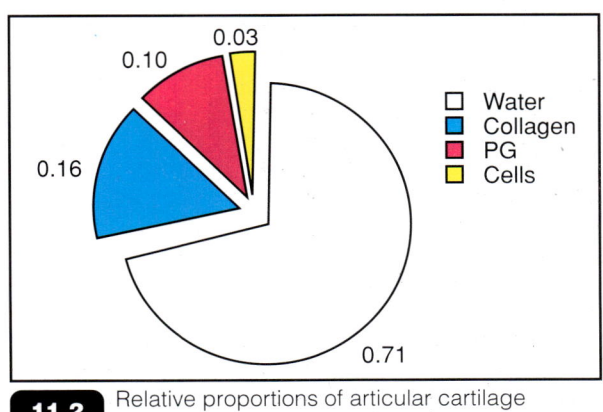

11.2 Relative proportions of articular cartilage constituents (PG, proteoglycan).

Chapter 11 Surgical biology of joints

> **Type II collagen provides the tensile stiffness of the articular cartilage. Once the collagen fibril is interrupted in injured articular cartilage, the hydration of the articular cartilage increases and it becomes mechanically inferior to normal articular cartilage. This structural damage is never reparable.**

> **Aggrecan is the critical proteoglycan for articular cartilage as it resists compressive load due to its ability to attract water osmotically. Aggrecan core protein degeneration inevitably compromises the mechanical integrity of the articular surface. Articular cartilage should never be desiccated during surgery.**

Proteoglycans, the other major solid component of the articular cartilage matrix, have one or more glycosaminoglycan chains (Figure 11.3). These chains have two regions: a linkage region, by which they are attached to a protein core (except in the case of hyaluronan); and a repeating disaccharide. Chondroitin sulphate, dermatan sulphate or keratan sulphate glycosaminoglycan chains are covalently linked to the core protein. Hyaluronan has a molecular weight of 300–2000 kD and is the only glycosaminoglycan that is not sulphated.

Aggrecan contains chondroitin sulphate and keratan sulphate side-chains. It forms large aggregates of many chondroitin sulphate proteoglycans non-covalently attached to hyaluronan (Luo *et al.*, 2000). The complex is stabilized by a glycoprotein called 'link protein'. As many as 100 aggrecan monomers aggregate with a single hyaluronan chain, so the molecular mass of the whole complex may be 200,000 kD.

The non-collagenous, non-proteoglycan glycoproteins (e.g. proteinases, growth factors, link proteins, fibronectins, cartilage oligomeric matrix protein (COMP), thrombospondin, tenascin) constitute a small, but important, portion of articular cartilage.

Microscopic structure

Articular cartilage varies in microstructure in different joints, in weightbearing *versus* non-weightbearing areas, and in young *versus* adult animals (Farquhar *et al.*, 1997). Three unmineralized zones (I–III) are delineated from the calcified cartilage (zone IV) by the 'tidemark' (Figure 11.4). The lower boundary of the mature calcified cartilage is the cement line formed at the maturation of the articular–epiphyseal complex and growth plate closure. The superficial layer appears to form a pre-stressed, wear-resistant protective diaphragm which can withstand tension in the plane of the articular surface. Collagen fibrils are more concentrated at the surface than in the deeper tissue.

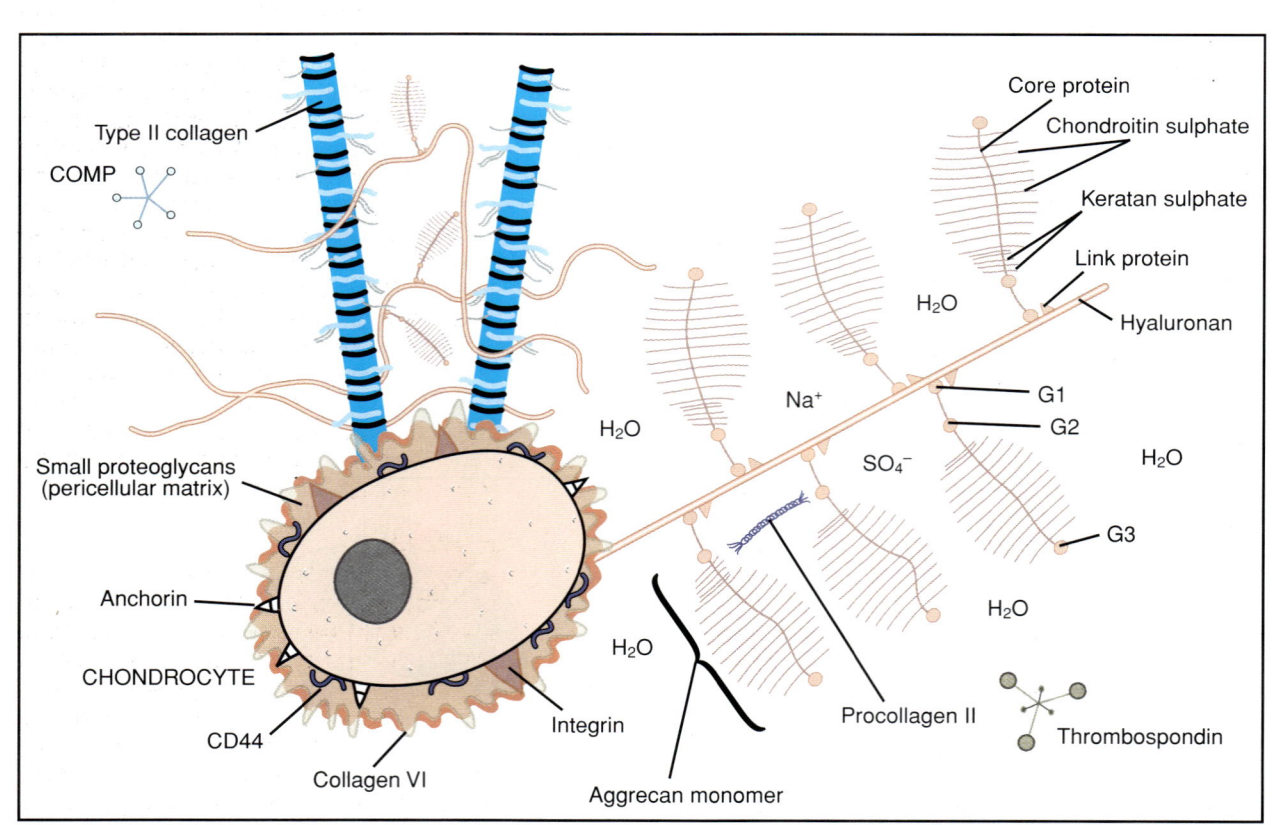

11.3 Diagrammatic representation of a complex extracellular matrix of collagens, proteoglycans and noncollagenous proteins. Scale varies throughout drawing. (COMP, cartilage oligomeric matrix protein; CD44, hyaluronan receptor; G1, G2, G3, globular domains along core protein)

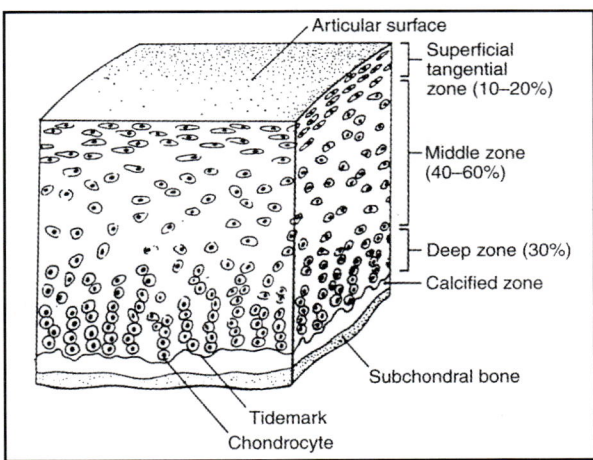

11.4 Diagram illustrating the arrangement of articular chondrocytes and collagen fibrils in non-calcified articular cartilage, calcified cartilage, subchondral plate and cancellous bone.

Zonal architecture enables the articular surface to resist tension, while the deeper zones, which contain proportionally more proteoglycan, resist compression. Once the articular surface is breached (even by laceration or scoring) and fibrillation is grossly apparent, the mechanical properties are irreversibly altered.

Matrix synthesis and turnover
Chondrocytes are the only cell type in adult articular cartilage and are solely responsible for maintenance of matrix metabolism. Nutrients, including glucose, oxygen and amino acids, diffuse from the synovial fluid. Generally, molecules larger than haemoglobin (69 kD) are excluded from diffusion into the matrix. Chondrocytes synthesize, organize and regulate the composition of a complex pericellular, territorial and interterritorial matrix to achieve net growth and modelling, remodelling or a balanced equilibrium. In adult canine articular cartilage, estimated collagen turnover time is 120 years (Akizuki *et al.*, 1987), while proteoglycan turnover is about 300 days (Maroudas, 1980).

Enzymatic cleavage of the collagen triple helix results in irreversible damage to the articular surface. Control of inflammation in the joint is therefore critical for maintenance of structural integrity of the articular surface. Induction of matrix metalloproteinase (MMP) activity by pro-inflammatory cytokines will eventually interrupt the collagenous architecture of the articular surface through proteolytic degradation.

Innervation of synovial joints
The nerve supply of diarthrodial joints originates from independent articular branches of peripheral nerves and related muscles; it controls proprioception and helps restrict joint motion to within physiological limits (Dee, 1978; Johnston, 1997). Nerves accompany blood vessels in synovial tissues. Joints have complex innervation; for example, the canine hip joint capsule receives innervation from the femoral, cranial gluteal and sciatic nerves.

The nerve fibres terminate in the joint capsule, fat pad, and meniscus and patellar, collateral, meniscal and cruciate ligaments. The elbow, shoulder, carpus and tarsus receive innervation from all the peripheral nerves that pass each joint. Each articular nerve contains small, medium and large myelinated and unmyelinated fibres. Nociceptive fibres, with free nerve endings, are present in the fibrous capsule, ligaments, fat pads, subsynovium, tendons and periosteum (Freeman and Wyke, 1967). Chemical mediators for nociception include prostaglandins, leucotrienes, substance P, bradykinin and cytokines (Dray, 1995). Prostaglandins sensitize nociceptors to algesic substances, such as bradykinin and histamine, and decrease the pain threshold. Proprioception is provided by a combination of slowly adapting mechanoreceptors (Pacinian-like corpuscles mostly located in the fibrous capsule), which signal changing pressure around the joint, and spindle receptors (Golgi tendon organs) in adjacent muscles, tendons, ligaments and meniscus (Zimny, 1988).

Inflammation causes pain when the joint is moved. Both stretching and compression of the joint capsule during flexion and over-extension cause pain. Flexion also reduces available intra-articular volume and exacerbates the capsular stretching caused by effusion in the joint.

Lubrication
At least 30 mechanisms for lubrication of the cartilage-on-cartilage surface have been proposed (Johnston, 1997). During compression, fluid is exuded from the cartilage; it is thought that a layer of fluid forms between opposing surfaces ('weeping lubrication') and decreases the coefficient of friction ('boosted lubrication'). Lubricin and associated phospholipids provide boundary lubrication at low loads. At high loads, lubricin is probably displaced from the articular surfaces and weeping lubrication may be more important. As the joint moves under load, fluid is probably exuded at the leading edge of cartilage contact, and imbibed at the trailing edge. The fluid is imbibed in response to the increased swelling pressure but stops flowing into the cartilage when the swelling pressure is resisted by the tension developed in the collagen network. Boundary lubrication of the synovial membrane is important to decrease resistance associated with joint movement. Hyaluronan in the synovial fluid allows the tissue to move easily (Davis *et al.*, 1978).

Load distribution
The stiffness of bone enables it to support large loads without substantial deformation. Structurally, subchondral bone is a mixture of trabecular and compact bone and, beneath it, is trabecular epiphyseal bone. Trabecular bone can deform to compressive strains of >50%. Trabecular bone can absorb considerable energy for large compressive loads while maintaining a minimum mass. The mechanical strength of trabecular bone decreases with age as anisotropy, mean marrow space volume and bone surface:volume ratio increase. The subchondral bone provides structural support to the overlying articular cartilage so that

Chapter 11 Surgical biology of joints

increases or decreases in subchondral bone stiffness outside the physiological range may result in articular cartilage injury (Radin and Rose, 1986). When axial loading is imposed, the subchondral plate bends, allowing congruent contact of the joint surfaces. This allows for stress dissipation across the joint surfaces.

Articular cartilage can undergo large volumetric and shear deformations during normal activity, which are fully recoverable in healthy tissue. Loading increases the contact area (reducing tissue stress levels) of the articular cartilage and increases joint conformity (providing additional stability). The mechanical properties of articular cartilage are controlled primarily by the ability of cartilage to maintain hydration under pressure, which is achieved through the low hydraulic permeability and the high osmotic pressure of the constituent proteoglycans. The osmotic pressure may contribute up to 50% of the compressive stiffness of the articular cartilage. This swelling pressure is balanced by the tensile stress of the collagen network.

> **Deterioration in the composition of articular cartilage inevitably renders the articular cartilage susceptible to mechanical injury. The mechanical properties of articular cartilage are directly related to its biochemical composition.**

Cartilage tissue is a heterogenous, fibre-reinforced composite saturated by a hydrated gel (Mow et al., 1999). In the laboratory, cartilage exhibits a soft, time-dependent response when subjected to load through a free-draining porous indentor. Fluid exudation is greatest initially, then gradually diminishes as the slow loss of water raises internal osmotic pressure and collagen fibril stress levels. Load-induced fluid motion may be important to nutrition of the chondrocyte. The simplest mathematical approaches to describing the constitutive modelling of articular cartilage can be divided into the following broad categories: elastic, viscoelastic or poroelastic.

Mechanical properties of articular cartilage are frequently measured in vitro (Setton et al., 1999). The tensile modulus and strength are measures of resistance to tensile loading and depend on the density and orientation of collagen fibrils and its crosslinking. Hydraulic permeability is a measure of matrix resistance to pressure-induced fluid flow.

> **The biomechanics of the joint are affected by the composition of the articular cartilage, joint anatomy and congruency of the articular surfaces. These factors then affect the response of a particular joint to developmental abnormalities, trauma and surgical intervention.**

Cytokines and growth factors

Cytokines and growth factors play critical roles in both health and disease. Articular cartilage contains stores of TGF and TGF-β receptors have been described. TGF-β increases the synthesis of several matrix constituents in a variety of cells including chondrocytes and mesenchymal stem cells, depresses proteinase activity and regulates cellular migration, proliferation, differentiation and apoptosis. Supraphysiological levels of TGF-β may induce synovial fibrosis, proteoglycan loss from cartilage and osteophyte formation, yet TGF-β can counteract the deleterious effects of interleukin-1 on cartilage metabolism.

Insulin-like growth factor-1 (IGF-1) has potent effects on articular cartilage metabolism, causing upregulation of proteoglycan and link protein synthesis, accompanied by inhibition of proteoglycan degradation. IGF-1 can counteract the proteoglycan-degrading and synthesis-inhibiting effects of IL-1, TNF-α and retinoic acid on articular cartilage.

Enzyme activities

The MMP family is a group of zinc-dependent endopeptidases that, when activated, degrade the extracellular matrix. The activity of MMPs is inhibited by tissue inhibitors of metalloproteinase (TIMPs) 1–5 (Brew et al., 2000). There is a slight excess of TIMPs over MMPs in normal articular cartilage.

Because of their roles in cartilage matrix degradation in OA, of particular interest are collagenases 1 and 3, stromelysin 1, and three isoforms of 'aggrecanase', members of the 'A Disintegrin and Metalloproteinase with Thrombospondin Motifs' (ADAMTS) family (Caterson et al., 2000).

> **Synovial and plasma cytokines, enzymes and matrix degradation products serve as potential biomarkers of the osteoarthritic process and their inhibitors serve as potential therapeutic targets.**

The response of joint tissues to injury and surgery

Healing and remodelling

Some joint tissues function adequately as scar tissue while others do not. The response to injury of each tissue therefore affects treatment and prognosis. The limiting factors to healing following joint surgery are:

- The age of the animal
- The extent of articular cartilage and subchondral bone injury
- Prior existence of OA.

Synovium and ligaments

The synovium has rapid regenerative capacity. Periarticular and intra-articular ligaments tend to recover slowly from injury but the fibrous tissue replacement often functions well, given sufficient healing time. The degree of ligament injury will affect the rapidity of healing and the long-term result but the degree of injury may be hard to assess clinically (Brinker et al., 1997). However, the strength of a transected medial collateral ligament may still be only half that of control ligaments almost a year after injury. Although injured ligaments are not acting in isolation, they become more lax under repetitive strain and promote joint degeneration over time.

Cartilage

Articular cartilage that opposes partial-thickness defects remains physically unchanged for at least 2 years. In contrast, marked alterations were found in measurements in cartilage opposing full-thickness defects. If the cartilage lesion is undermined or not attached firmly to subchondral bone, debridement is recommended to allow some repair, as the resultant fibrocartilaginous repair tissue may prove more durable. It has been recommended that, during debridement, the cartilage margin of the defect is made at right angles to the joint surface (Frenkel and Di Cesare, 1999).

Full-thickness articular cartilage defects that penetrate the subchondral plate heal through a process not unlike that of other tissues with a vascular supply. Almost all repair in full-thickness cartilage injury is extrinsic. The healing process is as follows:

1. A haematoma forms.
2. Activated platelets release platelet-derived growth factor (PDGF), a growth factor for mesenchymal cells, osteoblasts and endothelial cells and a chemoattractant for neutrophils and monocytes.
3. Necrotic cells are degraded; their degradation products attract neutrophils and monocytes.
4. There is phagocytosis and solubilization of the clot and necrotic tissue.
5. Some mesenchymal cells in the clot, together with local endothelial cells and mesenchymal cells proliferate (stimulated by PDGF and macrophage-derived growth factor) and invade the wound site from the bone marrow.
6. Extracellular matrix degradation occurs via MMPs from leucocytes, endothelial cells, osteoblasts and mesenchymal cells.
7. PDGF, IL-2 and prostaglandin E_2 promote cell migration into the damaged area. IGFs, TGF-β, fibroblast growth factors and bone morphogenetic proteins (BMPs) affect local differentiation of mesenchymal cells, which produce extracellular matrix. A vascular, fibroblastic repair tissue forms in the initial stages of healing.
8. During maturation, cartilage repair tissue becomes more cellular and less vascular. Fibrocartilage is a mixture of hyaline cartilage and fibrous tissue. The hyaline-like tissue is deep and the superficial articular surface is fibrous. The calcified cartilage and tidemark do not reform and there is poor integration of the repair tissue peripherally, which predisposes the tissue to mechanical disruption with repetitive use.

The timeline for healing of full-thickness defects in dogs can be extrapolated from experiments in horses (Convery et al., 1972):

- 1 month: granulation tissue;
- 6 weeks: cellular tissue with high synthetic activity but low glycosaminoglycan;
- 4 months: metaplasia to fibrocartilage (more abundant extracellular matrix);
- 6 months: 'imperfect' hyaline cartilage;
- 9 months: collagen content as control cartilage, although glycosaminoglycan lower.

Small lesions (up to 3 mm in diameter) heal with more hyaline cartilage than larger defects. Osteochondral defects showed replacement of fibrocartilage with fibrous tissue by 12 months after surgery (Hurtig et al., 1988). There is concern that such repair tissue would not withstand the mechanical forces of day-to-day wear and tear. Prognosis for functional recovery in dogs is affected by location of osteochondral defects. The humeral head seems to be more forgiving of focal deep articular cartilage lesions like osteochondrosis than are the stifle, elbow and talocrural joints. Currently, removal of loose osteochondral flaps, careful and limited debridement of subchondral bone and limited subchondral forage, or 'micropik', are recommended (Nixon, 2002).

> **Removal of loose osteochondral flaps and joint irrigation decreases synovitis. Limited debridement is recommended to reduce abnormal loading patterns at the articular surface and the depth of tissue that requires regeneration and repair. Subchondral forage and 'micropik' techniques encourage clot formation and migration of mesenchymal stem cells into the subchondral defect. This should result in the most mechanically suitable articular surface at the current level of our understanding and clinical surgical cabability.**

Because the intrinsic and extrinsic repair of articular cartilage results in a surface that degenerates over time, cartilage resurfacing has been attempted with a variety of grafts. Tissue engineering with native chondrocytes embedded in a plain matrix or in a matrix with exogenous growth factors is the current state-of-the-art technique (Frenkel and Di Cesare, 1999; Nixon, 2002). Most recently, chondrocytes transfected with growth factor genes under viral promoter control have been placed in full-thickness cartilage defects that may or may not penetrate the subchondral plate. Until such treatments are efficient and cost-effective, limited debridement of articular defects, subchondral forage and 'micropik' remain the treatment of choice.

Factors affecting the response

Genetics
Canine susceptibility to cartilage degeneration and OA is largely dictated by the joint involved and the genes contributing to the heritable traits that may have different expression patterns among joints.

Obesity
If surgical intervention can be delayed in obese dogs, weight reduction before surgery may improve postoperative recovery. Postoperative weight reduction for osteoarthritic conditions is highly recommended.

Age
The developing chondroepiphysis, from which the synovial joint is established at maturity, grows by the process of endochondral ossification beginning at the articular–epiphyseal complex and surrounding the secondary centre of ossification. The articular surface

matures as the calcified layer of cartilage is deposited and the subchondral plate is formed. This occurs at approximately the same time as the growth plates close. It is generally thought that surgical intervention to treat joint conditions results in a more favourable long-term outcome if that intervention is undertaken prior to skeletal maturity.

Mechanical environment

Immobilization of joints causes degenerative changes (Kallio et al., 1988). In addition, the absence of functional loads promotes bone loss. Therefore, early return to function with rapid resolution of pain should result in optimal surgical outcome.

The response of the articular cartilage to an exercise training programme appears to be influenced by the state of the cartilage prior to the initiation of exercise, to the early intensity of the exercise and to species variability. Proteoglycan content and cartilage thickness are influenced by exercise intensity (Vassan, 1983; Jurvelin et al., 1986; Kiviranta et al., 1988). Collagen content and synthesis of cartilage do not appear to be affected by running exercise (Kiviranta et al., 1988).

Static loading of articular cartilage *in vitro* generally inhibits biosynthetic activity. Dynamic loading appears to have a more complex effect, depending on load direction, intensity, frequency, duty cycle and time in culture. Moderate cyclical load increases proteoglycan and protein synthesis above the level in unloaded cartilage, suggesting a positive adaptation to load. In contrast, heavier or prolonged periods of loading produce a dramatic inhibition of proteoglycan and protein synthesis, particularly in cartilage from anatomical sites which are not subjected to heavy loads *in vivo*.

References and further reading

Akizuki S, Mow VC, Muller F et al. (1987) Tensile properties of human knee joint cartilage. II. Correlations between weight bearing and tissue pathology and the kinetics of swelling. *Journal of Orthopedic Research* **5**, 173–186

Brew K, Dinakarpandian D and Nagase H (2000) Tissue inhibitors of metalloproteinases: evolution, structure and function. *Biochimica et Biophysica Acta* **1477**, 267–283

Brinker WD, Piermattei DL and Flo GL (1997) Principles of joint surgery. In: *Handbook of Small Animal Orthopedics and Fracture Repair*, pp. 201–220. WB Saunders, Philadelphia

Caterson B, Flannery CR, Hughes CE et al. (2000) Mechanisms involved in cartilage proteoglycan catabolism. *Matrix Biology* **19**, 333–344

Convery FR, Akeson WH and Keown GH (1972) The repair of large osteochondral defects: an experimental study in horses. *Clinical Orthopedics and Related Research* **82**, 253–262

Davis WH, Lee SL and Sokoloff L (1978) Boundary lubricating ability of synovial fluid in degenerative joint disease. *Arthritis and Rheumatism* **21**, 754–756

Dee R (1978) The innervation of joints. In: *The Joints and Synovial Fluid*, ed. L Sokoloff, p. 177. Academic Press, New York

Dray A (1995) Inflammatory mediators of pain. *British Journal of Anaesthesia* **75**, 125–131

Eyre D (2002) Collagen of articular cartilage. *Arthritis Research* **4**, 30–35

Farquhar T, Bertram J, Todhunter RJ et al. (1997) Variations in composition of cartilage from the shoulder joints of young adult dogs at risk for developing canine hip dysplasia. *Journal of the American Veterinary Medical Association* **210**, 1483–1485

Freeman MAR and Wyke B (1967) The innervation of the knee joint: anatomical and histological study in the cat. *Journal of Anatomy* **101**, 505–532

Frenkel SR and Di Cesare PE (1999) Degradation and repair of articular cartilage. *Frontiers in Biosciences* **4**, D671–D685

Henderson B and Pettipher ER (1985) The synovial lining cell: biology and pathobiology. *Seminars in Arthritis and Rheumatism* **15**, 1–32

Hurtig MB, Fretz PB, Doige CE et al. (1988) Effects of lesion size and location on equine articular cartilage repair. *Canadian Journal of Veterinary Research* **52**, 137–146

Johnston SA (1997) Joint anatomy, physiology, and pathobiology of osteoarthritis. *Veterinary Clinics of North America: Small Animal Practice* **27**(4), 699–723

Jurvelin J, Kiviranta I, Tammi M et al. (1986) Effect of physical exercise on indentation stiffness of articular cartilage in the canine knee. *International Journal of Sports Medicine* **7**, 106–110

Kallio PE, Michelsson JE, Bjorkenheim JM et al. (1988) Immobilization leads to early changes in hydrostatic pressure of bone and joint. *Scandinavian Journal of Rheumatology* **17**, 27–32

Kiviranta I, Tammi M, Jurvelin J et al. (1988) Moderate running exercise augments glycosaminoglycan and thickness of articular cartilage in the knee joint of young beagle dogs. *Journal of Orthopedic Research* **6**, 188–195

Luo W, Guo C, Zheng J et al. (2000) Aggrecan from start to finish. *Journal of Bone Mineral Metabolism* **18**, 51–56

Lust G, Beilman WT, Dueland DJ et al. (1980) Intra-articular volume and hip joint instability in dogs with hip dysplasia. *Journal of Bone and Joint Surgery American* **62**, 576–582

Maroudas A (1980) Metabolism of cartilaginous tissues: a quantitative approach. In: *Studies in Joint Disease, Vol. 1*, eds. A Maroudas and EJ Holborow, p. 59. Pitman, Tunbridge Wells

Mosesson MW and Umfleet RA (1970) The cold insoluble globulin of human plasma. *Journal of Biological Chemistry* **245**, 5728–5736

Mow VC, Wang CC and Hung CT (1999) The extracellular matrix, interstitial fluid and ions as a mechanical signal transducer in articular cartilage. *Osteoarthritis and Cartilage* **7**, 41–58

Newman B and Wallis GA (2002) Is osteoarthritis a genetic disease? *Clinical Investigative Medicine* **25**, 139–149

Nixon AJ (2002) Arthroscopic techniques for cartilage repair. *Clinical Techniques in Equine Practice* **1**(4), 257–269

Radin EL and Rose RM (1986) Role of subchondral bone in the initiation and progression of cartilage damage. *Clinical Orthopedic and Related Research* **213**, 34–40

Schurz J and Ribitsch V (1987) Rheology of synovial fluid. *Biorheology* **24**, 385–399

Setton LA, Elliot DM and Mow VC (1999) Altered mechanics of cartilage with osteoarthritis: human osteoarthritis and an experimental model of joint degeneration. *Osteoarthritis and Cartilage* **7**, 2–14

Simon SR and Radin EL (1997) Biomechanics of joints. In: *Textbook of Rheumatology, Vol. 1, 5th edn*, ed. WN Kelley et al., p. 86. WB Saunders, Philadelphia

Todhunter RJ et al. (1998) Composition of Labrador Retriever chondroepiphyses. Annual Meeting of the American College of Veterinary Surgeons, Chicago, IL [abstract]

Todhunter RJ and Johnston S (2003) Osteoarthritis. In: *Textbook of Small Animal Surgery*, ed. D Slatter, pp. 2208–2246. WB Saunders, Philadelphia

Vassan N (1983) Effects of physical stress on the synthesis and degradation of cartilage matrix. *Connective Tissue Research* **12**, 49

Zimny ML (1988) Mechanoreceptors in articular tissues. *American Journal of Anatomy* **182**, 16–32

12

Principles of articular surgery

Sorrel Langley-Hobbs

Introduction

For dogs and cats, life revolves around motion to be able to function, work, play and lead an acceptable quality of life. The tasks of veterinarians performing articular surgery are to try to relieve pain and to restore mobility and function to affected joints. In circumstances where a pain-free mobile joint is not achievable, the decision to perform a salvage procedure such as an arthrodesis or joint replacement may be the only way to minimize pain and optimize function.

The option of non-surgical therapy should always be considered but its effectiveness usually decreases with increased lesion severity and joint instability (Roy and Dee, 1994). This chapter will consider:

- Need for surgery – patient evaluation
- Goals of surgery
- Preparation for surgery
- Articular surgery techniques
- Post-operative management.

Patient evaluation

A complete and thorough clinical examination of the patient will precede any decision to perform articular surgery. This should include consideration of the signalment. For example, a 7-month-old Labrador Retriever with lameness of the thoracic limb and a painful elbow joint is most likely to be suffering from elbow dysplasia/osteochondrosis and the contralateral joint should be examined for the same disease.

The history taken should include a general history and then questions pertinent to the joint problem, including:

- How long has the patient been lame? A short duration of mild lameness may make a period of conservative treatment acceptable prior to the decision to operate
- Was the onset of lameness acute or insidious and, if acute, was there an observed associated incident or trauma? An acute onset of lameness may suggest a more serious problem such as a fracture, which would require more immediate investigation and treatment
- Has the animal had any prior treatment? If the condition is, or has been, responsive to non-steroidal anti-inflammatory medication previously then is continued conservative management appropriate?
- Is the condition progressive?

The general physical examination is of major importance. Many articular conditions can occur concurrently with other diseases that may necessitate altering the treatment or management of the condition.

The circumstances and expectations of the owner also require consideration here. Is there willingness, ability and time available to provide appropriate post-operative care and are funds available to finance any proposed treatment? Are the owner's expectations likely to be met if all goes well?

The orthopaedic examination should include evaluation of the gait, stance and the physical examination of the patient's joints, bones and muscles (see Chapter 1).

Goals of articular surgery

The goals of articular surgery can be categorized as one or a combination of the following: diagnosis, prevention, therapy, palliation, stabilization and salvage.

Diagnosis

Arthroscopy is commonly performed for diagnostic purposes in the shoulder, elbow, stifle and tarsus and, less commonly, in the carpus and hip. In the absence of arthroscopy, exploratory arthrotomy can occasionally be indicated but this should be the last resort in a stepwise diagnostic approach. Arthrotomy and arthroscopy can also be performed to obtain samples for histopathological analysis or culture of microorganisms and antimicrobial sensitivity testing. However, one study showed that culture of synovial fluid in blood culture media is as effective as culture of synovial membrane, and this should obviate the need for obtaining samples of synovium for bacteriology (Montgomery et al., 1989).

Prevention

Certain surgical procedures are performed in an attempt to prevent or retard joint disease, although the procedure itself may, in fact, be periarticular. For example, triple pelvic osteotomy may be performed in an attempt to decrease functional hip laxity and reduce the

Chapter 12 Principles of articular surgery

progression of osteoarthritis. Radial and ulnar osteotomies may be performed to improve limb alignment, correct angular and rotational abnormalities and improve joint congruency in cases of subluxation.

Therapy

Carefully planned and atraumatic articular surgery for the treatment of an injury, such as a fracture or dislocation, can be very successful, with animals often returning to athletic function after such therapy. In addition, rapid surgical intervention in the case of a septic joint may prevent infection becoming established, which might otherwise have caused irreversible cartilage degradation.

Palliation

Some articular conditions cannot be completely resolved but surgery may improve limb function by decreasing pain and therefore palliate or slow down the development of osteoarthritis. Examples include correcting patellar luxation and debridement of osteochondral fragments in osteochondritic joints.

Stabilization

Articular or periarticular surgery is often performed in an attempt to stabilize a joint. Joint laxity, subluxation and luxation are often associated with capsular stretching or ligament rupture. Stabilization may be achieved either by primary ligament repair or replacement with a prosthesis or autogenous tissue. An example of the latter would be transposition of the biceps tendon to act as a lateral collateral ligament for patients with lateral shoulder dislocation.

Normal joints are designed to allow a specified amount of motion in certain directions, with well defined limits. Certain diseases and injuries lead to acute or chronic laxity in the periarticular structures that require treatment to return the joint to normal function. Collateral ligament ruptures are common injuries that, dependent on the severity, may require surgical intervention. Ligament injuries can be classified as type I, II or III (Farrow, 1978) (see later). Type III and some of the type II injuries require surgical intervention to restore joint stability and this will be discussed later in this chapter. In some circumstances no attempt is made to repair the damaged ligaments and a salvage surgery, such as an arthrodesis, is performed as the treatment of choice, e.g. pancarpal arthrodesis for palmar carpal ligament rupture (see Chapter 19).

Salvage

Intractably painful joints result in chronic lameness, osteoporosis, muscle atrophy, fibrosis and contracture. Pain and dysfunction persist as long as motion remains in the joint. Failure to respond to medical or surgical therapy may require an assessment for salvage surgery. When salvage surgery is planned, there are three principal options:

- Total joint replacement
- Excision arthroplasty
- Arthrodesis.

Salvage procedures should only be performed when attempts to restore joint function by other means have been exhausted or the severity of the disease makes salvage surgery the most appropriate option. The most common conditions that may result in intractable joint pain include osteoarthritis, luxation or subluxation (degenerative, traumatic or congenital), irreparable, non- or malunion articular fractures or inflammatory joint disease (McKee, 1994).

There are some diseases that are not primarily painful, where salvage surgery is a recognized treatment option. An example would include arthrodesis after ligament rupture when the lameness is mechanically debilitating rather than particularly painful (e.g. palmar or plantar ligament rupture).

Preparation for surgery

An understanding of the structure and function of joints is an essential basis for surgery (see Chapter 11). Knowledge of the anatomy and surgical approach is essential, particularly with respect to any vital structures that may be situated close to a joint, to avoid iatrogenic damage. Many approaches are detailed in this Manual but for additional information the reader should refer to surgical approach or anatomical texts. The surgeon should have carefully thought through and planned the procedure, ensuring that all necessary equipment is available and sterile, prior to surgery.

The operating environment

The operating room or theatre should be an appropriate environment for aseptic surgery. Ideally, filtered clean air is supplied under positive pressure such that the movement of air is down over the patient towards the outer room and away into less clean areas. The room should be clean, with appropriate daily cleaning procedures in place. The operating personnel should respect the environment of the operating room and maintain these high standards of cleanliness at all times.

The operating table should be sturdy and large enough for giant-breed dogs. The height of the table should be adjustable for surgeon comfort. A table that can tilt and rotate can also be useful. Appropriate positioning aids should be available (e.g. rope ties, troughs, sandbags, adjustable limb holder, ceiling hook, drip stand).

It is essential to have good lighting when performing articular surgery so that the joint can be thoroughly examined through a small atraumatic approach. Two directable theatre lights are highly recommended (Figure 12.1). Another option is to use a head lamp (Figure 12.2).

For arthroscopy, room lighting may need to be dimmed to facilitate the surgeon's view of the image monitor. Thus there may be a need to block natural light in some operating rooms. The light for the arthroscope itself is a dedicated light source (see Chapter 15).

Chapter 12 Principles of articular surgery

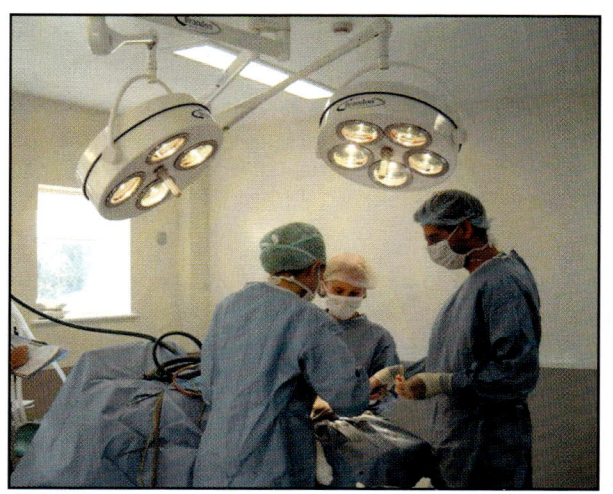

12.1 Use of two directable theatre lights with sterilizable handles greatly aids visualization of a joint, particularly the deeper structures.

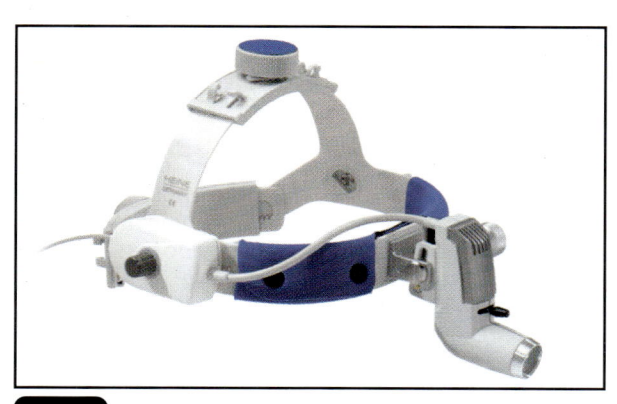

12.2 Headband-mounted LED headlamp.

Instrumentation

Appropriate instrumentation is essential and will contribute to the operative satisfaction and successful outcome of surgery (see Chapter 13). Often the incision and approach into the joint are necessarily small as they are limited by the desire to preserve important structures, such as ligaments. Therefore being able to retract the soft tissues or bones is essential in order to evaluate the joint fully. Gelpi retractors (Figure 12.3), small joint retractors and the self-retaining stifle distractor make visualization of a joint during an arthrotomy easier and more complete. For arthroscopy, dedicated instrumentation for small animals is required.

Surgical assistant

There are some arthrotomies where the presence of a surgical assistant is a useful, if not essential, addition to the surgical team. By stressing the joint in the appropriate direction, such as abduction and rotation, the deeper compartments can be visualized, ensuring, for example, that osteochondrosis flap removal is complete in the shoulder.

Surgeon preparation

For the start of surgery, the surgeon should be appropriately attired, wearing a clean scrub suit, hat, mask and shoes, prior to scrubbing for surgery. If there is a well trained surgical nursing team, the surgeon can prepare for surgery whilst the patient is being prepared and positioned; this can save valuable time. However, if the surgeon needs to supervise patient preparation and/or patient positioning, surgeon preparation should be delayed until the patient is ready for surgery.

Hands and arms should be thoroughly washed and then scrubbed using scrub soap, such as chlorhexidine or povidone–iodine.

> **PRACTICAL TIP**
> The duration of time that the surgical scrub solution is in contact with the skin is most important, this is not a part of the preparation to be rushed: a minimum of 5 minutes should be spent scrubbing up.

A sterile gown and gloves should be donned in a fashion that avoids any skin contact with the front of the gown and outer surface of the gloves.

Patient preparation

Infective organisms arise from three sources:

- The surgeon
- The patient
- The environment.

Through the use of theatre hats and masks, and donning sterile gloves and gowns after an appropriate scrubbing routine, the surgical team represents a relatively minor source of infective organisms. The same applies to the operating room environment, assuming routine cleaning procedures are followed on a frequent basis.

> **WARNING**
> The most important contributor of bacteria to the wound is the patient.

The primary sources from which patient-borne bacteria emerge are the hair and skin. Efforts must therefore be made to protect the patient from itself, by proper skin preparation, cleaning and by the use of sterile draping procedures to isolate the surgical field.

Other factors that influence infection rate (to a lesser extent than bacterial contamination) include:

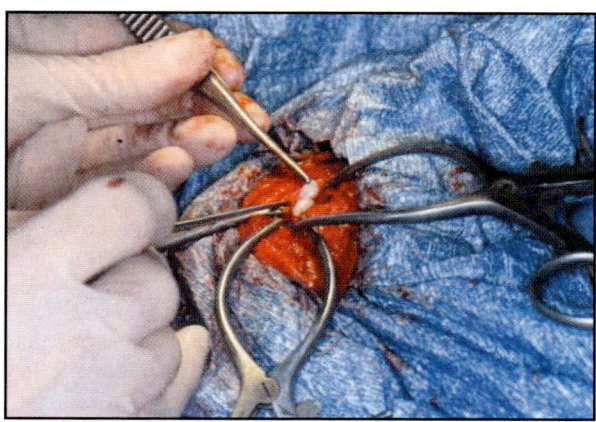

12.3 Gelpi retractors placed at ninety degrees to each other provide useful retraction of joint capsule and ligaments.

Chapter 12 Principles of articular surgery

- Tissue damage – necrosis, blood, bone sequestra and foreign bodies all create or enhance the environment conducive to bacterial growth
- Duration of surgery – for every additional hour of surgery the infection rate doubles
- General condition of the patient – age, obesity, malnutrition and comorbidity (e.g. diabetes mellitus) must all be considered.

Antimicrobial prophylaxis
In the absence of any obvious infection, the patient should be assessed as to the need for antibiotics. There is controversy regarding prophylactic antimicrobial therapy in clean procedures. The articular procedure itself will not increase the risk of infection compared with any other similar clean surgical procedure, if correct surgical principles are obeyed. However, septic arthritis can have a devastating effect if it is not rapidly recognized and treated appropriately; therefore an iatrogenic joint infection should be avoided by paying particular attention to aseptic technique.

If antibiotics are to be used, they are given to reduce the number of viable bacteria in the incision at the time of surgery to a level that normal defence mechanisms can handle, thereby preventing infection. Based on known concepts, the following prophylactic antibiotic regime would be pharmacologically ideal:

1. Administer a single intravenous bolus of drug 30–60 minutes prior to incision.
2. If surgery is prolonged, more than 2–4 hours, then give a maintenance dose of drug to sustain effective tissue levels.
3. In a primarily closed wound, the risk of contamination is present until a fibrin seal develops between wound edges (approximately 3–5 hours postoperatively). Just before the end of surgery, give another dose so that the effective plasma concentrations are present as long as the risk of bacterial contamination exists, and whilst the patient is compromised from the deleterious effects of anaesthesia and surgical stress.

> **In the absence of documented infection there is no rationale for continuing drug administration longer then 24–48 hours after surgery.**

The pathogenic bacteria that most commonly contaminate a surgical wound are *Staphylococcus* species, followed by *Escherichia coli*. Drugs active against the staphylococcal species should be used, such as penicillinase-resistant penicillins (e.g. oxacillin) and cephalosporins. The microbial resistance patterns that have developed against the natural penicillins and the aminopenicillins (amoxicillin and ampicillin) make these agents less attractive. For operations more likely to be associated with infections by Gram-negative bacteria, cephalosporins may be more effective (Riviere and Vaden, 1993).

Clipping
The area of skin prepared for surgery must be much larger than that of the intended incision, in general at least 15 cm beyond the surgical site in all directions. When performing surgery on the appendicular skeleton it is often useful to have the whole limb in the surgical field to allow limb manipulation and assessment of alignment intraoperatively; therefore it may be necessary to clip the whole limb free of hair, to the dorsal midline.

> **PRACTICAL TIP**
> Three principles that should be kept in mind when clipping hair: be neat; be gentle; and be thorough.

> **WARNING**
> Clipping inevitably leads to some epithelial damage and an increase in skin bacterial numbers. Hair should only be clipped close to the skin immediately prior to surgery. The incidence of postoperative surgical infection increases with the time interval between hair removal and surgery.

Positioning of the patient
The surgeon should consider what surgical approach will be performed and position the patient appropriately. In some situations repositioning may be necessary, perhaps when two joints are being operated upon, and so careful thought and planning are needed to achieve this aseptically without having to re-prepare and re-drape the patient, although in some circumstances this will be necessary. Use of sandbags, levers or adjustable arms can help maintain patient position, which is particularly useful for the surgeon without an assistant.

> **PRACTICAL TIP**
> Patient positioning is an underestimated part of surgery. Careful attention to patient positioning can be extremely helpful to the surgeon.

Aseptic patient preparation
After clipping the hair, the foot or distal appendage should be covered with an impervious barrier (e.g. tape and clean surgical glove, or cohesive bandage) so that no haired skin is exposed. The limb should then be suspended from a portable intravenous fluid stand, or similar device, and a surgical scrub performed. The patient is then transported to the operating room and positioned on the table with the leg still suspended. A final skin preparation is performed on the limb and the operative site is now ready for draping (Figure 12.4).

Draping
The purpose of draping is to protect exposed tissue from contamination by the surrounding skin during the surgical procedure; therefore, an attempt should be made to cover as much of the patient as possible. One way to achieve this when performing appendicular surgery is by use of an impervious stockinette:

1. The limb is aseptically prepared as discussed previously, with the haired foot covered with an impervious cover (Figure 12.5).

Chapter 12 Principles of articular surgery

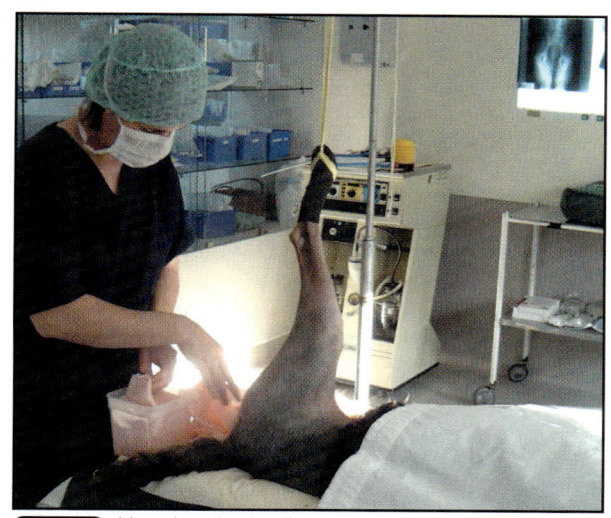

12.4 Hanging the leg from a drip stand aids skin preparation and helps maintain asepsis. This leg is being prepared for hip surgery: the whole limb has been clipped of hair and the foot is covered with a cohesive bandage to minimize contamination.

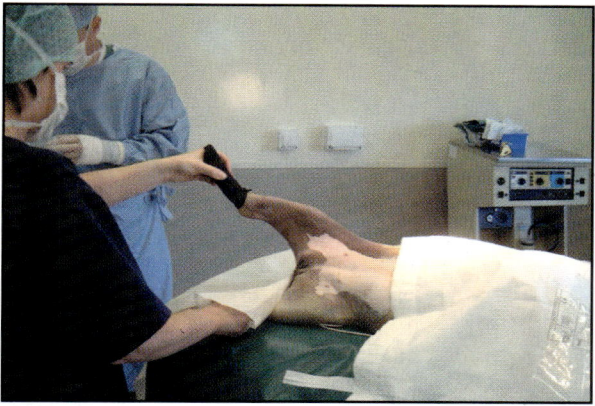

12.5 The limb has been clipped, scrubbed and prepared for surgery. The unclipped foot is covered with cohesive bandage. The nurse is holding the foot to allow the surgeon to apply the final skin preparation.

2. The surgeon places a sterile orthopaedic stockinette over the foot, rolls this down the aseptically prepared limb and then passes the whole limb through another fenestrated drape. The stockinette is cut along the proposed surgical incision site. The skin incision is made, taking care that the skin comes into contact only with the stockinette and not the sterile gloves.
3. Following minimal dissection of the subcutaneous tissue, the stockinette is attached to the subcutaneous tissue by a continuous suture placed in each skin edge so as to roll the stockinette over the skin edges.
4. The stockinette is then attached by a simple interrupted suture at the proximal and distal ends of the surgical site so that the incision can, if necessary, be extended in either direction without disrupting the secured skin edges (see Figure 12.3). The surgical field is now ready for deeper dissection with a minimal risk of contamination from the patient.

Alternatively, the limb can be prepared in a routine fashion with a sterile foot bag or drape and a single drape, or quadrant draping (Figure 12.6). Then an iodine-impregnated adhesive drape is placed on the leg, covering exposed skin, with the aim of minimizing any contact between skin and surgeon or deeper tissues (Figure 12.7). Another option is the use of a paper disposable drape that can also be incised and sutured to the wound edges as described for a stockinette.

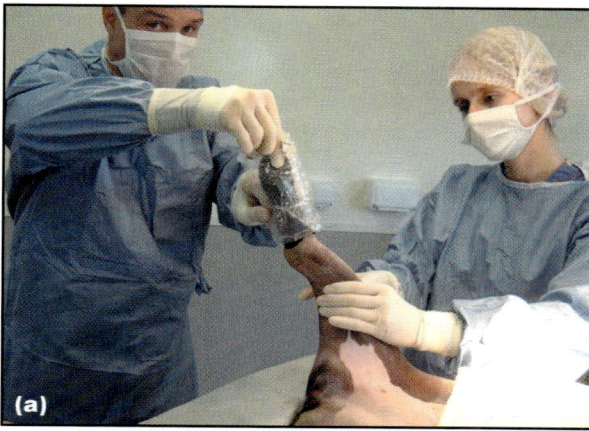

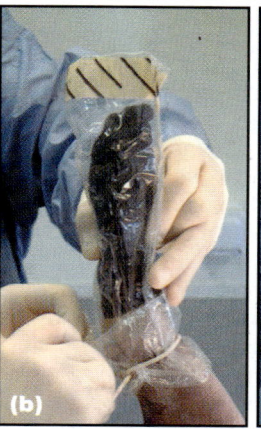

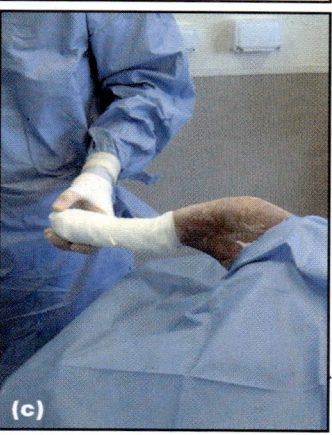

12.6 Application of a foot bag. **(a)** A transparent pre-sterilized autoclave bag is rolled down over the foot in an aseptic manner. **(b)** The sterile foot bag is secured in place with a sterilized piece of string or a towel clip. **(c)** The whole foot is then covered with a pre-sterilized cohesive bandage of a different colour.

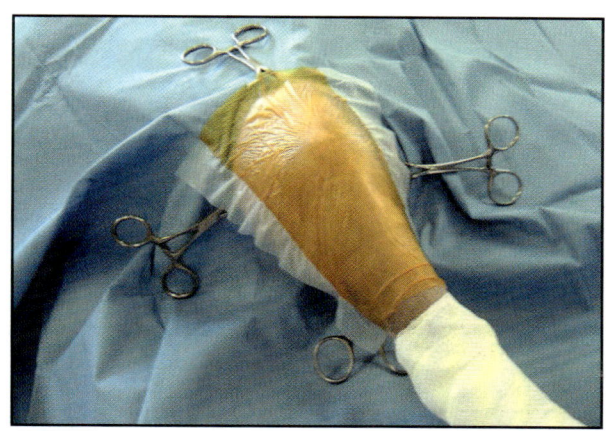

12.7 Use of an iodophor-impregnated adhesive drape to cover exposed skin on a draped leg.

155

Chapter 12 Principles of articular surgery

Articular surgery techniques

Halsted's principles of surgical technique (Figure 12.8) apply to articular surgery; some principles specific to articular surgery also apply.

Strict aseptic technique
Gentle tissue handling
Sharp anatomical dissection of tissue
Preservation of blood supply
Meticulous haemostasis
Careful approximation of tissue
Obliteration of dead space
Little or no tension across suture lines

12.8 Halsted's principles of surgical technique.

Arthrotomy

An arthrotomy is an incision into a joint. The incision should be made in a manner that will cause minimal damage to normal structures of the joint, tendons, ligaments and muscles, but maximize exposure of the desired area of the joint and provide adequate tissue margins to allow suturing.

During open surgery, flushing the wound frequently with sterile saline or Hartmann's solution will: aid inspection by removing blood and clots: decrease drying of the soft tissues and cartilage: dilute bacterial contamination: and remove small cartilage or bony fragments. Local irrigation of surgical sites with antibiotic solutions has not been shown to be superior to parenteral antimicrobial drug administration in controlled human trials (Riviere and Vaden, 1993).

Haemostasis will aid the surgeon's view and should therefore increase the speed and effectiveness of the procedure. It is important to remove large blood clots before closing the joint; blood provides an ideal environment for bacterial proliferation.

Surgical approach

Most arthrotomies are planned so as to avoid cutting collateral ligaments or tendons but in some situations it is necessary to increase articular exposure by cutting these structures in a planned manner. At the end of surgery it is then very important that they are repaired or sutured appropriately to maintain joint stability. Osteoarthritis secondary to surgically induced instability of the joint is an unfortunate sequel to many otherwise successful procedures (Piermattei and Flo, 1997a).

Alternatively, articular exposure is increased by performing an osteotomy of the origin or insertion of a ligament or tendon (Figure 12.9). An osteotomy will need repairing at the end of the surgical procedure, with a pin and tension-band wire technique, or lag screw, because an avulsion fracture has been created. The advantage of the increased exposure obtained by performing this more invasive approach may not outweigh the disadvantages because complications can occur. Articular fractures may be created inadvertently and postoperative immobilization may be necessary to allow the osteotomy to heal. The morbidity associated with these procedures varies according to anatomical location. For example, for the elbow, osteotomy of the medial epicondyle was found to offer the best combination of exposure and immediate postoperative stability in an experimental study (Suess *et al.*, 1994). However, a retrospective clinical study comparing medial epicondylar osteotomy or medial capsulotomy found that the percentage of complications requiring corrective surgery was significantly greater in the osteotomy group (Tobias *et al.*, 1994). Greater trochanteric osteotomies and olecranon osteotomies performed to reflect large muscle masses to increase exposure and visibility in order to achieve accurate fracture reduction are often successful, providing adequate care and attention are taken to reduce and stabilize the bone fragments at the end of surgery.

> **WARNING**
> Osteotomies performed to reflect a ligament are more likely to involve iatrogenic damage to the articular surface and result in complications, whereas osteotomies performed to reflect a tendon are generally more likely to be extra-articular and, with care, healing can be uncomplicated.

Incision into a joint often involves severing one or more fascial layers that function to stabilize the joint. These tissues are collectively known as retinacula; the fibrous joint capsule can also be considered part of the

Osteotomy	Tendon/ligament attachment	Joint exposure
Olecranon (extra-articular)	Triceps tendon	Caudal elbow joint
Greater trochanter (extra-articular)	Gluteal tendons (deep and middle)	Dorsal hip joint
Greater tubercle (extra-articular)	Supraspinatus tendon	Cranial shoulder joint
Tibial tuberosity (extra-articular)	Quadriceps tendon	Cranial stifle
Acromion (extra-articular)	Deltoid tendon	Lateral shoulder joint
Medial epicondyle humerus (articular)	Medial collateral ligament	Medial elbow joint
Medial epicondyle femur (articular)	Medial collateral ligament	Medial stifle joint
Medial malleolus tibia (articular)	Medial collateral ligament	Medial talar ridge

12.9 Osteotomies performed during articular surgery.

retinaculum (Piermattei and Flo, 1997a). These tissues can be sutured collectively, but in some cases they are better sutured individually in order to maintain function and increase the strength and tightness of the repair.

Osteophyte removal

There is debate about whether to remove osteophytes or not. Experimental work has indicated that this procedure has questionable value (Nesbitt, 1982). In experimental dogs, osteophytes returned to 60% of predebridement levels within 24–48 weeks and there was no measurable difference between treated and untreated dogs. However, these were research cases and there was minimal osteophyte production compared with clinical cases. It may be beneficial in some instances to remove osteophytes when they interfere with joint motion; for example, those at the proximal end of the femoral trochlear sulcus may interfere with gliding of the patella.

Ligament repair

Many arthrotomies will involve ligamentous repair, the injury either being iatrogenic, as part of the surgical approach, or traumatic. A *sprain* is an injury to a ligament.

Ligament injuries can be classified as first, second or third degree (Farrow, 1978):

- First-degree ligament sprains result from short-lived application of moderate force; damage is mild and minimal and no treatment is required
- Second-degree ligament injuries are more severe; although the ligament is grossly intact, long-term restoration of function is unlikely without treatment
- Third-degree ligament injuries are characterized by functional disruption of the ligament, or avulsion from bone and fracture fragments may be present; vigorous treatment is required to restore function and stability.

Surgical therapy for ligament injury consists of suture repair or prosthetic replacement or splinting. The locking loop (Kessler) and pulley suture patterns have proven most reliable (see Chapter 8a). Monofilament nylon or polypropylene in size 1 to 4 metric (5/0 to 1 USP) is most commonly used. If the ligament is badly damaged or shredded ('crabmeat-like' appearance) the suture tends to 'cheese-wire' through the tissue. In this situation the suture may need anchoring through a bone tunnel or around a suture anchor (see Chapter 14). It is important to try to place the anchor points as close to the origin or insertion of the ligament as possible.

If the ligament is avulsed close to bone it may be possible to reattach it using a screw and plastic spiked washer or a ligament bone staple.

Bony avulsions of ligaments can be reattached with small screws, with or without washers, divergent Kirschner wires, tension band wire or a stainless steel suture. Alternatively, the bone can be used as an anchor point for the suture: the bone fragment can be pulled down on to the bone taking the suture through a bone tunnel or around a screw and stainless steel washer (Piermattei and Flo, 1997a). The aim must be to restore joint stability and then protect the repair whilst it is healing (Figure 12.10).

Type of injury	Repair option
Stretched ligaments (second-degree injury)	Imbricate by suturing
Mid-substance torn ligaments	Suture incorporating joint capsule and use of prosthetic ligaments
Avulsed ligaments	Reattach close to original site by lag screw and spiked washer, or place suture in ligament and attach to bone screw or through bone tunnel
Bony avulsion of ligament	Lag screw with or without spiked washer, stainless steel wire suture or divergent Kirschner wires
Complete ligament destruction (shear injury)	Prosthetic replacement and immobilization. Fibrosis after application of a transarticular external skeletal fixator (TESF) may be sufficient in smaller patients
Any ligament injury	Can augment with transposition of adjacent fascia to add strength and fibroblastic elements

12.10 Surgical repair of ligaments. (After Piermattei and Flo, 1997a.)

The palmar carpal and plantar tarsal ligaments are not generally repaired (see Chapters 19 and 23). A healed ligament will never be as strong as the original and in these anatomical locations they are unlikely to withstand the forces of weightbearing. Arthrodesis is therefore considered the treatment of choice for injuries to these ligaments.

Closure

Although the capsule is usually sutured, complete closure is not essential to prevent synovial fluid leakage. Like the peritoneum, the synovium quickly seals itself by fibrin deposition and fibroplasia. Selection of suture material for joint capsule closure is a subject for debate and personal opinion but some general rules can be applied (see also Chapter 14).

- If the closure is tension-free and the capsule is not important in stabilizing the joint, a continuous suture pattern and a small-gauge absorbable material should be used. Suitable examples include a synthetic absorbable monofilament material, such as polyglecaprone or a more slowly absorbed monofilament material such as polydioxanone
- If the capsule is closed under tension and it is important for stability, a simple interrupted pattern should be used and a slowly absorbable or non-absorbable monofilament material such as polydioxanone (PDS II) or monofilament nylon. Non-absorbable braided materials, such as polyamide, have been associated with articular infections (Dulisch, 1981). Penetrating the joint capsule should be avoided, as the suture may rub on articular cartilage and cause erosion. Suture patterns such as the modified Mayo mattress suture cause imbrication by overlap.

Chapter 12 Principles of articular surgery

Arthroscopy
Arthroscopy is now commonly used for investigation and treatment of articular disorders in small animals; there are some principles of arthroscopy that differ significantly from traditional surgery. Arthroscopy is heavily dependent upon appropriate instrumentation (see Chapter 15a). During arthroscopy, fluid is moved continuously through the joint using a positive pressure system. The pressure of this system helps to reduce haemorrhage and bacterial contamination but it should not be set too high. Excessive pressure can lead to extra-articular fluid accumulation with resultant inward creep of periarticular tissues, leading to a reduced joint space and more difficult arthroscopy.

The operating environment
The operating room should be prepared to allow the surgeon to manipulate the arthroscope with ease whilst looking at the monitor on the arthroscopy tower. The position of the tower relative to the patient and table may vary according to which joint is being examined and whether a bilateral procedure is being performed. The room light should be dimmed so that the surgeon has a clear view of the monitor. Care should be taken to ensure that electrical cables to the tower do not run through areas that may become wet during the arthroscopy.

Patient preparation and draping
Arthroscopy is a minimally invasive technique; as the technique is performed through very small stab incisions, the area that needs to be clipped can be reduced to an area with a margin 15 cm from the site of arthroscopy portals. It should be remembered, however, that there may be a requirement to change the approach during the operation and wider clipping is indicated if this is thought at all likely. The operative site may be quadrant draped (shoulder, hip and, possibly, elbow) or the limb may be free draped (stifle, carpus, tarsus and, possibly, elbow). The use of impervious adhesive transparent sterile drapes is strongly recommended. Some of these may have integral fluid collection bags that can prevent some fluid spillage.

Arthroscopic technique
Although the detailed technique of arthroscopy will vary with the joint being examined and the portal being used, there are some important general principles that should be followed. These are described in Chapter 15.

Arthrodesis
The aims of arthrodesis are to achieve a solid bony union of the adjacent bones in a joint. Arthrodesis is a salvage procedure that should only be attempted as the last resort or where it is the recognized and recommended treatment for a specific condition, e.g. tarsal plantar ligament rupture. It is technically possible to arthrodese most joints in the body. However, in some situations, amputation may actually be a preferable option to arthrodesis of a joint. Fusion of the elbow and stifle will cause a significant gait abnormality and animals, particularly cats, may function better with three legs rather than have one mechanically abnormal, yet pain-free appendage (Moak et al., 2000). The surgical principles of arthrodesis are listed in Figure 12.11. Prior to performing an arthrodesis it is essential to evaluate the patient thoroughly to ensure that arthrodesis is the appropriate procedure to perform, and that there is no disease in other joints in the affected leg or in the other limbs that may contraindicate surgery.

Remove articular cartilage
Compress the debrided surfaces and rigidly fixate
Fuse the joint at an appropriate angle for weightbearing
Protect the joint from excessive motion until healing has occurred
Healing of arthrodeses is enhanced by cancellous bone grafting
(Johnson, 1981)

12.11 Basic surgical principles of arthrodesis.

Preoperative planning
For an arthrodesis to be successful the joint angle should be appropriate for weightbearing. Some average angles have been published (Figure 12.12) but individual breeds vary; where possible, it is preferable to measure the angle in the contralateral limb. Use of a goniometer, or pre-bending a pin to the appropriate angle and having it sterilized for use in surgery, is recommended. If it is necessary to remove a significant amount of bone, the angle of arthrodesis should be slightly increased to compensate for shortening. As well as paying attention to fusing the joint at an appropriate angle in the craniocaudal plane, care should also be taken not to introduce any rotation or angulation in the mediolateral plane.

Joint	Dogs	Cats
Carpus	5–10 degrees	10 degrees (Simpson and Goldsmid, 1994)
Elbow	120–145 degrees (Watson et al., 2003)	100–135 degrees (Moak et al., 2000)
Shoulder	110 degrees (Fowler et al., 1988)	–
Tarsus	135–145 degrees (Piermattei and Flo, 1997b)	115–125 degrees (Piermattei and Flo, 1997b)
Stifle	110–160 degrees (Cofone et al., 1992)	–

12.12 Angles for arthrodesis (guidelines only). It is preferable to measure the angle in the contralateral limb of the individual cat or dog.

Techniques for arthrodesis

- It is important to avoid rotational or angular deformity with an arthrodesis. Having adequate visibility of the rest of the limb and being able to flex and extend adjacent joints is highly recommended. Use of a piece of sterile adhesive drape around the foot maintains asepsis yet allows a better assessment of foot position (Figure 12.13).

Chapter 12 Principles of articular surgery

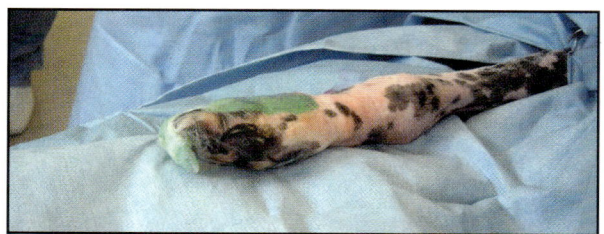

12.13 Application of a sterile adhesive transparent dressing to the foot allows correction of angulation or rotation prior to performing a carpal arthrodesis.

- The surgical approach must minimize damage to surrounding soft tissues, especially tendons and blood vessels. With distal limb procedures, an Esmarch bandage and tourniquet can be used to reduce haemorrhage and improve inspection of the tissues (Figure 12.14).
- All articular cartilage must be removed from what will be the contact surfaces at the fusion site. It is not necessary to remove cartilage from non-contact areas. Cartilage removal can be achieved by use of burrs, osteotomes, currettes or rongeurs, maintaining the contour of the underlying bone. Alternatively, an oscillating saw can be used to cut the surfaces flat, although this does result in some limb shortening. Either technique can be used as long as the surfaces are free of cartilage and there is good contact
- The arthrodesis site should be packed with autogenous cancellous bone. This will increase the speed of healing. A study performed by Johnson and Bellenger (1980) showed that osseous healing of a pancarpal arthrodesis was significantly greater at 12 weeks when bone graft was used.
- Rigid fixation of the arthrodesis site is mandatory, and compression of the bone surfaces should be the aim. Implants, such as plates, lag screws and tension band fixation, are usually most appropriate. External skeletal fixation can be useful in selected cases, particularly open injuries. The implants should generally be placed on the tension or convex surface of the joint. Kirschner wires can be used as temporary alignment devices.

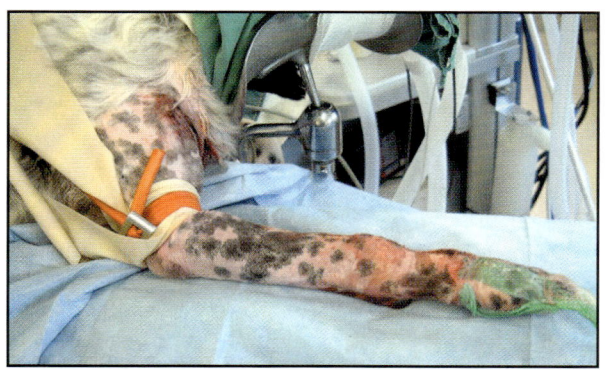

12.14 An Esmarch bandage and tourniquet were used on this dog to exsanguinate the limb and prevent or minimize blood flow during carpal arthrodesis surgery.

Postoperative management

The surgical incision should be protected from contamination immediately postoperatively until a fibrin seal has formed: this should usually occur within 3–5 hours. A self-adhesive dressing with a non-adherent patch (e.g. Primapore, Smith and Nephew; Figure 12.15) applied over the incision is useful both to avoid contamination and to deter interference by the patient.

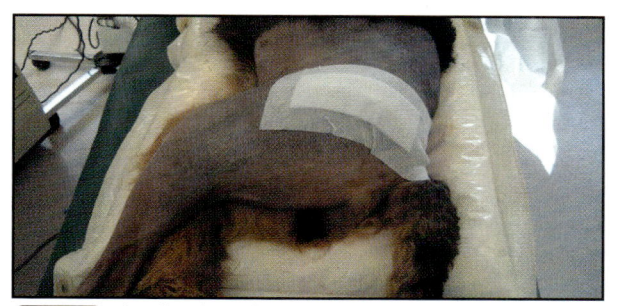

12.15 Application of a dressing to the surgical incision postoperatively prevents contamination and minimizes patient interference.

Postoperative management, including bandaging, is described in detail in Chapter 16. As a general rule appropriate auxilliary support, usually involving a splinted support dressing, cast, or external skeletal fixation after arthrodesis, is vital to achieve a good outcome.

To achieve a reduction in postoperative swelling the short-term application of a light bandage will be all that is necessary. After reduction of a dislocated joint, bandaging may be required for longer. Prolonged immobilization of certain joints, such as the elbow and stifle, should be avoided; these joints are prone to periarticular fibrosis. Alternatives to normal bandages that might be considered are flexion bandages of the hock and carpus, which can be effective in allowing motion whilst preventing weightbearing. Passive joint motion will assist in clearing postoperative haemarthrosis and inflammatory debris.

Restraint techniques may also be necessary in some patients to prevent self-trauma after articular surgery. These can include the use of Elizabethan collars, noxious topical agents to prevent licking and, possibly, sedation. Scratching of shoulder incisions by hind feet can be difficult to prevent; socks on the hind paws, hobbling the hind paws together or giving the patient a T-shirt or stockinette to wear over the torso have all been tried.

References and further reading

Alexander JW (1985) Preoperative and postoperative care. In: *Leonard's Orthopedic Surgery of the Dog and Cat*, 3rd edn, pp. 17–25. WB Saunders, Philadelphia

Campbell JR (1971) Luxation and ligamentous injuries of the elbow of the dog. *Veterinary Clinics of North America* **1(3)**, 429–440

Cofone MA, Smith GK, Lenehan TM and Newton CD (1992) Unilateral and bilateral stifle arthrodesis in eight dogs. *Veterinary Surgery* **21(4)**, 299–303

Dulisch ML (1981) Suture reaction following extra-articular stifle stabilisation in the dog – Part II: a prospective study of 66 stifles. *Journal of the American Animal Hospital Association* **17**, 573–571

Chapter 12   Principles of articular surgery

Farrow CS (1978) Sprain, strain and contusion. *Veterinary Clinics of North America* **8(2)**, 169–182

Fowler JD, Presnell KR and Holmberg DL (1988) Scapulohumeral arthrodesis: results in seven dogs. *Journal of the American Animal Hospital Association* **24**, 667–672

Johnson KA (1981) A radiographic study of the effects of autologous cancellous bone grafts on bone healing after carpal arthrodesis in the dog. *Veterinary Radiology* **22(4)**, 177–183

Johnson KA and Bellenger CR (1980) The effects of autologous bone grafting on bone healing after carpal arthrodesis in the dog. *Veterinary Record* **107(6)**, 126–132

McKee M (1994) Intractably painful joints. In: *Manual of Small Animal Arthrology*, ed. JEF Houlton and R Collinson, pp. 115–134. BSAVA Publications, Cheltenham

Moak PC, Lewis DD, Roe SC and de Haan JJ (2000) Arthrodesis of the elbow in three cats. *Veterinary Comparative Orthopaedics and Traumatology* **13**, 149–153

Montgomery RD, Long IR, Milton JL, DiPinto MN and Hunt J (1989) Comparison of aerobic culturette, synovial membrane biopsy, and blood culture medium in detection of canine bacterial arthritis. *Veterinary Surgery* **18(4)**, 300–303

Nesbitt T (1982) The effects of osteophyte debridement in osteoarthrosis. 17th Annual Meeting, American College of Veterinary Surgeons, San Diego

Piermattei DL and Johnson KA (2004) *An Atlas of Surgical Approaches to the Bones and Joints of the Dog and Cat, 4th edn.* WB Saunders, Philadelphia

Piermattei DL and Flo GL (1997a) Principles of joint surgery. In: *Handbook of Small Animal Orthopaedics and Fracture Repair*, ed. DL Piermattei, pp. 201–217. WB Saunders, Philadelphia

Piermattei DL and Flo GL (1997b) Fractures and other orthopaedic injuries of the tarsus, metatarsus and phalanges. In: *Handbook of Small Animal Orthopaedics and Fracture Repair*, ed. DL Piermattei, pp. 607–655. WB Saunders, Philadelphia

Riviere JE and Vaden SL (1993) Antimicrobial prophylaxis. In: *Disease mechanisms in small animal surgery, 2nd edn*, ed. MJ Bojrab, pp. 66–69. Lea and Febiger, Philadelphia

Roy R and Dee J (1994) Management of articular fractures, sprains and strains. In: *Manual of Small Animal Arthrology*, ed. JEF Houlton and R Collinson, pp. 55–61. BSAVA Publications, Cheltenham

Simpson D and Goldsmid S (1994) Pancarpal arthrodesis in a cat: a case report and anatomical study. *Veterinary Comparative Orthopaedics and Traumatology* **7**, 45–50

Suess RP, Trotter EJ, Konieczynski D, Todhunter RJ, Bartel DL and Flanders JA (1994) Exposure and post operative stability of three medial surgical approaches to the canine elbow. *Veterinary Surgery* **23**, 87–93

Tobias TA, Miyabayashi T, Olmstead ML and Hedrick LA (1994) Surgical removal of fragmented medial coronoid process in the dog: comparative effects of surgical approach and age at time of surgery. *Journal of the American Animal Hospital Association* **30**, 360–368

Watson C, Rochat M and Payton M (2003) Effect of weight bearing on the joint angles of the fore and hind limb of the dog. *Veterinary Comparative Orthopaedics and Traumatology* **16**, 250–254

13

Surgical instrumentation

John Lapish

Introduction

The limb joints of the dog and cat vary significantly in the amount of soft tissue overlay and in the available access to joint surfaces. Appropriate instrumentation aims to provide the surgeon access to the joint, bringing in light and some means of inspecting the articular and periarticular structures. Additional instruments are necessary to treat lesions. Surgical and arthroscopic solutions to these requirements are very different. Arthroscopy, and the equipment required, is discussed in Chapter 15.

Basic surgical kit

The exact components of a basic kit for joint surgery will be determined, at least to a degree, by personal preferences and patient size, but should contain a minimum of the elements shown in Figure 13.1.

Towel clamps

A minimum of six clamps is required to secure basic draping. Additional draping will require additional clamps.

Scalpels

A fresh scalpel makes the cleanest cut with a minimum of trauma. At the microscopic level even the sharpest of scissors cuts tissue with a crushing action. If the surgeon is knowledgeable and experienced, maximum use of the scalpel is preferred. Until this level of expertise is attained, more blunt dissection and scissor work is appropriate. A number 10 or 15 blade is preferred; and both fit the number 3 handle. The number 15 blade is the smaller of the two. Occasionally the sharp pointed number 11 can be useful (Figure 13.2).

For intra-articular procedures the Beaver-type blades are appropriate. Fitted into a Beaver-type handle, the 65 blade acts as a mini number 11 blade. The tip of the 64 blade is rounded and cuts along the tip and ventral and dorsal surfaces. It can therefore be pushed through the medial meniscus as part of the release procedure.

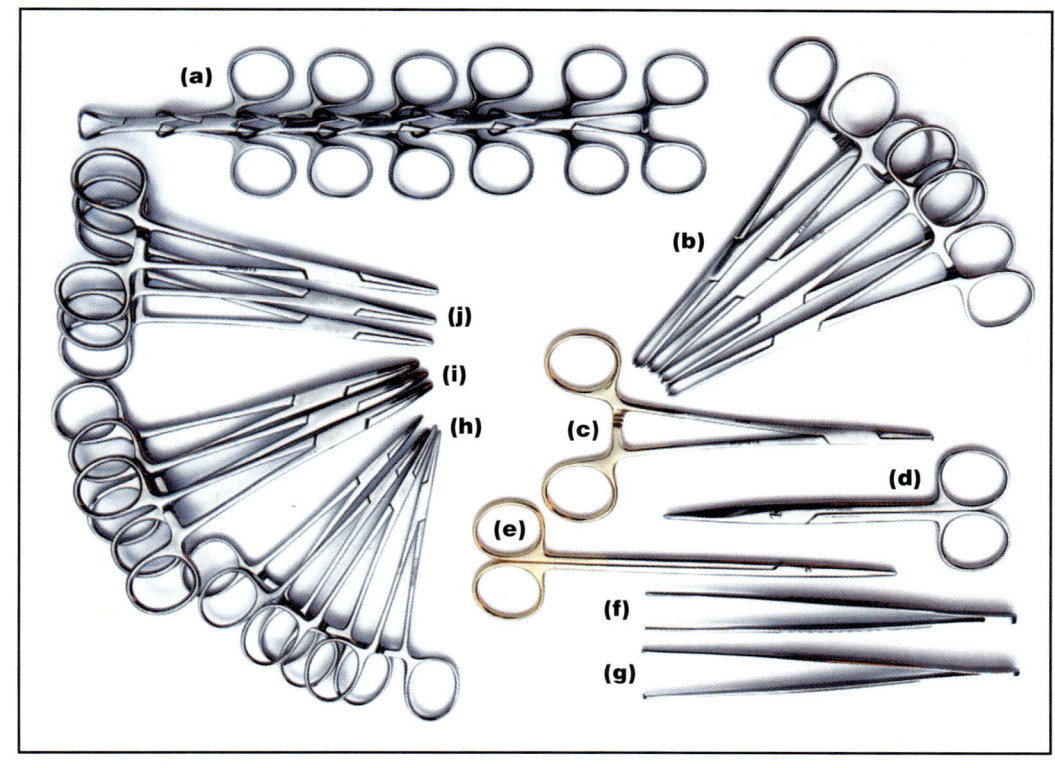

13.1 Basic joint surgery instruments: **(a)** Backhaus towel clips; **(b)** Allis tissue forceps; **(c)** Mayo–Hegar needle holder; **(d)** straight Mayo scissors; **(e)** straight Metzenbaum scissors; **(f)** DeBakey dissecting forceps; **(g)** rat-tooth dissecting forceps; **(h)** Halsted artery forceps; **(i)** curved Spencer Wells artery forceps; **(j)** straight Spencer Wells artery forceps.

Chapter 13 Surgical instrumentation

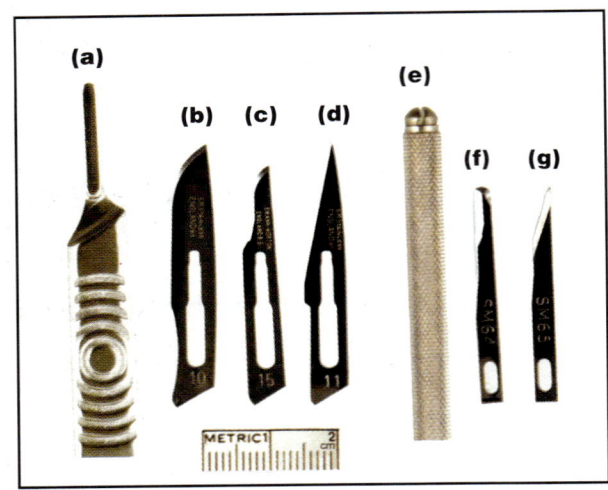

13.2 Scalpels: **(a)** no. 3 handle; **(b)** no. 10 blade; **(c)** no. 15 blade; **(d)** no. 11 blade; **(e)** Beaver-type handle; **(f)** no. 64 blade; **(g)** no. 65 blade.

Surgical scissors
Mayo or Metzenbaum are the standard surgical scissors. The more delicate Metzenbaum is preferred for joint surgery. Typically, the choice is between 14 cm Mayo and 18 cm Metzenbaum. A 14.5 cm version of the latter is available for smaller hands.

Dissecting forceps
A pair of rat-tooth forceps (e.g. Adson or Treves), usually one-into-two teeth and between 12.5 cm and 15 cm long, will be required for tougher tissues, particularly the skin. Dressing forceps with a serrated jaw or, preferably, atraumatic gripping forceps with a DeBakey tooth pattern are required for more delicate tissues. The DeBakey pattern grip was developed for vascular surgery.

Artery forceps
A combination of Spencer Wells and Halsted mosquito forceps will assist appropriate haemostasis for the range of blood vessels likely to be encountered in joint surgery. A combination of curved and straight forceps, 12.5 cm and 15 cm long, is useful.

Tissue forceps
Allis is the most commonly used type. All examples of this type have the same basic pattern but vary according to how many teeth are found along the tips. A broad grip of four or five teeth is preferred. They are used to hold and retract soft tissues. Some surgeons prefer Babcock forceps for use on skin margins. The weight of the instrument alone will create some retraction. If the forceps are held by an assistant the retraction is greater and directional. Allis tissue forceps are also very useful for securing electrocautery cables, air hoses, and suction and drainage tubes to the draping. This is safer than the use of pointed towel clips.

Needle holders
Repair of joint capsule incisions or tears will require the use of fine sutures and fine small needles. Accurate control can only be obtained by locking needle holders, preferably with tungsten carbide jaws. Use of Gillie-type instruments will result in needle slippage and frustration. The industry standard is the Mayo–Hegar, which is available in a wide range of sizes to suit all hands. The most common is the 16.25 cm (6.5 inch). Finer control may be obtained using a needle holder with a narrower jaw, such as the DeBakey, originally developed for vascular surgery. Inclusion of a needle holder requires the inclusion of suture cutting scissors in the surgical pack.

Retractors

In order to allow light and instruments into a joint it is necessary to retract overlying soft tissues. Instrumentation should be selected to maximize exposure while minimizing trauma to the soft tissues in general, and important structures in particular. Care must be taken to protect arteries, veins and, especially, nerves in the operative field.

Self-retaining retractors
Many veterinary surgeons work with minimal assistance; thus, self-retaining retractors, distracting tissues by some kind of self-locking system, can be invaluable. Self-retaining retractors are available in a large range of sizes and types. Very small and very large patients are over-represented in joint surgery lists, so a range of instruments is essential. The examples given below serve to illustrate the type. In general terms, the more superficial the need for retraction, the more prongs and the wider the 'spread' the retractor will have. At the joint capsule level, single retracting prongs are used to maintain a window for visualization or further instrumentation.

Multipronged retractors
These are illustrated in Figure 13.3.

- **Travers:** the multiple prongs and long flat arms create a wide aperture, making this type of instrument ideal for skin and superficial connective tissue. As with other retractors designed for human use, the instrument is intended to sit flat on the draped skin. However, in small veterinary patients, the handle part of the instrument may hang unsupported and may distort the incision. This style of retractor is available in a range of sizes from 16.5 cm (7 cm spread) to 20 cm (9 cm spread).

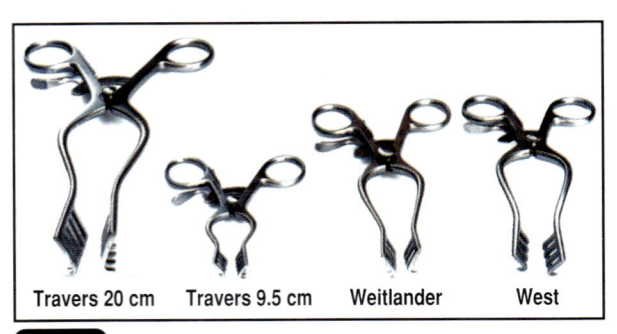

13.3 Multipronged self-retaining retractors. Travers 20 cm, Travers 9.5 cm, Weitlander, West.

Chapter 13 Surgical instrumentation

- **Weitlander:** 14 cm, smaller than, but similar to, the Travers. This retractor has flat arms and a smaller spread (6 cm) than the Travers.
- **West:** 14 cm, similar to the Weitlander but with curved arms that can sit neatly on smaller veterinary patients. Both Weitlander and West retractors may be used in conjunction with the bigger Travers in larger patients to retract deeper layers.

Gelpi-type retractors

This family of retractors (Figure 13.4), available in many variations of design and size, provides focal retraction, typically at the level of the joint capsule. The retractors are also useful to separate small muscle bellies, tendons and ligaments, for either access or protection. The Gelpi was developed as a human vulval retractor, and the long sharp tips on the standard human model make introduction into small spaces difficult. Numerous variations with shorter or overlapping tips are now available for veterinary use. Options are also available with reference to the shape of the arms and the reach of the retractor: some joint surgery procedures occur at significant depth, 8 cm or greater. Gelpis operating with small teeth on the ratchet offer better control of retraction at the joint capsule level.

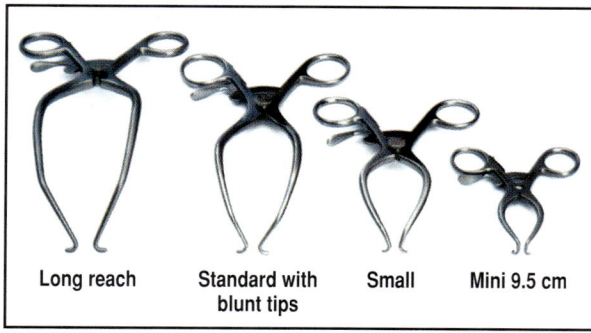

13.4 Gelpi-type retractors.

Hand-held retractors

Where assistance is available, hand-held retractors provide excellent focal retraction, particularly of muscle bellies (Figure 13.5). Langenbeck-type single-blade retractors are most commonly used, available in a range of sizes. The 6 mm and 13 mm blade widths are the most useful. Myerdings are heavier and appropriate for use around the hip joint of large dogs. The Senn is a smaller, double-ended instrument. One end is similar to a small Langenbeck, the other is sharp and multipronged and is often referred to as a 'cat's paw' retractor. It is commonly used to retract the stifle fat pad.

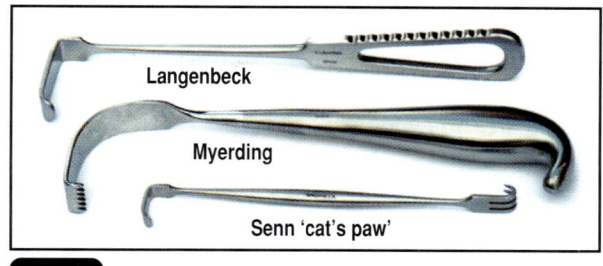

Hohmann retractors

This is a large family of retractors with over 20 variants. The instrument is designed as a combined retractor and elevator (Figure 13.6). The tip is used to elevate a bone or bone fragment by depressing and levering the wider blade portion of the instrument against a body of muscle. Thus, the skeletal element in question is elevated relative to surrounding muscles. This dual role makes the Hohmann particularly useful in exposing joint surfaces.

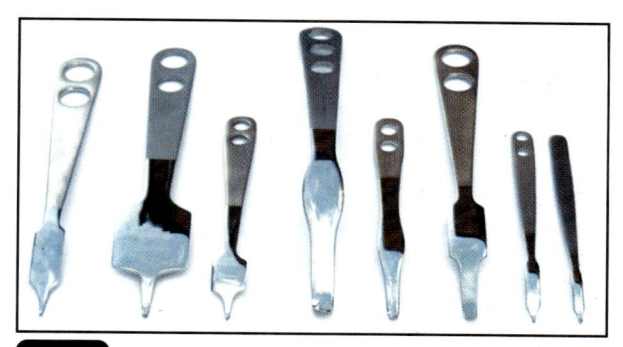

13.6 Hohmann retractors.

The most useful are the 12 and 18 mm versions, both with a short tip. Generally speaking, where the term Hohmann is used in a veterinary orthopaedic text, it is referring to the 18 mm with a short tip. Common applications include exposure of the fabella by retraction of the biceps femoris and the exposure of the femoral head and neck in a number of hip procedures. Small Hohmanns are very useful in the manipulation of bone fragments. Larger variants have the advantage of reducing the effort involved in hip procedures.

Penrose drains

The latex rubber Penrose drain, although technically not an instrument, is very useful at gently retracting nerves and other vital structures with a minimum of trauma. The drain is passed around the nerve, and its ends are clamped together using a pair of artery forceps or Allis forceps. The weight of the forceps sitting on the drape is usually sufficient to maintain gentle retraction. Penrose drains are available in 6 mm or 12 mm widths.

Specialist orthopaedic instruments

Graft passers

Graft passers are used to pull grafts or implants through joints or bone tunnels (Figure 13.7). A small-eyed passer is used to pull an implant directly, or a graft sutured to its eye. Straight graft passers are used for bone tunnels. Curved graft passers are almost exclusively used in and around the stifle joint to pass implants of grafts either through the joint, in a variant of the over-the-top cranial cruciate ligament

163

Chapter 13 Surgical instrumentation

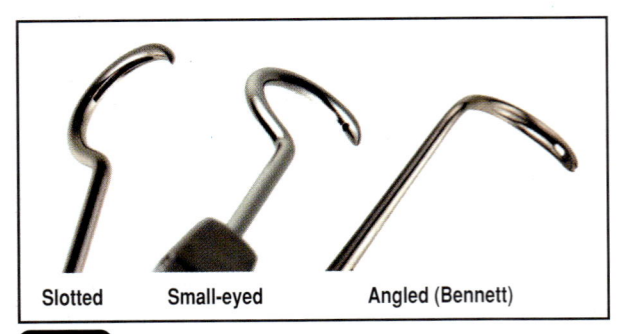

13.7 Graft passers.
Slotted — Small-eyed — Angled (Bennett)

procedure, or between the fabella and femur, as part of a variant of the lateral suture technique. A range of diameters, varying between 2 cm and 8 cm, is available to suit all breeds.

Resectors and disarticulators
Disarticulation of the femoral head is best achieved using a specialist instrument. Use of curved scissors is prone to failure, as the blades tend to slide off the ligament which is covered by synovial fluid. Unless the cut end of the round ligament is visible at the femoral fovea it is likely that it has not been completely resected. All resectors are typically curved or spoon-shaped to match the contours of the femoral head, and have a sharp edge or notch which engages and cuts the teres ligament (Figure 13.8). Substantial force may be required to cut and tear the teres ligament. Unless that is completely transected, the exposure required for excision of the femoral head and neck is extremely difficult to achieve.

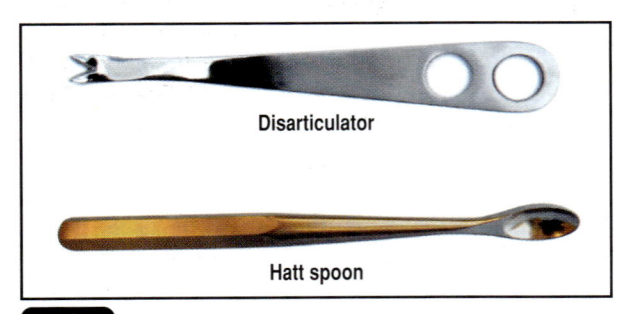

13.8 Resectors and disarticulators.
Disarticulator
Hatt spoon

Joint distractors
Stifle joint distractors work on the same principle as self-retaining retractors. As the handles are closed together, the working tips spread apart. Moving the fulcrum closer to the working tips increases the power of the distractor. Separation of the femur and tibia in a large dog, in order to view the medial meniscus, requires substantial force. The overlapping of the tips in the closed position minimizes articular cartilage trauma on insertion and removal. Distractor tips must significantly engage both the proximal tibia and distal femur in non-articular areas to avoid slippage. Distractors offer parallel distraction of joint surfaces. The distracted joint is maintained in the open position allowing inspection and treatment of meniscal lesions. Hohmann retractors may also be used to distract the tibia and femur but do not separate the joint surfaces quite as well. In addition, the Hohmann requires an assistant to maintain distraction for any treatment option. Smaller versions of stifle retractors are similar to small Gelpis but the overlapping tips facilitate insertion into very restricted areas to create small windows. Examples include the creation of a window for the meniscal release procedure caudal to the medial collateral ligament, and the creation of a joint capsule window during medial elbow arthrotomy.

Hand saws
Hand saw blades vary with respect to blade thickness, tooth size and flexibility (Figure 13.9). The tooth size dictates the depth of cut created with each pass of the blade. Smaller tooth sizes offer better control. The degree of 'saw set' (how much the tooth protrudes from the blade) dictates how wide the cut is and how much bone is removed.

Industrial small hacksaws are widely used in veterinary surgery. They are, however, not stainless steel and quickly deteriorate. The style of the hacksaw limits its use. It cannot be used in confined spaces. Hacksaw-type blades, both stainless and non-stainless, can be fitted into stainless steel handles, allowing their use for procedures in confined areas, such as femoral head and neck resection and tibial tubercle transposition. This type of saw is unsupported and so lacks directional control.

To increase control a blade can be stiffened along its length. This type of hard-backed saw is available in both stainless and non-stainless forms, with a range of tooth size. It is preferred for wedge trochleaplasty, where control over angle and direction of cut is important.

The Gigli saw is a cutting wire and is particularly useful where access is restricted. The saw may be threaded through very small spaces, and cuts only when placed under tension. Examples of use include proximal ulnar osteotomy and the ischial cut in the triple pelvic osteotomy procedure. Gigli saws always cut towards the hands of the operator, which can be contraindicated, such as in total femoral head and neck excision where use of the Gigli saw usually leaves a ventral spur.

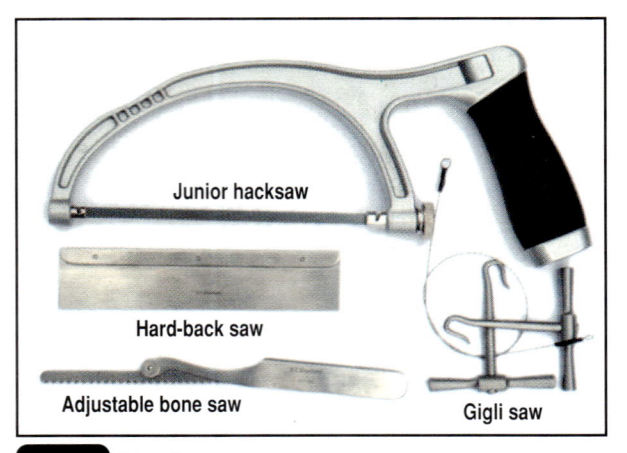

13.9 Hand saws.
Junior hacksaw
Hard-back saw
Adjustable bone saw
Gigli saw

Osteotomes

Osteotomes have a slim sharp blade designed to slice through bone; this is preferred for joint surgery (Figure 13.10). Chisels have a much heavier bevelled tip designed for more aggressive work elsewhere in orthopaedics. Osteotomes can be very effective in detaching ligamentous and tendinous attachments. No bone is lost compared with the various saw options. If re-attachment is anticipated, pre-placement of Kirschner wire holes is recommended prior to cutting. The osteotome width should be appropriate for the task, e.g. 6 mm for a small malleolus increasing to 20 mm for a femoral head and neck excision in a large dog. Use of an osteotome and mallet is very final and requires both confidence and experience.

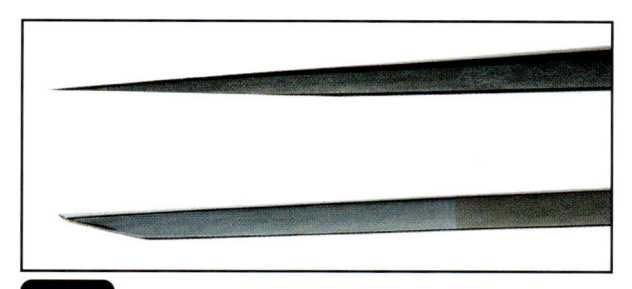

13.10 Osteotome (top) and chisel (bottom).

Rongeurs

Rongeurs (Figure 13.11) are designed to nibble bone incrementally. The spoon-type jaws enclose the bone fragment removed, which is withdrawn from the operative site. A large range is available, varying in bite size and angle of jaws. For most joint applications a combination of 5 mm angled bite and 2.5 mm straight bite (e.g. Lempert) is sufficient.

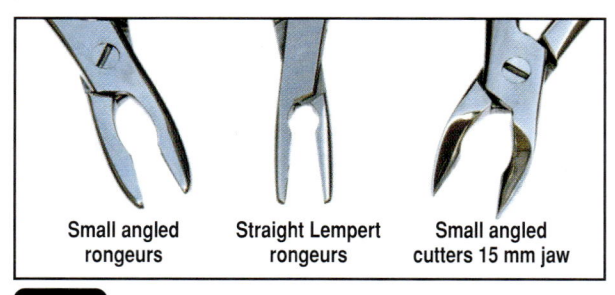

13.11 Rongeurs and cutters.

Small angled rongeurs | Straight Lempert rongeurs | Small angled cutters 15 mm jaw

Bone cutters

The jaws of bone cutters are designed to section and separate bone fragments (Figure 13.11). They are less sharp than osteotomes and tend to crush as well as cut. They are, however, more controllable than osteotomes and are widely used. A pair of angled cutters with 15 mm long cutting blades is particularly useful in miniature breeds to detach tibial tubercles and perform total femoral head and neck excisions.

Bone rasps

Rasps (Figure 13.12) are typically available in flat and tapering designs, and are useful to tidy up osteotomies. They are appropriate for the removal of bone spurs but are not appropriate for debulking bone. The bone debris created should be carefully flushed away prior to closure.

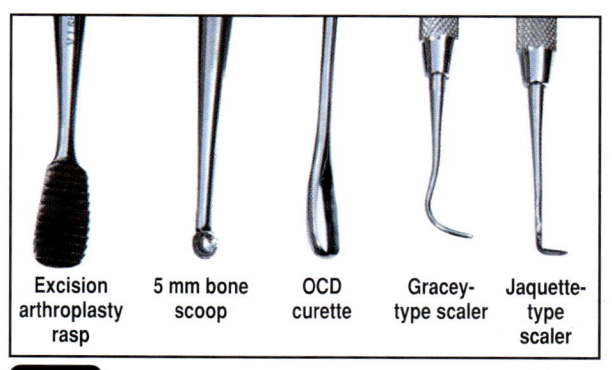

13.12 Rasps, scoops and curettes.

Excision arthroplasty rasp | 5 mm bone scoop | OCD curette | Gracey-type scaler | Jaquette-type scaler

Bone scoops and curettes

A 5 mm bone scoop is useful for the collection of cancellous bone for grafting and for the removal of cartilage in large joint arthrodesis. A purpose-designed curette is available for the treatment of osteochondritis dissecans (OCD) lesions in the shoulder. Small dental curettes and scalers have been used with success in the probing and treatment of OCD lesions in the elbow. Rasps, scoops and curettes are illustrated in Figure 13.12.

Powered instruments

Many joint surgery procedures require the use of powered instruments to create osteotomies or to drill holes for suture anchors, screws or bone tunnels. Modified and shrouded (or sterilized using ethylene oxide) industrial products can be both economical and effective, but are rather bulky. Dedicated orthopaedic power tools are typically autoclavable, air-driven and will take the form of either a stand-alone drill and saw or a modular system (Figure 13.13). A modular system will typically comprise

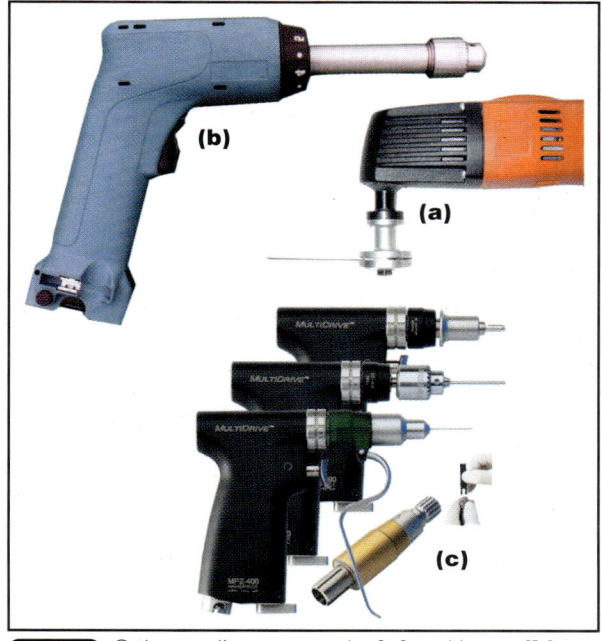

13.13 Orthopaedic power tools: **(a)** multi saw; **(b)** industrial-type drill; **(c)** Modular driver system.

Chapter 13 Surgical instrumentation

a handpiece with interchangeable attachments, usually including a chuck for drilling, an oscillating saw and a wire driver. Closing wedge tibial plateau levelling procedures may require blades up to 40 mm in length. If considering a purchase it is necessary to ensure that an appropriate range of blades is available. A high-speed burr is the most effective means of stripping articular cartilage prior to joint arthrodesis. Side-cutting burrs are more efficient than round burrs.

Periarticular implants and their insertion

Tissue anchors

Anchors are used to reattach ligaments or tendons, or to attach prosthetic supports (see Chapter 14), and are becoming commonplace in veterinary orthopaedics. The most basic form is a simple screw together with a spiked washer to retain the tissue or suture. More recently, modified screws have become available which have some means of passing a suture through the head. Placement will require appropriate drills and taps. Non-standard screw-type anchors all require dedicated drivers. True suture anchors are typically pre-threaded with the suture material and are placed below the bone surface where they cause minimal interference with overlying soft tissues. All the systems require dedicated insertion tools.

Kirschner and arthrodesis wires

Kirschner wires (K-wires) have a spatulate tip, which clears bone debris during insertion rather better than the arthrodesis wire, which is trocar tipped at both ends (effectively a mini Steinmann pin) (Figure 13.14). Although it cuts better, the long spatulate tip of the Kirschner wire reduces the amount of wire in final contact with the bone, thereby reducing pullout resistance. Most surgeons prefer the arthrodesis wire. Insertion is accomplished using a low-speed drill rather than a hand chuck. When drilling wires, the exposed end should be as short as possible to minimize bending and wobble. Dedicated wire drivers, either stand-alone or as part of a modular system, are best as they facilitate the incremental insertion of wires (Figure 13.15). The wire is effectively fed through the driver into the bone.

If it is desirable that the cut end of the wire should be under the bone surface (e.g. at an articular surface) the pin is partially cut using hard wire cutters. The partially cut area is driven beneath the bone surface and the wire is rocked at right angles to the partial cut. The wire will harden, become brittle at the partial cut and shear. It is not necessary to bend the wire aggressively, which may disrupt the repair. Alternatively, the wire may be cut at the bone surface and driven deeper using a pin punch. This technique is more traumatic to articular cartilage.

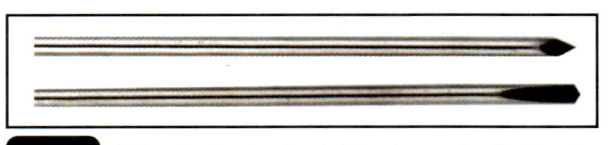

13.14 Arthrodesis wire (top); Kirschner wire (bottom).

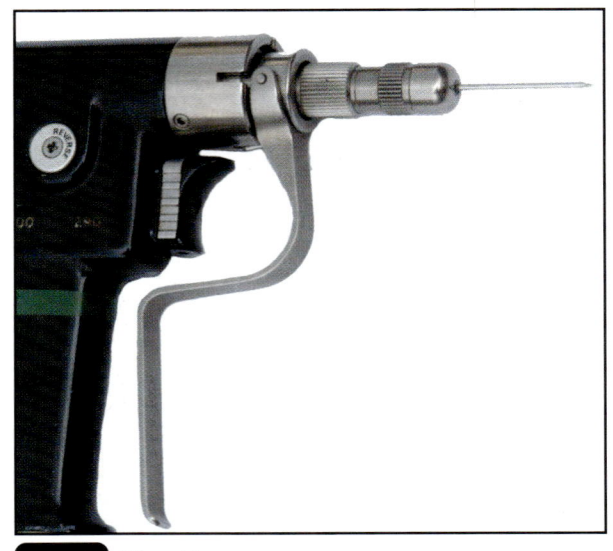

13.15 Wire driver.

In non-articular areas, or where the wires are to be used as anchorage for tension-band wires, the wires are deliberately cut long and bent. This will minimize soft tissue irritation and, to a degree, reduce the tendency to back out. It is important that the wire bends at, or close to, the bone surface. Bending below the bone surface will tend to open the osteotomy or fracture site; benders focus the bending forces at the bone surface, minimizing disruption of the repair (Figure 13.16).

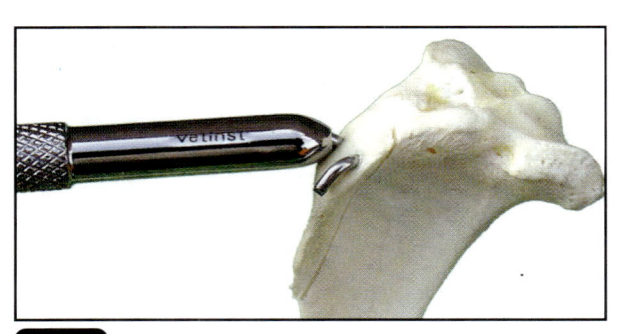

13.16 Kirschner wire bender.

Both Kirschner and arthrodesis wires are high tensile and require hard wire cutters, often surprisingly large, to cut them. Cutters designed to cut soft wire (cerclage) or bone will be damaged if used on hard wires.

Soft cerclage-type wire is necessary to create tension bands during the repair of osteotomies or avulsion fractures: 20 gauge (1.0 mm) wire is appropriate in most cases; for patients <5 kg, 24 gauge (0.6 mm) is appropriate; in very large dogs (>40 kg), 18 gauge (1.2 mm) is recommended.

Lighting

The surgical approach to any joint for investigation or treatment is designed to enable inspection of intra-articular structures; without appropriate lighting, even the best surgical approach will fail. A focal, adjustable light source is essential for most joint surgery. It is also

Chapter 13 Surgical instrumentation

desirable to keep radiant heat to a minimum to reduce desiccation. The 12-volt halogen-type sources are better in this regard than higher-powered light. If hot lights are used, appropriate irrigation of the tissues is essential. While focusing on the approach to the joint, it is important that attention is paid to exposed soft tissues.

Electrosurgery

Electrosurgery involves the passage of radio-frequency alternating current through body tissues to produce cutting and/or coagulation. In the radio frequency range (500,000–3,300,000 Hz), cutting and coagulation occurs without the potentially lethal effects of lower frequencies (50–60 Hz is the frequency of mains electricity). The electrosurgical effect is varied by adjusting voltage and the pulse rate of the electrical energy. Continuous low voltage will create a cutting effect; pulsed high voltage will cause coagulation; and blends of the two types will create intermediate effects. The different modes are selected from the control panel of the electrosurgical unit (Figure 13.17).

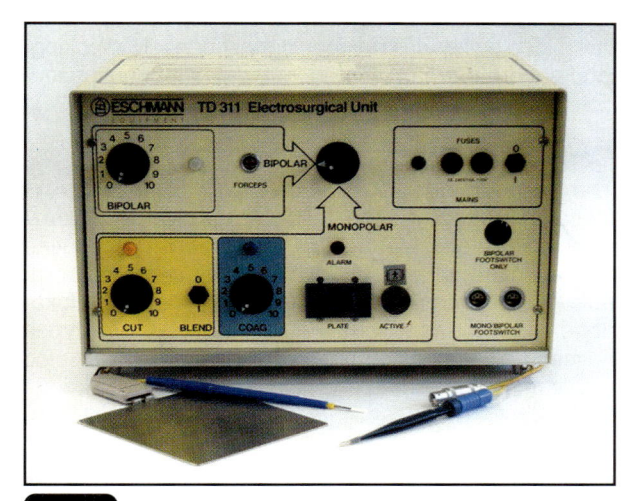

13.17 Electrosurgical unit.

The appropriate use of electrosurgical equipment for cutting and haemostasis will minimize visual obstruction of the surgical field and minimize loss of circulating blood volume. Monopolar units create heat at a single point as the electrical energy passes from the probe tip through the body to a large earth plate under the patient. The electrical energy thus affects a relatively large area until fully dissipated. Bipolar units, however, create heat as electrical energy passes between the similar sized tips of bipolar dissecting forceps. The effect of the electrical pulse is thus very localized. The use of bipolar equipment is recommended in the vicinity of nerves.

Suction

Use of suction will keep the operative site clear of blood and irrigating fluids. Use of an Adson/Frazier-type tip, which gives the user fine finger control of focal suction (Figure 13.18), is recommended. Most new suction units are supplied with a short silicone tube for attachment to a long disposable suction tube and tip.

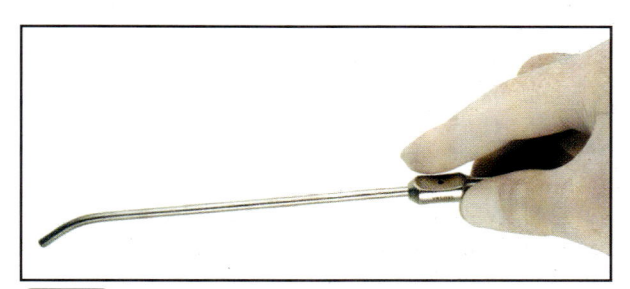

13.18 Adson suction tip.

> **PRACTICAL TIP**
> If autoclavable tips are being considered, at least an extra 2 metres of autoclavable silicone tubing should be purchased.

167

14

Biomaterials for joint surgery

Derek B. Fox

Suture materials and patterns

Most periarticular tissues hold sutures well because of the orientation and high concentration of collagen fibres. The strength of chosen suture materials should match the strength of the tissues involved with applications dictating appropriate suture size, longevity and tensile strength. Figure 14.1 shows the characteristics of commonly used suture materials. For general use in the periarticular environment, absorbable sutures are indicated. However, fascial and capsular imbrications, apposition of tendons and ligaments, and other applications aimed at maintaining reduction of sesamoid bones will require the use of more permanent sutures that retain their tensile strength for longer periods. Tendons, ligaments and fascia heal slowly, regaining as little as 50% of their strength over 6 weeks if immobilized (Montgomery, 1989). The loss of suture strength should be proportional to the gain in post-repair tissue strength (Smeak, 1997). Non-absorbable sutures are those classified as retaining the majority of their tensile strength for longer than 60 days and are thus often recommended for these applications.

Repair of severed tendons

A variety of suture patterns has been advocated for the apposition of severed tendons. Patterns that compromise blood supply least while providing the best tensile strength include the Kessler–Mason–Allen (locking-loop), modified Kessler and three-loop pulley. Research indicates that the three-loop pulley pattern provides more support, less tendon distraction and less tendon distortion than the locking-loop pattern (Jann et al., 1990). Furthermore, a recent study using cadavers showed that a modified three-loop pulley was mechanically superior to a locking-loop pattern for reattachment of the gastrocnemius tendon to the bone of the calcaneus (Moores et al., 2004).

Capsulorrhaphy

The most common use of sutures in articular surgery is for capsulorrhaphy, either following surgical arthrotomy or as part of open reductions of luxations. For routine closure following a capsulotomy, a long-lasting absorbable monofilament suture material, such as polydioxanone, is adequate. Certain multifilament suture types possess appropriate longevity and strength but also cause more tissue drag and have been linked with sinus formation and increased infection rates (Smeak, 1997).

Generic name	Trade names	Properties	Tensile strength loss	Completion of absorption	Relative tensile strength
Poliglecaprone 25	Monocryl	Monofilament Absorbable	50% by 7 days 80% by 14 days	91–119 days	Excellent
Polydioxanone	PDS II	Monofilament Absorbable	26% by 14 days 42% by 28 days	182 days	Excellent
Polyethylene	Polyethylene Ticron	Monofilament Non-absorbable	Slow loss over years	Not applicable	Excellent
Polyglactin 910	Vicryl	Multifilament Absorbable	50% by 14 days 80% by 21 days	60–90 days	Good
Polyglycolic acid	Dexon	Multifilament Absorbable	37% by 7 days 80% by 14 days	120 days	Good
Polyglyconate	Maxon	Monofilament Absorbable	19% by 14 days 80% by 28 days	180 days	Excellent
Polypropylene	Prolene Surgilene Fluorofil	Monofilament Non-absorbable	Not applicable	Not applicable	Good

14.1 Commonly used suture types. Adapted from Smeak (1997).

The author's preference is to close the joint capsule with a simple interrupted pattern to allow more accurate apposition of capsule edges and avoid the risk of complete re-opening or luxation of the joint following suture failure. Sutures should be placed close enough to one another that they result in the reformation of a tight seal; if possible, care should be taken not to engage the synovium during capsule closure, to prevent suture material being present within the joint. Although the risk is minimal, intra-articular suture material can abrade the articular cartilage or act as a nidus for infection.

Certain conditions that result in the formation of joint capsule redundancy, including patellar luxation and closure after total hip replacement, require capsular imbrication following arthrotomy. Because imbrication may place these tissues under higher tensile loads, a non-absorbable suture with prolonged degradation may be indicated. A popular method of joint capsule imbrication is the modified Mayo–mattress or 'vest-over-pants' pattern. Joint closure or imbrication should be completed carefully to avoid over-tightening. Over-tightening of the joint capsule can result in luxations in the case of the patella, decreased range of motion, pain or premature capsulorraphy failure.

Suture anchors

The reinsertion of various soft tissues, such as joint capsule, tendon and ligament, on to bone is a frequent demand on the orthopaedic surgeon. Traditionally, this has been accomplished through the use of bone tunnels, screw–washer combinations and staples. Complications with these procedures have included increased patient morbidity through greater required exposure and implant migration. However, with the advent of the suture anchor, soft tissue insertion on to bone has been revolutionized. Suture anchors, also called tissue anchors, are devices that insert into bone in a variety of different ways to act as insertion points for sutures, either fixating soft tissues or replacing the function of these structures. Suture anchors have the advantages, compared with older techniques, of possessing a lower profile with less subsequent surrounding tissue irritation, more precise placement in recreating isometric insertions, and quicker application (Beale, 2001). Anchors are intended to be temporary fixation devices, allowing soft tissues to heal to their original insertions or facilitating the formation of fibrous scar tissue over the course of their associated sutures, to help maintain appropriate joint integrity.

Many types of suture anchor are available and pullout strength is often regarded as the most critical criterion of effectiveness. Anchor strength is dependent on design, composition, size of drill hole, bone density and direction of applied load (Robinson, 2000). Most studies assessing the mechanical strength of anchors apply load perpendicularly or in parallel fashion to the long axis of the anchor, or both. The most common clinical relationship of anchor to suture is demonstrated by a tent peg analogy, in which the suture pulls on the anchor at an angle like the line of a rope, rather than directly along its axis, in which the anchor is at its weakest. This direction of load will result in higher pullout strengths. However, it is important to remember that within the anchor–suture–tendon combination, the suture–tendon interface is weakest (Barber et al., 1999).

There are over 75 different anchors available for human application but only a few systems have been specifically designed for veterinary use. Veterinary anchors are classified based on their positioning within the bone after application:

- *Subcortical anchors* are placed below the cortex of the bone through a drill hole. After insertion they change shape or diameter, and so resist being pulled out through the drill hole
- *Transcortical anchors* engage the *cis*-cortex of the bone and resist pullout by engaging the bone with threads of various types.

Subcortical anchors have the advantage of a lower profile and cause less interference in surrounding soft tissues (Figure 14.2). Transcortical screw-type anchors maximize pullout strength via an increased thread–bone interface at the expense of possessing a more prominent profile. Taylor (1992) and Edwards et al. (1993) first reported on the clinical use of suture anchors in veterinary medicine. They described the use of the Mitek (Norwood) Mini Generation II (G2) Anchor System, a subcortical prong-type anchor designed for human use, for the stabilization of tarsal and phalangeal collateral ligament injuries, a common calcaneal tendon avulsion, a coxofemoral luxation and

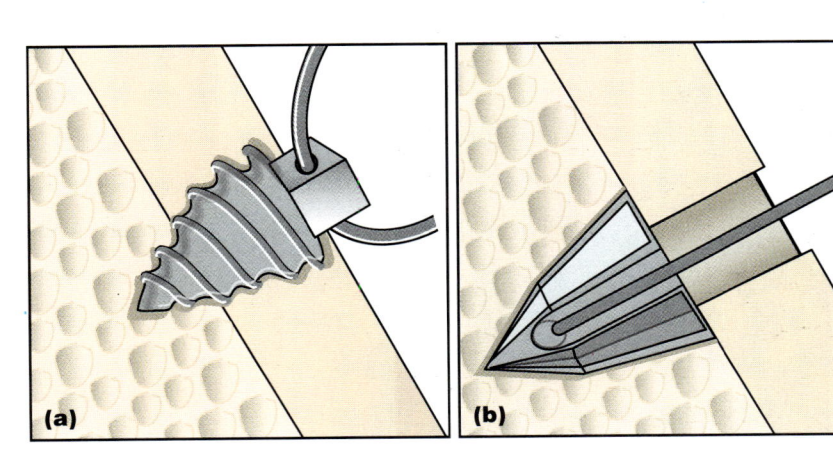

14.2 Suture anchors: **(a)** transcortical bone anchor; **(b)** subcortical anchor.

Chapter 14 Biomaterials for joint surgery

cranial cruciate ligament ruptures in a very small dog and cat with good results (Edwards et al., 1993). Robinson (2000) further described the use of the Mitek G2 tissue anchor system in a variety of similar clinical situations in small animals with very positive results. The Mitek G2 system uses nickel–titanium alloy, or Nitinol, prongs which deploy into cancellous bone upon complete insertion through the cortex. To ensure appropriate anchorage, a depth of 15 mm within the cancellous bone must be achieved through a drill hole 2.4 mm in diameter. When compared with other anchors, the Mitek GII failed less often when loaded in a perpendicular fashion and possessed a pullout strength of 82.5 N (Carpenter et al., 1993). An obvious disadvantage with the use of any anchor system intended for human application will be the cost of the implant and the required instrumentation.

The BoneBiter (Androcles Inc.) suture anchor, distributed by Innovative Animal Products, was the first anchor system to be manufactured for small animal veterinary applications. The BoneBiter anchor is subcortical and is available in two varieties, size 2 and size 5, which denote the largest suture size each can accommodate: 5 metric (2) and 7 metric (5), respectively (Figure 14.3). Pre-drilling is required prior to implantation. The size 2 anchor needs a 1.5 mm drill hole and the size 5 requires a 2.5 mm hole. Variations in bone density will occur with different anatomical locations and may require alterations in these sizes of drill holes. BoneBiter anchors are inserted in a subcortical fashion, requiring special instrumentation. In-house pullout strength testing of each size revealed average loads of 130 N and 160 N for perpendicular and parallel loading, respectively, for the size 2 anchor and 235 N and 341 N for perpendicular and parallel loading, respectively, for the size 5 anchor (Innovative Animal Products, 2003).

A new screw-type transcortical tissue anchor for small animal veterinary use is available from IMEX Veterinary Inc. IMEX anchors are available in two different thread diameters: 4.0 mm and 4.7 mm. Each is available in a short (6 mm) and long version (10 mm) (Figure 14.4). Pre-drilling is required; recommendations for drill hole sizes are 2.0–2.7 mm for the 4 mm anchor and 2.5–3.1 mm for the 4.6 mm anchor. Again, these drill hole sizes will need to be increased or decreased with variation in bone density. Cutting flutes present in the anchor sides allow a bone-clearing, self-tapping function. Insertion is completed with a custom driver. The author has used the IMEX anchors in numerous clinical cases of tarsal collateral injuries and coxofemoral joint capsule avulsions (Figure 14.5) with excellent results, both in ease of use and clinical outcome.

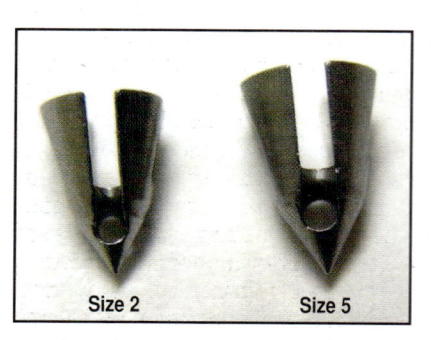

14.3 BoneBiter suture anchors.

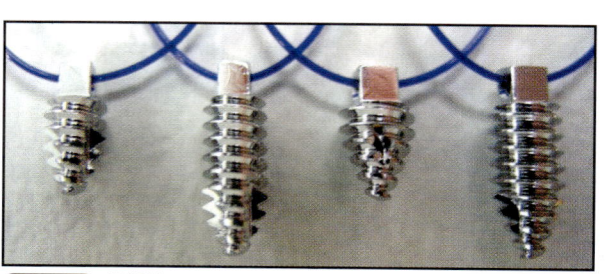

14.4 IMEX suture anchors; from left to right: 4.0 mm, short; 4.0 mm, long; 4.7 mm, short; 4.7 mm, long.

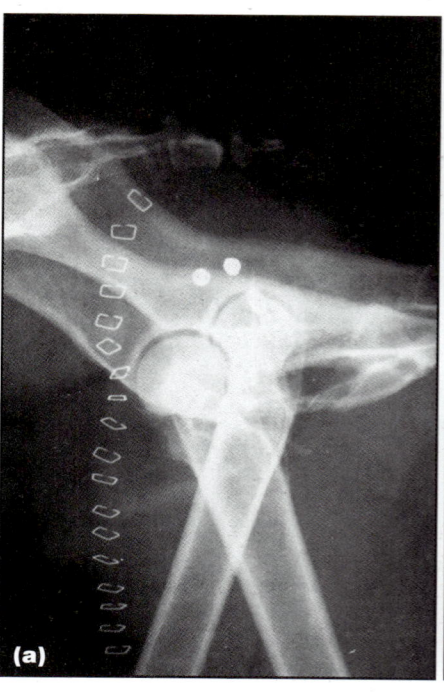

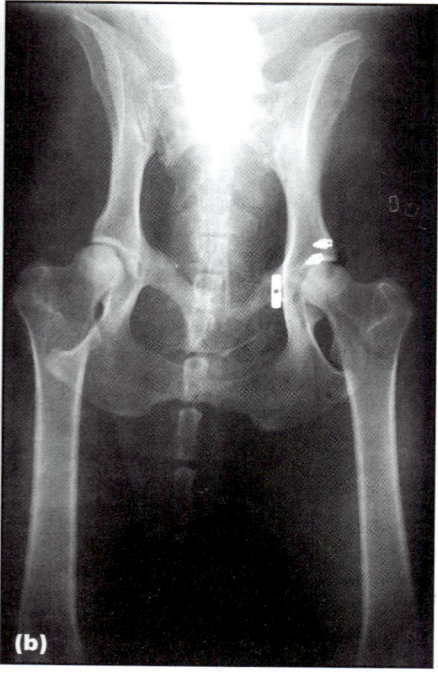

14.5 Lateral and VD postoperative radiographs of a repair of a canine hip luxation. Two IMEX suture anchors were used to secure an avulsed joint capsule and the luxation was repaired with an IMEX toggle pin.

Chapter 14 Biomaterials for joint surgery

Securos Veterinary Orthopedics Inc. also has a screw-type transcortical anchor intended for corticocancellous application. It comes in both 2.7 mm and 3.5 mm sizes with a single length of approximately 15 mm. The anchors possess a trochar tip and 'spindle' head which has a rounded groove intended to reduce suture fatigue at the eyelet. The Securos bone anchors use a unique delivery system. The anchors come attached to a longer rod of the same metal stock, called an 'insertion shaft', which is inserted into a common hand chuck. After pre-drilling and inserting the Securos anchor, the hand chuck is wobbled, thereby breaking free the insertion shaft from the anchor. Concerns with this system include premature disengagement of the insertion shaft during inadvertent over-torque and the need to apply a bending force to the anchor spindle after bone implantation.

A recent study investigated the pullout strength, ease of handling and general utility of several veterinary bone anchors compared with both cortical and cancellous screws. Results from the study indicate that IMEX anchors had similar pullout resistance to unicortical, 3.5 mm cortical and 4.0 mm cancellous screws and significantly higher loads to failure and ease of use compared with BoneBiter anchors (Robb et al., unpublished data).

Toggle pins

The toggle pin can be considered another type of suture anchor intended for application in a specific anatomical site. It does not engage cortical or cancellous bone in a subcortical fashion, but acts as a fixation point for suture placed through the femoral head and neck in the reduction of coxofemoral luxations. Its typical use involves drilling an appropriately sized hole in the acetabular fossa, and then feeding the toggle pin with associated suture through the hole into the pelvic canal. In this position, the pin will be pulled against the medial wall of the canal when the suture is tied at the level of the third trochanter. Current recommendations for the hand-manufacturing of toggle pins include small dogs to receive pins 9.5 mm (3/8 inch) long made from 0.9 mm (0.035 inch) Kirschner wire and large dogs to receive pins 15.9 mm (5/8 inch) long made from 1.1 mm (0.045 inch) Kirschner wire (Piermattei et al., 1997). To diminish the variability in hand-made toggle pins and reduce the risk of toggle-bending as a mode of failure, redesigned toggle pins (also called 'rods') have been manufactured and investigated. These consist of a thicker piece of metal through which a cross hole is bored to accommodate the desired suture. In one study, the mechanical properties of the toggle rod were not different from the conventional toggle pin, although the mode of failure of the rods was most commonly breakage, whereas the pins typically unfolded (Baltzer et al., 2001). Therefore, ease of use of prefabricated toggles was the main advantage. Variations of the newly designed toggle pin or rod are currently available.

Ligament prostheses and joint stabilizing materials

Traumatized or damaged ligaments (collateral ligaments) can sometimes, if caught very early, be repaired primarily with the use of non-absorbable sutures in similar fashion to repair of tendons. However, with time, degradative enzymes associated with the inflammatory process macerate ligament remnants, thereby making primary repair impossible. Many biomaterials have been investigated and are currently used as prosthetic devices in the replacement or reinforcement of injured stabilizing articular components, such as ligaments and joint capsule. Some of the specific applications include extra-articular and intra-articular materials in the cranial cruciate-deficient stifle, replacements or reinforcements of deficient collateral ligaments in a variety of joints, and intra-articular stabilization of coxofemoral luxations. Numerous studies have focused on the relative strengths of these materials, and the subsequent effects of different sterilization and fixation techniques. The objective of this section is to provide the reader with current recommendations according to the recent scientific literature regarding the various applications of prosthetic joint materials.

Cranial cruciate ligament disease is one of the most common canine orthopaedic disorders. Regardless of aetiology, the resulting joint instability necessitates surgical intervention. The implantation of extracapsular prostheses for the purposes of eliminating cranial draw has persisted as a surgical option for the treatment of this disease for many years. Most commonly, the prosthetic sutures will be placed from behind one (or both) fabella to a hole placed in the tibial crest. Although a number of different suture materials have been used for fabellotibial sutures, monofilament nylon fishing materials have been shown to exhibit excellent strength with minimal plastic deformation or tissue reactivity (Sicard et al., 2002). Among fishing materials, various sizes of both monofilament nylon fishing line (MFL) and monofilament nylon leader line (MLL) have been evaluated extensively (Figure 14.6). The most common products studied and used clinically are 27 kg (60 lb) test and 36 kg (80 lb) test Ande fishing line (Ande monofilament (premium), Germany) and Mason leader line (Mason hard type leader, Mason Tackle Co). Fishing lines are typically copolymers of nylon 6 and nylon 66, and leader line is composed of nylon 612; the result of this differing composition equates to leader line being less hygroscopic with a better dimensional stability (Caporn and Roe, 1996). This is particularly important with respect to sterilization techniques. It is believed that the absorption of water during steam sterilization of MFL results in its elongation and relatively poorer mechanical performance. Therefore several studies advocate the use of ethylene oxide sterilization of fishing materials (Lewis et al., 1997). Furthermore, Mason MLL is the safest material to sterilize in this fashion because it retains a higher strength and stiffness after sterilization when compared with other fishing lines (Caporn and Roe, 1996; Lewis et al., 1997; Sicard et al., 2002). Piermattei et al. (1997a) recommend matching the weight of the dog in

171

Chapter 14 Biomaterials for joint surgery

Study	Sterilization method assessed (if more than one)	Fixation method assessed (if more than one)	Materials tested	Main clinical implications
Lewis *et al.* (1997)	Ethylene oxide Steam	NA	Mason (MLL) 36 kg test No. 2 polypropylene No. 5 polybutylate-coated multifilament polyester	MLL is suitable for use; should sterilize with ethylene oxide
Anderson *et al.* (1998)	Ethylene oxide Steam	Slip knot Crimp clamp	Mason (MLL) 27 kg test	Crimp clamps provide superior *in vitro* loop fixation compared with slip-knot fixation
Nwadike and Roe (1998)	NA	Slip knot Square knot	Ande (MFL) 27 kg test Mason (MLL) 27 kg test	MLL secured with a slip knot recovered resting tension after cycling the best
Caporn and Roe (1996)	Ethylene oxide Steam	Square knot Clamped square knot	Ande (MFL) 27 kg test Ande (MFL) 36 kg test Mason (MLL) 27 kg test Mason (MLL) 36 kg test	MLL 27 kg test loops were unaffected by sterilization technique and had higher failure loads and stiffness than MFL. MLL 27 kg is most suitable for extra-articular stabilization
Sicard *et al.* (1999)	Ethylene oxide Steam	NA	Ande (MFL) 36 kg test Three other types of 36 kg test fishing line	Of MFL choices, Ande 36 kg test is the nylon material of choice when ethylene oxide is used. Steam elongated all MFL
Huber *et al.* (1999)	NA	Square knot Surgeon's knot Slip knot Clamped square knot	Ande 27 (MFL) kg test Mason (MLL) 27 kg test No. 2 nylon No. 2 polybutester No. 2 polypropylene	Clamping square knots of MLL increases its stiffness. Surgeon's knots should not be used with MFL or MLL because of reduction in stiffness and tension. Slip knots should not be used with MLL because of reduction of load
Sicard *et al.* (2002)	Ethylene oxide Steam	Square knot Crimp clamp	Ande 36 (MFL) kg test Mason (MLL) 36kg test Three other types of 36 kg test fishing material	Mason MLL has the least elongation and greatest strength when ethylene oxide is used. Crimped Mason MLL results in less elongation than knotted Mason MLL

14.6 Synopsis of studies assessing materials for extra-articular stifle stabilization in the recent literature. (NA, not assessed; MLL, monofilament nylon leader line; MFL, monofilament nylon fishing line)

pounds to the necessary size Mason MLL to use (between 9 kg (20 lb) and 36 kg (80lb) test). For smaller dogs (<5 kg) and cats, the author suggests the use of single or multiple strands of large polypropylene suture (3.5–5 metric (USP 2/0).

When considering methods of using large-diameter fishing material for extra-articular stifle stabilization, a number of different methods have been evaluated (Figure 14.6). Regardless of fixation technique, MLL appears to be superior to MFL. Studies show that surgeon's throws should be avoided with MLL, however, because they can result in a loss of stiffness and tension (Huber *et al.*, 1999). Contradicting reports exist regarding the safety of using the slip knot or sliding half hitch with MLL. Nwadike and Roe (1998) advocated the use of the slip knot, claiming a better recovery of resting tension after cyclic loading, while Huber *et al.* (1999) documented the slip knot as a cause of declining load in MLL. Both Caporn and Roe (1996) and Huber *et al.* (1999) do, however, recommend the use of instrument clamping of the standard square knot to maintain tension on the MLL and report a higher subsequent stiffness. Crimp clamping with a 316L surgical stainless steel tube has also been reported to be a superior method of fixation for large-diameter fishing materials; it results in increased strength and resistance to elongation when compared with slip knots or clamped square knots (Anderson *et al.*, 1998; Sicard *et al.*, 2002). Crimp clamping systems designed for this purpose are available from various manufacturers.

Monofilament failure typically occurs over time with any biomaterial chosen. The mode of failure for the majority of implants is breakage within 3 mm of the knot or clamp. This typically does not result in stifle instability, as long as the suture has remained intact long enough to facilitate the formation of periarticular fibrosis. Occasionally, any large fishing material may cause extracapsular irritation which will necessitate the removal of the implant(s).

The utility of a variety of other biomaterials as prosthetic devices has been investigated for the cranial cruciate ligament, teres (round) ligament of the hip, medial collateral ligament of the stifle and medial glenohumeral ligament of the shoulder. Various prosthetic replacements of the severed teres ligament in the luxated coxofemoral joint have been investigated extensively. These applications typically utilize the previously described toggle pin or rod. One study was unable to document a difference in the sustainable load between 5 metric (2 USP) braided polyester and 22.7 kg (50 lb) test monofilament nylon, but speculated that the higher stiffness of polyester sutures would be more favourable in this application (Flynn *et al.*, 1994). Another investigation suggests that 5 mm woven polyester possesses a longer life to fatigue during cyclic testing than 22.7 kg (50 lb) monofilament polybutester and 1 metric (5/0) braided polyester. The stabilized joints, however, could tolerate yield and maximum loads of only 41% of the intact joints and the woven polyester lengthened by 14% during cyclic loading, which might make it unable to maintain reduction during joint capsular healing (Baltzer *et al.*, 2001). Other concerns with the intra-articular use of woven or braided polyester include persistent infection, tissue reaction and sinus formation (Piermattei *et al.*, 1997b; Baltzer *et al.*, 2001). This author currently uses either 27 kg or 36 kg test MLL in conjunction with toggle rods in medium-sized and larger dogs that are acceptable open reduction candidates.

Polyester suture and polypropylene mesh have been evaluated for their effectiveness in replacing the medial collateral ligament of the canine stifle (Robello *et al.*, 1992); findings suggested that the polypropylene mesh resulted in a more stable and biomechanically natural prosthetic ligament than the polyester. Additionally, 18 kg (40 lb) test nylon monofilament has been used successfully as a prosthetic replacement for damaged medial glenohumeral ligaments in shoulder luxations and subluxations (Fitch *et al.*, 2001). Braided polyester, polyester tapes, woven Dacron (with and without fascial autografts), copolymer-coated carbon fibres and porcine small intestinal submucosa (SIS) have each been evaluated in research animals as intra-articular prostheses for the cranial cruciate ligament; there has been little further development for clinical application in small animals. Limiting factors have included questionable durability, tissue reaction and cost.

Total joint arthroplasty

Currently, total joint arthroplasty is limited to the hip and elbow in small animal patients. Total joint arthroplasty represents the most extensive use of intra-articular biomaterials used in small animal orthopaedic surgery. Total hip arthroplasty is discussed in detail in Chapter 21; however, a brief discussion of the composition of the main elements of hip and elbow prostheses is given here.

Hip prostheses

All available veterinary total hip replacement systems use a metallic femur on plastic acetabular configuration (Figure 14.7). Depending on the specific type of implant, the femoral endoprosthesis comprises titanium, cobalt chrome or 316L stainless steel. Cobalt chrome is currently the material of choice for femoral stems. The chromium constituent contributes to improved wear resistance compared with titanium, and improved corrosion resistance over that of stainless steel (Schulz, 2000). The plastic deformation experienced by cobalt chrome implants during articulation and load bearing results in increased strength; a phenomenon called 'work-hardening' (Gilbert, 1998). The combination of a titanium stem and cobalt chrome head is available in a European total hip model. This specific combination of metals resists galvanic corrosion through a process of self-passivation (Litsky and Spector, 1994; Schulz, 2000). All available acetabular components are constructed of ultra-high molecular weight polyethylene (UHMWPE). Current research indicates that cross-linking the UHMWPE improves wear, elongation and hardness (Wright and Li, 2000). Both cemented and cementless total hip replacement systems are currently available.

Elbow prostheses

Prostheses for total elbow replacement are under current investigation. Conzemius and colleagues have described the creation of an isometric humeral endoprosthesis manufactured from 316L stainless steel, which articulates in a non-constrained fashion with a radioulnar component made from UHMWPE (Conzemius *et al.*, 2003). Each half is cemented in place. The most recent report suggested that 16 of 20 dogs diagnosed with elbow osteoarthritis treated using the total elbow prosthesis had satisfactory outcomes (Conzemius *et al.*, 2003).

Implant failure

Aseptic loosening is one of the major causes of implant failure in total joint arthroplasty. Although aseptic loosening is multifactorial, foreign body reaction to wear products from the metal, plastic or cement components of total joint prostheses represents a major cause for loosening. Mechanical wear of these components leads to formation of particles which can be phagocytosed by macrophages and multinucleated giant cells located in the fibrous tissue of the regenerated capsule. Additionally, reticuloendothelial cells from the adjacent bone marrow may also become involved in the foreign body reaction (El-Warrak *et al.*, 2001). The macrophages are stimulated to release osteolytic cytokines, which lead to loosening of the implants (Hukkanen *et al.*, 1997). Subsequent formation of an interface membrane ensues which is composed of different layers:

System	Modular?	Cemented?	Stem composition	Head composition	Cup composition	Manufacturer
BioMedtrix	Yes	Yes	Cobalt chrome	Cobalt chrome	UHMWPE	BioMedtrix
Richards II	No	Yes	Cobalt chrome	Cobalt chrome	UHMWPE	No longer made
Mathys	No	Yes	316L stainless steel	316L stainless steel	UHMWPE	Mathys
Bardet	Yes	Yes	Titanium	Cobalt chrome	UHMWPE	J-F Bardet
New Generation	No	Yes	Cobalt chrome	Cobalt chrome	UHMWPE	New Generation
Zurich	Yes	No	Titanium	Titanium	Titanium and UHMWPE	Kyon

14.7 Canine total hip replacement systems and their composition. (UHMWPE, ultra-high molecular weight polyethylene)

a synovial-like layer at the cement surface, conglomerations of histiocytes and giant cells in a middle layer and a fibrous layer blending into the bone (Goldring et al., 1983; El-Warrak et al., 2001). The histology of this tissue will vary with the nature of the wear particles.

Polymethylmethacrylate

Polymethylmethacrylate (PMMA) is a polymer bone cement used for various applications in the articular environment and is available from a number of different manufacturers (Figure 14.8). It is used for cemented total joint replacement systems, as an internal fixation device for some articular fractures (acetabulum) and as a delivery system for antibiotics in cases of severe osteomyelitis. With most types, the cement is made at the time of surgery by combining a liquid and powdered solid together. The liquid is a methylmethacrylate monomer containing a polymerization inhibitor, hydroquinone. The solid is typically a powdered blend of PMMA, the initiator dibenzoyl peroxide and either barium sulphate or zirconium dioxide, which allow radiographic visualization. Some formulations include copolymer blends of PMMA and polystyrene or methacrylic acid, to provide greater wear resistance. The polymerization process is an exothermic reaction whose temperature rise is dictated by the thickness and amount of the cement and heat transfer to surrounding areas. Whereas non-implanted PMMA can achieve *in vitro* curing temperatures of between 60°C and 100°C, the actual temperature within bone has been reported to be as low as 40°C; this is below the temperature at which bone undergoes necrosis (47°C) (Wright and Li, 2000). PMMA is available in a variety of viscosities, ranging from a low-viscosity injectable liquid form to a high-viscosity dough type. Mixing low-viscosity PMMA under centrifugation or vacuum has been reported to decrease the porosity by as much as 50%, leading to an increase in tensile strength of about 44% when compared with hand-mixed cement (Wright and Li, 2000). The cure rate is dependent on the specific product in addition to the room and patient temperature, but typically occurs within 10–15 minutes. Ultimate strength is achieved at 24 hours.

Antimicrobial agents can be mixed with PMMA to avoid orthopaedic infection at 'clean' surgery sites already employing bone cement, as with total joint arthroplasty or fracture repairs, or as a delivery vehicle for antibiotics in existing severe osteomyelitis. Potential alteration of the mechanical properties of the PMMA by the antibiotic is obviously of great concern for the first application. It is now known that the use of liquid antimicrobials in PMMA mixtures will compromise the strength of the bone cement and should be avoided. However, the use of 2 g or less of antibiotic powder per 40 g of cement does not significantly alter the mechanical strength of the PMMA, and is therefore considered safe (Morris and Einhorn, 2000). Current recommendations for canine total hip arthroplasty are for the addition of 1 g of cefazolin to each full dose of PMMA (Schulz, 2000). Antibiotic-impregnated PMMA beads can also be used for implantation into sites of active infection. Commercial products are available that already contain the antimicrobial agent, or they can be made by hand. Elution of the antibiotic is bimodal, with the most rapid release occurring in the first 24 hours after implantation, followed by a continuous release lasting weeks to years. Various factors affect the elution rate of the antibiotics from the PMMA, including site of implantation, cement pore size, permeability, implant size and surface area, and the amount of antimicrobial agent added (Streppa et al., 2001). The typical delivery of antibiotics to the implanted site is very concentrated and often several times higher than the minimal inhibitory concentration. The impregnated beads are non-biodegradable and thus require removal, and they can invoke inflammatory reactions and subsequent fluid accumulation. Alternatives to non-biodegradable antimicrobial delivery systems include antibiotic-impregnated collagen sponges; these have been arthroscopically implanted within joints to treat septic arthritis in large animals with success (Hirsbrunner and Steiner, 1998; Summerhays, 2000).

Cement type	Manufacturer	Viscosity	Notes
Simplex P	Stryker Howmedica International Ltd	Medium	Exhibits very high ultimate tensile strength and deep bone penetration with subsequently high shear strength at cement–bone interface
Palacos	E. Merck	High	Exhibits high tensile strength and moderate bone penetration, but shows more plastic deformation under load than Simplex and CMW
Zimmer dough type	Warsaw, IN	High	Less tensile strength than Simplex P, Palacos and CMW 1 & 3
Zimmer Osteobond	Warsaw, IN	Low	Moderately high tensile strength, shorter working time than with Simplex P, cannot mix components from different lots
Zimmer LVC	Warsaw, IN	Low	Vacuumed product failed 4.4 times sooner than Simplex P when cycled
CMW 1	DePuy Ltd	High	
CMW 2	DePuy Ltd	High	Extremely short set time ~6 minutes
CMW 3	DePuy Ltd	Medium	Moderately high tensile strength, close to Simplex P in function
SmartSet MV Endurance	DePuy Ltd	Medium	Cannot mix components from different lots

14.8 Commonly used types of PMMA with manufacturer, viscosity and pertinent notes regarding the products. Data from package inserts and Harper and Bonfield (2000).

The future of biomaterials in veterinary arthrology

The future use of biomaterials in small animal articular surgery may be focused largely on articular cartilage and fibrocartilage repair or regeneration in cases where the integrity of these tissues is compromised or completely lost. Conditions such as osteochondrosis dissecans and osteoarthritis typically result in partial or full thickness erosions in articular cartilage. Nearly 50% of dogs diagnosed with cranial cruciate ligament disease will experience significant meniscal damage, requiring meniscectomy. Loss of function of these articular structures is a part of a process that inevitably leads to degenerative joint disease. The healing potential of articular cartilage and meniscal fibrocartilage is extremely limited. Currently, a tremendous research effort is geared toward the production of implantable biomaterials that can facilitate the regeneration or repair of these cartilages.

Some of the biomaterials being investigated include various forms and mixtures of polyglycolic and polylactic acid, and different forms of type I collagen, periosteum and perichondrium. Many of these investigations are conducted on research dogs for the ultimate purpose of human application. However, if cost prohibitions can be overcome with the formation of specific veterinary products, these could eventually become a part of the small animal orthopaedic surgeon's arsenal. For example, articular applications of porcine SIS in the facilitation of meniscal regeneration are being studied (Cook *et al.*, 2001; Fox *et al.*, 2004). SIS is an acellular type I collagen biomatrix harvested from swine intestine, which has shown promising tissue regenerative potential in various orthopaedic and general surgical applications, including ligament, tendon and muscle. The use of SIS to facilitate human meniscal regeneration in a clinical trial is currently being reviewed in the US by the Food and Drug Administration.

Determining the 'magic' combinations of scaffolds, cells, bioactive factors and mechanical stimuli in the pursuit of tissue repair and regeneration, otherwise known as tissue engineering, will probably hold significant importance in the future of small animal orthopaedic surgery.

References and further reading

Anderson CC, Tomlinson JL, Daly WR *et al.* (1998) Biomechanical evaluation of a crimp clamp system for loop fixation of monofilament nylon leader material used for stabilization of the canine stifle joint. *Veterinary Surgery* **27**, 533–539

Baltzer WI, Schulz KS, Stover SM, Taylor KT and Kass PH (2001) Biomechanical analysis of suture anchors and suture materials used for toggle pin stabilization of hip joint luxation in dogs. *American Journal of Veterinary Research* **62**, 721–728

Barber FA and Herbert MA (1999) Suture anchors: update 1999. *Arthroscopy* **7**, 719–725

Beale BS (2001) Suture Anchors and Prosthetic Ligament Reconstruction. In: *Proceedings of the District of Columbia Academy of Veterinary Medicine Meeting*. Washington, DC. www.dcavm.org/01nov.htm

Caporn TM and Roe SC (1996) Biomechanical evaluation of the suitability of monofilament nylon fishing and leader line for extra-articular stabilisation of the canine cruciate deficient stifle. *Veterinary and Comparative Orthopaedics and Traumatology* **9**, 126–133

Carpenter JE, Fish DN, Huston LJ and Goldstein SA (1993) Pull-out strength of five suture anchors. *Arthroscopy* **9**, 109–113

Conzemius MG, Aper RL and Corti LB (2003) Short-term outcome after total elbow arthroplasty in dogs with severe, natural occurring osteoarthritis. *Veterinary Surgery* **32**, 545–552

Cook JL, Tomlinson JL, Arnoczky SP *et al.* (2001) Kinetic study of the replacement of porcine small intestinal submucosa grafts and the regeneration of meniscal-like tissue in large avascular meniscal defects in dogs. *Tissue Engineering* **7**, 321–334

Edwards MR, Taylor RA and Franceshi RA (1993) Clinical case applications of Mitek® tissue anchors in veterinary orthopaedics. *Veterinary and Comparative Orthopaedics and Traumatology* **6**, 208–212

El-Warrak AO, Olmstead ML, von Rechenberg B and Auer JA (2001) A review of aseptic loosening in total hip arthroplasty. *Veterinary and Comparative Orthopaedics and Traumatology* **14**, 115–124

Fitch RB, Breshears L, Staatz A and Kudnig S (2001) Clinical evaluation of prosthetic medial glenohumeral ligament repair in the dog (ten cases). *Veterinary and Comparative Orthopaedics and Traumatology* **14**, 222–228

Flynn MF, Edmiston DN, Roe SC *et al.* (1994) Biomechanical evaluation of a toggle pin technique for management of coxofemoral luxation. *Veterinary Surgery* **23**, 311–321

Fox DB, Cook JL, Arnoczky SA *et al.* (2004) Fibrochondrogenesis of free intra-articular small intestinal submucosa scaffolds. *Tissue Engineering* **10**, 129–137

Gilbert JL (1998) Metals. In: *The Adult Hip*, 1st edn, ed. JJ Callaghan *et al.*, pp. 123–134. Lippincott–Raven, Philadelphia

Goldring SR, Schiller AL, Roelke M *et al.* (1983) The synovial-like membrane at the bone-cement interface in loose total hip replacements and its proposed role in bone lysis. *Journal of Bone and Joint Surgery [Am]* **65**, 575–584

Harper EJ and Bonfield W (2000) Tensile characteristics of ten commercial acrylic bone cements. *Journal of Biomedical Materials Research (Applied Biomaterials)* **53**, 605–616

Hirsbrunner G and Steiner A (1998) Treatment of infectious arthritis of the radiocarpal joint of cattle with gentamicin-impregnated collagen sponges. *Veterinary Record* **142**, 399–402

Huber DJ, Egger EL and James SP (1999) The effect of knotting method on the structural properties of large diameter nonabsorbable monofilament sutures. *Veterinary Surgery* **28**, 260–267

Hukkanen M, Corbett SA, Batten J *et al.* (1997) Aseptic loosening of total hip replacement. Macrophage expression of inducible nitric oxide synthase and cyclo-oxygenase-2, together with peroxynitrite formation, as a possible mechanism for early prosthesis failure. *Journal of Bone and Joint Surgery* **79**, 467–474

Innovative Animal Products (2003) *BoneBiter™ Suture Anchor System Size 2 and Size 5 Testing data*. www.innovativeanimalproducts.com/androcles/Testing.html

Jann HW, Stein LE and Good JK (1990) Strength characteristics and failure modes of locking-loop and three-loop pulley suture patterns in equine tendons. *Veterinary Surgery* **19**, 28–33

Lewis DD, Milthorpe BK and Bellenger CR (1997) Mechanical comparison of materials used for extra-capsular stabilisation of the stifle joint in dogs. *Australian Veterinary Journal* **75**, 890–896

Litsky AS and Spector M (1994) Biomaterials. In: *Basic Orthopedic Science*, ed. SR Simon, pp. 447–486. American Academy of Orthopedic Surgeons, Columbus

Montgomery RD (1989) Healing of muscle, ligaments and tendons. *Seminars in Veterinary Medicine and Surgery: Small Animal* **4**, 304–311

Moores AP, Comerford EJ, Tarlton JF and Owen MR (2004) Biomechanical and clinical evaluation of a modified 3-loop pulley suture pattern for reattachment of canine tendons to bone. *Veterinary Surgery* **33**, 391–397

Morris CD and Einhorn TA (2000) Principles of orthopedic pharmacology. In: *Orthopedic Basic Science: Biology and Biomechanics of the Musculoskeletal System*, 2nd edn, ed. JA Buckwalter *et al.*, pp. 217–237. American Academy of Orthopaedic Surgeons, Columbus OH

Nwadike BS and Roe SC (1998) Mechanical comparison of suture material and knot type used for fabello-tibial sutures. *Veterinary and Comparative Orthopaedics and Traumatology* **11**, 47–52

Piermattei DL, Flo GL and Brinker WO (1997a) The hip joint. In: *Handbook of Small Animal Orthopedics and Fracture Repair*, 2nd edn, ed. WO Brinker *et al.*, pp. 422–468. WB Saunders, Philadelphia

Piermattei DL, Flo GL and Brinker WO (1997b) The stifle joint. In: *Handbook of Small Animal Orthopedics and Fracture Repair*, 2nd edn, ed. WO Brinker *et al.*, pp. 416–580. WB Saunders, Philadelphia

Robello GT, Aron DN, Foutz TL and Rowland GN (1992) Replacement of the medial collateral ligament with polypropylene mesh or a polyester suture in dogs. *Veterinary Surgery* **21**, 467–474

Robinson A (2000) Clinical application of prong-type tissue anchors in small animal surgery. *Journal of Small Animal Practice* **41**, 207–210

Schulz KS (2000) Application of arthroplasty principles to canine

Chapter 14   Biomaterials for joint surgery

cemented total hip replacement. *Veterinary Surgery* **29**, 578–593

Sicard GK, Meinen J, Phillips T and Manley PA (1999) Comparison of fishing line for repair of the cruciate deficient stifle. *Veterinary and Comparative Orthopaedics and Traumatology* **12**, 138–141

Sicard GK, Hayashi K and Manley PA (2002) Evaluation of 5 types of fishing material, 2 sterilization methods, and a crimp-clamp system for extra-articular stabilization of the canine stifle joint. *Veterinary Surgery* **31**, 78–84

Smeak DD (1997) Selection and use of currently available suture materials and needles. In: *Current Techniques in Small Animal Surgery, 4th edn*, ed. MJ Bojrab, pp. 19–26. Willams & Wilkins, Baltimore

Streppa HK, Singer MJ and Budsberg SC (2001) Applications of local antimicrobial delivery systems in veterinary medicine. *Journal of the Veterinary Medical Association* **219**, 40–48

Summerhays GE (2000) Treatment of traumatically induced synovial sepsis in horses with gentamicin-impregnated collagen sponges. *Veterinary Record* **147**, 184–188

Taylor RA (1992) Clinical utilization of the Mitek® tissue anchor. In: *Proceedings of the Veterinary Orthopedic Society, 19th Annual Meeting*. Keystone, Colorado

Wright TM and Li S (2000) Biomaterials. In: *Orthopedic Basic Science: Biology and Biomechanics of the Musculoskeletal System, 2nd edn*, ed. JA Buckwalter et al., pp.181–215. American Academy of Orthopedic Surgeons, Columbus OH

15a

Arthroscopic equipment

John Lapish and Bernadette Van Ryssen

Introduction

Arthroscopy may be considered expensive in terms of both the dedicated instrumentation required and the time and money involved in training, but it is recommended that sufficient resources are allocated to purchase good quality equipment at the outset. Equipment failures are very frustrating and ultimately very expensive.

The arthroscope

The arthroscope (Figure 15.1) is an optical instrument, comprising a cylinder with several lenses, which collects and transmits an image from the tip of the instrument along the shaft to an eyepiece or camera. A light post close to the eyepiece allows light to be passed into the shaft and down optic fibres surrounding the lens system to illuminate the subject area at the tip. The choice of 'scope depends on its intended use. The 'scope may be required only for use in joints, or it may be required for other forms of endoscopy, such as rhinoscopy or cystoscopy. Where multiple uses are envisaged, a second or third purchase may be required to complete an arthroscopy set. Individual manufacturers' patterns may vary slightly and components are not usually interchangeable.

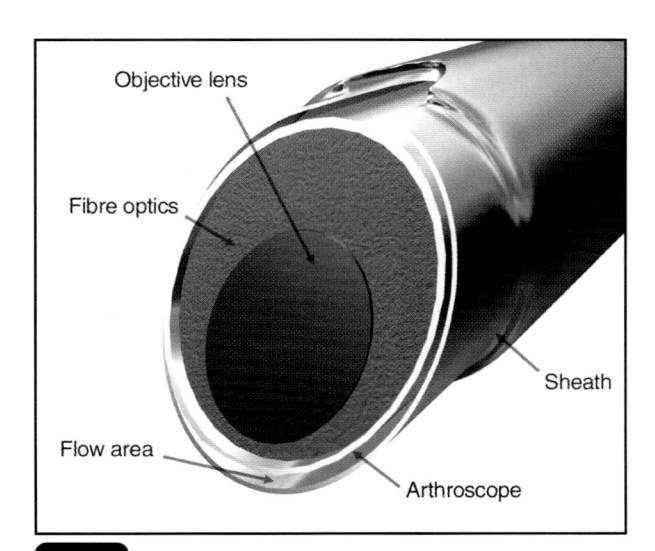

15.1 Arthroscope.

Diameter

Three sizes are commonly used in small animals: 2.7 mm, 2.4 mm and 1.9 mm, referring to the outside diameter of the unsheathed shaft of the 'scope. As the diameter becomes smaller, there is less space for optical fibres, which has implications for light transmission and image size. Recent improvements in construction, such as the use of rod–lens systems as opposed to optical fibres, have improved the performance of the smaller arthroscopes. Additionally, the smaller arthroscopes are fragile; care must therefore be exercised to avoid damage in use, cleaning and storage.

The effective diameter is enlarged by 0.5–1 mm by the arthroscopic sleeve.

Viewing angle

The viewing angle is that angle between the lens face and a line drawn at right angles to the long axis of the arthroscope (Figure 15.2). A 0-degree 'scope views straight ahead from the front of the lens, while a 90-degree 'scope sees an image at right angles to its long axis. The larger the viewing angle, the wider the field of view that can be achieved by turning the arthroscope around its axis (Figure 15.3); with this, however, the image is more distorted, and orientation within the joint becomes difficult. Most veterinary arthroscopes have a viewing angle of 30 degrees, which is a compromise between field of view and distortion.

The user needs to be aware which way the lens is pointing. The light post is used as a reference point and is positioned opposite the angle of view. Rotating the scope along its long axis will allow the surgeon to view a large area within the joint with minimal repositioning. A 0-degree scope looking straight ahead would require much repositioning to view the same area. An oblique viewing angle offers the surgeon a limited ability to 'see around corners'.

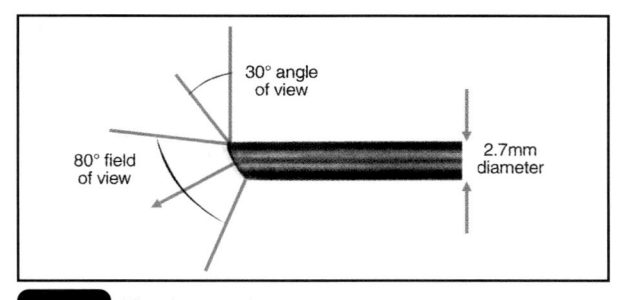

15.2 Viewing angle.

177

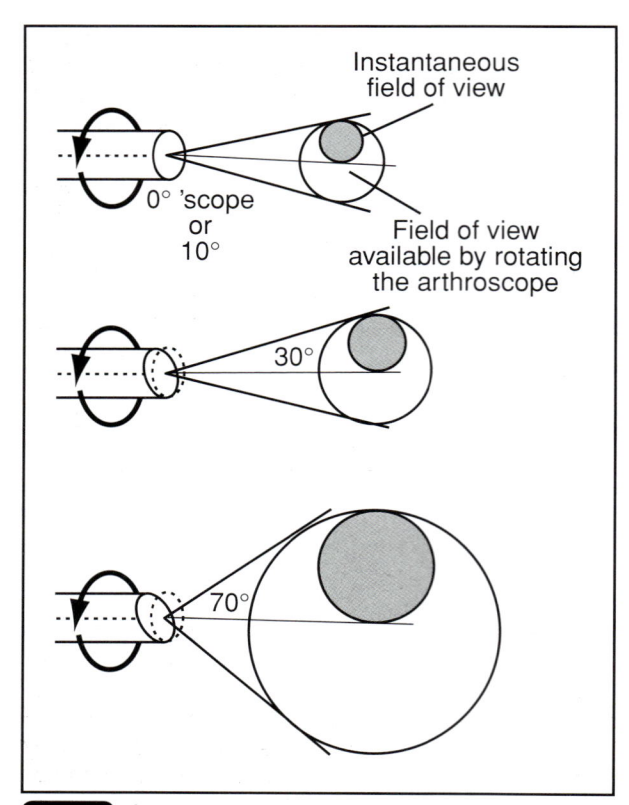

Chapter 15a Arthroscopic equipment

15.3 Fields of view with different viewing angles.

Field of view
This is limited by the size of the objective lens, which is, in turn, limited by the arthroscope's diameter. A 2.7 mm diameter 'scope typically has a field of view of 80 degrees. In the 1.9 mm 'scope, this falls to 65 degrees. The brightness of the image is also decreased in a thinner 'scope (Figure 15.4) and in older models. Many arthroscopes have an arrow in their view, indicating the view direction.

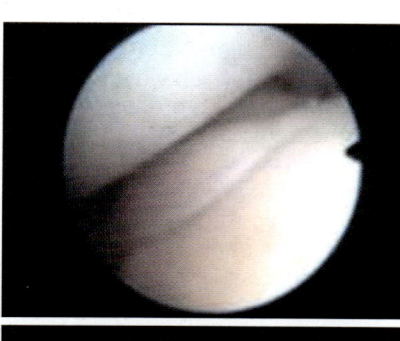

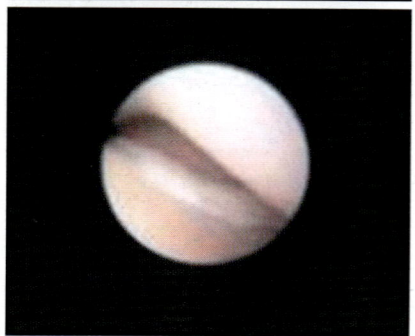

15.4 Arthroscopic views through a 2.4 mm (top) and a 1.9 mm arthroscope. The black triangle indicates the direction of view.

Working length
The working length of the arthroscope ranges from 8 to 18 cm and is usually related to diameter. The 1.9 mm diameter arthroscopes are short (approximately 11 cm) while the 2.7 mm arthroscopes are usually 14 cm. Longer versions are available.

Sheath and trocar
Each arthroscope requires a dedicated sheath (also called a 'trocar sleeve') to protect it from bending or breaking and to deliver fluid to the tip via a stopcock with a luer-lok. Sheaths offering a high rate of flow are preferable. The sheath reduces the effective working length of the 2.7 mm 'scope to 12 cm and the 1.9 mm to approximately 8.0 cm. Conversely, the sheath will increase the working diameter of the arthroscope: 2.7 mm becomes 3.8 mm and 1.9 mm becomes 2.8 mm.

Each sheath has a dedicated trocar that prevents blocking of the sheath when creating a viewing portal into the joint. Most sheaths are supplied with blunt and sharp trocars (Figure 15.5). A locking system attaches the arthroscope or trocar within the sheath.

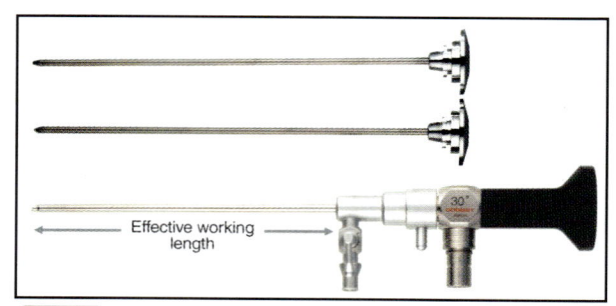

15.5 Arthroscope sheath with blunt and sharp trocars.

WARNING
Care should be exercised using the sharp trocar when approaching articular surfaces.

Light source and cables
A light source can be equipped with a halogen or a xenon lamp. Halogen light is yellow and less bright. Xenon provides bright and white light, but units are more expensive to buy and to maintain. Xenon light sources are essential if the unit is to be used for laparoscopic work but halogen can be used successfully in most joint investigations. Some light sources have an automatic intensity control. An intensity of 100–150 W is sufficient for joints. When used for other forms of endoscopy (gastroscopy, laparoscopy, thoracoscopy), the intensity should be increased up to 400 W.

Both xenon and halogen bulbs have a limited lifespan (xenon typically 500 hours, halogen typically 2000 hours) and bulb failure is, at best, embarrassing, so a spare should always be available. Modern units will indicate the remaining bulb life.

A light cable connects the light source to the arthroscope at its light post. The cable carries light from the source to the arthroscope through fibreoptics. Each cable has dedicated connectors to couple with the light source and the arthroscope. Connections on both light source and arthroscope vary from manufacturer to manufacturer. Converters are available for both light source and arthroscope but it is wise, if possible, to purchase the appropriate cable for the system.

Flexible glass fibre cables are commonly used. They are available in different diameters and should be adapted to the arthroscope. A small animal arthroscope requires a thin light cable to prevent the loss of light. Decreased light capacity is due to glass fibre breakage. The cable should not be bent or wound too tightly to prevent damage to its fibres. Fluid-filled cables are less flexible, but allow more light and are often used in industrial endoscopy.

Camera

Direct viewing of a joint through the arthroscope eyepiece is possible but practicality and the issue of contamination dictate that a camera system is an essential part of the equipment. Most cameras are universal and fit the head of most arthroscopes. Arthroscopic cameras work in a very similar fashion to video cameras in common usage. The image at the eyepiece of the arthroscope is focused on a light-responsive electronic chip(s). The signal created is transferred to a camera controller, which processes the image into a signal recognized by the monitor and/or recording system. Most veterinary cameras have a single chip, which is sufficient for most users (Figure 15.6). Many medical systems have three-chip cameras, which can produce a better image, provided the rest of the equipment is of a sufficiently high standard. However, the image from a new one-chip camera is frequently better than that of an old or damaged three-chip camera. Three-chip systems are bulky and heavy, particularly older models obtained from ex-hospital sources.

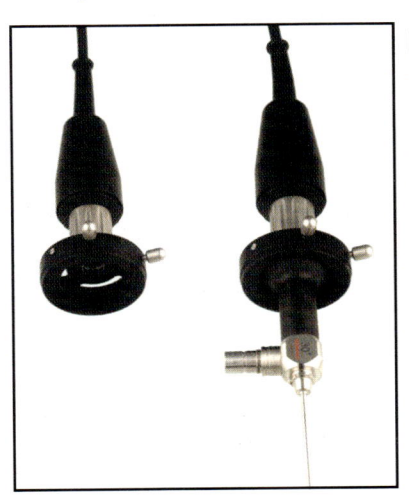

15.6 Single-chip camera head, clip-on style: without arthroscope (left) and with an arthroscope locked into postion (right).

Surgeons considering purchasing pre-owned equipment should be aware that each camera will produce a unique signal type which varies from country to country. European cameras generate a PAL signal, while American cameras work to the NTSC standard. The two standards are not compatible, which means that all ancillary equipment must match the camera, e.g. monitors and recording equipment. Some dual-standard equipment is available. The connection of the camera head to the eyepiece of the arthroscope is also variable. To maximize the choice and longevity of the instrumentation it is advised that a clip-on camera head, compatible with DIN standard eyepieces, be selected. More secure, direct coupling systems reduce the incidence of fogging and movement between the camera and the arthroscope but will tie the user into one supplier.

To ensure that tissue colours are accurately represented it is essential that the camera is 'white-balanced' before each procedure.

A soakable/immersible camera is water-resistant and can be sterilized with fluid (see below). If not soakable, sterile impermeable hoses are available to cover the camera.

Monitor

Professional monitors (Figure 15.7) offer a better image than domestic screens, as they have a better resolution. However, a combination television and recorder from the company that makes most of the monitors can offer a reliable, entry-level monitoring and recording system. It is important that the components of a system match in terms of quality: a very highly specified camera coupled with a cheap monitor, or the other way around, will disappoint.

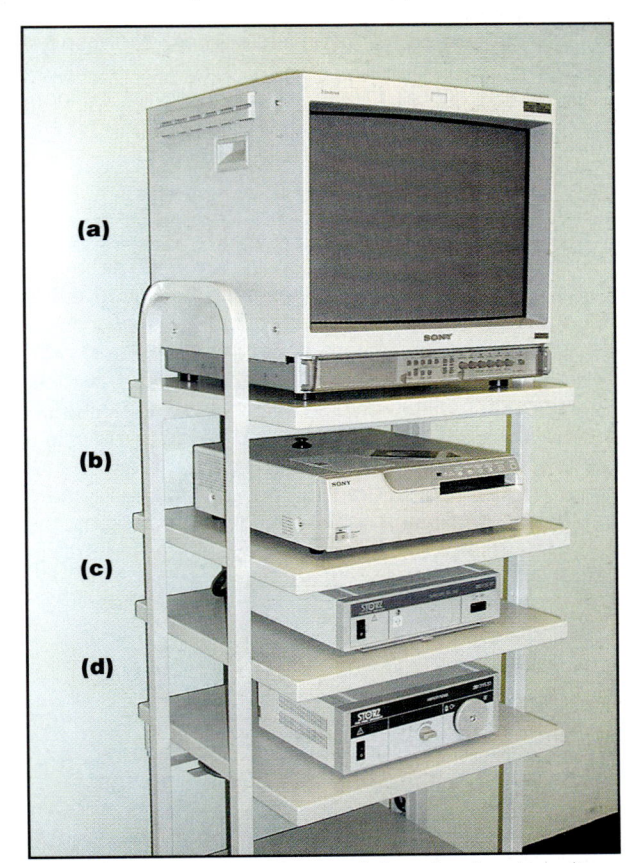

15.7 Fully equipped tower: **(a)** professional monitor; **(b)** image capture; **(c)** camera controller; **(d)** xenon light source.

Chapter 15a Arthroscopic equipment

Recording

Documentation of images is important for teaching, research, patient data and client information. Domestic video recorders will create a permanent record of a procedure but the data are relatively crude and difficult to manipulate. Still video printers capture an image from a video stream which can then be printed on to photographic paper; since digitalization, this system has become obsolete. Digital video and data storage technology now allows the surgeon to record and store very large amounts of data in a digital format; the digital information can then be manipulated by appropriate computer software to create both still and moving images in a variety of formats for storage or display. If clinical presentations are anticipated, a digital system is very desirable. Domestic DVD or combined DVD/hard drive recorders offer huge storage capacities at reasonable prices. The data are stored as digital video (DV) which can be converted into many other formats. The major arthroscopy companies offer sophisticated data storage systems that are able to capture and store still and movie files via sterile touch screens or camera finger controls. Permanent records are maintained on DVD discs or computer hard drives.

Arthroscopic instruments

Some basic surgical instruments are necessary for an arthroscopic approach. The surgeon may wish to convert the arthroscopic investigation into a surgical one, so it is suggested that the same basic kit as described in Chapter 13 is made available. In addition, a selection of appropriately sized sterile hypodermic needles (18 gauge) and syringes (5 ml and 10 ml) should be available.

Instrument cannulae

In order to examine the joint fully, it may be necessary to manipulate some intra-articular structures. The instruments used must be small and are introduced either directly through the periarticular soft tissues or via a dedicated cannula. Where serial insertions and withdrawals or a range of instruments are required, particularly through multiple layers of soft tissue, a cannula is preferred as it will minimize trauma. Trying to relocate a portal without one can be frustrating. Instrument cannulae are available in different diameters and have a sharp or blunt trocar to insert and re-insert the cannula into the joint. The use of an instrument cannula during arthroscopic surgery has several advantages:

- Allows easy access into the joint
- Enables thorough irrigation to flush out small fragments and debris
- Helps to prevent soft tissue trauma and periarticular fluid accumulation, particularly important in the shoulder, elbow and tarsus.

Sets of cannulae dedicated to the most common joints are now available (Figure 15.8). Initially, a small-diameter cannula is inserted using a trocar. The portal may then be enlarged by the use of a guide rod or

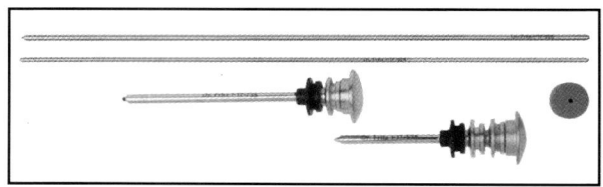

15.8 Working cannula set by van Bree for shoulder and elbow.

'switching stick'. Using a 'switching stick' and cannulae of different sizes (1.5–3.5 mm), the cannula diameter can be changed according to the thickness of the instruments and the size of the fragment. The stick is inserted into the joint through the small cannula, which is then withdrawn. Larger cannulae may be slid down the switching stick and introduced into the joint. Exchanging a small cannula for a larger one can be surprisingly difficult without such an aid.

Disadvantages of using an instrument cannula include limited mobility of the instruments and the restricted diameter of the instruments or size of the fragments that can pass through it. In human and equine arthroscopy, an instrument cannula is not used routinely since the most frequently treated joints in people (knee) and horses (carpal and hock joints) are large and superficial. As they are not covered with a muscular layer, passage of instruments through a stab incision is easy.

Intra-articular hand instruments

Hand instruments are designed to move or retract intra-articular structures. Where intra-articular surgery or sampling is involved, additional cutting instruments will be required. Sets are available which comprise a single handle and a selection of interchangeable blunt and sharp probes (Figure 15.9).

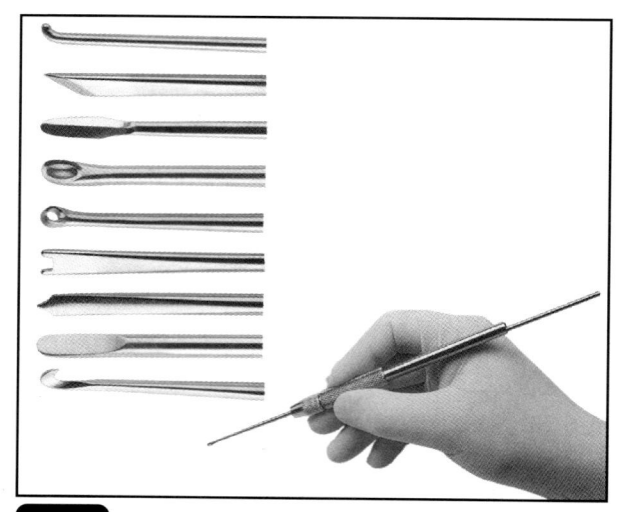

15.9 Instrument handle and tip options.

Several hand instruments (2–3.5 mm diameter) are available for the arthroscopic treatment of canine joints (15.10):

- Hooked probe
- Sharp spoon or curette
- Eye curette

Chapter 15a Arthroscopic equipment

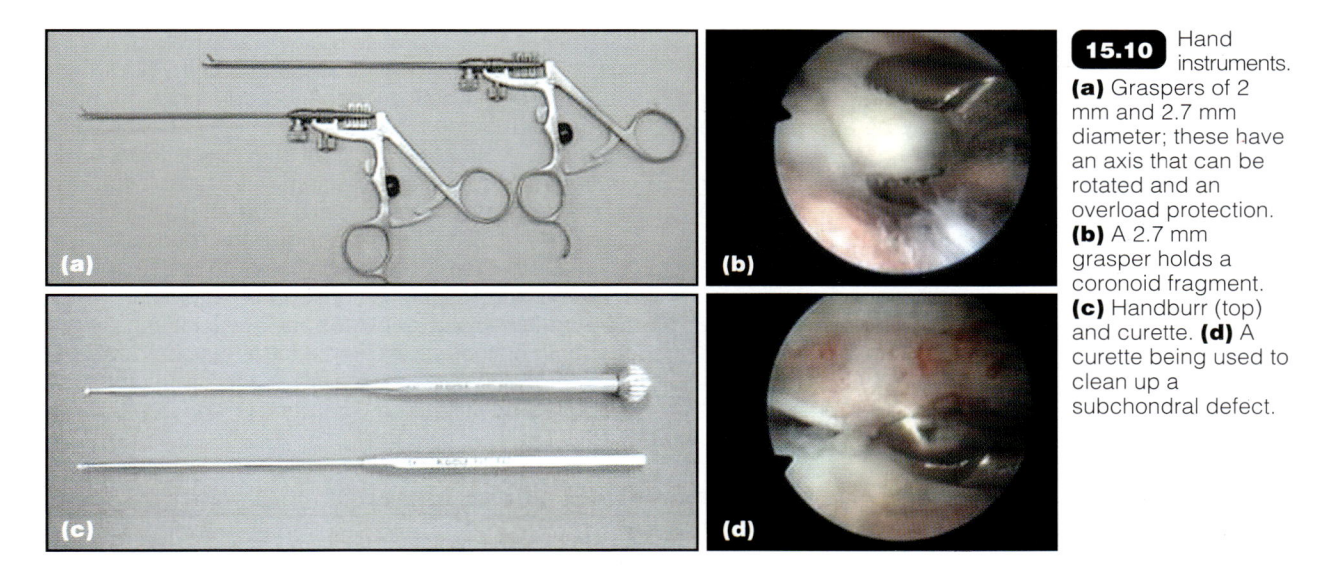

15.10 Hand instruments. **(a)** Graspers of 2 mm and 2.7 mm diameter; these have an axis that can be rotated and an overload protection. **(b)** A 2.7 mm grasper holds a coronoid fragment. **(c)** Handburr (top) and curette. **(d)** A curette being used to clean up a subchondral defect.

- Hand burr
- Graspers of different diameter (2 mm, 2.7 mm and 3 mm), strength and type of mouth.

Good grasping forceps have a small diameter to permit insertion into the narrow joint space but should be strong enough to grasp and remove osteochondral fragments. Some forceps can be rotated around their long axis, thus changing the direction of the mouth. An overload protection prevents breakage of the forceps when the applied forces are too high. Various designs are available for grasping, cutting or nibbling intra-articular structures (Figure 15.11).

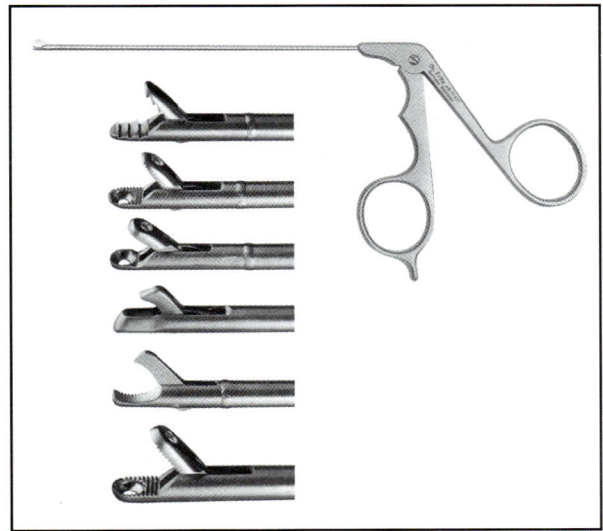

15.11 Arthroscopic punches, biopsy forceps, rongeurs and grasping forceps.

Arthroscopic forceps should be selected according to patient and portal size. A very small pair of grasping or cutting forceps will fit any portal but will be easily damaged if used on large fragments.

Hand instruments are useful for the debridement of cartilage and bone. They are somewhat slow to remove material but are inexpensive, uncomplicated to set up, and operate well in comparison with powered systems.

A further advantage of hand instruments is the accuracy that can be obtained using controlled and fine movements. The availability of suitable instruments is important for a successful procedure.

Powered instruments

In joints with a large fragment or tough subchondral bone, a motorized burr, termed a 'shaver', is very useful for removing a fragment rapidly (Figure 15.12). It may be used to debride cartilage, bone or soft tissues. For stifle arthroscopy, a shaver with a rotating blade is indispensable for visualizing the complete joint.

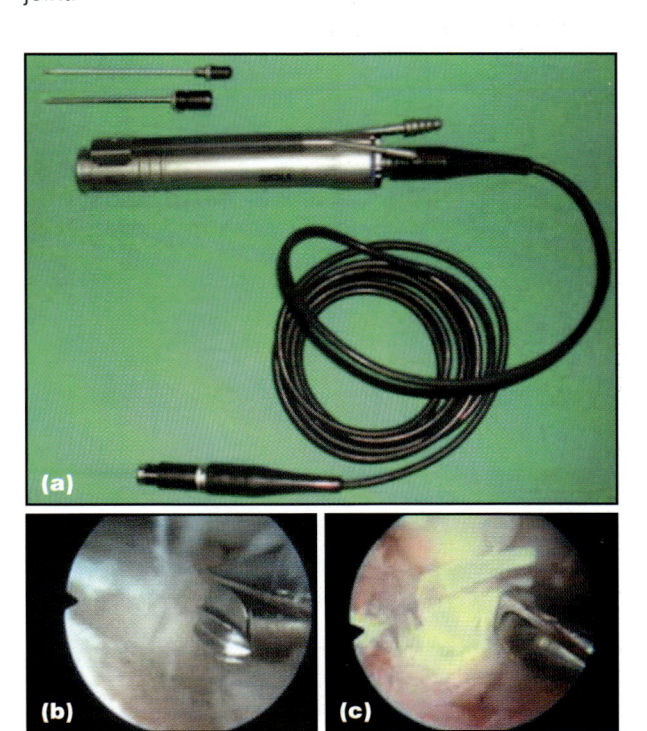

15.12 Shaver for small animal arthroscopy. **(a)** Shaver and blades. **(b)** Motorized burr used in a left elbow to remove the medial coronoid process. **(c)** Shaver used in a stifle to remove the fat pad and remnants of the cruciate ligament.

Chapter 15a Arthroscopic equipment

A range of tips of different designs and sizes is available to manage the different tissues. Tips designed for soft tissues are typically larger and more aggressively toothed. Suction may be applied to the cutting tip via the hand piece to remove debris. The hand piece is driven by a control box operated by finger or foot controls. The speed and direction of cut are selectable. The tips are usually designed to be disposable, however, with careful use, cleaning and re-sterilization, they may be re-used.

Arguments against motorized instruments are the cost of the equipment, the longer, more complicated set-up and the potential to cause iatrogenic damage. In the author's experience [BVR], a shaver is useful, but seldom indispensable for shoulder or elbow arthroscopy. This means that the relatively high cost of motorized equipment does not necessarily have to be incurred before starting arthroscopic surgery.

Aiming device

During the development of small animal arthroscopy, one major problem appeared to be the triangulation procedure. It can be difficult to bring a needle into the field of view as the first step in the insertion of an instrument cannula, particularly in the shoulder. An aiming device can help to guide a Kirschner wire towards the tip of the arthroscope. Once this has been achieved, the aiming device can be removed, and an instrument cannula can be inserted along the K-wire. In experienced hands, the fixed triangulation position determined by the aiming device can be a limitation, but for learning arthroscopists it is a very helpful tool. The Lehman shoulder aiming device is available for all the standard arthroscopes and works very well for both caudal and cranial approaches to the shoulder (Figure 15.13).

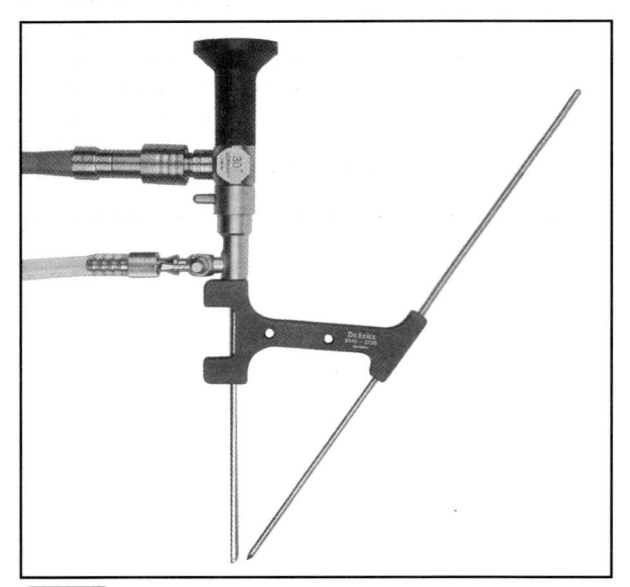

15.13 Lehman triangulation device.

Electrocautery

Arthroscopic electrocautery or radiofrequency devices focally create heat by intermolecular friction within the tissues to create haemostasis or debridement, or to shrink the joint capsule in selected cases of instability. Long fine insulated probes are available, which may be powered by standard surgical electrocautery units. Tips are available in both monopolar and bipolar formats. The tips are bathed in fluid at all times but essentially the same processes occur at the tissue level as in surgical electrosurgery. Radiofrequency ablation dissolves intra-articular tissues at a relatively low temperature. The resulting debris is removed by suction. The technique is therefore an alternative to the shaver for removing soft tissues. At least one manufacturer supplies combined shaver blades and ablator wands which offer both options on the same intra-articular device.

Radiofrequency devices are especially useful in the shoulder and stifle (see Chapters 17 and 22).

Care of equipment

Sterilization

This can be achieved by several methods. The quickest and least expensive is 'cold sterilization' where the instruments are immersed in a sterilizing fluid. Glutaraldehyde solutions are safe for the instruments and guarantee sterility. Their major disadvantages are environmental pollution and their carcinogenic properties. Alcohol (70%) is a cheap and safe alternative for veterinary medicine. It does not cause corrosion and guarantees sterility. Since it is not virotoxic it is not used in human medicine. Autoclaving is a safe method for most instruments but is not suitable for light cables, cameras and most arthroscopes. Gas sterilization is safe but expensive and not widely available.

Maintenance, cleaning and storage

Arthroscopic instruments should be cleaned gently with non-aggressive products. The arthroscope and camera are easily damaged by ultrasonic cleaning. Storage should provide a safe environment to avoid bending or breakage of the arthroscope. The light cable and camera cable should not be bent or wound too tightly.

Generally it is important to have a working knowledge of the technical aspects of the procedure. Successful arthroscopy relies on all aspects of the equipment functioning satisfactorily. Thus it is important to be able to identify and correct malfunctions quickly if the procedure is to be performed efficiently.

Joint distension and irrigation

Joint distension and irrigation has several goals:

- Distension of the joint capsule before penetration with an instrument
- Expansion of the joint space
- Evacuation of debris and blood to obtain a clear view
- Lavage of the joint after treatment.

Several types of fluid can be used, such as sodium chloride, lactated Ringer's solution or glycine. Although glycine is the least harmful *in vitro*, no difference has been experienced in clinical cases. Irrigation pressure

Chapter 15a Arthroscopic equipment

and the volume of the inflow fluid depend on the capacity of the tubes and the arthroscope. It should reach 20–100 mmHg.

Fluid under pressure may be obtained by either gravity-feed systems or a pump. Gravity may be sufficient provided the fluid bags can be lifted high enough, but greater, more controllable pressure may be obtained by use of a fluid compression bag inflated using a hand or machine pump (automatic rapid intravenous infuser) (Figure 15.14). The simplest system is an inflatable pouch put around a 1, 3 or 5 litre plastic fluid bag, the inflow tubes being simple intravenous infusion sets. Without careful monitoring, hand inflation systems offer erratic pressure levels, and use of a regulated pump offers much better control. A carbon dioxide-powered pump may be used to pressurize a compression bag or infuse carbon dioxide directly into the joint. Dedicated roller pumps are able to maintain a constant line pressure over extended periods but they may require dedicated tubing, are expensive to purchase, and are more prone to breakdown. Top-of-the-range units are able to regulate intra-articular pressure exactly by controlling both inflow and outflow.

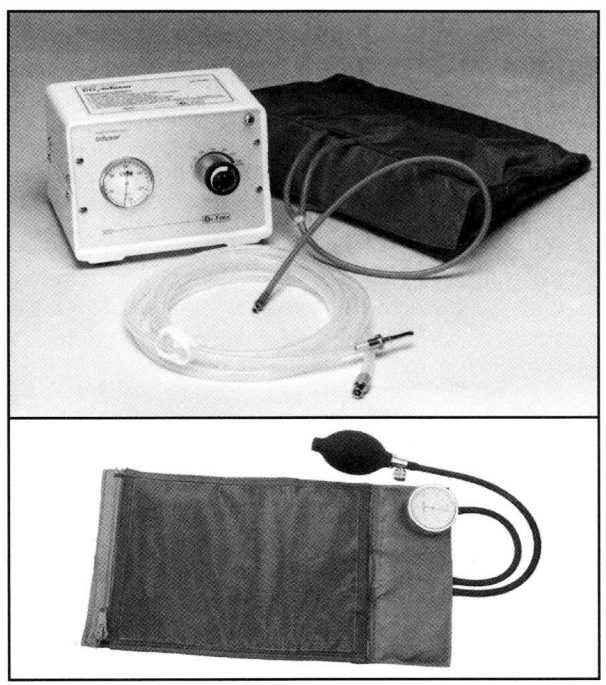

To create fluid flow through the joint, appropriate fluid outflow or egress must be maintained. Efficient drainage of irrigation fluid promotes a clear intra-articular view. This is particularly important in the stifle, where haemorrhage occurs frequently and synovial villi easily block the outflow of fluid. In the smaller joints (elbow, hock and hip), a large-bore hypodermic needle may be sufficient. In the larger joints (shoulder, stifle) where greater volumes of fluid are involved, dedicated multifenestrated egress cannulae may be necessary (Figure 15.15). If an instrument cannula is used, a drainage cannula is not necessary. The waste fluid may be collected by bag systems or suction devices.

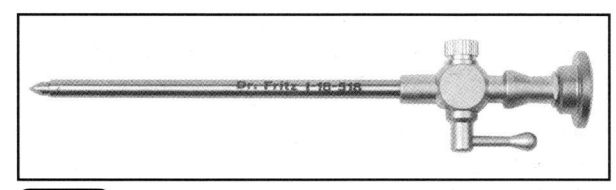

15.14 Infusion pressure bags: with carbon dioxide pressure system (top); with hand pump (bottom).

15.15 Egress cannula.

Apart from an impaired view, inefficient outflow will also cause extravasation and periarticular fluid accumulation.

Use of direct carbon dioxide infusion is indicated in some inflamed joints where inflammatory synovial villi obstruct the visual field. The villi are flattened under gas pressure rather than floating free in infused fluid. In addition, use of carbon dioxide increases the field of view and image clarity of the arthroscope; the gas is usually used intermittently with fluid to allow for flushing.

183

15b

Principles of arthroscopy

Bernadette Van Ryssen

Introduction

Arthroscopy is a minimally invasive technique used in the diagnosis and treatment of joint disorders. Since its introduction in the 1960s, arthroscopy has become a widespread procedure in human medicine. Thanks to the continuous development and improvement in instrumentation (especially the arthroscope and the light source) and the development of new techniques and their applications, the subject has evolved rapidly. This technical evolution is due to advances not only in the medical field but also in industrial endoscopy, a branch less known, which allows the internal inspection of machinery and aircraft without dismantling them. Several advanced techniques are now used in human medicine, such as osteochondral grafts, laser surgery, and arthroscopically assisted joint replacement.

Arthroscopy has been used in horses and in dogs since the 1970s. In the horse, it is now a well established technique that has replaced most arthrotomies. In the dog, much progress has been made though the subject is still developing. A book on small animal arthroscopy has been published (Beale et al., 2003) and basic and advanced arthroscopy courses are offered on a regular basis. More and more specialized centres offer arthroscopy as a routine diagnostic and surgical technique.

The success of arthroscopy can be explained by several advantages over other diagnostic and surgical modalities. The diagnostic advantages include:

- The minimally invasive nature of the technique, which enables a quick recovery and avoids scar tissue formation
- Improved visibility within the joint. The detailed view and magnification of the intra-articular structures and lesions, and the extended field of view by positioning the arthroscope in various compartments increases the diagnostic possibilities (Figure 15.16). Not only can discrete lesions be seen arthroscopically, but early lesions that cannot be detected radiographically can be diagnosed. In bilateral cases, the prognosis for the contralateral side can be estimated by arthroscopic inspection and, if necessary, a bilateral treatment can be performed
- A second look by arthroscopy in previously treated joints provides invaluable data in some cases. *However, second-look arthroscopy must be justified in terms of potential benefit to the patient.* It is not acceptable to perform it merely for scientific curiosity, even if owner consent is obtained. Nevertheless, it can be extremely useful to determine why progress is slower than anticipated or in formulating the next step in the management protocol.

Arthroscopy should always be preceded by a thorough clinical and radiographic examination and should never replace it. Indeed, an appreciation of the clinical evidence is mandatory if correct treatment decisions are to be made. Care should be taken to avoid overuse, disuse or abuse.

A certain scepticism about arthroscopy in small animals still exists and it cannot be denied that arthroscopy has a long learning curve. Not only does one have to become familiar with the instruments and technique, but the interpretation of the lesions and treatment decisions are built on the experience of several years. Failure to insert the instruments correctly, disorientation within the joint, breakage of

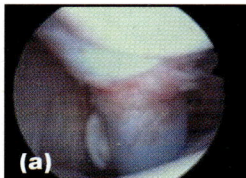

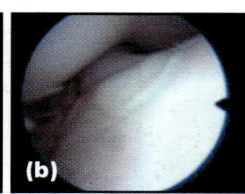

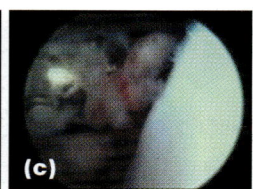

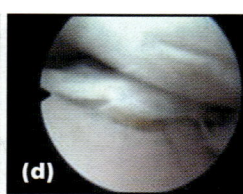

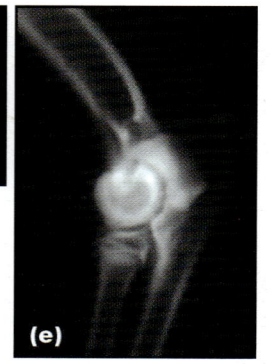

15.16 Diagnostic arthroscopy. **(a)** Left shoulder: the attachment of the biceps tendon to the supraglenoid tubercle. A 'joint mouse' is visible at the entrance of the tendon sheath. **(b)** Right elbow: fissure of the medial coronoid process. **(c)** Right shoulder: hypertrophic synovial villi, with biopsy forceps. **(d)** Left elbow: a large loose fragment of the coronoid process, moderate kissing lesions on the opposite humeral condyle. **(e)** Radiographic view corresponding to (d): the minimal changes (new bone on the anconeus and a small step) do not demonstrate the pathology as clearly as the arthroscopic image.

Chapter 15b Principles of arthroscopy

instruments, iatrogenic damage, impatience of the surgical team, and the need to convert to an open arthrotomy can discourage the learning surgeon. Nevertheless, the advantages of the technique, particularly for orthopaedic surgery, make it well worth persevering.

Image quality depends on several factors and each element of the arthroscopy system should function optimally to obtain the best result. These elements include the arthroscope, its light cable, the light source, camera and monitor. The view obtained of the joint will also depend on joint irrigation, the degree of haemorrhage and the intra-articular position of the arthroscope (Figure 15.17). If one of the elements is inadequate, visualization, orientation, interpretation and surgery will be either difficult or impossible. Optimizing the system is part of the learning curve.

The video cart, patient and surgeon should ideally be in one line (Figure 15.18a). This helps hand/eye coordination and right/left control. The camera should be kept in a fixed position towards the animal to maintain the correct orientation. This means that the structures seen left and right on the screen are also localized left and right to the arthroscope. The arthroscope can be twisted around its axis by moving the light post (Figure 15.18b).

Patient preparation

Anaesthesia

Arthroscopy requires general anaesthesia for complete relaxation. Although the puncture wounds are small, intra-articular treatment of painful joints requires anaesthesia that is sufficiently deep, not only for the welfare of the animal and the surgeon, but also to avoid instrument breakage by unexpected movements.

Positioning

Manipulation of arthroscopes and instrumentation inside a joint via an image on a monitor screen can be very demanding; therefore, careful positioning of the patient and the surgeon is essential. An operating table, fully adjustable for height and tilt, is a prerequisite for good arthroscopy.

The position of the patient depends on the type of joint and type of approach (Figure 15.19). Elbow arthroscopy is performed with the dog in lateral recumbency, with the joint being treated on the table. Shoulder and hip arthroscopy may either be performed with the patient in lateral recumbency with the treated joint uppermost, or by a hanging limb technique. Tarsal

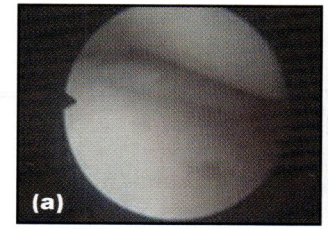

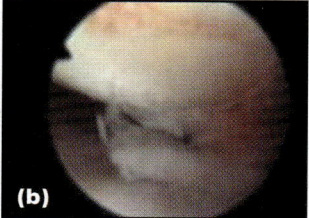

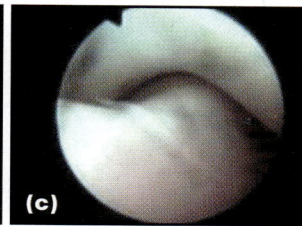

15.17 Examples of poor arthroscopic images due to (a) fogging of the tip of the arthroscope, (b) poor positioning of the 'scope, and (c) spots on the tip.

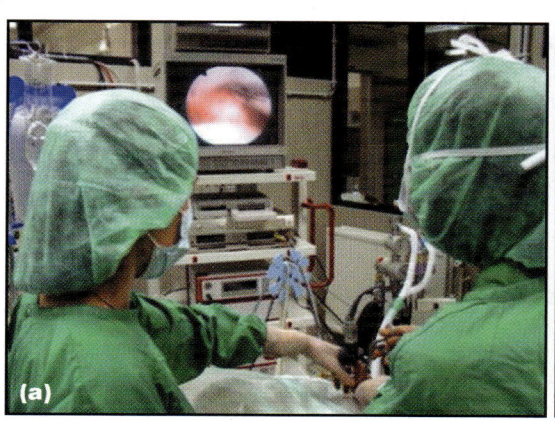

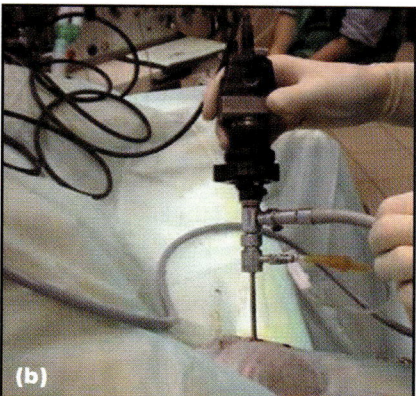

15.18 Orientation of monitor, patient, surgeon and camera. (a) The dog should be in a straight line with the monitor and surgeon. (b) The camera is fixed in the right position; the view direction is changed by moving the light post.

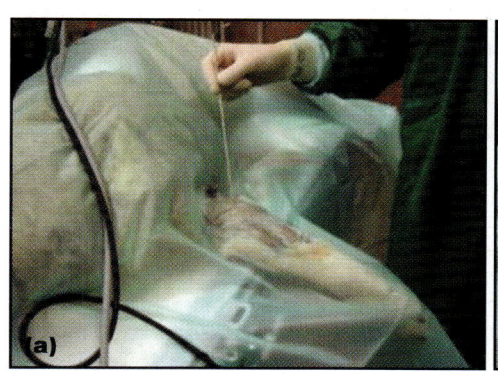

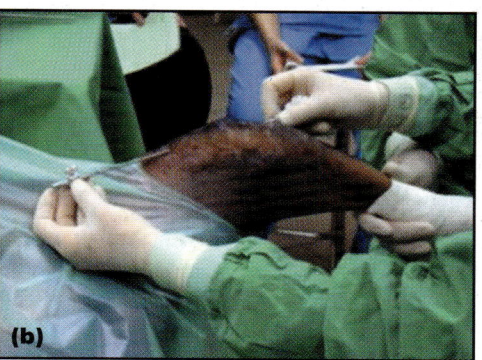

15.19 Positioning and draping. (a) For elbow arthroscopy the dog is positioned in lateral recumbency with the affected joint on the table. A medial field is prepared and draped with an adherent spray and plastic drape. (b) For stifle arthroscopy the dog is positioned in dorsal recumbency.

Chapter 15b Principles of arthroscopy

arthroscopy is performed in sternal recumbency for a plantar approach and in dorsal recumbency for a dorsal approach.

Once fully draped, orientation around a limb can be difficult. Full use should be made of channels, ties and sandbags to fix the overall position of the patient. A leg holder or support is useful to hold the leg in a fixed position and to distract the joint or apply forces to it. Distraction devices are widely utilized in human arthroscopy. Their employment in the dog has been reported (Schultz *et al.*, 2004), but their use would appear to be less widespread.

Sandbags may also be necessary to act as a fulcrum to open a joint maximally for investigation, such as in arthroscopy of the elbow. A multi-arm positioning device is available to provide multiple fixed positioning during an investigation; when attached between the distal limb and the table it may be locked into a range of positions (Figure 15.20). An optional accessory allows the stifle to be positioned accurately for an investigation.

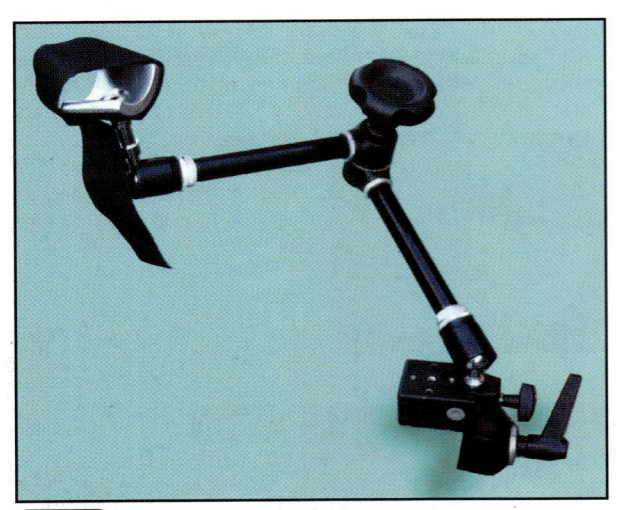

15.20 Multi-arm positioning device. (Courtesy of Dr Fritz)

Preparation of the operative field
Clipping, scrubbing and disinfection are standard as for conventional joint surgery.

Several methods can be used to drape the operation field. General principles dictate that the draping should be impermeable and allow sufficient mobility of the limb. A simple and quick system is the use of an adherent operating drape that is either self-adherent (i.e. it has an adherent window) or is applied with the use of a sterile spray (see Figure 15.19). If an adherent drape is used, the surgical field should be dried well before applying the drape or spray. In this way, only a limited field needs to be prepared while good mobility of the limb is guaranteed. *This system may not be sufficient if the arthroscopic procedure has to be converted into an arthrotomy.*

General arthroscopic procedure
An arthroscopic procedure consists of three different steps, which may vary from joint to joint and from surgeon to surgeon.

1. A needle is inserted into the joint to aspirate synovial fluid and to inject irrigation fluid. Thus, the joint capsule is distended, which facilitates the next step of the procedure. For the stifle and carpus, this step can be skipped.
2. The arthroscope is inserted. To determine its correct position and direction, a needle is inserted in the joint where the arthroscope should be positioned. The needle is positioned correctly if it has the expected inclination (direction) and depth, and if irrigation fluid exits from it. Insertion of a needle prior to insertion of the arthroscopic sleeve helps to localize the most advantageous position and to prevent iatrogenic damage. The arthroscopic sheath is inserted into the joint via a stab incision. Depending on the type of joint and the preference of the surgeon, the stab incision can be limited to the skin or it may puncture the joint capsule. A sharp or blunt trocar is contained within the sheath during its insertion and afterwards replaced by the arthroscope.
3. The operating instrument or instrument cannula is inserted. The puncture site and direction are determined with a needle under arthroscopic guidance. The instrument is inserted directly into the joint via a stab incision or via the instrument cannula.

The surgical team
Arthroscopy is a demanding procedure, not only because of the learning curve, but also because of the need for a well trained team. Although some surgeons prefer to work alone it is very helpful to have an assistant to hold the camera. Movements can be more controlled and an extra hand can open up the joint space to facilitate the procedure. The surgeon should be patient and gentle and show ability for precise surgery. The operating team should be receptive to new techniques and willing to invest time. During the learning phase, the team should also encourage the surgeon who, however experienced he or she is in surgery, will be confronted with failures and prolonged operation times.

Postoperative care
Local anaesthetic (bupivacaine) can be injected into the joint through the egress needle, prior to its removal at the end of the procedure. The wounds are sutured. A light bandage reduces swelling and bleeding. Most animals can be discharged the same day if required. Postoperative care generally consists of anti-inflammatory drugs and exercise control. For further details, the reader is referred to individual chapters and procedures.

Diagnostic possibilities
Arthroscopy allows a detailed and extensive examination of the intra-articular structures due to the magnification, illumination and irrigation of the joint. By positioning the arthroscope in different joint compartments, areas and structures are visible which would not be possible during arthrotomy without major surgical trauma.

Chapter 15b Principles of arthroscopy

Visible intra-articular structures and their appearance

Cartilage

Normal cartilage has a smooth, white and glistening surface.

Primary lesions (Figure 15.21): The most important primary lesions of cartilage are those of osteochondritis dissecans (OCD). A fissure, chondromalacia (seen as soft discoloured irregular cartilage often covering abnormal subchondral bone), or one or multiple fragments containing subchondral bone may be seen. A cartilage flap is also generally present. The cartilage of a fragment or flap is usually intact, i.e. white and smooth, as if it were resistant to inflammation and degeneration. 'Joint mice' are formed when part of, or an entire flap breaks off. Traumatic lesions are rare and usually involve cartilage as well as subchondral bone. The lesions look like fresh fractures and are often covered with blood. In rare cases, zones of cartilage are replaced by ingrowing tumour tissue, as seen in cases of synovial cell sarcoma.

Secondary lesions (Figure 15.22): Secondary lesions of cartilage are induced by mechanical forces. They may be caused by pressure from a fragment, by microtrauma due to a limb deformity or joint incongruency, or by chronic synovitis altering the composition of the synovial fluid and thus its nutritional capacity. Secondary changes can be limited to a small zone or may extend over a large area. They can be seen as rough zones, discoloration of the cartilage (turning more yellow), fibrillation (which may be very discrete to extremely obvious), small fissures, 'cracks' and erosions. Erosions may be superficial or full thickness. The latter may appear as stripes, patches, nude bone, irregular bone or as broad tracks. (See also Subchondral bone, below.)

Findings that may be clinically insignificant (Figure 15.23): Not all arthroscopic findings are of clinical significance and a great deal of experience is required to be sure which are incidental findings and which represent significant pathology. For instance, the synovial membrane, originating at the transition of cartilage to bone, is often seen as an indistinct margin, creating zones without cartilage but covered with synovial membrane. This can be the case in both normal and diseased joints. These zones may look like aggressive lesions when the synovial membrane is inflamed, particularly in the elbow and stifle.

Pannus may be seen as a component of the primary joint disease or it can be seen as hypervascular tissue covering cartilage, menisci, ligaments or tendons secondary to joint incongruency and severe inflammation. In the latter instance, treatment of the primary problem may result in resolution of the secondary condition. In chronic inflammation, intra-articular ligaments and the joint capsule may show light to severe secondary fibrillation. These secondary lesions should not be confused with a rupture.

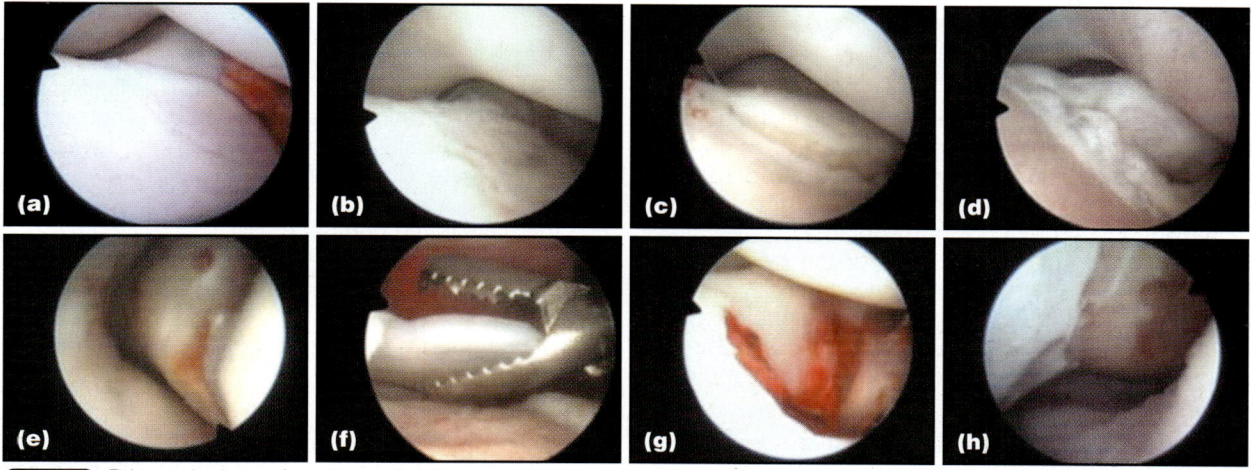

15.21 Primary lesions of cartilage. **(a)** Fissure. **(b)** Chondromalacia. **(c)** Fragment, no kissing lesions. **(d)** Fragment and erosions. **(e)** Loose anconeal process. **(f)** OCD flap and grasper. **(g)** Traumatic fracture of the medial coronoid process. **(h)** Synovial cell sarcoma.

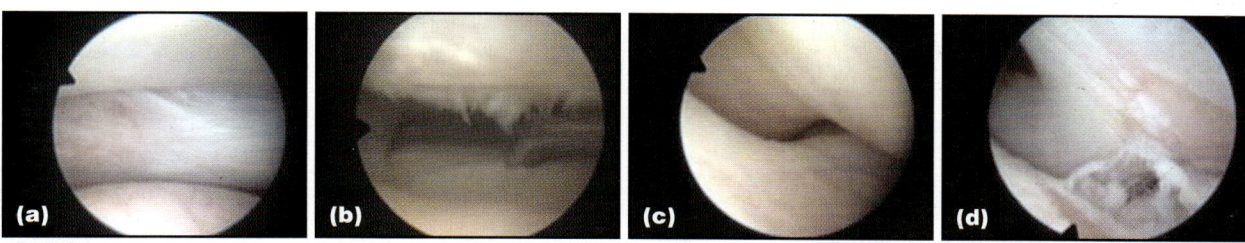

15.22 Secondary lesions of cartilage. **(a)** Shoulder: 'cracks' on the humeral head. **(b)** Stifle: fibrillation of the cartilage of the medial femoral condyle. **(c)** Elbow: partial thickness kissing lesions (stripes). **(d)** Elbow: full thickness kissing lesions (erosions plus stripes).

Chapter 15b Principles of arthroscopy

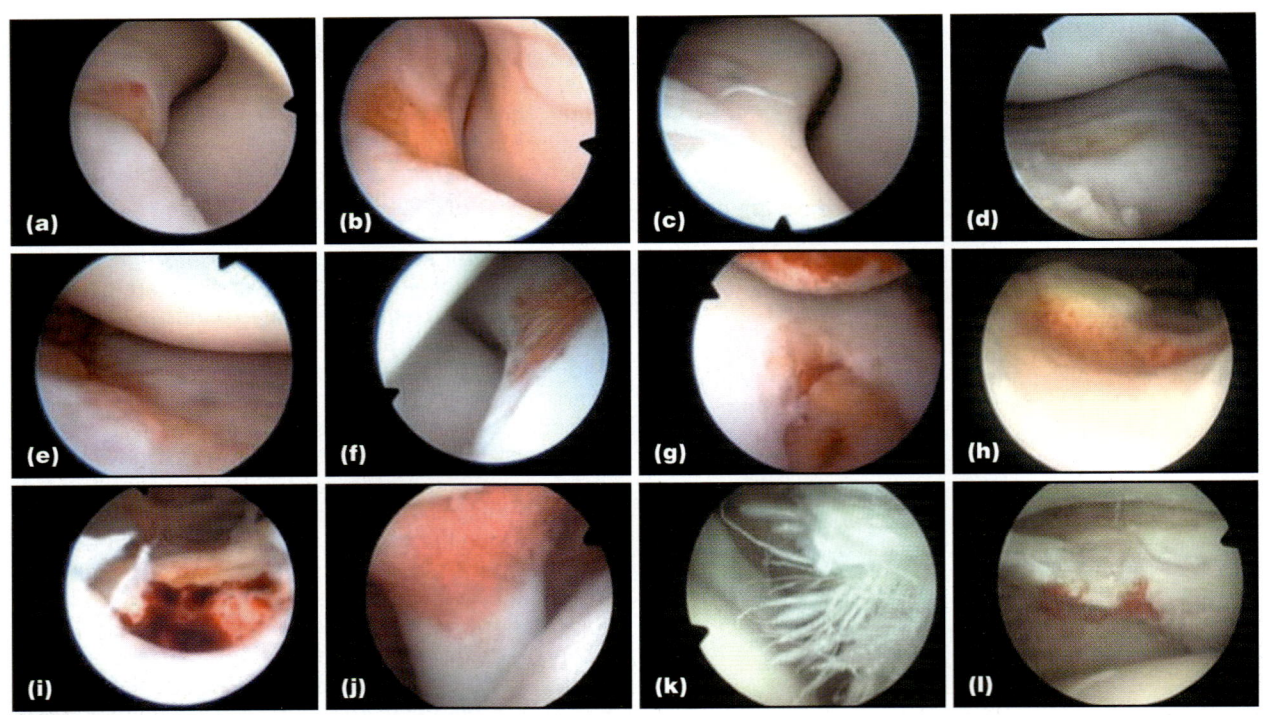

15.23 Arthroscopic findings that may be clinically insignificant. **(a)** Elbow, trochlear notch of the ulna: depression without cartilage, filled with synovial villi. **(b)** Elbow, trochlear notch of the ulna: irregular cartilage, partially covered with pannus. **(c)** Elbow, trochlear notch of a sound joint: smooth cartilage. **(d)** Elbow: pannus and irregular cartilage covering the radial head. **(e)** Elbow: pannus and irregular cartilage covering the step in an incongruent elbow joint. **(f)** Elbow: pannus with clear blood vessels covering the medial part of the trochlear notch of the ulna. **(g)** Stifle: red, inflamed synovial membrane at the distal pole of the patella. **(h)** Stifle, transition of synovial membrane to cartilage at the proximal site of the patellar groove: zones covered with pannus. **(i)** Stifle showing severe inflammation and local haemorrhage (zones are sometimes very red because of severe synovitis). **(j)** Shoulder: biceps tendon covered with hypertrophic synovial membrane. **(k)** Shoulder: chronic synovitis with fibrillation of the joint capsule and intracapsular ligaments. **(l)** Shoulder: partial tear of the medial glenohumeral ligament.

Osteophytes

In osteoarthritis, osteophytes are visible at the border of the cartilage. They originate at the transition between cartilage and synovial membrane and appear as irregular new bone covered with cartilage. Particularly in the shoulder, this irregularity is often misinterpreted as a cartilage lesion at the caudodistal border of the humeral head. Other typical sites for osteophytes are the caudal rim of the glenoid cavity in the shoulder, the lateral border of the humeral condyle in the elbow and along the femoral condyles in the stifle (Figure 15.24).

Synovial membrane

The extent of the synovial membrane that can be inspected is limited, but changes usually affect the entire membrane and are seen all over the joint. In normal joints, the number of synovial villi is limited and they are thin and short. The number of villi is not equally distributed; typically, some areas in the joint have more villi than others. Pathological changes include:

- Increase in the number of villi
- Alteration of colour of villi (red or white)
- Changes in vascularization of villi (avascular or hypervascular)
- Differing forms of villi (elongated, thickened or 'branches') (Figure 15.25).

Small red villi indicate an acute inflammation, while hyperplastic large white villi suggest a chronic process. Often a mixture of different forms is found.

Primary changes of the synovial membrane can be seen in cases of capsular tumour when increased

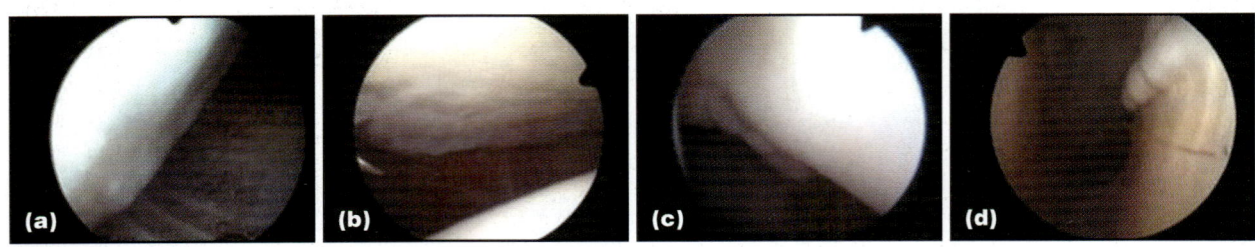

15.24 Osteophytes. **(a)** Shoulder: caudodistal part of the humeral head. **(b)** Shoulder: caudal border of the glenoid cavity. **(c)** Elbow: lateral ridge of the humeral condyle. **(d)** Stifle: lateral ridge of the femoral condyle.

Chapter 15b Principles of arthroscopy

15.25 Pathological changes of the synovial membrane. **(a)** Stifle: tumoral changes. **(b)** Stifle: infection. **(c)** Shoulder: acute, light inflammation. **(d)** Elbow: moderate chronic inflammation. **(e,f)** Shoulder: acute, severe inflammation. **(g)** Elbow: severe chronic inflammation. **(h)** Shoulder: villi surrounding 'joint mouse'. **(i)** Stifle: chronic inflammation and discoloration. **(j)** Stifle: synovial villi at the inner border of the meniscus.

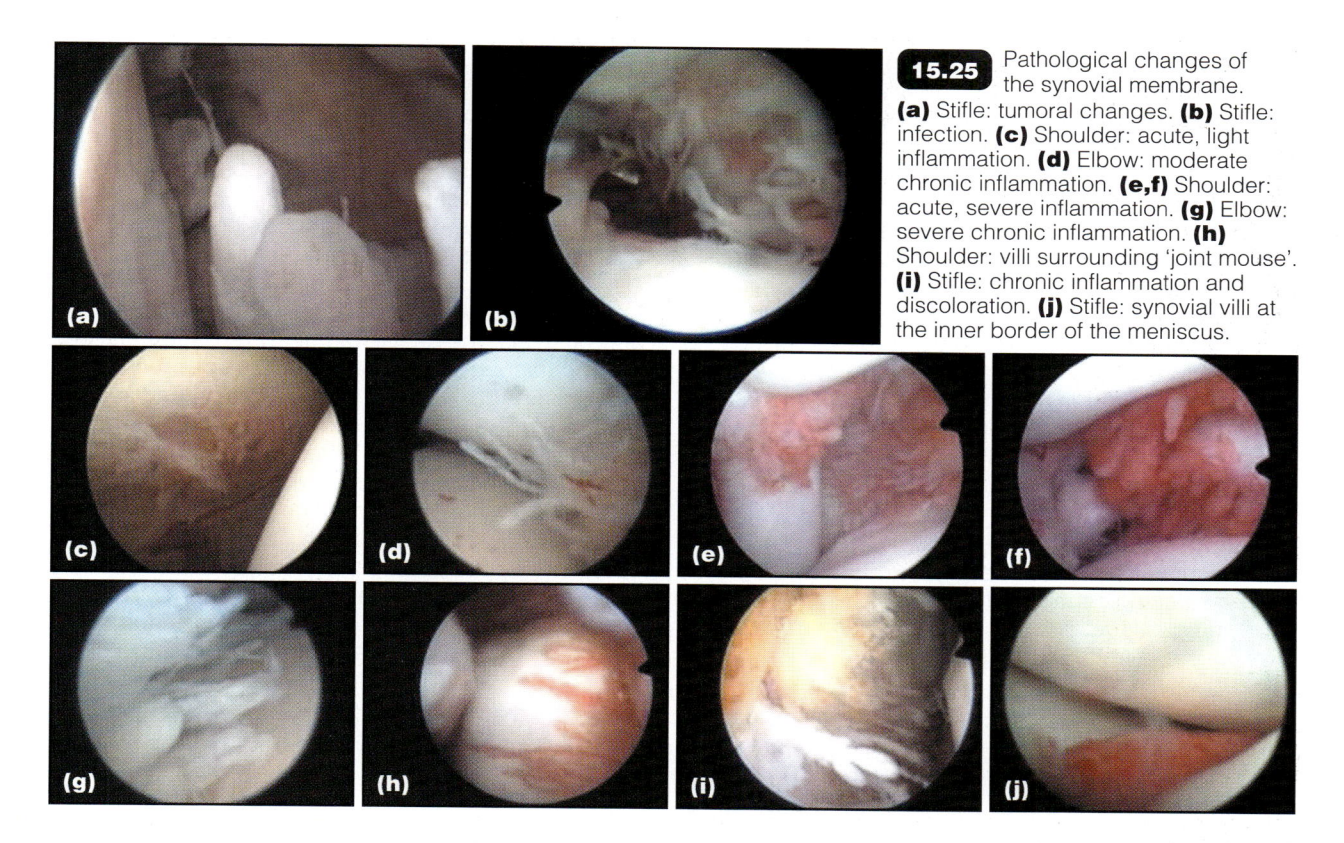

numbers of thickened discoloured villi can easily be seen. In cases of infection, the villi are hypertrophic and hyperaemic. In chronic cases they have a hyperplastic appearance. Often fibrin rafts adhere to the joint capsule and cross the joint space. Autoimmune disorders present as a severe inflammation, but are not characterized by specific changes.

Secondary changes are seen in association with other primary processes, such as osteochondritis, ligamentous problems, (micro-) trauma, etc. The changes always involve the entire joint, but may be more prominent in the proximity of the primary problem.

Ligaments and tendons

Several ligaments and tendons occur intracapsularly, surrounded by synovial membrane. These can be inspected arthroscopically. The biceps tendon, subscapularis tendon and medial glenohumeral ligaments can be inspected in the shoulder; the medial collateral ligament, annular ligament (medial and lateral part) and the proximal part of the distal biceps tendon in the elbow; the cruciate ligaments, meniscal ligaments and long digital extensor tendon in the stifle; the deep flexor tendon in the hock joint; the teres ligament in the hip joint; and several ligaments within the carpus (Figure 15.26).

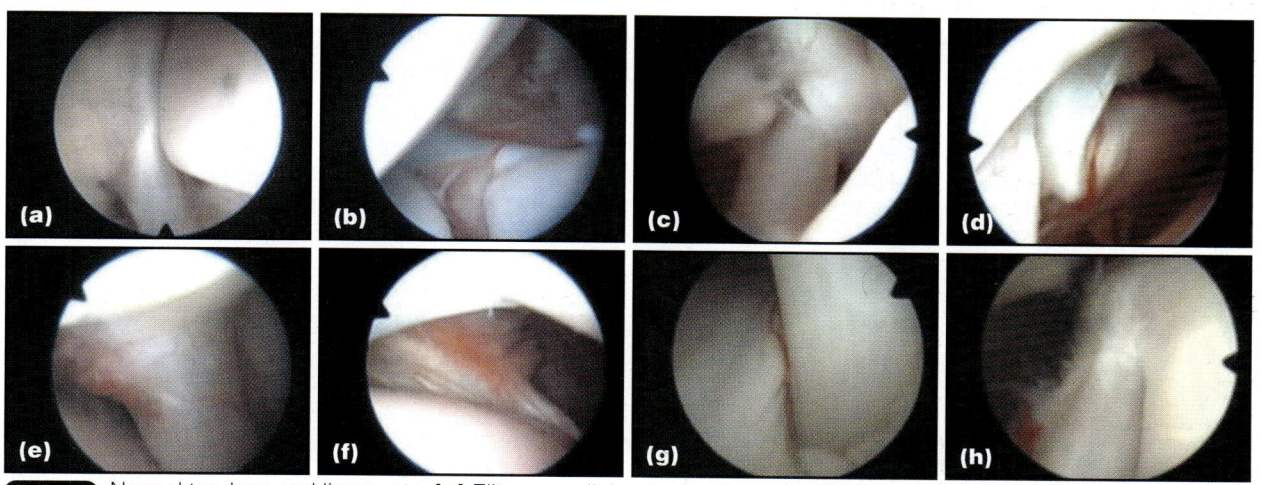

15.26 Normal tendons and ligaments. **(a)** Elbow: medial collateral ligament. **(b)** Elbow: annular ligament, attachment at the lateral coronoid process. **(c)** Elbow: crossing of medial collateral ligament and distal part of biceps tendon. **(d)** Carpus: intra-articular ligaments. **(e)** Shoulder: biceps tendon. **(f)** Shoulder: medial glenohumeral ligament. **(g)** Stifle: cruciate ligaments. **(h)** Stifle: origin of the long digital extensor tendon.

Chapter 15b   Principles of arthroscopy

The normal aspect of a tendon or ligament is smooth, white and glistening. Primary and secondary lesions appear similar and present as thickening, discoloration, fibrillation and partial or complete ruptures, with hypertrophy and calcification of the remnants (Figure 15.27). Only rarely can haemorrhage be seen in a ruptured tendon. Primary ligamentous lesions are frequently accompanied by a severe secondary synovitis in the author's experience. Common primary disorders include partial or complete rupture of the cranial cruciate ligament and partial or complete rupture of the biceps tendon. A controversial subject is shoulder instability in which fibrillation and partial or complete rupture of the medial glenohumeral ligament and/or subscapularis tendon is involved (see Chapter 17).

Subchondral bone

Subchondral bone is not visible in sound joints. It is only seen in pathological joints when there is damage to the overlying cartilage, such as when a fragment, flap or erosion is present (Figure 15.28).

Bone can also be visible as a part of a fragment. Most often the bone has a different colour, being more yellow or white, and is of a soft consistency. The bone belonging to a fragment or delineated by a fissure is often not vascularized, but in some cases it bleeds during removal, which indicates growth potential. Indeed in several cases with large fragments in the elbow, the fragment was vascularized, while the smaller fragments were not. After removal of an OCD flap or fragment, the underlying subchondral bone becomes visible. Usually the bone just underneath the fragment is soft, granular and easily detachable. In some cases, several brown spots are visible. After removal of the fragment and superficial curettage of the defect, sound bone is visible as pink, relatively hard bone. In young dogs, the subchondral bone bleeds easily after curettage.

Nude subchondral bone in connection with kissing lesions is often pink and hard. These kissing lesions occur at the site opposite the lesion, or can surround a lesion. In the author's experience, bleeding barely occurs even when this type of lesion is foraged or micropicked. The appearance of these kissing lesions

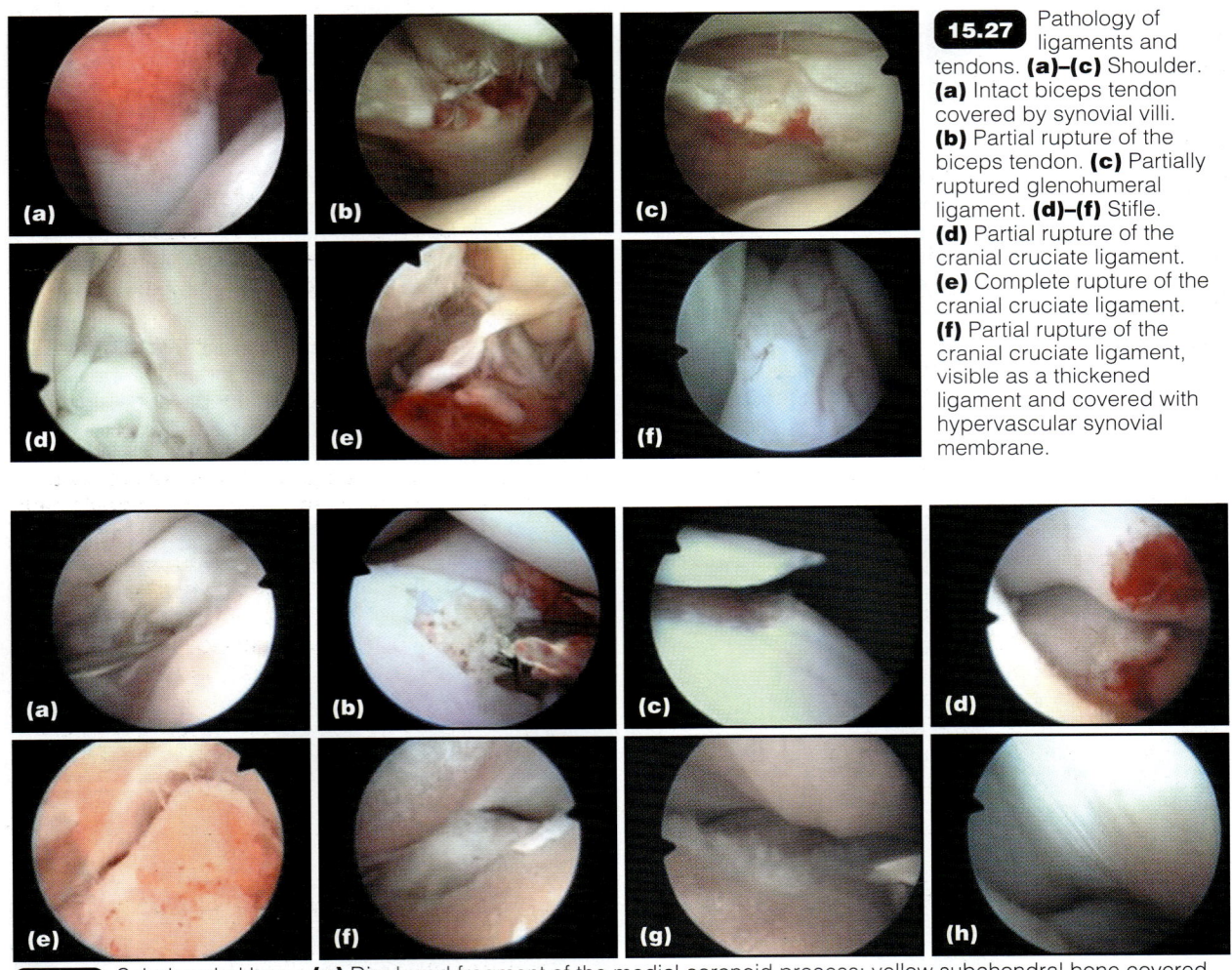

15.27 Pathology of ligaments and tendons. **(a)**–**(c)** Shoulder. **(a)** Intact biceps tendon covered by synovial villi. **(b)** Partial rupture of the biceps tendon. **(c)** Partially ruptured glenohumeral ligament. **(d)**–**(f)** Stifle. **(d)** Partial rupture of the cranial cruciate ligament. **(e)** Complete rupture of the cranial cruciate ligament. **(f)** Partial rupture of the cranial cruciate ligament, visible as a thickened ligament and covered with hypervascular synovial membrane.

15.28 Subchondral bone. **(a)** Displaced fragment of the medial coronoid process: yellow subchondral bone covered by white cartilage. **(b)** Soft bone visible during motorized shaving of a coronoid fragment. **(c)** OCD flap, subchondral bone is visible underneath. **(d)** OCD of the elbow: large bleeding defect of the medial humeral condyle. **(e)** Defect after removal of a large fragment of the talus, the distal part of the tibia is eroded too. **(f)** Complete erosion of the medial compartment of the elbow joint. A fragment is visible in the middle of the picture. **(g)** A kissing lesion due to rubbing against a fragment or idiopathic elbow joint incongruity. **(h)** Superficial lesions of the cartilage.

can differ. Usually there is one smooth surface, but some lesions are covered with white foci, and in other cases, tracks are visible.

Menisci
The menisci are fibrocartilaginous structures that are not visible on plain radiographs unless they are calcified; this is a rare finding. Primary changes occur as tears in different forms and at different locations. The medial meniscus is most commonly involved. Both menisci may also show secondary changes as a result of inflammation or microtrauma. These secondary changes are fibrillation or thickening of the inner border, synovial growth on the external and internal borders and an irregular, striated surface (Figure 15.29). The arthroscopic diagnosis of meniscal lesions is not always easy because the view of them may be obstructed by synovial villi and remnants of a ruptured cruciate ligament.

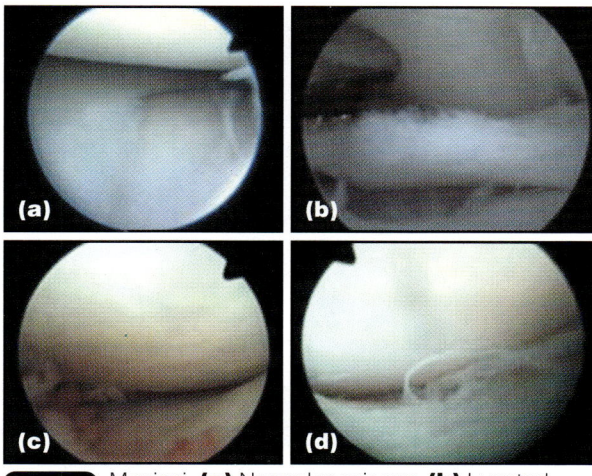

15.29 Menisci. **(a)** Normal meniscus. **(b)** Luxated medial meniscus. **(c)** Synovial villi covering the inner border of the meniscus. **(d)** Fibrillation of the inner border of the meniscus.

Indications for diagnostic arthroscopy
Arthroscopy is particularly useful in those cases where lameness is associated with little or no clinical or radiographic evidence of pathology. Lesions involving articular cartilage, synovial membrane and intra-articular ligaments or tendons may be seen arthroscopically when other imaging modalities are either inferior or inappropriate. Arthroscopy can also be used to confirm suspected lesions such as a fragmented coronoid process or a partial rupture of the cranial cruciate ligament. It can be used to provide a prognosis, as in severe or chronic cases of osteoarthritis, or to evaluate the status of a previously treated joint, e.g. in the evaluation of tissue ingrowth.

Semi-surgical indications include joint lavage in cases of infection and biopsy in synovial disorders.

Limitations
Although some colleagues claim that an animal weighing < 15 kg is not suitable for the procedure, arthroscopy of cats and small-breed dogs can be performed. Nevertheless, the talocrural joint remains a small joint, even in large- to giant-breed dogs.

Contraindications for arthroscopy are the same as those for general anaesthesia. Arthroscopy may also introduce infection into a joint if the arthroscope or instruments are passed through infected periarticular tissues.

Complications and problems
Arthroscopy in small animals is a difficult procedure and even an experienced surgeon will encounter problems from time to time. There are two reasons why small animal arthroscopy is difficult. First, the joints are very small compared with human or equine joints. Secondly, the most frequently affected joints in the dog have specific anatomical difficulties:

- The shoulder is covered with a larger muscular layer
- The elbow has a narrow joint space
- Visualization of the stifle is difficult because of the fat pad, synovial villi and ligamentous remnants
- The hock joint has a very small joint space, which easily collapses.

In addition to the specific difficulties associated with each of the joints, there are several general problems or complications that can cause a delay or even failure of the intervention. The most common problems are related to technique. These include:

- Difficulties with instrument insertion
- Poor positioning of the arthroscope, resulting in limited mobility and decreased field of vision
- Difficulties with the triangulation technique
- Collapse of the joint space due to periarticular fluid accumulation
- Dislodging the arthroscope out of the joint
- Instrument breakage
- Synovial villi obstructing the view.

Although these problems can occur at any time, most will be solved after gaining more experience.

The most frequent complication is iatrogenic cartilage damage. This is caused during insertion of the instruments and their subsequent manipulation. Small iatrogenic lesions do not have any clinical consequences but they should be avoided as much as possible. Other complications include fluid extravasation into the periarticular tissues, haemorrhage and loss of an osteochondral fragment. The incidence of postoperative sepsis and neurovascular injuries is negligible. The more experienced the surgeon becomes, the less frequently problems and complications will occur.

References and further reading

Beale B, Hulse D, Schulz K and Whitney W (2003) *Small Animal Arthroscopy*. WB Saunders, Philadelphia

Kivumbi CW and Bennett D (1981) Arthroscopy of the canine stifle joint. *Veterinary Record* **109**, 241–249

Lewis DD, Goring RL, Parker RB *et al.* (1987) A comparison of diagnostic methods used in the evaluation of early degenerative joint disease in the dog. *Journal of the American Animal Hospital Association* **23**, 305–315

Chapter 15b Principles of arthroscopy

McGinty JB (1996) Preface. In: *Operative Arthroscopy*, 2*nd* edn, Lippincott–Raven, Philadelphia

Miller CW and Presnell KR (1985) Examination of the canine stifle: arthroscopy versus arthrotomy. *Journal of the American Animal Hospital Association* **21**, 623–629

Person MW (1986) Arthroscopy of the canine shoulder joint. *Compendium on Continuing Education for the Practicing Veterinarian* **8**, 537–546

Person MW (1985) A procedure for arthroscopic examination of the canine stifle joint. *Journal of the American Animal Hospital Association* **21**, 179–186

Person MW (1989a) Arthroscopic treatment of osteochondritis dissecans in the canine shoulder. *Veterinary Surgery* **18**, 175–190

Person MW (1989b) Arthroscopy of the canine coxofemoral joint. *Compendium on Continuing Education for the Practicing Veterinarian* **1**, 930–935

Siemering GB (1978) Arthroscopy of dogs. *Journal of the American Veterinary Medical Association* **172**, 575–577

Schulz KS, Holsworth IG and Hornof WJ (2004) Self-retaining braces for canine arthroscopy. *Veterinary Surgery* **33(1)**, 77–82

Van Ryssen B and van Bree H (1992) Arthroscopic evaluation of osteochondrosis lesions in the canine hock joint: a review of two cases. *Journal of the American Animal Hospital Association* **28**, 295–299

Van Ryssen B and van Bree H (1997a) Arthroscopic findings in 100 dogs with elbow lameness. *Veterinary Record* **40**, 360–362

Van Ryssen B and van Bree H (1997b) Diagnostic and surgical arthroscopy in osteochondrosis lesions. *Veterinary Clinics of North America* **28(1)**, 161–189

Van Ryssen B, van Bree H and Missinne S (1993) Successful arthroscopic treatment of shoulder osteochondrosis in the dog. *Journal of Small Animal Practice* **34**, 521–528

Van Ryssen B, van Bree H and Simoens P (1993) Elbow arthroscopy in clinically normal dogs. *American Journal of Veterinary Research* **54(1)**, 191–198

Van Ryssen B, van Bree H and Vyt P (1993a) Arthroscopy of the canine hock joint. *Journal of the American Animal Hospital Association* **29**, 107–115

Van Ryssen B, van Bree H and Vyt P (1993b) Arthroscopy of the shoulder joint in the dog. *Journal of the American Animal Hospital Association* **29**, 101–105

16

Postoperative management and rehabilitation

Darryl L. Millis

Introduction

Many sophisticated surgical procedures have been developed for joint conditions. Despite these advances, the postoperative management of joint surgery is often overlooked. Appropriate aftercare of joint surgeries can have a great influence on the ultimate outcome for the patient. Perioperative pain management, bandaging and coaptation, early physical rehabilitation, and appropriate follow-up and recheck evaluations all play a role in return to function of the patient. An individual time-scaled plan should be devised for each surgical patient and discussed with the client preoperatively, and detailed at the time of the animal's discharge back into their care. This should take into account the signalment, temperament and intended function of the animal, in addition to the suitability of its home environment for recovery and rehabilitation, and the commitment and capabilities of the client.

Pain management in dogs

Appropriate peri- and postoperative management is an essential component and can be a critical factor in ensuring a successful outcome (see the *BSAVA Manual of Canine and Feline Anaesthesia and Analgesia*). Recognition of behaviours that indicate pain is important (Lamont *et al.*, 2000). Initially, pain may be indicated by howling and thrashing, and abnormal cardiovascular and respiratory patterns and parameters during recovery. Pain behaviour 24–96 hours postoperatively may be indicated by reluctance to rise, lying quietly in the cage or run, and carrying the affected limb in a flexed, guarded position. A dog with less pain may rise to greet the handler, vocalize for attention and carry the limb in a more extended position.

Inadequate treatment may lead to excessive discomfort and delay early use of the limb, resulting in a delayed or incomplete return to function. Muscle atrophy, joint stiffness, cartilage degeneration and joint dysfunction may all follow from delayed limb use as a result of excessive pain. In addition, uncontrolled pain has potential adverse sequelae, including: increased sympathetic activity; endogenous corticosteroid production and release; inflammatory mediator and cytokine production; and impaired immune function. All these events may slow wound healing and increase the likelihood of postoperative infection (Trim, 1999). The appropriate use of physical techniques in combination with pharmaceutical agents is necessary to achieve adequate pain control.

Medication

Many medications and techniques are available to provide effective pain control in the peri- and postoperative periods, including opiate analgesia, alpha-2 agonists, epidural analgesia, local anaesthetics, sedatives and non-steroidal anti-inflammatory drugs (NSAIDs). Many of these are controlled substances or are injectable and should be administered by a veterinary surgeon.

Pre-emptive analgesia

There is much evidence that analgesics are more effective when administered prior to surgery, to prevent the 'wind-up' effect of surgical pain (Shafford *et al.*, 2001). Pre-emptive analgesia reportedly decreases spinal sensitization to painful stimuli and results in improved efficacy. Lower doses of analgesics may be given when administered prior to a painful stimulus, which reduces the cardiopulmonary depressant effects of anaesthetic agents. Using a combination of analgesics and delivery techniques, a technique known as balanced analgesia, improves analgesia with fewer side effects than might result from large doses of a single agent.

Some surgeons advocate the application of transdermal fentanyl patches the day before surgery. Premedication with opioid medication, such as butorphanol, morphine or methadone, in combination with a tranquillizer such as acepromazine, also helps to prevent sensitization of pain pathways and reduces the concentration of inhalant anaesthetics needed during surgery.

NSAIDs may be administered prior to surgery to help prevent or limit the production of prostaglandins, and amplification of pain signals. In the UK, carprofen or meloxicam may be administered parenterally. In the USA, these medications or deracoxib may be administered orally prior to surgery. It is advisable to ensure that intraoperative intravenous fluids are administered to support renal function. It is important to use only one anti-inflammatory medication in a patient, including corticosteroids, and to avoid combining two or more NSAIDs. Although the newer NSAIDs have no or little effect on platelet function in normal animals, caution is advised in using NSAIDs in patients with known bleeding disorders. In addition, there may be an increased risk of postoperative vomiting or diarrhoea in dogs treated with NSAIDs if the patient experiences undue stress as a result of anaesthesia and surgery.

Epidural opioid administration is becoming more popular, especially for procedures that are expected to be very painful. Epidural opioids provide profound analgesia for 12–24 hours. Contraindications to epidural injections include local infection, neurological dysfunction, marked obesity (difficult to palpate landmarks), hypovolaemia and hypotension. It is best to perform epidural injection during preparation and clipping of the patient. In some patients, an indwelling epidural catheter may be secured so that medication may administered repeatedly. Care must be taken to be certain that the patient cannot remove or chew at the catheter.

Injection of local anaesthetics, such as bupivacaine or carbocaine, into the affected joint prior to surgery helps to reduce intraoperative pain and the amount of anaesthetic agents needed during surgery. An additional injection into the joint at the conclusion of surgery provides an additional 2–4 hours of analgesia, and also blocks pain pathways that are different from those blocked by opioid medications. Morphine has also been administered intra-articularly, and may be combined with a local anaesthetic.

Postoperative analgesia

The period of most pain for complex surgical procedures is the first 24–72 hours after surgery. Patients may be maintained in the hospital during this time and receive supplemental analgesic medication, such as butorphanol, morphine or methadone, given by injection at regular appropriate intervals. NSAIDs effectively control mild postoperative pain and are generally the agent of choice during the early postoperative period and for home administration (Lascelles et al., 1994, 1998; Budsberg et al., 1996; Cross et al., 1997; Millis et al., 2002). Fortunately, most patients appear to be more comfortable after 24–72 hours and usually do not require potent opiate analgesics. NSAIDs are often adequate to provide pain relief, and these are easily administered by owners. The analgesic effects of NSAIDs are partly attributed to inhibition of the cyclo-oxygenase (COX) enzymes and the subsequent production of prostaglandins. These are mediators of inflammation and amplify nociceptive input and transmission to the spinal cord via sensory afferents in peripheral nerves. Although NSAIDs exert analgesic effects mainly at peripheral sites, there are also central sites of action. Although paracetamol (acetaminophen) is not a classic NSAID, it may provide some analgesia to the central nervous system, particularly when it is combined with an opioid, such as codeine. In addition to their peripheral and central analgesic effects, NSAIDs help to reduce tissue oedema.

Some precautions are necessary in using NSAIDs in the perioperative period. Patients with renal disease should generally not receive NSAIDs for perioperative analgesia. In addition, NSAIDs should not be administered to patients with gastrointestinal disease, vomiting or diarrhoea. The surgeon should be familiar with the pharmacokinetics of drugs so that appropriate dosing strategies may be planned to take advantage of peak drug effects, either alone or in combination with other analgesics, for managing postoperative pain. Medication is often continued for 7–14 days after surgery, but sometimes for considerably longer. Medication is discontinued if vomiting, diarrhoea or decreased appetite occur. NSAIDs administered in the early postoperative period allow rehabilitation to begin sooner.

In the UK, aspirin with codeine (Empirin) may be considered several days after surgery. This combination should not be administered sooner than this because of its inhibitory effect on platelet function, which may result in unwanted haemorrhage into joints. It should not be used in combination with any other anti-inflammatory medications, or if the patient has any vomiting or diarrhoea.

Tramadol is also useful for treating perioperative pain. It has a dual mode of action, including μ agonism (although it is not an opioid) and monoamine reuptake inhibition (principally serotonin and norepinephrine), which enhances endogenous spinal inhibitory mechanisms and produces mild anti-anxiety effects. Although the degree of μ agonism is relatively weak, the monoamine reuptake inhibition allows for synergistic action, with analgesia comparable to meperidine or codeine. Tramadol can be combined with other analgesics, resulting in multimodal analgesia. Tramadol should not be given with tricyclic antidepressants or monoamine oxidase inihibitors because of its action as a monoamine reuptake inhibititor.

Cryotherapy

In addition to medications, cryotherapy (the application of cold) is important in the immediate postoperative period. Cryotherapy decreases blood flow and reduces pain, swelling, inflammation, haemorrhage and metabolic activity. In general, cryotherapy is applied for the first 72–96 hours, for 20 minutes, three to six times daily following surgery. The first application is administered immediately after surgery while the patient is recovering from anaesthesia. Cryotherapy may be beneficial for up to 2 weeks after surgery. A light pressure wrap between sessions may help limit oedema.

Ice packs, commercial cold water circulating units or commercial cold packs wrapped in a towel may be used. Crushed ice may be placed in a sealed plastic bag wrapped in a towel. The heat will transfer better if the towel is moistened with cold water, and a wrap placed around the cold pack to add compression is effective in transferring heat and limiting oedema. Cryotherapy should not be used in individuals who are cold-sensitive or have had previous frostbite. Caution should be exercised when applying cryotherapy around superficial peripheral nerves because of possible cold-induced nerve palsy. Cold should not be used in patients with generalized or localized vascular compromise, over open wounds, over areas of poor sensation, or in very young or old dogs.

Chapter 16 Postoperative management and rehabilitation

Pain management in cats

The principles of perioperative pain management in cats are similar to those in dogs, with some exceptions (Lamont, 2002). **Paracetamol should NOT be used in cats.** It is also beneficial to administer analgesic agents pre-emptively to prevent sensitization of pain pathways, and to use multiple agents to accomplish this. Opioid agents are excellent analgesic agents in cats. Prior concerns about unwanted dysphoria and excitement after administration may be avoided by using conservative doses and combining these agents with a tranquillizer or sedative, such as acepromazine or diazepam. Although cats are generally more sensitive to NSAIDs, as a result of differences in metabolism compared with dogs, several have been used in the treatment of postoperative pain, most notably carprofen and meloxicam. Carprofen is approved in the UK as a single injection, and the use of meloxicam should be restricted to 3–5 days after surgery. Local anaesthetic agents may also be used, but the correct dose must be carefully calculated to avoid toxicity in cats. Ketamine is also a useful postoperative analgesic by virtue of its ability to act as an *N*-methyl-D-aspartate receptor antagonist in the central nervous system, and by blocking glutamate, an excitatory amino acid.

Cryotherapy may be used in cats to help provide anti-inflammatory and analgesic effects. Cats may be more sensitive to cryotherapy than dogs, so it is important to place a towel between the cat and the cold pack for comfort. Cold may be applied for 20–30 minutes, 3 to 6 times per day.

Support and bandaging

Coaptation and bandaging are useful devices in the early postoperative period to help support tissues, limit joint motion, maintain tissues in an appropriate position and help limit oedema and swelling. The most common bandage placed immediately after the application of cryotherapy following surgery is a soft padded bandage, sometimes called a modified Robert Jones bandage (see Technique 16.1). In general, this bandage is placed for only 24–48 hours.

On occasion, a non-weightbearing device is necessary to prevent applying force to a limb with a tenuous repair. In the forelimb, a carpal flexion bandage or Velpeau sling may be used. The Velpeau sling provides greater restriction to movement of the forelimb, while the carpal flexion bandage prevents weightbearing, but allows nearly full range of motion of all joints except the carpus and digits. A Velpeau sling is sometimes useful for reducing motion of the shoulder joint. A carpal flexion sling is useful to reduce weightbearing, yet allow motion of the elbow joint following repair of complex fractures, such as a bicondylar or 'Y' fracture of the elbow.

An Ehmer sling or Robinson sling may be used to prevent weightbearing of a rear limb. The Ehmer sling is especially valuable to immobilize all joints of the rear limb, and to maintain the femur in an abducted and internally rotated position to maintain hip reduction, such as following repair of a comminuted fracture of the acetabulum or coxofemoral joint luxation (Figure 16.1). The Robinson sling allows motion of the hip, stifle and tarsus, while preventing weightbearing.

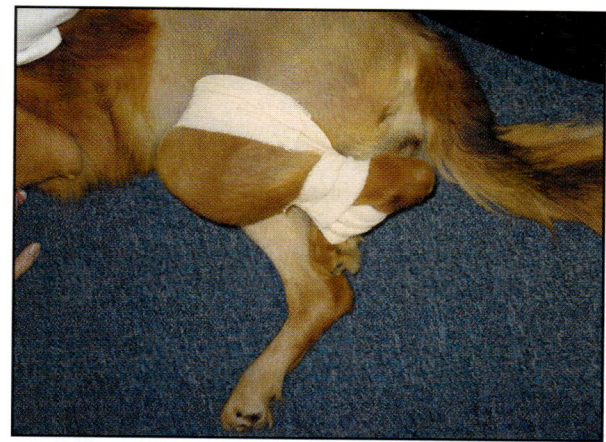

16.1 An Ehmer sling on a pelvic limb. Correct placement results in internal rotation of the coxofemoral joint and external rotation of the tuber calcis.

In some situations it is beneficial to maintain the joint in a certain position to maintain the periarticular tissues in a stretched or elongated position. One example is following repair of distal femoral physeal fractures in puppies. In these cases, the stifle and hock are placed in a 90-degree flexed position for 1–3 days following surgery, until swelling and oedema begin to resolve and the patient begins weightbearing; this helps to maintain the soft tissues of the cranial femur and stifle in a stretched position to prevent quadriceps contracture. After swelling and pain begin to resolve, and the patient begins to bear weight, it is better to allow active motion of the stifle.

In some situations, prolonged external coaptation is necessary following joint surgery. It is important to understand the changes that tissues undergo when joint motion is prevented, including capsular tightness, adaptive shortening of muscle groups, and atrophy of articular cartilage, muscle, ligaments, tendons and bones. It is critical to remobilize tissues over a period of time, and to avoid attempts to increase joint range of motion suddenly and forcibly. Also, a 2-week period is necessary to reverse the process of musculoskeletal tissue atrophy, although several weeks to months may be necessary to regain relatively normal tissue structure and function.

If coaptation devices are maintained for too long, contracture of tendons, muscles and joint capsule may result in joint stiffness, reduced range of motion (ROM) and, occasionally, inability to attain a normal standing posture. If contracture has occurred following prolonged immobilization, ROM and stretching exercises are indicated. In rare instances, it may be necessary to provide prolonged chronic stretch of tissues. One method is to use half of a bivalved cast moulded to the normal contralateral limb. The affected limb is wrapped in cotton padding, the half cast is placed on the limb, and gauze is wrapped around the limb and cast with tension to pull the contracted portion of the limb toward the cast. The bandage is changed once or twice daily, with gradually increasing amounts of tension until the tissues are stretched and

195

Chapter 16 Postoperative management and rehabilitation

the limb contracture is no longer present. Unfortunately, if the contracture is too chronic or severe, complete restoration of tissues may not be possible, although some improvement may occur.

Proper bandage care is essential to a successful outcome. The bandage must be kept clean and dry, and the patient should be kept indoors. A plastic bag may be placed over the foot while walking outside, especially if the ground is wet. The plastic bag should be removed when the dog is inside. The toes should be checked two or three times daily to be certain that there is no swelling of the toes and that the foot is warm to the touch. The position of the bandage should be checked to be certain that it is not slipping. If the bandage becomes wet or soiled, or if it slips or is too tight, it should be changed immediately. If no open wounds are present under the bandage, it may be changed every 7–10 days. It is helpful to mark the date that a bandage change is anticipated directly on the bandage with an indelible ink pen. If open wounds are present, the bandage should be changed as needed, sometimes several times daily.

Care of Ehmer and Velpeau slings is similar to that for Robert Jones bandages. In addition, it is critical to assess the toes several times daily to be certain that the sling does not result in venous stasis and swelling of the foot. The medial surface of the thigh should be checked if an Ehmer sling is applied, especially if the adhesive from the tape is in direct contact with the skin. This area is sensitive and irritation may occur; in some cases, superficial wounds on the thigh develop.

Re-examination schedules and follow-up

An appropriate recheck schedule allows adequate evaluation of the patient, assessment of healing at different stages of recovery, and the opportunity to provide appropriate intervention if necessary. For most joint surgeries, examination should take place 10–14 days after surgery at the time of suture removal; the patient is evaluated for limb use, abnormal articular or periarticular swelling or oedema, joint range of motion and evidence of infection. Other follow-up evaluations are typically made at 4, 8 and sometimes 12 weeks after surgery to be certain that the patient is progressing as expected, weightbearing is increasing, joint range of motion is maintained and that no surgical complications or failure of repair have occurred. In cases of articular fractures, radiographs are taken at these intervals to be certain that fracture healing is progressing.

In general, younger patients require recheck evaluations at more frequent intervals following joint surgery. Young dogs tend to have a vigorous healing response and periarticular fibrosis is generally greater, potentially resulting in decreased joint range of motion. Early intervention is critical to help prevent permanent loss of joint motion. In skeletally immature patients with articular fractures, bones heal more rapidly and clinical fracture union occurs much earlier than in mature patients. In addition, bone mineral content is less in immature dogs, and implants may be more prone to migrate as a result of the softer bone.

> Patients less than 5 months of age with articular fractures should be checked every 10–14 days. Dogs between 5 and 10 months old should be checked every 2–4 weeks, and those that are more than 10 months old should be checked every 3–4 weeks. Recheck evaluation should generally include radiographs to be certain that healing is progressing as expected and that implants are not migrating.

Physical rehabilitation

Rehabilitation is very important in the immediate postoperative period. Joint effusion and tissue oedema should be minimized to decrease reflex inhibition of active joint movement. Efforts are also made to re-establish normal range of motion within a few days of surgery, otherwise some dogs may permanently lose some joint range of motion following surgery. For example, if normal motion is not established by 2 weeks after surgery for cranial cruciate ligament rupture, some dogs have permanent loss of full stifle extension, and there is an association between decreased range of motion and lameness during recovery (Millis et al., 1997).

Efforts must also be made to minimize muscle atrophy as much as possible and to regain lost muscle mass as soon as possible. Normal dogs undergoing cruciate ligament transection and immediate stifle stabilization have only two-thirds of their preoperative muscle mass 5 weeks after surgery, and regain only a small amount of the lost muscle mass by 10 weeks with no rehabilitation (Millis et al., 2000). Physical rehabilitation reduces the amount of muscle atrophy that occurs (Millis et al., 1997).

Immediate postoperative period

Pain management for the first 7 days after surgery is important to reduce inflammation and oedema, improve joint motion and encourage early active limb use. This is generally accomplished with an NSAID which is administered 30–60 minutes prior to the first rehabilitation session of the day. Gentle massage therapy, ROM exercises and cryotherapy are started the day after surgery. Neuromuscular electrical stimulation (NMES) may also be initiated. Activities that increase pain and discomfort should be avoided because they slow return to function by increasing the degree of reflex inhibition. Animals should be muzzled prior to any manipulations to prevent injury to the therapist.

Massage therapy

Massage therapy should include gentle manipulation of soft tissues superficially and, over time, more deeply, to minimize adhesions and to reduce oedema and joint stiffness. Vigorous cross-fibre frictional massage may be used in the deeper tissues to help prevent adhesions of muscles, fascia, tendons or ligaments during later sessions when the animal is more comfortable, usually by days 5–7. It is performed by using small, deep strokes with the tip of one finger. The massage is performed in the direction of tissues or in circular strokes, moving skin

Chapter 16 Postoperative management and rehabilitation

and underlying tissue together to loosen tissue. Transverse friction massage is performed perpendicular to tissues, such as a tendon sheath.

If the purpose of the massage is to relax the patient and prepare for ROM or therapeutic exercises, a 5–10 minute superficial massage is probably adequate immediately preceding these activities. If deep tissue massage, such as transverse friction massage, is necessary to help prevent or break down adhesions between tissues, the massage should be performed for 5–10 minutes, two to four times daily.

Range of motion and stretching exercises

In the acute injury phase and immediately following surgical procedures, local oedema, joint effusion and pain may restrict full, active joint motion.

> **It is important to re-establish full range of motion as soon as possible because animals may have permanent loss of motion in as little as 2 weeks after some surgical procedures; this will ultimately limit an animal's functional ability (Grauer et al., 1987).**

Range of motion (ROM) and stretching exercises are very important to achieve improved motion after joint surgery, including increase in flexibility, prevention of adhesions between soft tissues and bones, remodelling of periarticular fibrosis and improvement of soft tissue extensibility (Salter et al., 1984). Tissues limiting passive ROM include joint capsule, periarticular soft tissues, muscles, ligaments, tendons and skin. Surgical incisions may result in adhesions and fibrosis between tissues, limiting their ability to glide over one another. Musculotendinous tissue may also be relatively shortened as a result of spasm or contracture.

ROM (see Technique 16.2) and stretching exercises must be performed properly to be effective (Madding et al., 1987).

> **WARNING**
> **Under no circumstances should the animal experience pain or discomfort from forcible flexion or extension of joints; this would result in reflex inhibition, delayed limb use, tissue fibrosis and, ultimately, decreased joint motion.**

Each joint in the affected limb should be placed through its comfortable ROM. Application of superficial heat or therapeutic ultrasound prior to stretching may improve tissue extensibility. Joints are slowly flexed to the point where the animal first begins to experience mild discomfort and held for 20–30 seconds to allow stretching of tissues. Following flexion, the joint should be slowly extended to the point where the animal first begins to experience mild discomfort and held stretched for 20–30 seconds. After stretching two or three times, joints should be passively placed through their available ROM 15–20 times. The motion should be smooth, slow and steady with joint motion occurring by moving the distal limb and holding the proximal limb steady. These manoeuvres may be repeated two to six times daily. The goal of stretching and ROM exercises should be to stretch and realign soft tissues and immature collagen, rather than tearing and destroying soft tissues. It may take several days to weeks to regain complete ROM.

In some situations, muscles that cross two joints may be especially restricted, such as the rectus femoris and biceps brachii muscles. In these situations, it is beneficial to put an individual joint through a stretching session, and then place the other joint through a stretching session. As ROM and flexibility improve, both joints may be simultaneously placed through stretching and ROM exercises. For example, the hip and stifle joints may be simultaneously stretched in extension.

Caution should be exercised when performing ROM exercises in patients with unstable fractures, ligament or tendon injuries. Caution should also be exercised to prevent overstretching, which is the elongation of tissues beyond normal limits. If stretching occurs within the normal physiological limits of the tissue, elastic deformation occurs in which the tissues return to their normal resting length after the stretch is completed. If the tissue is stretched beyond its limits, plastic deformation occurs, in which permanent deformation of the tissue(s) remains after the stretch is completed.

In some situations, prolonged mechanical stretching may be necessary to treat difficult contractures. Splints or other coaptation devices may be applied to provide prolonged stretch to tissues. An attempt is made to stretch the affected limb to a contoured splint with bandage material used to apply mild tension, applying controlled prolonged gentle stretch to the tissues. When the splint is replaced, additional stretch may be applied by increasing the tension on the tissues with the bandaging material.

Neuromuscular electrical stimulation

In the early postoperative period, when the animal is unwilling to bear weight and actively use the limb, electrotherapy may be instituted to attenuate muscle atrophy (Technique 16.3). NMES has a wide variety of benefits, including increasing muscle strength and joint ROM, decreasing oedema and pain, promoting wound healing, and restoring function. In clinical patients recovering from cranial cruciate ligament surgery, daily NMES for 15 minutes, ROM exercises and early use of the limb for 2 weeks resulted in attenuation of muscle atrophy in the affected limb following surgery.

Pulsed alternating current, low-frequency units are the most widely used neuromuscular electrical stimulators for therapeutic applications. Precautions should be taken to avoid injury to the handler and animal. A muzzle should be applied prior to initiating NMES. The animal is placed in lateral recumbency. Sedation may be necessary if the patient is anxious. Treatment should be administered under the supervision of personnel trained in its proper use.

NMES is used most frequently in the immediate postoperative period (first 2 weeks). It may be used for selective strengthening of a muscle group or groups. It may be applied to one or two muscle groups. If two muscle groups are treated together, they may be contracted sequentially or together (co-contraction). Muscles are generally treated for 10–20 minutes, three to seven times a week. Caution should be exercised when first initiating NMES by placing a muzzle on the animal, because some patients may find the treatment uncomfortable initially; the majority of patients generally accept treatment after several sessions. In addition, it is important not to overtreat because of the possibility of creating muscle soreness after several treatments. If this occurs, the treatment is shortened to 10 minutes every other day. Contraindications to NMES include:

- Stimulation directly over the heart
- Use in animals with pacemakers
- Use in animals with seizure disorders
- Stimulation over areas of thrombosis, infected areas or neoplasms
- Stimulation over the carotid sinus
- Any time active motion is contraindicated
- Use over the trunk in pregnant animals.

Following ROM exercises and NMES, additional massage may be beneficial. Finally, cryotherapy should be administered for 15 minutes after a session. A bandage may be applied if necessary to minimize swelling.

Heat

After 72–96 hours, heat applied to the area following surgery may be beneficial prior to performing massage and ROM exercises. Heat increases blood flow, tissue extensibility and general relaxation, while it decreases pain, muscle spasms and joint stiffness. Superficial heating typically affects superficial tissues to a depth of 1–2 cm. Commercially available hot packs, circulating warm water heating blankets or towels moistened with warm water may be applied to the affected area for 10 minutes prior to instituting therapy. Caution should be used in applying heat too early prior to the resolution of acute inflammation as this may worsen swelling and oedema. Heat should also not be used over areas of subcutaneous or cutaneous haemorrhage or thrombophlebitis, or over malignant tissue. Superficial heat should be used with caution in patients with poor thermoregulatory capacity or impaired circulation, or over open wounds.

Although warm packs or towels are effective for superficial heating, deeper heating may be desired. Therapeutic ultrasound may be useful in these situations. Ultrasound is capable of heating tissues up to 5 cm deep to temperatures of 40–45°C. In addition to the benefits of heating tissues, ultrasound may also increase collagen deposition, wound closure and wound breaking strength. Other non-thermal effects include increased cell membrane permeability, calcium transport across cell membranes, nutrient exchange and phagocytic activity of macrophages.

Therapeutic ultrasound units usually have frequencies of 1 MHz and 3 MHz, with different sized transducers. Most ultrasound units have continuous and pulsed modes. The continuous mode is used for heating. Caution must be exercised to avoid overheating areas with little soft tissue covering, such as the distal radius and ulna, and over peripheral joints, including the carpus, elbow, tarsus, stifle and digits.

> **WARNING**
> Heat should not be applied if acute inflammation, swelling or oedema are present.

The indications, contraindications and physiological effects of therapeutic ultrasound must be thoroughly understood.

To perform ultrasound treatment, the hair is clipped and ultrasound gel is applied liberally to the site. The proper size transducer head, and proper frequency for the tissue depth are selected. Power settings are typically 1–1.5 watts/cm^2. Most units have a timer that stops the ultrasound after treatment. The treatment area should be equivalent to twice the diameter of the sound head. Larger areas will not have effective tissue temperature increases. The ultrasound head is slowly and continuously moved over the treatment area in an overlapping circular or grid pattern. The animal should be observed for discomfort, such as pulling the limb away, which may indicate overheating, especially over joints or bony surfaces. The time of tissue temperature elevation is relatively short, so stretching and ROM exercises should be performed either during the latter half of the treatment or immediately after, to take full advantage of tissue extensibility (Warren et al., 1976; Wessling et al., 1987; Taylor et al., 1990; Draper et al., 1998; Reed et al., 2000; Loonam et al., 2003). In general, ultrasound is used for 10 minutes once daily. As the condition improves, treatment may be administered less frequently.

Early postoperative period

As oedema, inflammation and pain begin to subside, additional exercises may be added to the rehabilitation protocol. The goals of therapeutic exercise should be to reduce body weight, increase joint mobility and increase function though the use of non-weightbearing or low-impact exercises designed to improve muscle strength (Kisner and Colby, 1990; Brody, 1999). Muscles act as shock absorbers for joints and also help to provide stability to prevent unwanted arthrokinematic movements. Therapeutic exercises, such as weightshifting (Technique 16.4), walks at slow speeds to encourage weightbearing, treadmill walking, walking up and down inclines, climbing stairs, wheelbarrowing (to encourage use of forelimbs) and 'dancing' (to encourage use of hindlimbs) may be initiated as the animal's condition allows. Other methods to encourage active limb use include playing ball, sit-to-stand exercises (for hindlimbs) and taping a bottle or syringe cap to the bottom of the contralateral normal foot. It is important to consider muzzling the animal when recommending new exercises (especially 'dancing') to prevent injury to the handler. The animal should not be forced to exercise during times of increased pain and decreased limb use because overly vigorous exercise may increase inflammation and lameness.

Therapeutic exercises

Walks on a lead provide good low-impact aerobic forms of exercise. The length of walks should be titrated so there is no increased pain after activity. Also, it is better to divide the exercise time into several smaller segments during the day rather than a single session. Initially, walks should be approximately 5 minutes in length. Over the course of several weeks, the exercise periods may be gradually increased to provide three 20-minute walks each day.

> **PRACTICAL TIP**
> The walks should be brisk and purposeful, minimizing stopping. In prescribing the activity, owner compliance must be considered, and an exercise prescription should accommodate the owner's schedule and benefit the animal.

Walking up and down inclines or stairs are also good low impact activities that are easily incorporated into a walking programme to improve muscle strength and cardiovascular fitness as the patient improves. For additional muscle strengthening, 0.5–1 kg strap-on weights may be fastened to the lower limbs.

The amount and speed of therapeutic exercises may be gradually increased. Light jogging on grass may be added as the dog tolerates increased activity. Faster trotting may be added as endurance and lameness improve. More active ROM activities, in which the patient provides muscle contraction and active motion of a joint, may be achieved by instituting exercises designed to more completely use the full available ROM, including swimming, walking in water, tall grass, snow or sand, climbing stairs, crawling through a tunnel or negotiating cavaletti rails as the animal nears recovery.

Following exercise, a 10-minute warmdown period is recommended to allow muscles to cool down. The first 5 minutes may be spent walking at a slower pace after a brisk walk or swimming. ROM exercises may be repeated for the next 5 minutes. Finally, ice may be applied to painful areas for 15–20 minutes to control post-exercise inflammation.

Some dogs that have recovered from joint surgery may have near normal function, while others, particularly those with moderate to severe osteoarthritis, require a regular exercise programme to maintain fitness. It is extremely important to maintain a consistent level of activity on a daily basis. More harm may come to the animal by overdoing activity 1 or 2 days a week with relatively no activity during the rest of the week, because sudden exercise that is too vigorous may increase joint inflammation. Although consistent daily exercise is essential, a rehabilitation programme must account for exacerbations and remissions during recovery. The level of exercise must be prescribed for each individual based on the type of surgery, response to concurrent therapy, the patient's pain tolerance and the owner.

Hydrotherapy

After the incision is sealed, aquatic activity may be instituted. Aquatic exercises are incorporated with other therapeutic exercises to ensure a functional recovery. Walking in an underwater treadmill (Technique 16.5) allows weightbearing exercise in a buoyant environment and is the aquatic therapy of choice in the early postoperative period. Joints typically undergo a greater ROM when walking in water, with most of the increased range being in flexion, and maintenance of essentially normal joint extension.

> **WARNING**
> Full swimming is generally not recommended for the first 3–6 weeks after most joint surgeries because of the greater stress placed on the joint compared with walking in water. As the patient enters the chronic phase of recovery, swimming may be instituted.

An underwater treadmill allows active use of muscles, appropriate gait patterning with limited weightbearing and enhanced cardiovascular fitness, while taking advantage of the buoyant effects of aquatic therapy to reduce weightbearing stress on bones and joints. The depth of the water may be adjusted to alter the buoyancy that the patient experiences, and the speed of the treadmill may be altered. The length of time and speed of walking may be gradually increased as the patient's recovery allows. Initially, patients may walk at a very slow pace for 2–3 minutes twice daily. As function improves, a reasonable goal is 20–30 minutes at a brisk walk twice daily.

A pool or clean lake is ideal for stepping up activity to swimming. Self-contained tubs with whirlpool action are also available for smaller patients. Some dogs do not tolerate swimming and there is some risk in damaging tissues if the animal thrashes excessively. However, swimming is an excellent means of improving muscle strength and joint mobility in a non-weightbearing environment. Careful patient monitoring and assistance are important to prevent excessive thrashing. Fear of water must be addressed to avoid injury. Initially, dogs may swim for 1–3 minutes once daily, for 3–7 days per week. As strength and stamina improve, dogs may swim 5–20 minutes per session. When done carefully, swimming is an effective, functional exercise.

Chronic management of the postoperative patient

In the weeks to months following surgery, the goal should be to restore the animal to as normal use of the limb as possible. Depending on the situation, full return to function may not be a realistic goal. For example, the presence of severe osteoarthritis at the time of surgery for cranial cruciate ligament rupture may not allow full return to function. Strategies should be designed to encourage increased weightbearing of the limb, enlarge and strengthen muscles and increase the speed and power of activity. Appropriate exercise and training following surgery are important to:

- Regain muscle strength and endurance
- Maintain stability of the joint by enhancing supporting periarticular muscles, ligaments and joint capsule
- Maintain cardiovascular fitness
- Improve articular cartilage health.
- Anti-inflammatory medications given prior to activity may help limit inflammation and pain following exercise. While increasing the activity level (step-up activity), careful attention should be paid to be certain that the animal is not experiencing additional pain and discomfort as a result of increasing the level of activity.

Chapter 16 Postoperative management and rehabilitation

Specific considerations

Stifle
Stifle arthrotomies are particularly common, generally for rupture of the cranial cruciate ligament. The severity of arthritis, presence or absence of meniscal injury, degree of joint ROM, the method of joint exploration and the type of surgical procedure affect postoperative rehabilitation (Millis et al., 1997). Moderate to severe pre-existing arthritis slows recovery in the early postoperative period. It is unlikely that a dog with severe arthritis will have as near-complete recovery compared with one with no or mild arthritic changes. Many dogs with delayed diagnosis and treatment of cranial cruciate ligament rupture have reduced ROM, especially extension, prior to surgery. It is unlikely that complete joint motion can be achieved in these patients.

The method of joint exploration may affect postoperative recovery. Performing a full arthrotomy increases morbidity, including pain and joint swelling. Arthroscopic evaluation and joint debridement, although initially more difficult and time consuming, results in less pain and swelling, and earlier return to limb use (Hoelzler et al., 2004). Limb use may be impressive following arthroscopic joint debridement, necessitating restriction of activity in some patients during early rehabilitation.

The type of surgical procedure affects the aggressiveness of postoperative rehabilitation. In general, extracapsular repairs, such as the modified retinacular imbrication (fabellotibial suture) technique, provide excellent immediate stability if performed properly. Intracapsular repairs which rely on autogenous graft material, such as the under and over technique, undergo a period of weakening prior to the return of adequate graft strength. The tibial plateau levelling osteotomy (TPLO) procedure results in dynamic rather than static stability of the stifle joint, and because the biomechanics of the stifle are acutely altered, care must be taken to allow adequate time for the osteotomy to heal and for tissues to remodel before instituting aggressive rehabilitation to avoid problems with patellar ligament desmitis or avulsion of the tibial tuberosity.

Although technically not an articular fracture, distal femoral physeal fractures may have profound effects on the stifle joint if managed inappropriately (Bardet, 1987). Long-term external coaptation of these injuries is absolutely contraindicated because coaptation may result in fracture disease and quadriceps contracture. Following adequate internal fixation stabilization, cryotherapy is applied immediately postoperatively, followed by a light pressure wrap to limit oedema. Alternatively, a flexion sling may be applied for 2–3 days after surgery. ROM exercises and massage are commenced the day after surgery. Methods of initiating early limb use, including treadmill walking and placing a syringe cap on the bottom of the contralateral foot, in combination with very slow lead walks, are initiated. It is important to continue treatment of swelling and ROM exercises until normal stifle ROM is achieved and the dog is walking very well on the limb, usually by 10–14 days after surgery.

Hip
In cases of acetabular fracture repair or stabilization of a coxofemoral joint luxation, an Ehmer sling may be placed postoperatively. After sling removal, there may be loss of hip extension. ROM and stretching exercises are important to regain motion. Depending on the stability of the repair, incline walking, stair climbing, 'dancing' and aquatic exercise may be instituted at appropriate time intervals.

Following triple pelvic osteotomy, exercise to limit muscle atrophy should be instituted. However, care should be used to avoid excessive stress on the repair. Lead walks, sit-to-stand exercises and aquatic exercise are all useful to help attenuate muscle atrophy. Total hip replacement provides a different challenge because these dogs often feel less pain soon after surgery and it is important to restrict activity during tissue healing. In some cases, there is restricted hip extension and it is important to provide gentle ROM and stretching exercises to help improve hip mobility. Rehabilitation following femoral head and neck ostectomy is challenging because these patients are often in pain and success hinges on early return to function. Cryotherapy is initiated immediately after surgery, and the hip is slowly placed through continuous full ROM while the dog is recovering from anaesthesia, until the dog shows signs of discomfort. Appropriate analgesia is very important to help limit reflex inhibition and encourage early limb use. ROM and stretching exercises are important, especially in extension. Early limb use should be encouraged with a ground treadmill, slow lead walks, and aquatic exercises. Stair climbing and sit-to-stand exercises should be initiated when the dog is ambulating well. For dogs that are reluctant to use the limb, weightshifting activities and a syringe cap placed under the contralateral foot are useful to help encourage weightbearing.

Elbow
Fortunately, most fractures of the lateral aspect of the humeral condyle recover quite well with relatively little rehabilitation, assuming that repair is adequate. Limiting postoperative swelling and initiating early ROM and walking exercises are the key to re-establishing a functional joint. The situation is not as simple with bicondylar, or 'Y', fractures of the distal humerus. It is vital that adequate postoperative rehabilitation is performed on these cases because elbow stiffness and reduced limb function typically occur after repair without rehabilitation. The use of limited surgical approaches and avoiding an osteotomy of the olecranon (if possible) result in less tissue trauma and swelling postoperatively and should be used whenever possible. Cryotherapy and a pressure wrap help limit immediate postoperative swelling. ROM and stretching exercises are initiated the day after surgery and are performed a minimum of four times per day. Underwater treadmill activity is particularly beneficial in these cases because weight is unloaded from the fracture site, the hydrostatic pressure of the water helps to limit swelling and dogs have greater joint excursion during walking underwater, resulting in active ROM exercise.

Return to function

Many factors affect the return to function. The primary factor is the underlying condition that requires surgery and its severity. For example, a comminuted articular fracture would probably not have as complete a return to function as a two-piece fracture which is adequately reduced and compressed. Another factor affecting return to function is the pre-existing condition of the joint. Dogs with moderate to severe osteoarthritis of the elbow joint have a more prolonged recovery from surgery for fragmented medial coronoid process and may not have as complete a recovery as young dogs with early disease and minimal osteoarthritis. Younger animals generally heal more rapidly than older patients. The type of repair may have a profound influence on the return to function. Large dogs receiving a total hip replacement for hip dysplasia generally have greater function and more normal use of a limb than those receiving a femoral head and neck excision. Individual variation is an unpredictable factor in the return to function of patients. Some seemingly hopeless cases have very good function following joint surgery, while an occasional patient with a routine surgical condition may have poor limb function after recovery.

A thorough knowledge of the phases of tissue healing as they relate to specific forms of joint surgery will help establish a realistic recovery timetable. Although it is not possible to determine the exact time of healing and return to function, general expectations for healing are apparent from clinical and research experiences. Appropriate physical rehabilitation with gradual challenges to tissues should enhance healing and help patients return to their optimal function.

References and further reading

Bardet JF (1987) Quadriceps contracture and fracture disease. *Veterinary Clinics of North America: Small Animal Practice* **17**, 957–973

Brody LT (1999) Mobility Impairment. In: *Therapeutic Exercise: Moving Toward Function*, ed. CM Hall and LT Brody, pp. 87–111. Lippincott, Williams & Wilkins, Philadelphia

Budsberg SC, Johnston SA, Schwarz PD, DeCamp CE and Claxton R (1999) Efficacy of etodolac for the treatment of osteoarthritis of the hip joints in dogs. *Journal of the American Veterinary Medical Association* **21(4)**, 206–210

Cross AR, Budsberg SC and Keefe TJ (1997) Kinetic gait analysis assessment of meloxicam efficacy in a sodium urate-induced synovitis model in dogs. *American Journal of Veterinary Research* **58(6)**, 626–631

Dhert WJ, O'Driscoll SW, VanRoyen BJ and Salter RB (1988) Effects of immobilization and continuous passive motion on postoperative muscle atrophy in mature rabbits. *Canadian Journal of Surgery* **31**, 185–188

Draper DO (1998) Immediate and residual changes in dorsiflexion range of motion using an ultrasound heat and stretch routine. *Journal of Athletic Training* **33**, 141–144

Grauer D, Kabo JM, Dorey FJ and Meals RA (1987) The effects of intermittent passive exercise on joint stiffness following periarticular fracture in rabbits. *Clinical Orthopedics* **220**, 259–265

Halbertsma JP, van-Bolhuis AI and Goeken LN (1996) Sport stretching: effect on passive muscle stiffness of short hamstrings. *Archives of Physical Medicine and Rehabilitation* **77**, 688–692

Hoelzler MG, Millis DL, Francis DA and Weigel JP (2004) Results of arthroscopic versus open arthrotomy for surgical management of cranial cruciate ligament deficiency in dogs. *Veterinary Surgery* **33**, 146–153

Kisner C and Colby LA (1990) Range of motion. In: *Therapeutic Exercise: Foundations and Techniques*, 2nd edn, ed. C Kisner and LA Colby, pp. 19–59. FA Davis Company, Philadelphia

Lamont LA et al. (2000) Physiology of pain. *Veterinary Clinics of North America: Small Animal Practice* **30(4)**, 703–728

Lamont LA (2002) Feline perioperative pain management. *Veterinary Clinics of North America: Small Animal Practice* **32**, 747–763

Lascelles BD, Butterworth SJ and Waterman AE (1994) Postoperative analgesic and sedative effects of carprofen and pethidine in dogs. *Veterinary Record* **134**, 187–191

Lascelles BD, Cripps PJ, Jones A and Waterman-Pearson AE (1998) Efficacy and kinetics of carprofen, administered preoperatively or postoperatively, for the prevention of pain in dogs undergoing ovariohysterectomy. *Veterinary Surgery* **27**, 568–582

Loonam J, Millis DL, Stevens M and Moyers T (2003) The effect of therapeutic ultrasound on tendon heating and extensibility. *Proceedings of Veterinary Orthopedic Society*, Steamboat Springs, Colorado, p.69

Magnusson SP (1998) Passive properties of human skeletal muscle during stretch maneuvers. A review. *Scandinavian Journal of Medicine and Science in Sports* **8**, 65–77

Madding SW, Wong JG, Hallum A and Medeiros JM (1987) Effect of duration of passive stretch on hip abduction range of motion. *Journal of Orthopedic and Sports Physical Therapy* **8**, 409–416

McNamara PS, Johnston SA and Todhunter RJ (1997) Slow-acting, disease-modifying osteoarthritic agents. *Veterinary Clinics of North America: Small Animal Practice* **27(4)**, 863–867

Millis DL, Levine D and Taylor RA (eds) (2004) *Textbook of Small Animal Rehabilitation and Physical Therapy*. Elsevier, Philadelphia

Millis DL, Levine D, Brumlow M and Weigel JP (1997) A preliminary study of early physical therapy following surgery for cranial cruciate ligament surgery in dogs. *Veterinary Surgery* **26**, 434

Millis DL, Levine D, Mynatt T and Weigel JP (2000) Changes in muscle mass following transection of the cranial cruciate ligament and immediate stifle stabilization. *Proceedings of the 27th Annual Conference of the Veterinary Orthopedic Society*, Val d'Isere, France, p.3

Millis DL, Weigel JP, Moyers T and Buonomo FC (2002) The effect of deracoxib, a new COX-2 inhibitor, on the prevention of lameness induced by chemical synovitis in dogs. *Veterinary Therapeutics* **3**, 453–464

Noyes, FR, Mangine RE and Barber SD (1992) The early treatment of motion complications after reconstruction of the anterior cruciate ligament. *Clinical Orthopedics* **217**, 217–228

Olson VL (1987) Evaluation of joint mobilization treatment. A method. *Physical Therapy* **67**, 351–356

Reed BV, Ashikaga T, Fleming BC and Zimny NJ (2000) Effects of ultrasound and stretch on knee ligament extensibility. *Journal of Orthopedic Sports Physical Therapy* **30**, 341–347

Salter RB, Hamilton HW, Wedge JH et al. (1984) Clinical application of basic research on continuous passive motion for disorders and injuries of synovial joints: a preliminary report of a feasibility study. *Journal of Orthopedic Research* **1**, 325–342

Schollmeier G, Sarkar K, Fukuhara K and Uhthoff HK (1996) Structural and functional changes in the canine shoulder after cessation of immobilization. *Clinical Orthopedics* **323**, 310–315

Seymour C and Gleed R (eds) (1999) *BSAVA Manual of Small Animal Anaesthesia and Analgesia*. BSAVA Publications, Cheltenham

Shafford HL (2001) Preemptive analgesia: managing pain before it begins. *Veterinary Medicine*, **96**, 478–491

Streppa HK, Jones CJ and Budsberg SC (2002) Cyclooxygenase selectivity of nonsteroidal anti-inflammatory drugs in canine blood. *American Journal of Veterinary Research* **63(1)**, 91–94

Taylor DC (1990) Viscoelastic properties of muscle–tendon units. The biomechanical effects of stretching. *American Journal of Sports Medicine* **18**, 300–309

Trim CM (1999) Postanesthetic care and complications. In: *Manual of Small Animal Anesthesia*, ed. RR Paddleford, pp. 196–226. WB Saunders, Philadelphia

Warren CG, Lehmann JF and Koblanski JN (1976) Heat and stretch procedures: an evaluation using rat tail tendon. *Archives of Physical Medicine and Rehabilitation* **57**, 122–126

Wessling KC, DeVane DA and Hylton CR (1987) Effects of static stretch versus static stretch and ultrasound combined on triceps surae muscle extensibility in healthy women. *Physical Therapy* **67**, 674–679

Chapter 16　Postoperative management and rehabilitation

TECHNIQUE 16.1
Soft padded bandage

Positioning
The dog is placed in lateral recumbency with the limb placed so that the joints mimic a functional standing position.

Assistant
Useful to help restrain the patient and hold the limb in the proper position while the bandage is placed.

Supplies
Adhesive tape; cast padding or cotton roll; conforming gauze; outer wrap, such as self-adherent non-adhesive wrap or an adhesive wrap.

Application
With the patient in lateral recumbency, the joints of the limb are placed in a functional weightbearing position. Two strips of adhesive tape are placed on the distal limb on the dorsal and palmar (plantar) or medial and lateral surfaces to the level of the carpus (tarsus) (Figure 16.2a).

> **PRACTICAL TIP**
> A tongue depressor may be placed between the two strips to prevent them from sticking to one another.

If an incision or wound is present, a dressing may be placed directly over the wound or incision. Beginning distally, the cast padding or cotton roll is spiralled up the limb, overlapping layers by 50% (Figure 16.2b). The bottom of the bandage should be at the level of the nail beds of the middle toes. The proximal portion of the bandage should generally extend to above the elbow (stifle) joint (Figure 16.2c). The conforming gauze should be applied next, following the same placement used for the cotton layer (Figure 16.2d). The gauze should be placed snugly, but not so tight as to result in venous stasis and swelling of the toes. One technique is to compress the cotton with the fingers and hand of one arm, while stretching the gauze and placing it over the compressed cotton. The gauze should not extend beyond the level of the cotton to prevent constricting the limb (Figure 16.2e). The tape stirrups are separated from the tongue depressor, each strip is rotated 180 degrees, and the tape is placed proximally on the bandage material to help keep it from slipping. The outer layer is then applied, going from distal to proximal, being certain to cover the cotton and gauze (Figure 16.2f, g). The outer layer should not be pulled tightly at the ends of the bandage; rather, the covering should be pulled free of the roll, the tension should be released from the material, and the material simply placed over the cotton and gauze. Finally, an indelible marking pen is used to write the date the bandage was placed and the date the bandage should be changed.

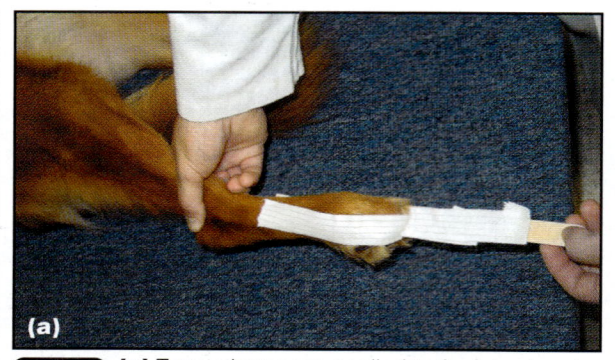

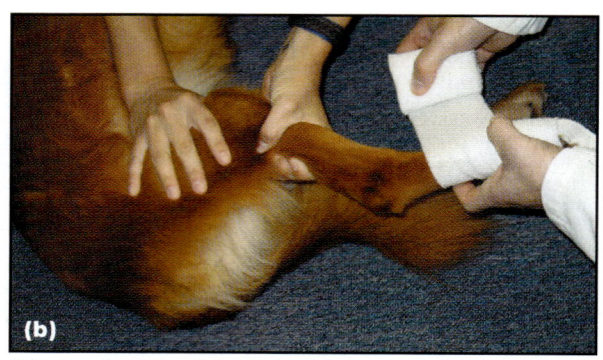

16.2 **(a)** Tape stirrups are applied to the lateral and medial aspects of the distal limb. **(b)** Cast padding is applied, beginning distally at the level of the digits. The limb is placed with the joints in a functional walking position and the cotton is overlapped 50% as it is applied. (continues)

Chapter 16 Postoperative management and rehabilitation

TECHNIQUE 16.1 continued
Soft padded bandage

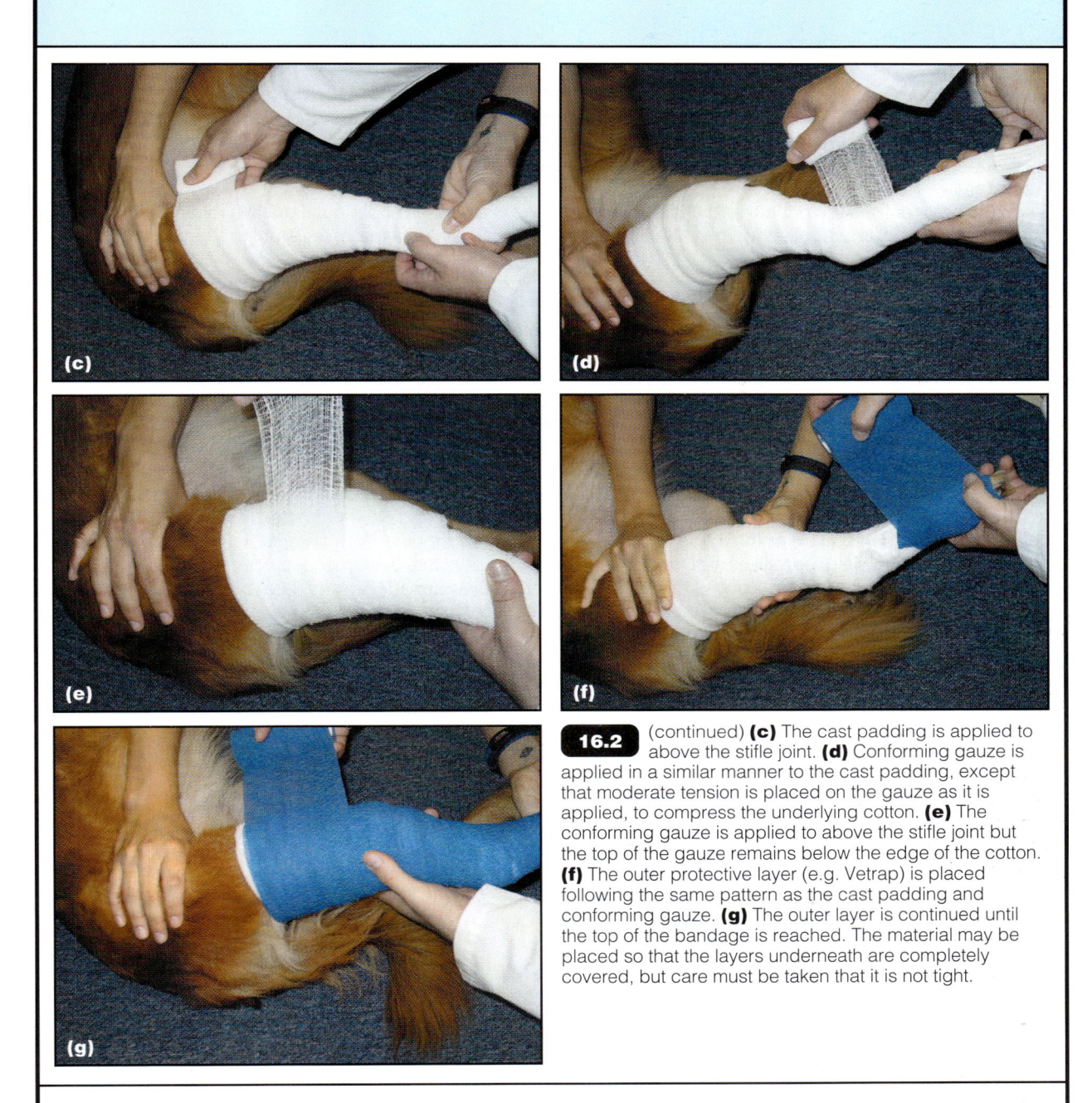

16.2 (continued) **(c)** The cast padding is applied to above the stifle joint. **(d)** Conforming gauze is applied in a similar manner to the cast padding, except that moderate tension is placed on the gauze as it is applied, to compress the underlying cotton. **(e)** The conforming gauze is applied to above the stifle joint but the top of the gauze remains below the edge of the cotton. **(f)** The outer protective layer (e.g. Vetrap) is placed following the same pattern as the cast padding and conforming gauze. **(g)** The outer layer is continued until the top of the bandage is reached. The material may be placed so that the layers underneath are completely covered, but care must be taken that it is not tight.

Aftercare
The bandage should be monitored twice daily for swollen toes, warmth, wetness, soiling or slippage, and changed if necessary. The bandage must be kept clean and dry, and the patient should be kept indoors. A plastic bag may be placed over the foot while the patient is walking outside if the ground is wet. The plastic bag should be removed when the dog is indoors. If no open wounds are present under the bandage, it may be changed every 7–10 days. If open wounds are present, the bandage should be changed as needed, sometimes several times daily.

Chapter 16 Postoperative management and rehabilitation

TECHNIQUE 16.2
Passive range of motion (ROM) exercises

Positioning
The dog is placed in lateral recumbency. The treatment should be administered in a quiet and comfortable area, away from distractions, such as loud noises, other pets and other people that are not helping with the treatment. This will allow the patient to be calm, relaxed and more receptive to the treatment.

Assistant
Useful to help restrain the patient and assist supporting the limb in the proper position. It is recommended that patients have a muzzle applied for the initial treatments, and if they are in pain, resistant to treatment or overly anxious.

Technique
After the animal has relaxed, both hands are placed gently on the injured limb and a very gentle massage is begun to help further relax the patient. This massage is performed for 2–3 minutes, and then one hand is gently moved to the portion of the limb above the joint. The other hand is placed on a portion of the limb below the affected joint. The entire limb must be supported to avoid any undue stress to the involved joint. If joint stiffness is present, heat may be applied to the soft tissues around the joint to help with extensibility of tissues (however, heat should not be applied within the first 72 hours after surgery or after acute inflammation has occurred).

After the hands are in the correct position and the limb is supported, the treated joint is flexed slowly and gently. The other joints of the limb should be allowed to remain in a neutral position (a position as if the animal was standing). One should try not to move the other joints while working on the affected joint. Some joints may be restricted by the position of the joints above or below the target joint. For example, maximal hock flexion cannot be obtained while the stifle is maintained in an extended position. In this case, placing the stifle in a flexed position allows more complete flexion of the hock. The joint is slowly flexed (Figure 16.3a) until the patient shows initial signs of discomfort, such as tensing the limb, moving, vocalizing, turning the head towards the therapist or trying to pull away; undue discomfort should not be caused.

With the hands maintained in the same positions, the joint is slowly extended (Figure 16.3b). Again, one should try to keep the other joints in a neutral position and minimize any movement of the other joints. The joint is slowly extended until the patient shows initial signs of discomfort.

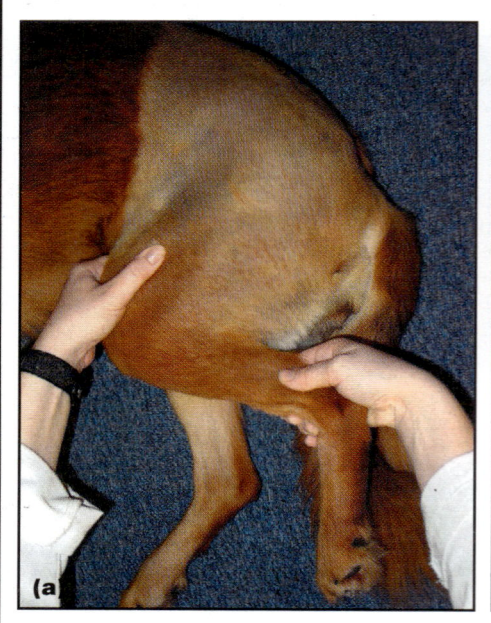

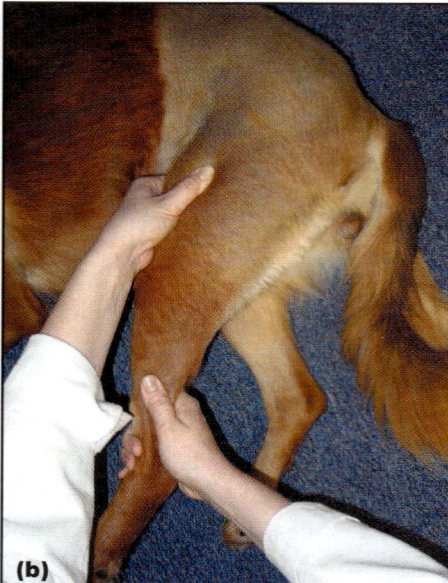

16.3
Stifle joint.
(a) Placement of hands to perform passive flexion. The joint is slowly flexed until the dog first indicates mild discomfort. Note that the limb is supported and that only the stifle joint is flexed; the other joints are placed in a neutral position. **(b)** The joint is then slowly extended until the dog first indicates mild discomfort.

→

Chapter 16 Postoperative management and rehabilitation

TECHNIQUE 16.2 *continued*
Passive range of motion (ROM) exercises

Alternatively, a number of joints may be placed through ROMs simultaneously, a technique sometimes referred to as 'ROM through functional patterns' (Figure 16.4). This form of ROM exercises may be appropriate as an animal nears active use of a limb. Flexing and extending all of the joints of a limb in a pattern that mimics a normal gait pattern may also be beneficial for neuromuscular re-education.

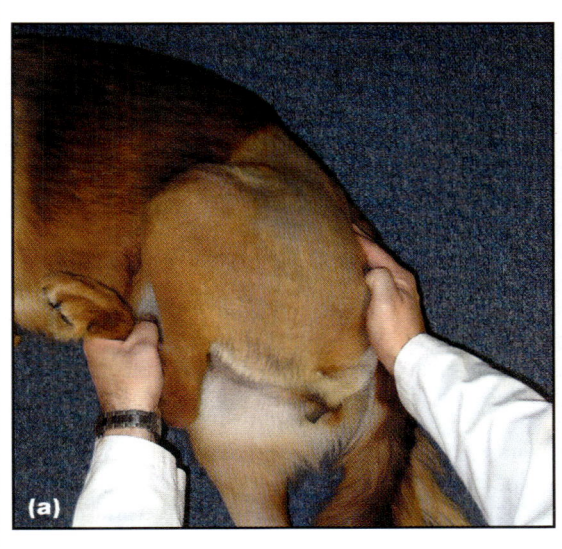

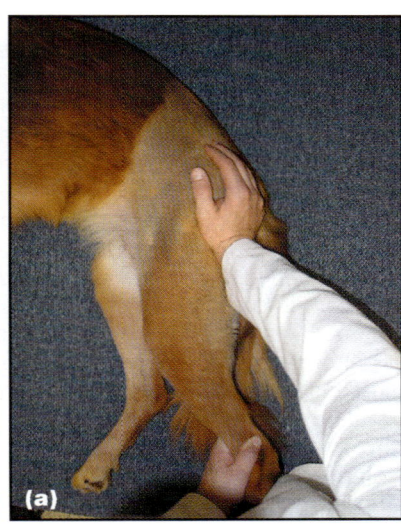

16.4 Placement of joints through a functional ROM. **(a)** Flexing the joints of the pelvic limb. **(b)** Extending the joints of the pelvic limb.

It is also important to maintain normal ROM in the other joints of the affected limb. After completing ROM exercises of the affected joint, the limb is kept in a neutral position and the hands are slowly moved distally to the digits (or if already working on the digits, hands are moved proximally). The injured joint must be supported. Performing ROM exercises of the digits requires additional consideration because it is difficult passively to flex and extend a single joint at a time because of the proximity of the other joints of each digit. In addition, it is more efficient to perform ROM exercises in all joints simultaneously. The fingers or palm are placed on the pads of the patient's foot and the toes are slowly extended until the point of initial discomfort. Then the fingers or palm are placed on the dorsal surface of the digits and the digits are slowly flexed until the point of initial discomfort. After performing ROM exercises on the digits, ROM exercises are performed on the other joints.

Frequency of treatment
The number of ROM repetitions and the frequency of the treatments depend on the condition treated. In general, for most routine postoperative conditions, 15–20 repetitions, performed 2–4 times per day are probably adequate. As the range of motion returns to normal, the frequency may be reduced. For more challenging conditions, such as articular fractures, physeal fractures in young dogs, joints with contracture or joints which have been immobilized for a period of time, an increase in the number and frequency of repetitions may be necessary.

After ROM exercises
The ROM session may be ended with a gentle slow massage to the injured limb for approximately 5 minutes. This helps to maintain a relaxed state. An ice pack may be applied to the injured joint after the ROM exercises and massage.

Chapter 16 Postoperative management and rehabilitation

TECHNIQUE 16.3
Neuromuscular electrical stimulation (NMES)

Positioning
The dog is placed in lateral recumbency. The treatment should be administered in a quiet and comfortable area, away from distractions. For initial treatments, and for anxious patients, a properly fitted muzzle should be placed to avoid injury to the therapists.

Assistant
Necessary to restrain the patient and assist supporting the limb in the proper position.

Preparation and electrode placement
The hair over the area to which electrical stimulation will be applied must be clipped to lower impedance. The skin should be cleaned with alcohol prior to treatment. Alternatively, special electrodes with multiple fine metal tines may be used in animals with short, but not clipped hair. It will be necessary to wet the hair and skin to allow conduction of electricity. The motor point (the area where the motor nerve enters the muscle) must be located, so that an adequate contraction is obtained with as low a current as possible to minimize discomfort to the patient. Electrodes may be placed solely on one or two muscle groups to cause a contraction, and motion at the joint the muscles act upon, or placed on opposing muscle groups to cause a co-contraction which may simulate an isometric contraction and result in little or no joint movement.

Motor point location is performed by first applying electrode gel to the skin, and then placing one electrode over the general area of the motor point. The other electrode is placed further distally over the muscle. As an example, for stimulation of the caudal thigh muscles (semitendinosus, semimembranosus and biceps femoris muscles), one electrode is placed proximally just distal to the region between the ischiatic tuberosity and greater trochanter where the sciatic nerve enters these muscles, and the other electrode is placed over the distal aspect of the muscles. Contact gel is applied to the skin. With the unit on, the electrode may then be moved around until a good contraction is achieved. Setting the frequency at 1 Hz will help in motor point determination because the twitch contraction will be more obvious and will become stronger as the electrode moves closer to the motor point. An indelible marking pen is then used to draw a circle around the electrode. This allows the electrode to be placed in the same area during subsequent treatments, without having to repeat the process of motor point location.

Technique
The unit is adjusted to the proper settings. The therapist is encouraged to consult other references and professionals to obtain additional information. The frequency should be adjusted to the desired setting (25–50 Hz) before beginning the actual treatment.

A symmetrical biphasic waveform is typically used for muscle strengthening. Ampage may be increased to the tolerance level of the animal, and reduced if the animal displays any signs of distress, including turning its head in recognition of the stimulus or becoming agitated. In general, alternating contraction of opposing muscle groups is performed. As an example, electrodes may be placed on the quadriceps and caudal thigh muscle groups following surgery for cranial cruciate ligament rupture (Figure 16.5). Co-contraction of opposing muscle groups should be considered if no joint motion is desired.

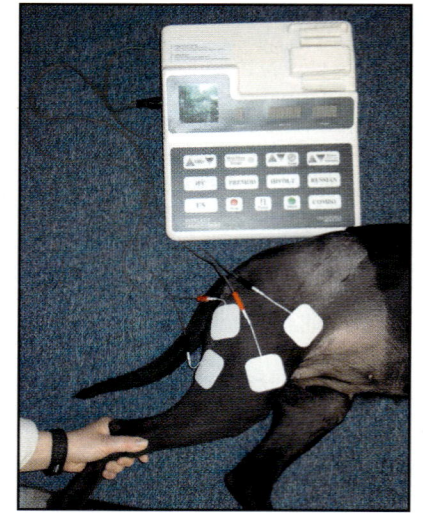

16.5 NMES is applied to the quadriceps and caudal thigh muscle groups. The patient is placed in lateral recumbency. The hair has been clipped and the skin cleaned with alcohol. Electrodes have been placed, with one set on the quadriceps muscles, and the other on the caudal thigh muscles. The proximal electrodes of each set are placed in the region of the motor points (area where the nerve enters the muscles) for the femoral and sciatic nerves.

→

TECHNIQUE 16.3 continued
Neuromuscular electrical stimulation (NMES)

Treatment time and frequency
Although the optimum time of treatment and the frequency of treatment are unknown, most clinicians believe that NMES should be applied to the desired area(s) for 15–20 minutes, three to seven times a week. Occasionally, a patient may experience muscle soreness early in the treatment programme if electrical stimulation is used too frequently, for treatment periods that are too long or with application of current that is too great (muscle contraction is too strong). In these cases, skipping treatment for a day or two and resuming treatment with reduced treatment time, frequency or strength of contraction, is usually adequate to resolve the problem. When the animal begins active use of the limb, the use of NMES may be phased out.

Chapter 16 Postoperative management and rehabilitation

TECHNIQUE 16.4
Weightshifting exercises

Positioning
The dog is placed in a standing position, with the four limbs placed squarely and symmetrically. Some patients may only touch the affected foot to the ground, or may even be non-weightbearing. Weightshifting exercises may be performed if the foot is within 3–6 cm of the ground, but if the limb is held in a tightly guarded flexed position, additional efforts should be made towards pain control, reducing swelling and passive range-of-motion exercises before attempting weightshifting exercises.

Assistant
Useful to help provide support to a weak patient and to help prevent sudden loss of balance and falling.

Supplies
Rubber mats or carpet to provide adequate footing. Low-calorie treats or a ball may be used to help encourage weightshifting. A balance board or platform may also be useful.

Technique
While the animal is standing, a treat may be used to encourage weightshifting. The interested dog will follow the treat from side to side and up and down. One should start with small movements, and progress to larger, more challenging movements. The movement of the head causes the dog's centre of gravity (COG) to shift. As the COG shifts, the dog must shift its weight to maintain its balance. The animal is required to use strength, coordination and balance. This form of weightshifting is especially useful for the forelimbs.

If the dog is motivated by ball play, a more challenging form of this exercise is close-distance ball tossing from above and the sides. During early attempts at these exercises it may be necessary to have someone available for standby assistance because the dog may be over-challenged, lose its balance and fall.

The handler may also attempt to disturb the animal's balance by gently pushing the animal at the hips or shoulder or lifting the unaffected contralateral limb (Figure 16.6). The goal is to disturb its balance just enough so the animal can recover, being careful not to push with a force that may cause the animal to fall. Generally, pushing the animal to the more affected side challenges the animal sufficiently to allow the activity to have the desired effect. Some dogs become conditioned to this activity, however, and shift their weight towards the therapist to prevent being pushed to the affected side. In this case, a rebound weight shift may be effective. For this manoeuvre, the therapist gently pushes the animal towards the affected side. When the animal shifts its weight to resist the movement, the therapist suddenly releases pressure, and simultaneously pushes gently toward the unaffected side. This results in a sudden unbalancing. The animal initially shifts its weight toward the unaffected side, but to keep from falling, it immediately shifts its weight back toward the affected side. The dog may only shift the weight for a brief moment, but the goal of encouraging weightbearing on the affected limb is met.

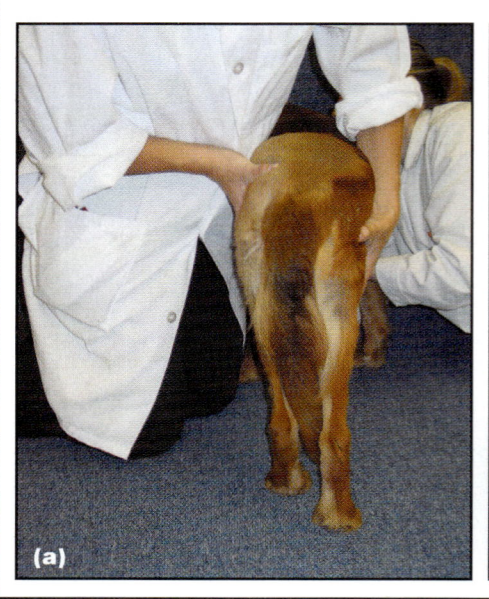

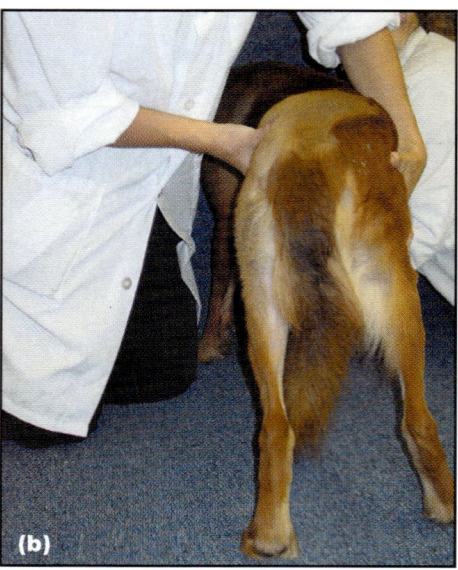

16.6 Weightshifting exercises. **(a)** The patient stands with all four limbs placed squarely on the ground. **(b)** Weight is slowly shifted over to the affected limb, in this case the left hind, to encourage increased weightbearing on the limb. In some cases, it is beneficial to place pressure over the dorsum to further increase the force placed on the limb.

→

TECHNIQUE 16.4 continued
Weightshifting exercises

Additional challenges may be added by slowly moving a supporting towel back and forth, in a motion similar to polishing a shoe, to force the dog to shift its weight back and forth.

Weight shifts may also be performed during walking. As the animal is walked in a straight line, the handler gently pushes the animal to one side to challenge the dog to maintain its balance. Caution should be used to tailor the force of the push with the animal's stage of recovery to avoid falls and injury.

Lifting and holding a single limb off the ground while the dog is standing causes a shift in the animal's COG. If the animal is unable or unwilling to perform this exercise, it will not shift its weight properly, but instead will bear the weight on the handler's hand or collapse to the ground. A technique to avoid bearing all of the weight on the handler is to abduct the raised limb slowly, which allows transfer of weight from the handler to the desired limb to avoid falling.

A platform on rockers may be used to rock the dog forward and backward, side to side, diagonally, and through 360 degrees. A balance board for humans may be used to help the animal practise proprioceptive positioning on just the thoracic or pelvic limbs by placing the desired limbs on the board while the other limbs remain on the ground. If the goal is to have the animal exercise using all four limbs, then a specially made platform must be used to accommodate quadrupeds. It is important to have one person help support the dog while another person slowly and gently rocks the platform to allow the animal an opportunity to shift its weight and exercise its proprioceptive mechanism and shift weight to the affected limb.

Therapeutic exercise balls and rolls may also be used to improve balance, coordination and strength. The thoracic limbs are placed on the ball and supported by the handler, requiring the dog to maintain static balance of the caudal trunk and hindlimbs. Dynamic balance may also be challenged as the ball or roll is slowly moved forwards, backwards, and side to side, challenging the hindlegs to maintain balance while movement occurs. To address the cranial trunk, head, neck and thoracic limbs, the pelvic limbs are placed over the ball as the forelimbs are asked to balance the body weight during both stance (static) and gentle movements (dynamic). A very challenging activity is to place all four limbs on an exercise roll, and, with support from an assistant, attempt to balance the dog's weight on the roll.

Frequency of treatment
The type and frequency of weightshifting exercises depend on the severity of the condition. In general, for most routine postoperative conditions, 5–10 minutes of activity, two to three times per day are likely adequate. As use of the limb, balance and proprioception return to normal, the level of challenge may be increased.

Chapter 16   Postoperative management and rehabilitation

TECHNIQUE 16.5
Underwater treadmill exercise

Preparation
Dogs may be exercised on an underwater treadmill if they are ambulatory and the incision is sealed, with no gaping of the incision, and no drainage, discharge or infection present. The patient should be clean and brushed prior to hydrotherapy. The dog is allowed to walk into the treadmill in preparation for exercise. For elective surgical procedures, such as cruciate ligament surgery, it is beneficial to introduce the patient to water prior to surgery.

Assistant
An assistant is usually not necessary.

Technique
Walking in the water is an excellent way to allow a dog to exercise more comfortably following joint surgery due to the buoyancy provided by the water. This type of exercise may be used as a progression to swimming.

In addition to the buoyancy effects of walking in water, joint kinematics are also altered during hydrotherapy. For example, one study comparing walking over ground *versus* walking on an underwater treadmill found that joint flexion and overall active joint ROM were greater in underwater walking, while joint extension was similar to walking over ground. Because the water level may be adjusted, the relative degree of buoyancy and resistance to walking in water may also be adjusted. In addition, adjustment of the water level to the level of various joints may further influence joint kinematics because those particular joints must gain the necessary momentum and force to break through the water surface and overcome surface tension of the water.

Commercially available underwater treadmills have an exercise chamber, the treadmill, a water storage chamber, chlorinator, heater, filters and pumps. The dog is walked into the empty chamber, the door is sealed, and water is pumped into the chamber. It is important not to allow the water to get much higher than the elbow joint because the dog may sometimes panic when it makes the transition between standing and swimming. After the appropriate water level is reached, the treadmill is started. Most dogs readily walk on the treadmill (Figure 16.7). Occasionally, an attendant may be needed to assist the movement of the animal's limbs. In most cases, the treadmill is started at a slow walking speed.

Following exercise, the water is drained from the chamber, and the animal is dried with a towel or air dryer.

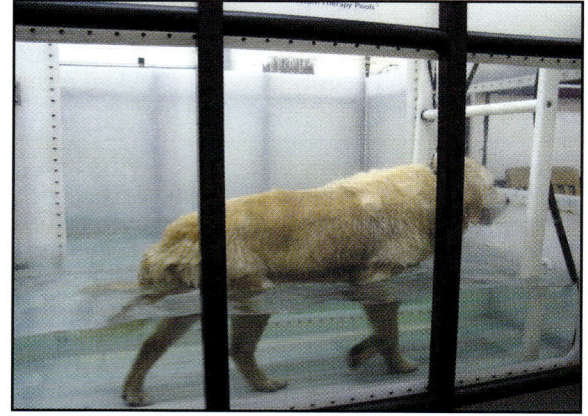

16.7 Underwater treadmill exercise. Note the flexion of the carpus and elbow joints, which is typically greater than when walking over ground. The top of the water level is typically near the elbow.

Frequency of treatment
Initially, 3–5 minutes twice daily is generally adequate to accustom the dog to the underwater treadmill and to begin the rehabilitation programme. As the dog develops more stamina, pain resolves and use of the limb improves, the amount of time during each session and the speed of walking may be gradually increased until the dog is walking very rapidly or trotting for 20–30 minutes twice daily.

Consideration should be given to the type and severity of the animal's condition. Patients recovering from joint surgery, especially cranial cruciate ligament rupture, may begin treatment 4–10 days after surgery depending on the condition of the incision. The treadmill should be at a speed that is a slow walk for the dog, beginning for 3 minutes twice daily, and increasing approximately 1–2 minutes per session, depending on the progress of the dog. By the second week, the speed may be increased each day until a steady walk is achieved by the end of the second week. The patient should be carefully monitored to be certain that lameness is not worse following the session.

→

TECHNIQUE 16.5 continued
Underwater treadmill exercise

Precautions
Some dogs fear water and this must be considered before treatment, though dogs seem to fear underwater treadmill exercise less than swimming in a pool. If possible, dogs should be introduced to water before surgery. Preoperative evaluation is not possible for some traumatic injuries, such as fractures.

Dogs should never be left unattended in the water. To minimize the risk of infection, hydrotherapy should wait until after suture removal if there are no wound complications, such as discharge from the incision, gaping of the wound edges or evidence of infection. The cleanliness of the water is important, and commercially available systems have filters, automatic chlorinators and heaters. The cardiovascular fitness of the dog must also be considered because many dogs are initially unable to exercise more than a few minutes before fatiguing. Animals with respiratory conditions should not undergo hydrotherapy because hydrostatic pressure on the thorax may be detrimental.

17

The shoulder

Steve Butterworth and James L. Cook

Introduction

Diseases and disorders of the shoulder appear to be a frequent cause of lameness in dogs and can also be seen in cats. It is vital for the practitioner to have a comprehensive understanding of shoulder problems in order to distinguish between causes of thoracic limb lameness and allow optimal treatment and client education.

Fractures of the scapula and proximal humerus may be responsible for shoulder lameness; these are covered in the *BSAVA Manual of Small Animal Fracture Management and Repair*. Conditions that may cause shoulder lameness which are discussed in this chapter include:

- Congenital/developmental
  - Luxation of the scapulohumeral joint
  - Scapulohumeral dysplasia
  - Osteochondrosis: osteochondritis dissecans (OCD) of the humeral head; un-united caudal glenoid
- Acquired
  - Luxations: scapulohumeral luxation; dorsal luxation of the scapula; medial luxation of the biceps brachii tendon of origin
  - Muscle-related: contracture of the spinatus muscles; teres minor myopathy
  - Tendon- or ligament-related: biceps brachii tendinitis/tenosynovitis; rupture of the biceps brachii tendon sheath; supraspinatus mineralizing tendinopathy; infraspinatus bursal ossification; medial or lateral collateral instability; biceps brachii tendon rupture/avulsion
  - Osteoarthritis
  - Inflammatory arthritis; infective; immune-mediated
  - Neoplasia: osteosarcoma; synovial sarcoma; other sarcomas (chondrosarcoma, fibrosarcoma, haemangiosarcoma); brachial plexus tumours.

Anatomy

The scapulohumeral joint is an enarthrodial joint formed by the articulation of the scapular glenoid with the humeral head (Figure 17.1). The scapula is made up of a flat blade, lying in the sagittal plane. The scapular spine arises on its lateral aspect; it projects almost perpendicularly from the blade and ends distally as the acromion process. Distally, the scapular blade becomes narrower, creating the scapular neck, before expanding to form the glenoid with its cranial prominence, the scapular tuberosity and its concave articular surface. The latter articulates with the convex surface of the humeral head. Cranially, the proximal humerus possesses two tubercles, the greater tubercle, positioned laterally, and the lesser tubercle, placed medially. The intertubercular groove lies between them.

The joint capsule is attached to the rim of the glenoid and to the humeral head and has several outpouchings. The most significant of these are the caudal pouch and

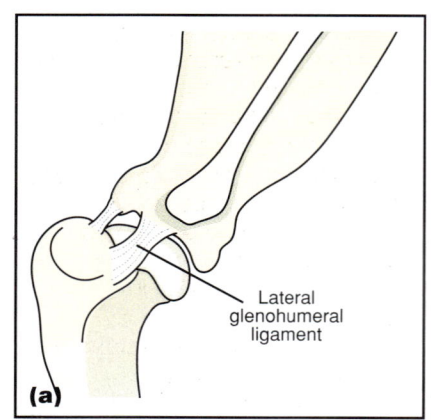

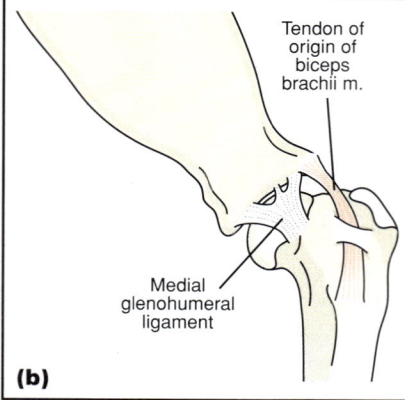

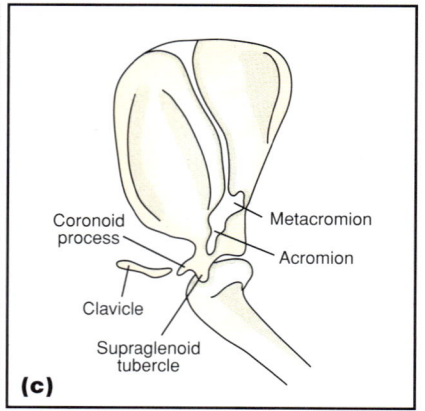

17.1 Surgical anatomy of the shoulder. **(a)** Syndesmology, lateral aspect, in the dog. **(b)** Syndesmology, medial aspect, in the dog. **(c)** Shoulder joint of the cat, lateral aspect. (continues) ▶

Chapter 17 The shoulder

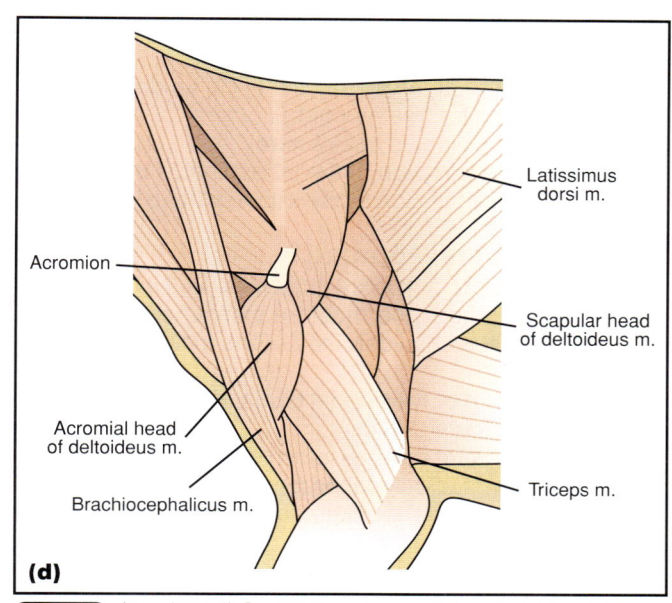

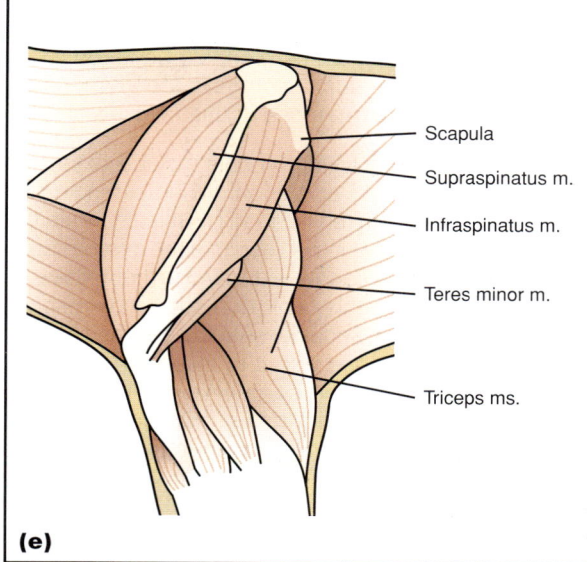

17.1 (continued) Surgical anatomy of the shoulder. **(d)** Superficial muscles over the lateral aspect of the shoulder, in the dog. **(e)** Deep muscles over the lateral aspect of the shoulder, in the dog.

the cranial extension, which forms a tendon sheath around the tendon of origin of the biceps brachii muscle as it passes through the intertubercular groove. Within the joint capsule are lateral and medial thickenings which make up the glenohumeral ligaments.

Additional support for the joint comes from the adjacent ('cuff') muscles. The supraspinatus and infraspinatus muscles arise from the scapular blade, cranial and caudal to the scapular spine, respectively, and insert on the cranial and lateral aspects of the greater tubercle. Medially, the subscapularis muscle arises from the scapular blade and inserts on the lesser tubercle; cranially, the biceps brachii muscle arises from the scapular tuberosity and passes through the intertubercular groove, underneath the intertubercular ligament. The tendons of all these muscles have very close associations with the joint capsule. In addition, there are several other muscles, such as the deltoid, teres minor and major and coracobrachialis, which lend some support to the joint without such intimate contact with the capsule.

Joint stability is dependent on the capsule, with its lateral and medial thickenings, and also on the 'cuff' muscles. An *in vitro* analysis of shoulder stability (Vasseur *et al.*, 1982) showed that removal of all the 'cuff' muscles had little effect on the static stability of the joint, although these were thought to serve an important function *in vivo*, and that it was necessary to damage the capsule itself before increased laxity could be detected. Another *in vitro* study (Sidaway *et al.*, 2004) reported that the biceps brachii tendon contributes to passive shoulder joint stability, and that the medial glenohumeral ligament is important to medial stability in dogs.

Neurovascular structures to be borne in mind when contemplating surgery around the shoulder are few but comprise:

- The omobrachial vein (a branch of the cephalic vein), which passes across the craniolateral aspect of the joint
- The cranial circumflex artery and vein and the axillary nerve, which cross the caudal aspect of the joint capsule
- The suprascapular nerve, which courses from cranial to caudal under the tendons of insertion of the suprascapular muscles and the acromion of the scapula.

> When dealing with cats it is important to bear in mind their different osteology (Figure 17.1c). The metacromion is located on the distal scapular spine and extends caudally, the coracoid process forms a prominent extension from the rim of the glenoid craniomedially and a clavicle is present.

Clinical examination

As with other joints, patients with lameness relating to the shoulder will show particular features on clinical examination:

- Gait may be altered in a characteristic way (e.g. in cases of infraspinatus contracture) but in most the only abnormality may be the reduced weightbearing associated with any thoracic limb lameness. Although a reluctance to extend the joint fully may cause a shortened cranial phase to the stride, this can be difficult to appreciate
- Palpation may reveal atrophy of the spinatus muscles; this can be seen as part of a generalized proximal limb muscle atrophy associated with any chronic thoracic limb lameness, but it is often seen sooner and more prominently in cases with shoulder pain
- There may be an abnormal relationship of anatomical landmarks, for example in a case of luxation

- The finding of 'point pain' on palpation of specific structures, such as the biceps tendon of origin, can be important, but care should be taken in over-interpreting such findings in the absence of a good deal of experience in this field.

Manipulation of the joint should include extension, flexion, abduction and adduction. When extending the joint, care should be taken not to stress the elbow also, as pain from this joint might then confuse the interpretation. However, the elbow can be extended without stressing the shoulder and so this confusion should be resolved readily. Flexion of the shoulder should be carried out with the elbow in flexion and with it in extension. This may provide useful information since flexion of the shoulder with the elbow extended creates more tension in the biceps tendon of origin and so pain from this structure should be exacerbated by shoulder flexion with concurrent elbow extension. Palpation should also be undertaken during manipulation so that any changes in anatomy can be appreciated, e.g. scapulohumeral luxation or displacement of the biceps tendon of origin. Manipulation should also test joint stability to reveal such problems as luxation. The scapulohumeral joint is an enarthrodial joint and so has a large range of motion. Care should be taken not to mistake joint laxity for instability; if doubt exists, a comparison should always be made with the non-lame limb. Joint subluxation has been proposed as a cause of lameness resulting from instability (Bardet, 1998; Cook, 2003) and, although the clinical tests used to detect such instability are not universally accepted as reliable, the evidence for this and the condition as an entity is growing (Cook et al., 2005a,b).

Finally, a neurological evaluation is imperative as brachial plexus pathology can produce a thoracic limb lameness associated with pain on shoulder manipulation. In such cases, axillary pain may be suggestive but neurological deficits, such as a reduced withdrawal reflex, radial carpal extensor test, absent panniculus reflex ipsilaterally, or Horner's syndrome, are very suggestive of a brachial plexus problem.

Surgical approaches

Craniomedial approach

The craniomedial approach (see Operative Technique 17.1) is used relatively infrequently but is indicated for the following procedures:

- Exposure of the biceps brachii tendon of origin for treatment of:
  - Tendon rupture (partial or complete)
  - Medial displacement due to rupture of the transverse humeral ligament
  - Bicipital tenosynovitis
  - Traumatic shoulder luxation by means of bicipital transposition
- Exposure of the scapular tuberosity for treatment of avulsion fractures.

Craniolateral approach

Indications for a craniolateral approach (see Operative Technique 17.2) are limited but include:

- Exposure of the proximal humerus and scapular neck for treatment of scapulohumeral luxations
- Exposure of the spinatus muscle tendons of insertion for treatment of:
  - Infraspinatus contracture
  - Mineralization of the infraspinatus bursa
  - Mineralization of the supraspinatus tendon.

Caudolateral approach

The caudolateral approach (see Operative Technique 17.3) is perhaps the most frequently used open approach to the shoulder. Indications include:

- Exposure of the caudal humeral head for treatment of OCD
- Exposure of the caudal rim of the glenoid for treatment of osteochondrosis (osteochondral fragmentation) or fragmented osteophytes.

Arthroscopy

Indications

Arthroscopy is used increasingly in the shoulder joint. Advantages for arthroscopy of the shoulder include increased viewing of intra-articular structures, increased access, decreased morbidity and, with practice, decreased surgery time. Disadvantages are the necessary investment in equipment and expertise and the increased operative time when the operator is inexperienced. Indications for arthroscopy of the shoulder include:

- Diagnosis and treatment of OCD
- Diagnosis of shoulder instability syndrome
- Treatment of shoulder instability syndrome by thermal capsulorrhaphy
- Diagnosis of ruptures of biceps brachii tendon of origin
- Biceps brachii tenotomy or tenodesis
- Diagnosis and treatment of caudal glenoid osteochondral fragmentation
- Synovial biopsy.

Equipment and technique

For small dogs a 2.4 mm 25–30 degree foreoblique arthroscope is used, but for most dogs a 2.7 mm arthroscope is preferred (see Chapter 15a for details of equipment). In giant breeds, a 4 mm arthroscope can provide some advantages. The use of an instrument cannula is preferred, to facilitate instrument passage through the soft tissues lateral to the joint, and a selection of grasping forceps is useful for joints of different size. A radiofrequency unit is required for the thermal capsulorrhaphy (capsular shrinkage) technique for instability syndrome and also for tissue ablation (e.g. for biceps tenotomy).

The egress cannula is usually placed craniolaterally. In most cases, e.g. for diagnosis and treatment of OCD, a lateral arthroscopic portal is established with a caudolateral instrument portal. However, sometimes (e.g. for diagnostic arthroscopy in adult dogs with suspected soft tissue injury) a slightly more caudal ('laterocaudolateral') portal can provide better inspection of the craniolateral soft tissue structures. Occasionally, a craniomedial portal may need to be established using a push-through technique, although particular patient positioning with dorsiflexion of the dog's cervical spine is necessary to avoid interference between the arthroscope and the dog's head. Some surgeons are starting to use a suspended position for shoulder arthroscopy so that the joint is under distraction. The technique is described in Operative Technique 17.4.

Congenital/developmental scapulohumeral luxation

Although this condition is rare, there does appear to be a breed predisposition, with Toy Poodles and Shetland Sheepdogs being over-represented alongside some of the other toy breeds.

Affected dogs are usually presented for recurrent lameness, which develops at 3–10 months of age. Occasionally they will be presented after reaching skeletal maturity, following minor trauma. Patients characteristically adopt a begging posture, with the joint held partially flexed. In some cases the problem is bilateral and such dogs may be found to have much better developed hindquarters or even a tendency to try to walk upright on their pelvic limbs. The direction of luxation is invariably medial. This can easily be appreciated, as the acromion is much more prominent than normal owing to its lateral displacement.

Caudocranial radiographs will confirm medial luxation, while mediolateral projections will demonstrate a flattened or convex glenoid and a relatively large and flattened humeral head (Figure 17.2).

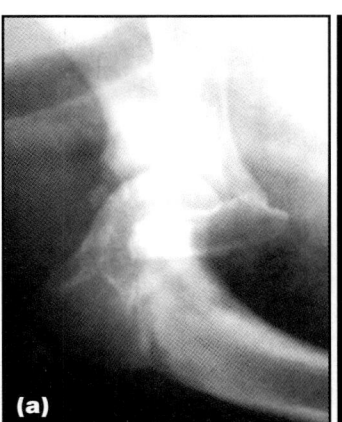

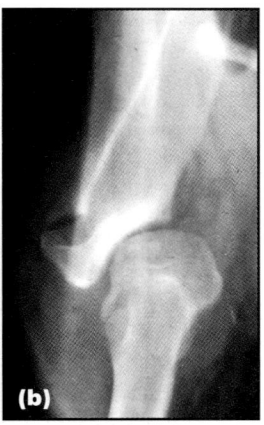

17.2 Congenital shoulder luxation. **(a)** Mediolateral and **(b)** caudocranial radiographs of the shoulder of a 9-month-old Keeshond, showing medial luxation. There is gross deformity of the articular surfaces, making the joint inherently unstable. (Courtesy of C Gibbs)

This type of luxation is not amenable to reduction because of the misshapen epiphyses. Attempts to try to stabilize the joint are prone to failure, due to this inherent incongruity. However, if the problem is diagnosed early, reduction may be possible and successful treatment by application of a closed pinning technique has been described (Read, 1994). In cases where reduction cannot be achieved, conservative measures are advisable. The joint tends to stabilize and the degree of lameness/incapacity improves as the dog matures. In general it may be anticipated that, by 1 year of age, these dogs will be somewhat disabled but pain-free and able to lead normal lives. If lameness persists, salvage procedures, such as excision arthroplasty or arthrodesis, should be considered.

Shoulder dysplasia

Shoulder dysplasia is a condition described as excessive joint laxity and has been documented as a cause of lameness in two single case reports, one involving a 3.5-year-old Collie and the other a 10-month-old Labrador Retriever. From such scant reports it is to be expected that, as a condition, it is quite rare. However, one of the authors has seen several dogs of chondrodystrophic breeds, most notably Bassett Hounds, presented for non-specific thoracic limb lameness with mild discomfort on shoulder extension. Radiographically they were found to have shallow glenoids and flattened humeral heads, as expected for the breed (Figure 17.3). No other abnormality could be found clinically or radiographically. The lameness was successfully managed by conservative means and, in the case of immature dogs, improvement seemed to occur as they reached skeletal maturity. Obviously this observation cannot establish shoulder dysplasia as a cause of thoracic limb lameness in these dogs but all other likely diagnoses were ruled out as far as possible.

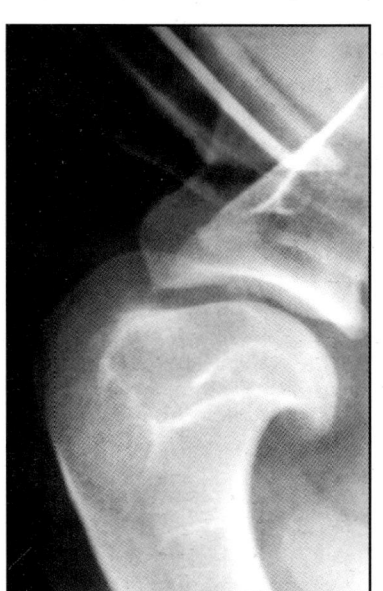

17.3 Shoulder dysplasia. Mediolateral radiograph of the left shoulder of a 3-year-old Bassett Hound that showed intermittent lameness associated with shoulder pain. The glenoid appears shallow and the humeral head flattened.

Osteochondrosis

Osteochondrosis generally involves the articular cartilage covering the medial aspect of the caudal third of the humeral head although, uncommonly, the caudal rim of the glenoid may also be involved (see later). The under-run cartilage of the humeral head may split vertically, causing flap formation, whereupon the term

215

Chapter 17   The shoulder

osteochondritis dissecans (OCD) becomes appropriate. If such a flap is formed, it may become mineralized and thus visible radiographically. In addition, it may break free and form a 'joint mouse', which can absorb nutrients from the synovial fluid, grow and possibly become mineralized. Occasionally such 'fragments' will migrate later in life into the biceps tendon sheath and cause lameness necessitating their late removal. Once the flap has become detached the defect may fill in with granulation tissue which is then converted into fibrocartilage.

Signalment and history
The condition shows a breed predisposition, with giant breeds such as Great Dane, Pyrenean Mountain Dog and Irish Wolfhound being over-represented. However, medium-sized breeds such as Labrador Retriever, Golden Retriever and Bernese Mountain Dog are also affected, as are some smaller breeds such as Border Collie. Although the ratio of males to females varies between reports, there is a general consensus that more males are affected clinically. One large retrospective study (Rudd et al., 1990) gave a male:female ratio of 2.24:1. In clinical cases the condition is found to be radiographically bilateral in just over 50% of cases.

The lameness usually begins when the dog is between 4 and 7 months of age, although the owners may delay presentation of the patient because the onset is somewhat insidious. This age of onset might be expected since it is the period of most rapid growth. However, in one study, 36% of dogs were over 1 year of age at the time of diagnosis (Rudd et al., 1990). Thus, the condition should not be excluded as a cause of shoulder lameness simply because a dog is older than 12 months. The degree of lameness varies but is usually mild to moderate and may be intermittent. The owner will usually report that the lameness deteriorates with exercise and that there is stiffness after rest, particularly following exercise. Restriction of exercise tends to improve the lameness.

Clinical findings
A weightbearing lameness is generally evident, although if both shoulders are clinically affected the dog might show more of a stiff shuffling thoracic limb gait rather than an overt lameness. Disuse atrophy, especially of the spinatus muscles, may be present and make the scapular spine more prominent. Pain is usually elicited on extension of the joint.

Diagnosis
Diagnosis is generally confirmed by radiography. A mediolateral projection of the extended shoulder will usually suffice (Figure 17.4) but occasionally inwardly and/or outwardly rotated views may prove necessary to skyline the lesion. Changes that may be observed on plain radiographs in cases involving the humeral head include:

- A subchondral defect with flattening of the caudal humeral head
- A sclerotic margin to any such defect
- The presence of a cartilage flap (only visible if mineralized)

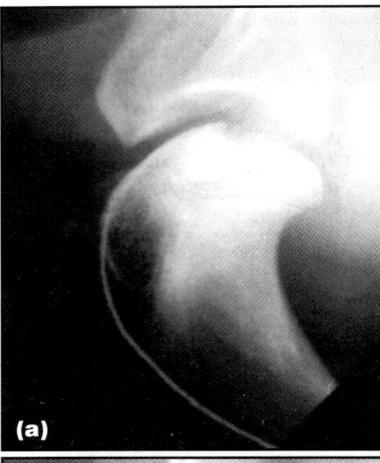

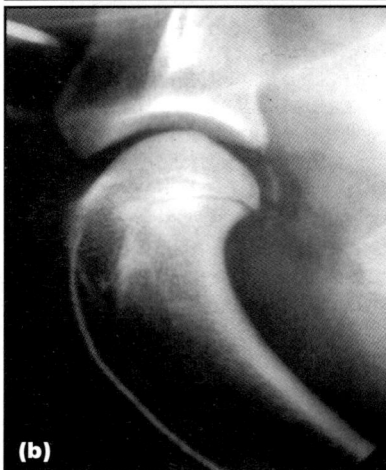

17.4 Radiographic appearance of shoulder OCD. **(a)** Mediolateral radiograph of the shoulder of an 11-month-old Great Dane. A subchondral defect is clearly present in the caudal humeral head, with a sclerotic margin. **(b)** Mediolateral radiograph of the shoulder of an 11-month-old Border Collie. The caudal humeral head appears flattened and a mineralized cartilage flap is evident in the caudal joint space.

- The presence of 'joint mice' (only visible if mineralized), most commonly found in the caudal recess of the joint
- Secondary osteoarthritis, most often seen as osteophyte formation on the caudal borders of the glenoid and/or the humeral head.

It is always worth radiographing both shoulders as the problem is often bilateral. This may be helpful in cases that have suffered subclinical osteochondrosis in one shoulder and then developed a clinical lameness due to the same problem in the second limb. The changes in the latter may not yet have developed or be quite subtle, and finding changes in the 'normal' limb helps to reinforce the clinical picture with respect to diagnosis of osteochondrosis in the lame limb.

In addition to the above changes, van Bree (1992) has described the 'vacuum phenomenon' in shoulder osteochondrosis. This refers to the appearance of gaseous collections in the articular space, creating an image resembling a negative arthrogram. This change was noted in 20 of 100 radiographs of shoulders affected by osteochondrosis and never in 30 radiographically normal contralateral joints; it could not be induced in 36 normal shoulder joints radiographed in full extension. The phenomenon is found in addition to other radiographic changes and so should be added to the list of other possible findings rather than being considered as a separate entity.

Chapter 17 The shoulder

Positive contrast arthrography (Figure 17.5) may help to assess whether a non-mineralized cartilage flap or 'joint mouse' is present. Some reports have suggested that the findings might help determine whether a case should be treated conservatively or surgically. To date there are no clear data to suggest that arthrography can predict the outcome in a joint causing clinical problems. In the case of bilateral osteochondrosis, arthrography has been shown to be of some use in predicting the likely outcome for the clinically 'silent' joint, i.e. the shoulder showing radiographic signs but no clinical lameness at the time of initial diagnosis following surgical treatment of the lame shoulder (van Bree, 1992). Of those dogs with a detectable, loose cartilage flap in the 'silent' joint, 50% became lame at a later date and required surgery on that limb. No surgery was required in those joints that had no cartilage flap or where one had detached and fallen into the caudal pouch of the joint. It is still questionable whether this information helps very much, since a 'wait and see' policy with respect to the second limb would produce the same long-term results.

Arthroscopy may be used to examine the articular surface and, as well as confirming radiographically diagnosed OCD (Figure 17.6), it may detect fissures in the cartilage that are not evident on arthrography.

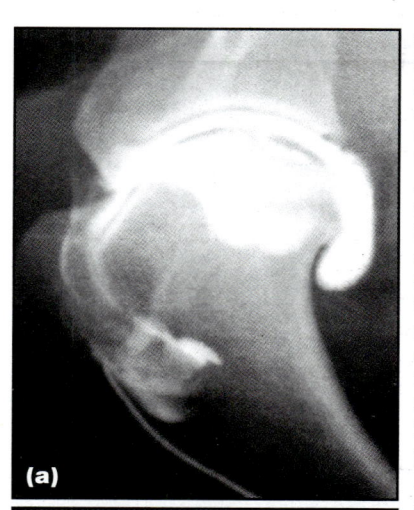

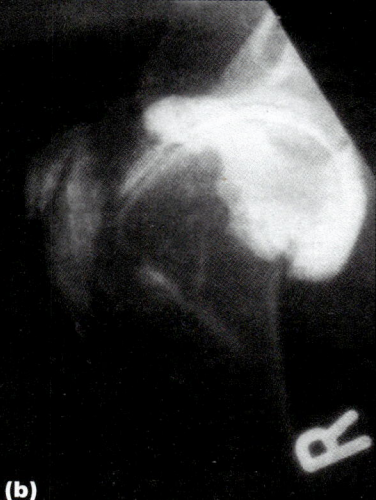

17.5 **(a)** Mediolateral arthrogram of the Great Dane in Figure 17.4. A low dose of contrast medium is required, otherwise the articular surface of interest becomes obliterated; with such a low dose the tendon sheath of the biceps brachii is often poorly filled. **(b)** A low-dose normal arthrogram for comparison. Note the intact cartilage line over the humeral head.

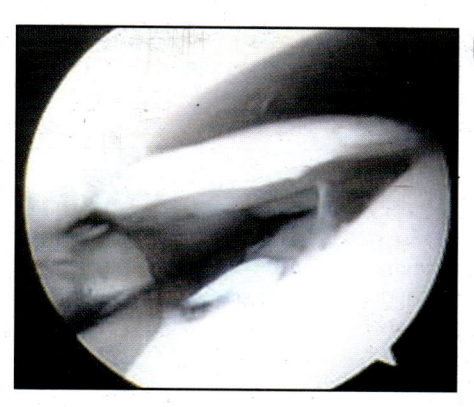

17.6 Arthroscopic view of an OCD lesion.

Conservative treatment

Conservative treatment will resolve the lameness in some cases, and 6–8 weeks of controlled (lead) exercise may be worth trying in the first instance. Although it could be argued that cases with small subchondral defects and/or no evidence of flap formation on arthrography might be more likely to respond to such measures, there is no documented evidence to support such a concept. If such measures are continued then the majority of cases will eventually become sound, but this may take several months and the resulting secondary osteoarthritis might be more pronounced. Whilst these dogs are being rested it may be necessary to prescribe a non-steroidal anti-inflammatory drug (NSAID) to prevent excessive discomfort. Some authors advocate a regime of vigorous exercise for these dogs, with the aim of promoting detachment of the cartilage flap and resolution of the lameness once the subchondral defect has filled in with fibrocartilage. The results following conservative measures are poorly documented but in one report by Vaughan and Jones (1968), of 22 dogs treated in this way only 12 became sound. The use of polysulphated glycosaminoglycan preparations, such as sodium pentosan polysulphate, has been advocated, but there has been no documented evidence that it produces an improvement beyond those expected with restricted exercise alone.

Surgical treatment

Surgical treatment is indicated if a positive diagnosis has been reached and 6–8 weeks of conservative management have failed to resolve the lameness. Surgery is preferred to further conservative management because the success rate is high and the period of convalescence relatively short. The majority of patients will be sound by 6–8 weeks after surgery but some, seemingly those with very large lesions, have been known to take up to 4–5 months to become sound. In bilateral lameness the contralateral limb may be treated simultaneously or surgery may be staged, with a 6–8 week interval. In many instances the contralateral lameness appears to resolve during the period of convalescence that follows the initial surgery, possibly because there is increased weightbearing on the limb and this encourages detachment of the cartilage flap.

The aim of surgery is to remove the detached articular cartilage; this can be achieved by arthrotomy or arthroscopically. A caudal approach to the joint provides good exposure of the affected portion of the humeral

Chapter 17 The shoulder

head. Arthroscopic removal of shoulder OCD lesions was first described by Van Ryssen et al. (1993). Arthroscopy reduces the morbidity of the procedure and hence aids recovery. In addition, arthroscopy allows for a greater inspection of the joint and retrieval of joint mice from unusual positions (e.g. biceps tendon sheath, medial to glenoid or caudal joint recess). It has been advocated in some reports as being less invasive than arthrotomy, so having a lower incidence of postoperative seroma formation and producing a more cosmetic result, whilst achieving the same long-term results (Meyer-Lindenberg et al., 2002). The disadvantages of arthroscopy are the increased equipment costs and the expertise required. Although the inexperienced arthroscopist may take longer with arthroscopic removal of OCD lesions compared with open surgery, the technique becomes just as quick, if not quicker, with practice.

Removal of the cartilage flap with curettage of the resulting subchondral defect is aimed at facilitating repair of the defect. Such repair is generally in the form of fibrocartilage and the cells responsible for this are pluripotential mesenchymal cells that come from subchondral bone. Hence, curettage is aimed at producing a bleeding bed in the defect to facilitate cell migration.

Arthrotomy
A caudolateral approach is used. If 'joint mice' have been identified elsewhere in the joint, additional approaches may be required but such a situation is rare. The technique is described in Operative Technique 17.5. Bilateral arthrotomies can be performed under the same general anaesthetic, if required, but this is not commonly indicated.

Arthroscopy
A lateral arthroscopy portal is used with a caudolateral instrument portal and craniolateral egress portal. Once the instrument portal is established, the use of an instrument portal cannula is optional. Grasping forceps are introduced and a section of the cartilage flap is grasped. The forceps are twisted to break this section of cartilage from the remainder of the flap; grasping forceps that have long jaws can expedite this process. It can be tempting to try to remove the whole flap having grasped its edge, but this can often lead to the flap breaking as it is drawn through the joint capsule. If this occurs, the loose flap can be difficult to grasp as it floats around the joint. Once the flap is removed, a curette or manual shaver is used to subject the defect to light curettage. The joint recesses are checked for joint mice prior to removal of the arthroscope. It is perfectly possible to perform bilateral shoulder arthroscopies under one anaesthetic if required.

Postoperative care
Following open surgery or arthroscopy, the dog should be restricted to lead exercise and room rest for 6–8 weeks whilst healing of the cartilage defect takes place. The distance walked is governed only by what does not make the patient significantly worse (in terms of degree of lameness or stiffness after rest). After that period most patients will be sound and can be returned to normal exercise over the following month.

Prognosis
Following removal of an OCD flap and any resulting 'joint mice', Clayton Jones and Vaughan (1970) reported that 28 of 29 cases recovered full use of their operated limb with no lameness, whilst Rudd et al. (1990) found that 30 of 40 dogs treated surgically became sound.

Un-united caudal glenoid

In some cases with the signalment and clinical features given for osteochondrosis, radiography will show lack of fusion of the centre of ossification relating to the caudal rim of the glenoid (Olivieri et al., 1999). Arthroscopy may be used to confirm the presence of a separate mobile part of the glenoid (Figure 17.7). Surgical removal appears to resolve the lameness if conservative measures fail to do so.

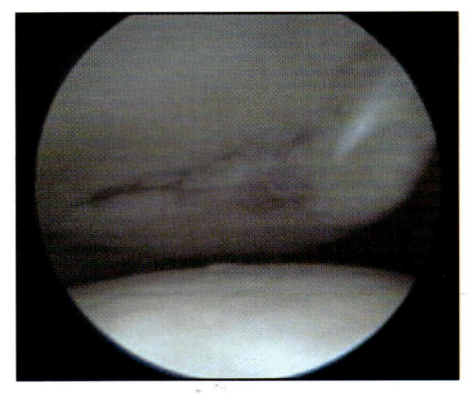

17.7 Arthroscopic view of a displaced, un-united centre of ossification of the caudal rim of the glenoid in a dog.

Luxations

Scapulohumeral luxation
Luxation of the shoulder is an uncommon condition. It may be overdiagnosed because on manipulation of the normal shoulder joint an audible click may be misinterpreted as joint laxity. Scapulohumeral luxation results in loss of joint function, a decreased range of joint movement and pain on manipulation, which decreases as the condition becomes chronic.

Acquired luxations are usually associated with a fall or knock, particularly when a dog turns at speed. The direction of luxation is generally lateral or medial. It has been said that the smaller breeds tend to suffer medial luxation whilst lateral luxations are seen more in the larger breeds. However, a review of the literature suggests there is no correlation and each case should be judged on its own merit. Cranial and caudal luxations are rarely encountered. Cranial luxations may be associated with rupture of the transverse humeral ligament allowing displacement of the biceps brachii tendon and loss of cranial support (see Medial luxation of the biceps brachii tendon).

Clinical findings
Affected dogs will be presented with a history of acute-onset severe (usually non-weightbearing) thoracic limb lameness as a consequence of moderate to severe trauma. The elbow is held flexed and adducted, with the distal limb held abducted in cases of medial luxation and

Chapter 17 The shoulder

adducted if the luxation is lateral. There may be palpable asymmetry between the acromion and greater tubercle when compared with the contralateral limb. In more longstanding cases, especially those with recurrent luxation that reduce spontaneously and cause an intermittent lameness, muscle atrophy may be noted. Manipulation will reveal a reduced range of movement and pain on extension or flexion. In some cases the luxation will reduce spontaneously on manipulation of the joint, particularly when the patient is positioned for radiography. It is, therefore, important not to rely on radiography for a definitive diagnosis but, rather, to evaluate the joint stability clinically. This is done by holding the scapula in a fixed position whilst the joint is flexed, extended, rotated, abducted and adducted. It is imperative that any suspected abnormality is evaluated by comparison with the contralateral limb as instability can easily be misdiagnosed, particularly when the dog is sedated or anaesthetized for radiography.

The possibility of concurrent injuries should be considered. Crepitation might suggest a fracture, while neurological deficits might indicate brachial plexus involvement (particularly in lateral luxations).

Diagnosis
Standard mediolateral and caudocranial radiographic projections (Figures 17.8) are used to assess the direction of luxation, the contour of the joint surfaces, osteophyte formation and the existence of concurrent fractures. Since shoulder luxations have a tendency to reduce spontaneously during positioning for radiography, plain radiographs may show no abnormality. If the instability is clearly evident clinically radiography might be used simply to screen the joint for complicating factors. If, however, radiographs are required to demonstrate the instability, then stressed views may be required. These can be difficult to obtain and views of both limbs must be taken for comparison as the range of 'normal' appearance is great.

Arthrography might be employed to establish whether leakage of contrast medium occurs and to determine the site of joint capsule tearing. Some care should be taken in the interpretation of such films, as there are normal capsular extensions under the tendons of the cuff muscles and some of the contrast often leaks back along the needle. It must be stressed that the most reliable test for instability is clinical manipulation; radiography should be used, in this respect, only as a last resort.

The direction of luxation is important in determining the method of stabilization. If the luxation is longstanding then the joint surfaces may show remodelling, in which case stability may be more difficult to establish, or osteophytes may be present indicating secondary osteoarthritis. Both these will tend to make the prognosis worse. If concurrent fractures are present they may interfere with reduction or inherent stability and indicate the need for open reduction and fixation.

Conservative treatment
This is generally successful where luxation has not previously occurred and there are no concurrent fractures. Closed reduction is generally possible, followed by external support. A Velpeau sling (see Figure 17.9) should be employed in medial luxations, as this creates lateral pressure on the humeral head, thus maintaining the reduction. A non-weightbearing sling (see Figure 17.10) is used for lateral luxations or in cases where the direction is uncertain. Alternatively a body cast may be used. This is best fitted in the conscious dog with the limb in a weightbearing position so that the cast can be closely applied, otherwise it may not serve its purpose and/or be uncomfortable for the dog. Whichever method is used, the joint should always be re-radiographed following application of the sling or cast to ensure that reduction has been achieved and maintained. The external support is maintained for 2–6 weeks to allow the soft tissues to heal, and exercise is restricted for a further 2–4 weeks after removal of the support.

Surgical treatment
Surgical treatment is required if the luxation is recurrent or a fracture fragment has to be re-attached or removed. There are several techniques described in the literature, all of which aim to re-establish collateral support for the joint (see Operative Techniques 17.6, 17.7 and 17.8).

For restoration of both lateral and medial support, a combination of lateral and medial shoulder stabilization may be used by combining Operative Techniques 17.6 and 17.7. However, it is possible for one prosthesis to serve both functions. A craniolateral approach is used, but with elevation and cranial retraction of the supraspinatus muscle. A need to reflect the acromial head of

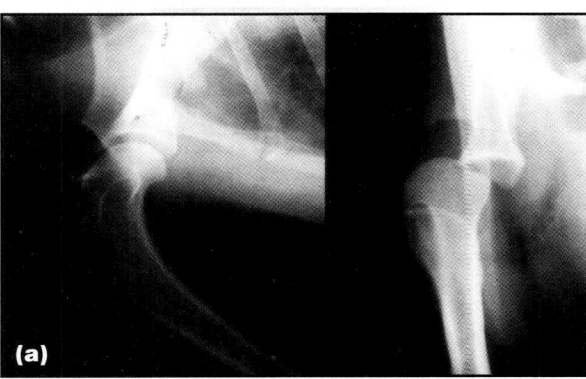

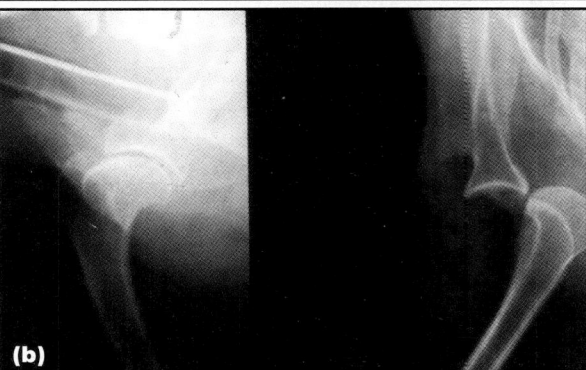

17.8 Acquired shoulder luxation. **(a)** Mediolateral and caudocranial radiographs of the shoulder of a 2-year-old Yorkshire Terrier, showing lateral luxation as a result of being attacked by another dog. Note the 'normality' of the joint in the mediolateral view. (Courtesy of ARS Barr) **(b)** Mediolateral and craniocaudal radiographs of a shoulder of a 12-year-old Shetland Sheepdog, showing medial luxation resulting from the dog being 'extracted' from under an armchair.

Chapter 17 The shoulder

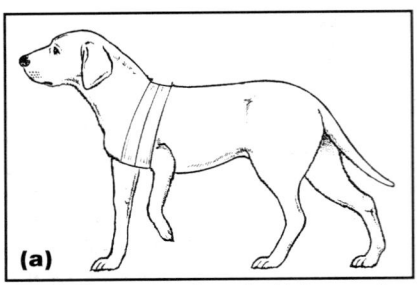

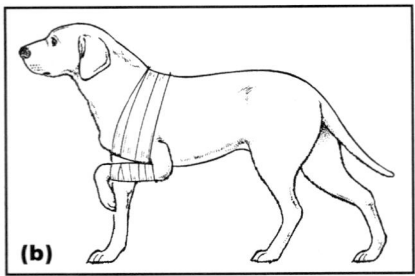

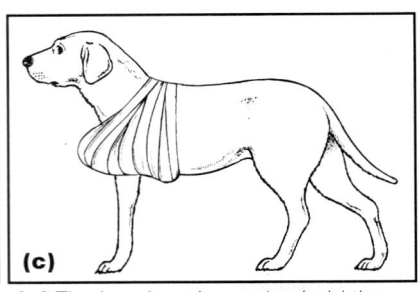

17.9 Application of a Velpeau sling for treatment of medial shoulder luxations. **(a)** The bandage is used to hold the distal humerus adducted against the chest wall. **(b)** Cotton wool is placed around the antebrachium for padding. **(c)** The entire limb is enclosed in the bandage, including the cranial aspect, so that the dog does not step out of the sling. Reproduced from the *BSAVA Manual of Small Animal Arthrology*.

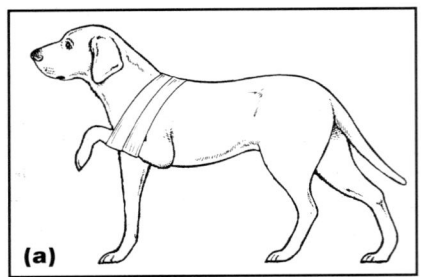

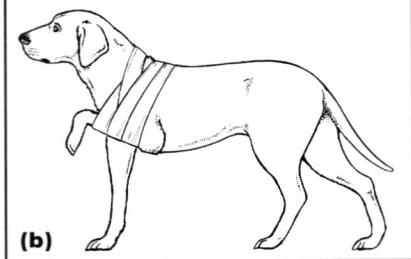

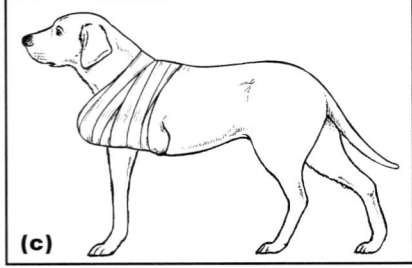

17.10 Application of a non-weightbearing sling for treatment of lateral shoulder luxations. **(a,b)** The distal limb is flexed and the antebrachium bandaged to the body. **(c)** The entire limb is enclosed, including the cranial aspect, so that the dog does not step out of the sling. Reproduced from the *BSAVA Manual of Small Animal Arthrology*.

the deltoid muscle by tenotomy or acromial osteotomy is often stated but is not often necessary. Transverse tunnels are then created in a lateral to medial direction through the scapular neck (cranial to the scapular spine and avoiding the suprascapular nerve) and through the greater tubercle (starting at a point close to the insertion of the teres minor tendon). With the aid of wire loops, the prosthesis is placed from lateral to medial through the scapula, and then from medial to lateral through the humerus (see Operative Technique 17.6). Access to the medial ostia of the bone tunnels is facilitated by cranial retraction of the supraspinatus muscle; it can be improved further by osteotomy of the greater tubercle, but this is usually avoidable. The prosthesis is then drawn tight, but not too tight (during tightening, any restriction of flexion or extension is repeatedly checked and avoided), and secured with either a knot or a crimp. Closure is as described in Operative Technique 17.2. If osteotomy of the greater tubercle has been performed then reattachment using a lagged bone screw, crossed Kirschner wires or a pin and tension band wire is required.

Although it is often considered appropriate to restore the lateral support in medial luxations and medial support in lateral luxations (or both in either), one of the authors [SB] routinely replaces only the lateral support for luxations in either direction unless the joint is grossly unstable on reduction.

Following surgery, the dog should be restricted to lead exercise and room rest for 6–8 weeks, whilst fibrosis around the prosthesis becomes established. The distance walked is governed only by what does not make the patient significantly worse (in terms of degree of lameness or stiffness after rest). After that period most cases should be sound and can be returned to normal exercise over the following month.

Prognosis

Maintaining reduction of an acquired shoulder luxation may be problematical. If conservative measures fail, surgery should be undertaken but the prognosis remains only fair to good for a return to complete normality, particularly in cases with medial luxation. In general it is often found that if surgery has failed to maintain reduction then revision surgery is also prone to failure, unless a definite reason for failure has been identified. In these cases, it may be more appropriate to consider a salvage procedure, such as arthrodesis or excision arthroplasty. One potential method of helping to prevent reluxation after surgery to recreate collateral support is to place a transarticular pin across the joint from distal to proximal for a period of 4–6 weeks (Figure 17.11).

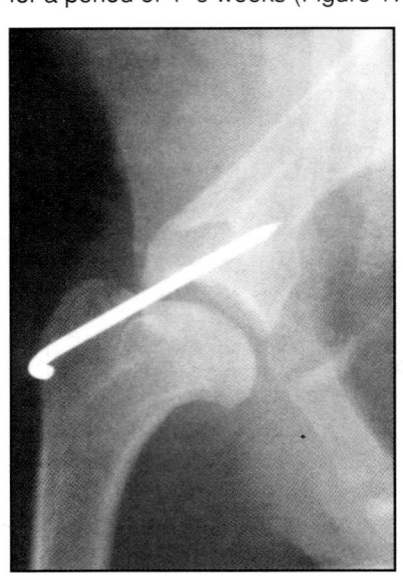

17.11 Mediolateral postoperative radiograph of a 9-year-old Toy Poodle following placement of a transarticular pin to stabilize a medial subluxation after revision surgery to replace a collateral prosthesis. The first prosthesis used had failed after 2 weeks. The pin was left in place for 4 weeks and the shoulder remained stable.

Chapter 17 The shoulder

Dorsal luxation of the scapula
This is an uncommon condition, which is invariably a result of trauma causing rupture of the serratus ventralis muscle and possibly additional tearing of the trapezius, rhomboideus, teres major and latissimus dorsi muscles. Diagnosis is based on the clinical appearance of dorsal displacement of the scapula which is clearly evident on weightbearing.

Treatment requires a caudolateral approach to allow re-apposition of the torn muscles and reattachment of any avulsed muscles to the scapula using sutures of stainless steel wire or nylon by way of bone tunnels. Further support is usually required and the caudal edge of the scapula may be attached to one or more of the underlying ribs using stainless steel wire. Postoperatively, the limb is supported in flexion for 2–3 weeks and exercise is restricted for 6 weeks. The prognosis appears to be reasonably good.

Medial luxation of the biceps brachii tendon
This is an uncommon cause of lameness that has been reported in racing Greyhounds, a German Shepherd Dog, an Afghan Hound and a Border Collie (Bennett and Campbell, 1979; Goring *et al.*, 1984; Fox and Bray, 1992; Boemo and Eaton-Wells, 1995). Lameness is gradual in onset and worsens with exercise. There may be evidence of pain and/or crepitus on shoulder manipulation. As the shoulder is flexed the tendon may be felt to 'pop' out of the intertubercular groove in a medial direction and then return to its normal position on extension of the joint. There may be an associated luxation of the shoulder joint due to loss of cranial support (Figure 17.12a).

This displacement of the biceps tendon follows rupture of the transverse humeral ligament. Treatment involves relocation and retention of the tendon in the intertubercular groove (Figure 17.12b) using a cranial approach. A recently suggested technique involves placement of a partially threaded bone screw in the lesser tubercle, medial to the tendon (McKee and Macias, 2004). The shank of the screw and the ensuing fibrous reaction prevent re-luxation of the tendon.

The prognosis for a return to full work has to be guarded.

17.12 Medial displacement of the biceps brachii tendon of origin. **(a)** Mediolateral radiograph of a 3-year-old Border Collie's shoulder after he had collided with another dog whilst working. Cranial displacement of the humerus (cranial subluxation) is evident and was associated with medial displacement of the biceps brachii tendon. **(b)** Postoperative radiograph following relocation of the tendon in the intertubercular groove and the use of orthopaedic wire to replace the restraining transverse humeral ligament. (Courtesy of HR Denny) Alternatively, the biceps tendon can be replaced through a craniomedial approach and stabilized by placement of two bone screws around which are anchored several sutures.

Muscle-related disease

Contracture of the infraspinatus (or supraspinatus)
This uncommon condition may involve dogs of any breed or age, but most cases are in medium-sized working dogs or particularly active pets (Bennett, 1986). The infraspinatus is affected much more frequently than the supraspinatus (Vaughan, 1979). A traumatic aetiology is suspected, since histological examination shows evidence of haemorrhage, degeneration, atrophy and fibrosis. On careful questioning, the owner will often reveal that the dog had a previous acute onset lameness, usually starting at or soon after exercise, which improved over the following few days. The current progressive lameness then developed a few weeks later.

Clinical findings
Dogs do not show discomfort and are still keen to exercise. When they are standing, the limb may be positioned normally, though in chronic cases it may be held slightly adducted at the elbow with abduction of the foot (Figure 17.13). At a walk and trot there is

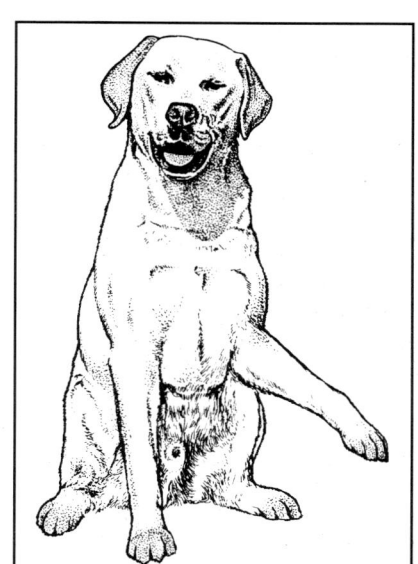

17.13 Patients with contracture of the infraspinatus muscle may adopt this typical posture when sitting. The elbow is held adducted with the distal limb externally rotated. Reproduced from the *BSAVA Manual of Small Animal Arthrology*.

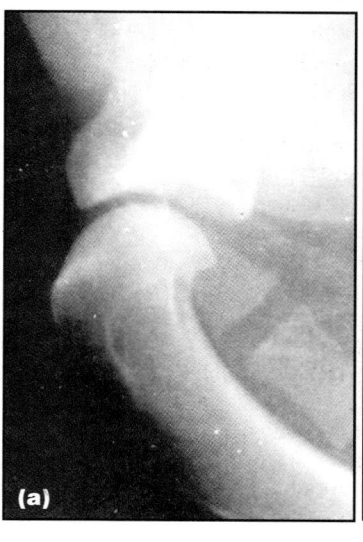

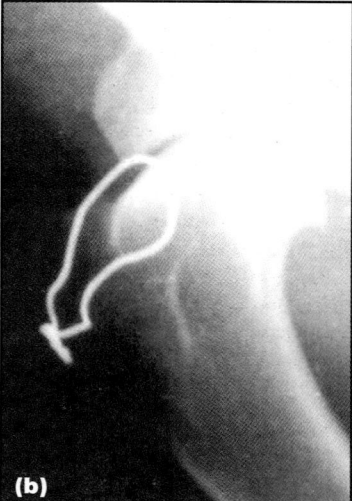

Chapter 17 The shoulder

obvious circumduction of the limb on protraction and a flip-like extension of the paw as the limb moves forwards. Manipulation of the joint causes no pain but flexion is reduced. If the whole limb is flexed up, the antebrachium tends to deviate laterally from the body instead of remaining in a straight line. Palpation will normally reveal atrophy of the suprascapular muscles and possibly similar changes in other shoulder muscles. The condition may be bilateral.

Radiography
The mediolateral radiographic view may show a relative reduction in the width of the caudal joint space. In the caudocranial view there may be a reduction in the distance between the acromion or the rim of the glenoid and the greater tubercle of the humerus (Figure 17.14). It is useful to take similar views of the contralateral shoulder for comparison.

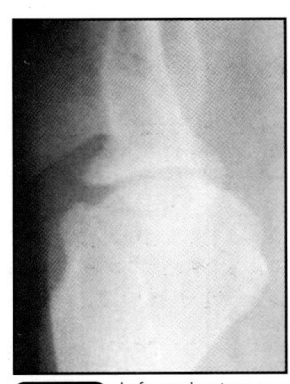

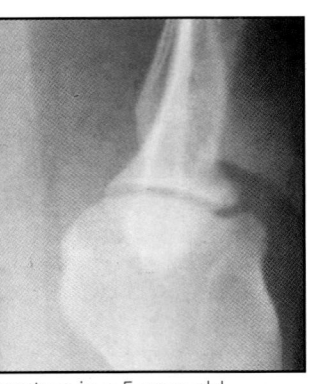

17.14 Infraspinatus contracture in a 5-year-old Labrador Retriever. Caudocranial radiographs of right and left shoulders. The dog had developed an acute-onset lameness several months previously, which had resolved, but then a gait abnormality consistent with infraspinatus contracture had developed over several weeks. The radiograph shows a reduction in the distance between the greater tubercle and the rim of the glenoid in the affected left shoulder.

Treatment
Treatment involves tenotomy of the affected tendon to restore a normal thoracic limb action. A lateral approach to the greater tubercle provides good exposure of the tendon, which appears scarred and fibrotic. The tendon is sectioned at its insertion; elevation from the joint capsule may require the breakdown of adhesions. Following this, normal movement of the joint should be restored immediately. The dog should be rested until the skin sutures are removed and then rapidly returned to a normal exercise regime to prevent the formation of adhesions. Following surgery the prognosis is favourable for a return to normal function. No recurrences have been recorded.

Teres minor myopathy
Lameness associated with shoulder pain was recorded in a 5-year-old working Labrador Retriever (Bruce *et al.*, 1997). Ultrasonography suggested pathology in the teres minor muscle. After conservative management failed to improve the lameness, surgical excision of the muscle led to complete recovery. Histopathology confirmed a diagnosis of teres minor myopathy.

Tendon/ligament-related disease

The aetiology of these conditions is poorly understood but is thought to be related to trauma, often of a repetitive nature. Another possibility would be that it is a manifestation of osteoarthritis of the shoulder, particularly in the case of bicipital tenosynovitis, whereby adhesions form between the tendon and the joint capsule in the region of the intertubercular groove as a part of the overall arthropathy.

The conditions are generally seen in the older, medium- to large-breed dogs although smaller breeds may sometimes be affected. The onset of lameness may be acute (following a particularly active period of exercise) or more chronic and insidious. The dogs affected often lead active lives, e.g. they may have a habit of digging or scrambling up canal banks. The owners will often report a lameness that deteriorates with excessive exercise but improves with rest, although there may be some stiffness for a few minutes on rising.

The degree of lameness may range from mild to quite severe and pain will be evident on manipulation of the shoulder. Flexion of the joint stresses the biceps tendon, especially if the elbow is kept extended, and may exacerbate the pain. Full extension of the joint also seems to cause discomfort, but this may be because of the pressure applied to the cranial aspect of the proximal humerus when such a manipulation is performed. Direct pressure applied over a particular tendon or ligament may produce evidence of 'point pain' that can help to determine the likely structure involved. Evaluation of instability in cases suspected of having collateral insufficiency is probably best reserved for the anaesthetized patient. Patients vary in their 'normal' reactions to such manipulations and a comparison of both thoracic limbs should always be made.

Conservative treatment, with strict rest for 4–6 weeks, may improve the clinical signs. Systemic NSAIDs may help during this period. If such measures fail, the injection of 20–60 mg of methylprednisolone (40 mg for a dog of about 30 kg) either around the tendon itself or into the joint under strict asepsis, followed by 4 weeks' strict rest and then a gradual return to normal exercise, may alleviate the signs. The response to such an injection is usually quite rapid, although the patient may be more uncomfortable for a few days following investigation and injection. In one study (Butterworth, 2003) about 50% of cases treated for non-specific shoulder lameness (where the clinical and radiographic features were consistent with those described above but a definitive diagnosis was never made) showed long-term improvement. In other cases there may be temporary improvement, which still serves to confirm the shoulder is the source of lameness. When a specific tendon is implicated on clinical examination, personal observation suggests that some dogs respond better to peritendinous injection of methylprednisolone whilst others respond more favourably when it is administered intra-articularly.

Bicipital tendinitis/tenosynovitis
The clinical diagnosis of bicipital tendinitis/tenosynovitis is difficult (Lincoln and Potter, 1984), particularly with respect to differentiation of this from such conditions

Chapter 17 The shoulder

as glenohumeral ligament pathology and mineralizing supraspinatus tendinopathy (see below).

Plain radiographs may demonstrate new bone deposition superimposed on the greater tubercle, which may be located within the intertubercular groove (Figure 17.15a,b). In some instances minor lucencies may be observed superimposed on the greater tubercle. The significance of these changes has been brought into question by the fact that many normal dogs, without clinical lameness, show similar changes.

Arthrography may demonstrate poor filling of the tendon sheath due to adhesions and confirm the diagnosis (Figure 17.15c,d). Unfortunately, as in human patients, radiographs (including arthrograms) may appear normal. This is not surprising when one considers that it is secondary changes that are being observed, rather than the primary problem.

Ultrasonography has been investigated as a diagnostic technique; although studies in the past (Rivers *et al.*, 1992) suggested it was less sensitive than arthrography, a more recent study (Kramer *et al.*, 2001) has suggested it can be used reliably to detect pathology of the biceps tendon.

Arthroscopy was first suggested as a means of evaluating the biceps tendon by Person (1986). Since then it has become the 'gold standard' for diagnosing bicipital tendinitis/tenosynovitis (Figure 17.16) as well as several other conditions of the shoulder joint (Bardet, 1999).

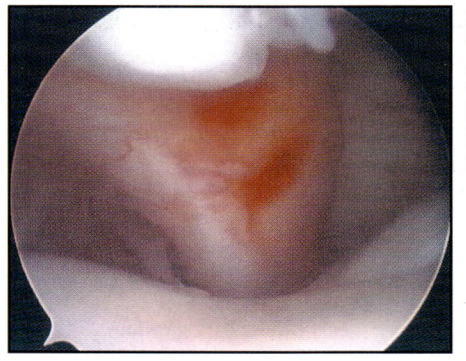

17.16 Arthroscopic view of biceps tendinitis/tenosynovitis.

Treatment
Surgical management should be considered if conservative measures (detailed above) fail. Tenodesis or tenotomy of the biceps brachii tendon of origin may be contemplated as a treatment for:

- Bicipital tendinitis/tenosynovitis when conservative measures have failed to improve the lameness
- Partial or complete rupture of the biceps tendon of origin, as the primary treatment in acute or chronic cases
- Displacement of the biceps tendon from the intertubercular groove as a result of rupture of the intertubercular ligament (tenodesis as an alternative to replacement of the ruptured ligament).

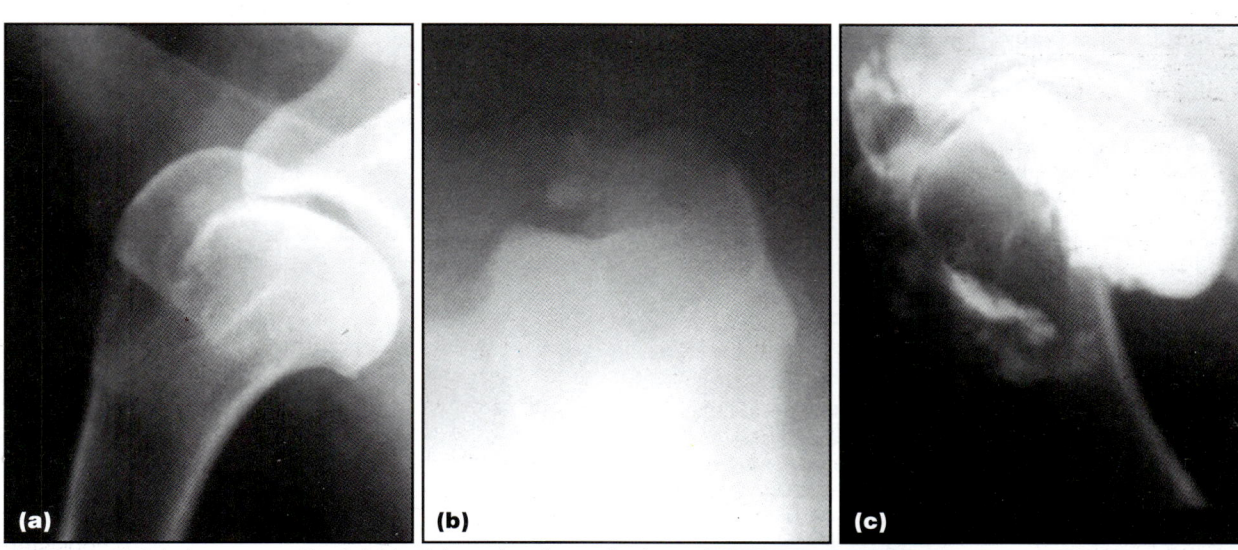

17.15 Bicipital tenosynovitis. **(a)** Mediolateral radiograph of a 12-year-old Border Collie with thoracic limb lameness associated with pain on shoulder extension or direct pressure applied over the biceps tendon. There is new bone deposition superimposed on the greater tubercle, possibly in the region of the intertubercular groove. **(b)** A tangential view shows osteophytes medial to the greater tubercle. **(c)** Mediolateral arthrogram (post-injection of 6 ml of contrast medium) of a shoulder of a 7-year-old Airedale that was showing similar signs to the dog in (a). There is poor filling of the bicipital tendon sheath. **(d)** A normal arthrogram for comparison.

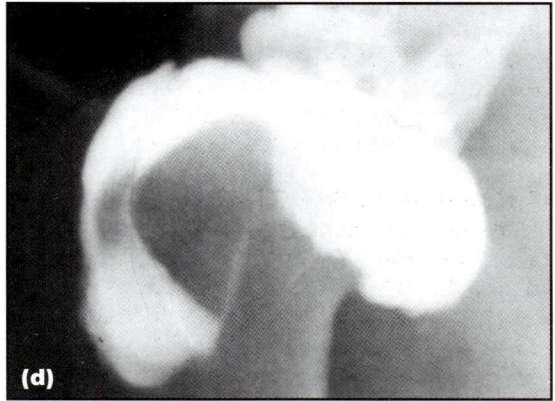

Chapter 17 The shoulder

The tendon is exposed using a cranial approach. Several methods exist (see Operative Technique 17.8) and there are insufficient numbers of cases recorded to establish which of the techniques, if any, is most appropriate. Advocates of tenodesis suggest that securing the biceps tendon proximally is likely to result in a more rapid and predictable return to function. It has also been reported that some dogs remain lame after tenotomy but improve after subsequent tenodesis. Stobie *et al.* (1995) reported excellent or good outcomes for all 14 dogs treated for this condition by tenodesis after medical treatment had failed.

The investigation and diagnosis of this disease will often involve arthroscopic examination of the biceps tendon (see Figure 17.16). Tenotomy can be achieved with standard camera and instrument portals (Holsworth *et al.*, 2002) and this has been reported to produce results comparable to tenodesis. The instrument portal is craniolateral, with a lateral arthroscope portal. The biceps tendon is transected using an arthroscopic blade (or a No. 11 blade) or a radiofrequency probe. Arthroscopic tenotomy and tenodesis have also been described (Cook *et al.*, 2004).

The dog should be rested for between 4 and 6 weeks after surgery.

Rupture of the biceps tendon sheath

In some dogs with clinical signs as described above, arthrography will show leakage of contrast agent from the distal portion of the tendon sheath (Figure 17.17). If conservative management (as described above) fails to improve the lameness, surgery to promote biceps tenodesis (see Operative Technique 17.8) has been reported to improve matters (Innes and Brown, 2004). No other pathology was recognized arthroscopically in either of the two cases but, in one, the resected tendon was submitted for histopathology and revealed concomitant bicipital tendinopathy. Given that tenodesis could improve lameness resulting from tendinopathy, the significance of the sheath rupture may be brought into question in terms of its association with lameness.

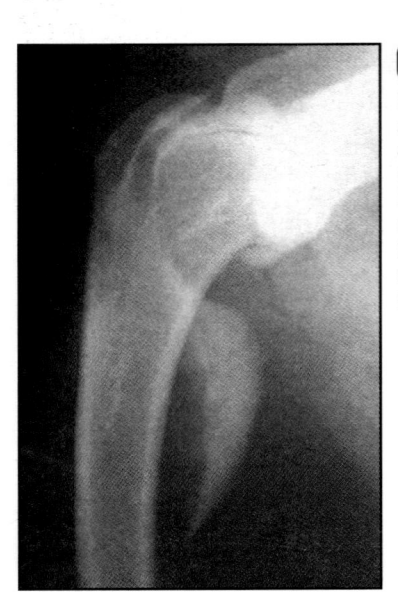

17.17 Mediolateral arthrogram from a 4-year-old Border Collie, showing leakage of contrast agent from the biceps tendon sheath, indicating rupture.

Supraspinatus mineralizing tendinopathy

In some dogs with clinical signs as described above, radiographs show new bone deposition along the cranial edge of the greater tubercle or superimposed on it (Figure 17.18a). This represents mineralization within the tendon of the supraspinatus muscle. Such changes may be seen in many clinically normal dogs but the associated tendinopathy has been reported as a cause of thoracic limb lameness (Muir and Johnson, 1994; Kriegleder, 1995). It is possible that when this condition is associated with lameness it is because of encroachment of the mineralized tissue on the biceps tendon or its sheath (Figure 17.18b). Of those cases that fail to improve with conservative management (as described above) some will improve after surgical removal of the mineralized tissue (Flo and Middleton, 1990; Muir *et al.*, 1996; Laitinen and Flo, 2000). A more recently suggested treatment involves extracorporeal shock wave therapy, but this has yet to be fully evaluated (Danova and Muir, 2003).

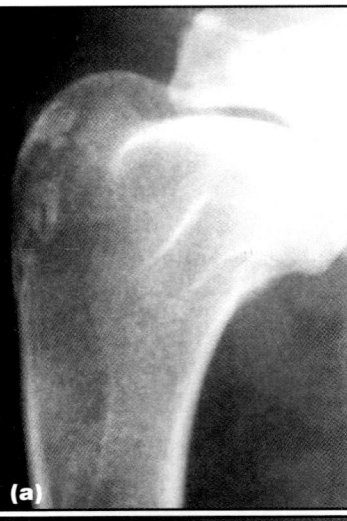

17.18 (a) Mediolateral radiograph from a 9-year-old German Shepherd Dog, showing mineralization over the cranial aspect of the greater tubercle in the vicinity of the supraspinatus tendon of insertion. There is also mineralization further caudally, which could involve the intertubercular groove. **(b)** Skyline radiograph of the greater tubercle, from a 2-year-old Neopolitan Mastiff, showing mineralization medial to the greater tubercle, which would be in the vicinity of the biceps tendon of origin.

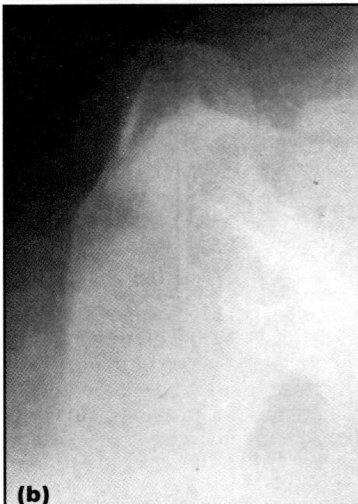

Infraspinatus bursal ossification

Radiographs may show evidence of ossification within the infraspinatus bursa. In the mediolateral view the density is superimposed on the greater tubercle, but in the caudocranial view the density lies lateral to the proximal humerus (McKee and Macias, 2004; Figure 17.19). These

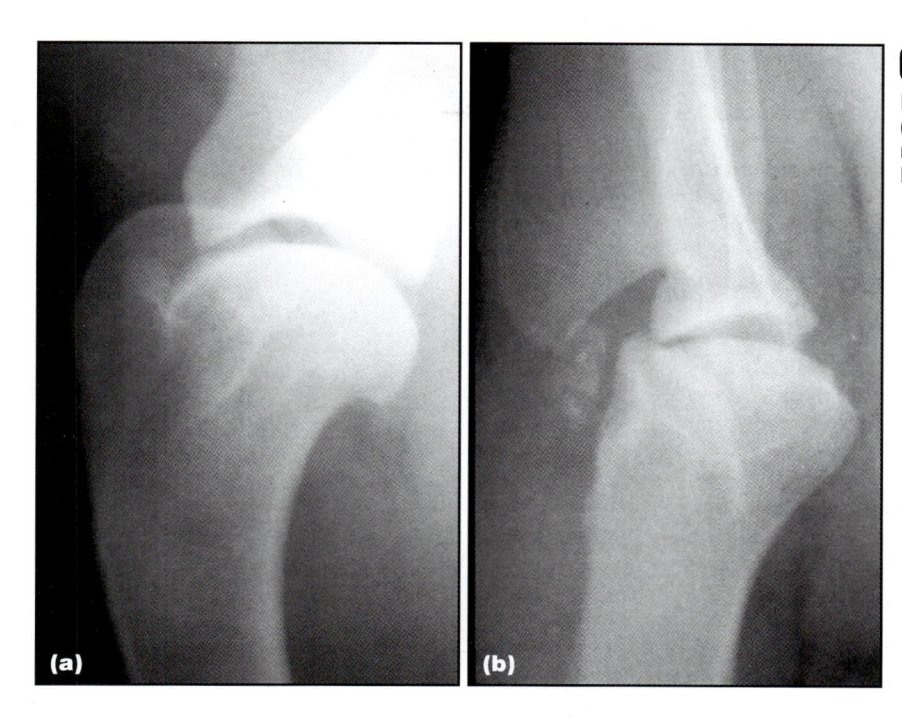

Chapter 17 The shoulder

17.19 Mediolateral (a) and caudocranial (b) radiographs, showing mineralization within the infraspinatus bursa. (Courtesy of WM McKee)

changes have been associated with clinical lameness in some dogs (McKee *et al.*, 2002) although in most of those where arthroscopy was performed other pathology was also recognized. Surgical resection of the ossified masses and release of the associated infraspinatus tendon has been advocated where conservative measures (as described above) fail.

Medial or lateral scapulohumeral instability
Shoulder instability appears to occur in two forms:

- Traumatic luxations (see Luxations, above)

- A chronic increase in shoulder laxity associated with loss of integrity of the soft tissue supporting structures of the shoulder. This has been recognized in recent years, with the advent of arthroscopy. Whilst there is still a poor understanding of this 'shoulder instability syndrome', it appears that the structures most commonly affected are the medial glenohumeral ligament and the subscapularis tendon of insertion (Bardet, 1998), and, less commonly, the lateral glenohumeral ligament (Mitchell and Innes, 2000) (Fig 17.20).

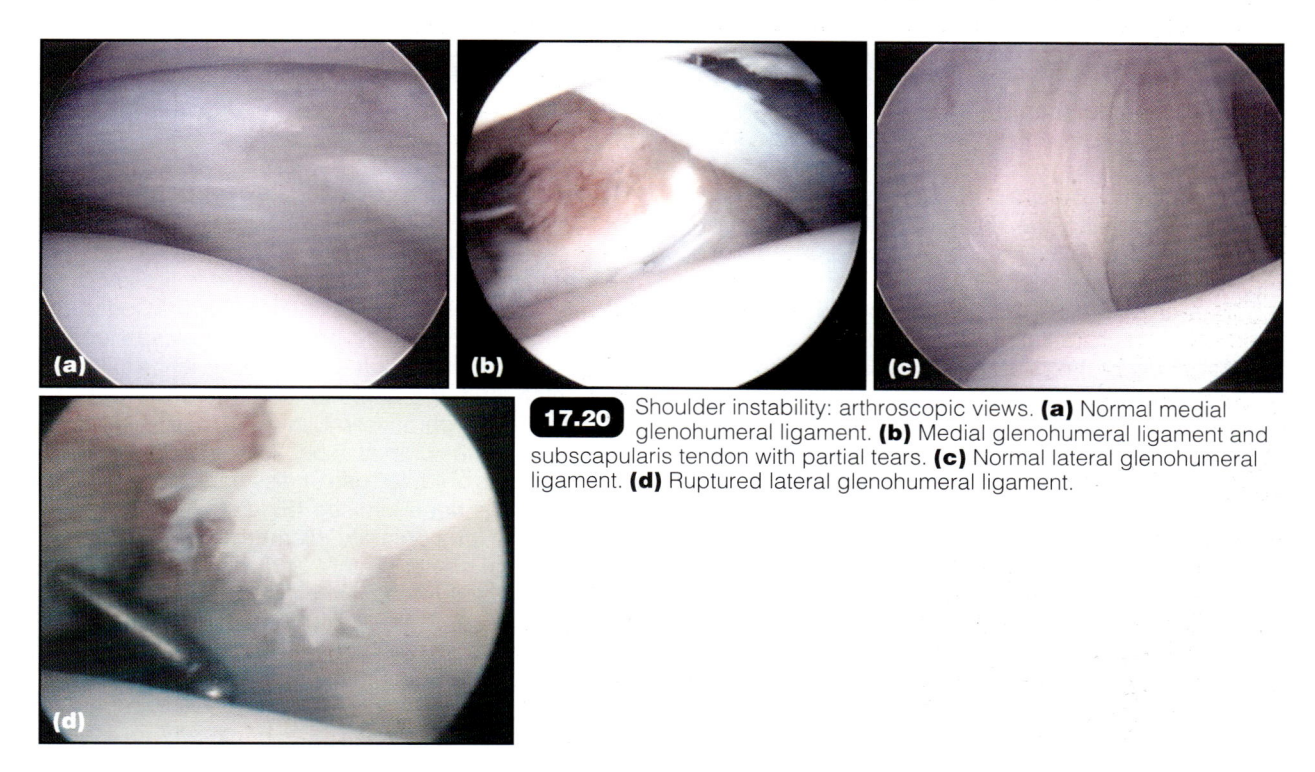

17.20 Shoulder instability: arthroscopic views. (a) Normal medial glenohumeral ligament. (b) Medial glenohumeral ligament and subscapularis tendon with partial tears. (c) Normal lateral glenohumeral ligament. (d) Ruptured lateral glenohumeral ligament.

Chapter 17 The shoulder

In some cases showing lameness associated with pain on shoulder manipulation, the cause may be pathology involving either the medial or lateral collateral support for the joint (Bardet, 1998). It has been suggested that insufficiency in the medial support (provided by the medial glenohumeral ligament and subscapularis muscle tendon of insertion) can be evaluated by assessing the angle of abduction through the shoulder when compared with the normal limb or what is considered 'normal' (Cook et al., 2005a). When measured with a goniometer, the angle of abduction in normal shoulders is about 33 degrees, whereas in those shoulders diagnosed as having medial shoulder instability the angle of abduction was about 54 degrees.

Radiographic findings are non-specific and the definitive diagnosis is based on the arthroscopic examination of the glenohumeral ligaments and subscapularis tendon. Separation of the glenohumeral ligaments from the labrum of the glenoid and mid-substance tears (in these ligaments or the subscapularis tendon) have been recognized (Cook et al., 2005a) (see Figure 17.20d). Unfortunately, the significance of these findings alone is somewhat unreliable since they are sometimes seen in combination with other shoulder pathology, and when the latter is treated the lameness may improve.

Surgical treatment
Surgery is considered where conservative measures (as described above) have failed to improve the lameness associated with suspected medial shoulder instability. This might involve placement of a medial prosthesis (Fitch et al., 2001; Ringwood et al., 2001) (see Operative Technique 17.7) or thermal modification ('shrinkage') of the joint capsule (Cook et al., 2005a). In the case of lateral glenohumeral ligament insufficiency that has proved unresponsive to conservative management, lateral capsulorrhaphy has been proposed for treatment (Mitchell and Innes, 2000).

Thermal capsulorrhaphy
This technique (O'Neill and Innes, 2004; Cook et al., 2005b) involves the arthroscopically guided use of a monopolar or bipolar radiofrequency probe (Figure 17.21a). The technique relies on thermal denaturation of collagen within the subsynovium at approximately 65°C; this causes loss of the intramolecular collagen cross-links with retention of the less labile intermolecular cross-links (Hayashi and Markel, 2001). The shrinking of the capsule provides a 'scaffold' for fibrosis during repair. However, the heat produced by the probe will also kill cells and so it is necessary to leave 'islands' or 'lines' of viable tissue. Thus surgeons often adopt a 'grid-iron' or 'paintbrush' approach to application of the probe to produce shrinkage with intervening viable tissue. The need for active repair and fibrosis on a shrunken capsule requires a period of 3–6 weeks of non-weightbearing to allow for new collagen formation and organization. A non-weightbearing sling (Figure 17.21b) is therefore applied after this surgery for a minimum of 3 weeks, followed by a carefully planned rehabilitation programme (see Chapter 16).

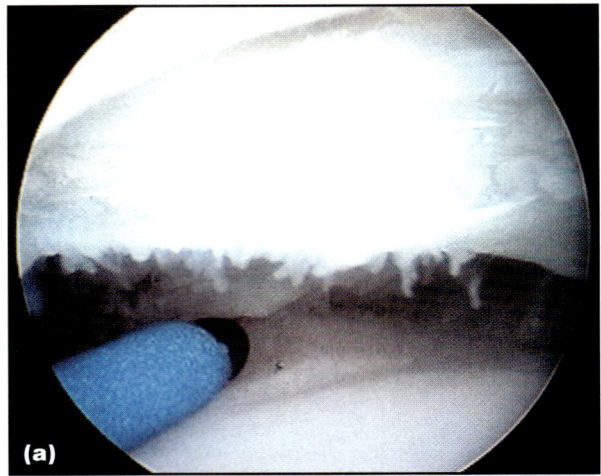

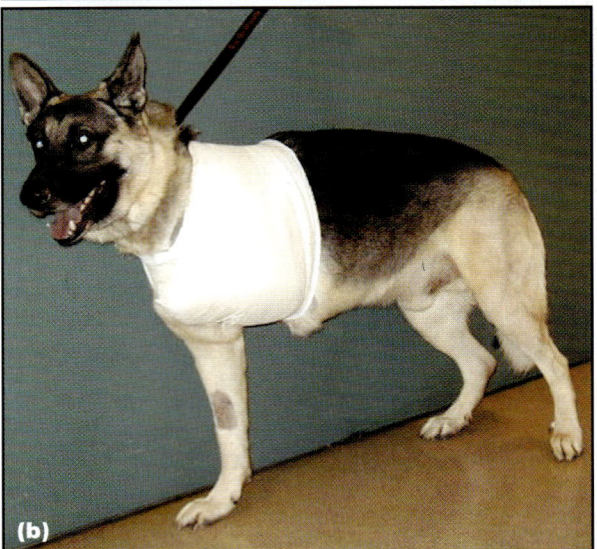

17.21 (a) Monopolar radiofrequency micro TAC-S probe (Oratec) placed against the medial joint capsule of the shoulder joint during thermal capsulorrhaphy. (b) Velpeau non-weightbearing sling for postoperative care following thermal capsulorrhaphy.

Rupture/avulsion of the biceps brachii tendon of origin
This is an uncommon injury but has been recorded in cases with shoulder luxation, particularly those occurring in a craniomedial direction (Bennett and Campbell, 1979). In such cases the possibility of biceps tendon injury should be investigated at surgery, since failure to recognize and repair such damage may lead to reluxation postoperatively. Clinically, there is swelling and pain over the cranial aspect of the shoulder. Plain radiography is of limited use unless part of the scapular tuberosity has been avulsed (Figure 17.22a). Arthrography may demonstrate disruption of the tendon sheath at the site of rupture and arthroscopy can be used to view the damage (Figure 17.22b).

If the shoulder is stable, conservative measures may be employed (see above). Should these fail, or if joint instability is present, the tendon may be exposed using a cranial approach. Wherever possible the tendon should be re-attached to its origin (Figure 17.23).

Chapter 17 The shoulder

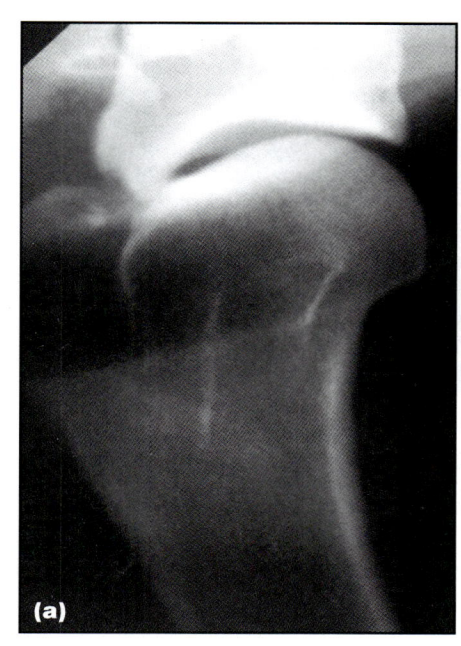

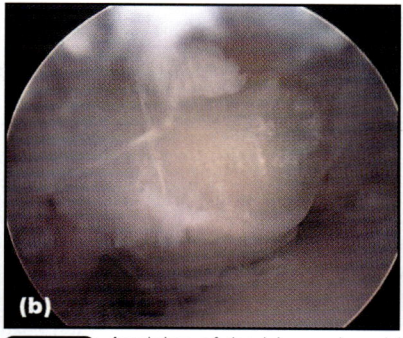

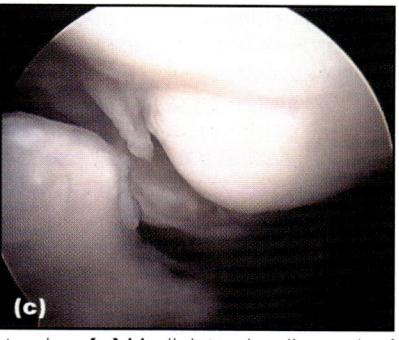

17.22 Avulsion of the biceps brachii tendon. **(a)** Mediolateral radiograph of the shoulder of a 4-year-old Irish Setter that developed an acute onset lameness. The biceps brachii tendon had avulsed from the scapular tuberosity, from which a small fragment of bone has also been avulsed. **(b,c)** Arthroscopic views of an avulsed biceps tendon.

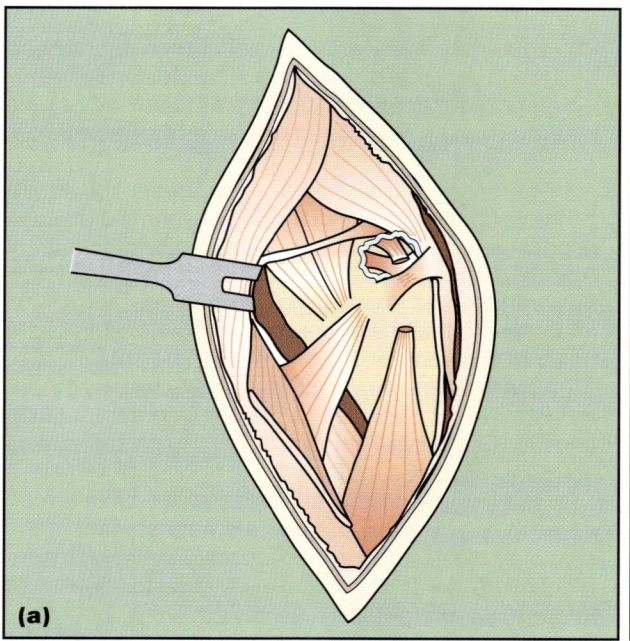

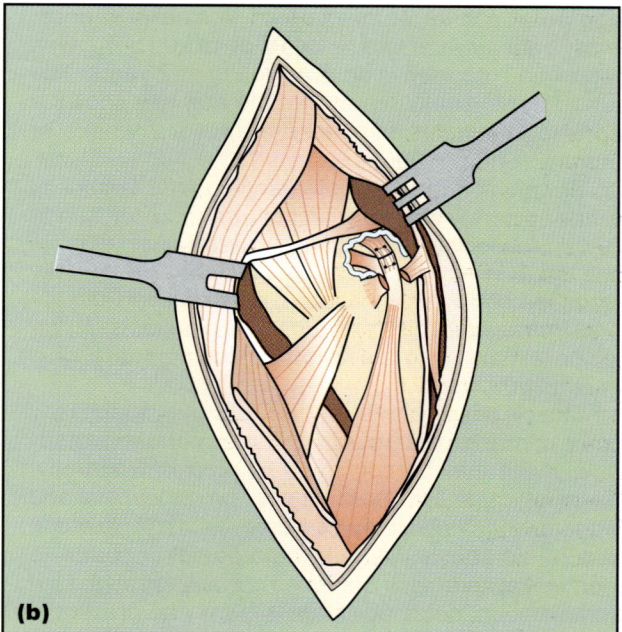

17.23 Surgical treatment of ruptured/avulsed biceps brachii tendon. **(a)** The biceps brachii tendon of origin is exposed by way of a craniomedial approach. **(b)** Repair of a 'mid-tendon' rupture using appropriate sutures (locking loop in this illustration). If the tendon has avulsed from the scapula it may be necessary to anchor the sutures through holes drilled in the tuberosity.

In some cases this might prove impossible and the tendon has to be relocated on the proximal humerus. Such relocation obviously removes the support that the biceps tendon contributes to shoulder stability, and this may have to be taken into account in choosing an appropriate surgical method to stabilize the joint.

Neoplasia

Shoulder lameness as a result of neoplasia is seen not infrequently in dogs. Musculoskeletal tumours are discussed in detail in Chapter 9 and also in the BSAVA *Manual of Canine and Feline Oncology;* brachial plexus conditions, including neoplasia, are further covered in Chapter 10.

Skeletal tumours

A neoplasm of the scapulohumeral joint itself is likely to be a synovial sarcoma. This is an infrequent cause of shoulder lameness in middle- to old-aged dogs and is associated with chronic progressive clinical signs. Pain is evident on shoulder manipulation and soft tissue swelling is usually palpable. Enlargement of the axillary lymph node may be present, possibly indicating lymphatic metastasis. Treatment may take

Chapter 17 The shoulder

the form of forequarter amputation but the prognosis is guarded due to the likely development of pulmonary metastasis.

Osteosarcoma of the proximal humeral metaphysis is the commonest neoplasm to affect the shoulder. In one review of osteosarcomas affecting the appendicular skeleton in 74 dogs (Gibbs et al., 1984) the lesion was located in the proximal humerus in 20% of cases. Lameness may vary from being very mild to very severe. Manipulation of the shoulder will reveal pain, particularly on extension, and palpation will often reveal muscle wastage. In the later stages of the disease, the tumour causes enlargement of the proximal humerus which may feel hot and swollen.

Other sarcomas, such as fibrosarcoma, chondrosarcoma and haemangiosarcoma (Erdem and Pead, 2000) may affect the proximal humerus or scapular blade.

Brachial plexus tumours

Brachial plexus tumours may cause an intractable lameness associated with shoulder pain. These tumours are usually seen in medium to large breeds of dog but it cannot be discounted in smaller breeds. Most patients are middle-aged or older, but cases have been reported in dogs as young as 2 years. The owners will usually report that the dog has shown a chronic intractable lameness for several weeks or months (Sharp, 1995).

A weightbearing and/or swinging limb lameness will be evident, with pain detectable on shoulder manipulation (especially extension) or axillary palpation. In some cases a mass may be detected, especially when the dog is anaesthetized, but lack of an identifiable mass does not preclude the diagnosis. If the lesion extends into the vertebral column, neck pain may be present.

Muscle atrophy is usually very obvious, particularly of the suprascapular muscles. This is neurogenic atrophy, which may be confirmed by electromyography. Neurological deficits such as poor proprioceptive and withdrawal reflexes may be noted, as may ipsilateral loss of the panniculus reflex and partial or complete Horner's syndrome. If the lesion is causing spinal cord compression, neurological deficits may be present in the pelvic limbs (Targett et al., 1993).

In the vast majority of cases, plain radiographs show no abnormality and serve only to rule out other potential causes of such a lameness. Occasionally, when the tumour involves the nerve root as it passes out of the vertebral column, there is evidence of enlargement of the corresponding intervertebral foramen. If vertebral canal involvement is suspected, myelography may show the presence of an intradural, extramedullary lesion. Although pulmonary metastases are rare in these cases, thoracic radiographs should be taken to evaluate such a possibility. Magnetic resonance imaging is able to detect some, but not all, of these lesions. Electromyography may detect denervation potentials in muscle groups within the limb, suggesting nerve root pathology.

If further confirmation of the diagnosis is required, surgical exploration of the brachial plexus, with or without biopsy, is possible by way of a craniolateral approach (Sharp, 1988) or of the vertebral canal by way of laminectomy.

The only practicable means of treatment involves forequarter amputation (Harvey, 1974). In cases where the lesion has spread to involve the vertebral canal, forequarter amputation and removal of the intradural component via laminectomy have been advocated.

The prognosis in these cases is very guarded since, although the rate of distant metastasis is quite low, the tumours are locally invasive. Complete removal may prove very difficult or impossible since the extent of the lesion may not be detectable on gross examination.

Arthrodesis of the scapulohumeral joint

As in all joints, arthrodesis of the scapulohumeral joint must be considered a salvage procedure and only undertaken when all other possible management options have failed or would be inappropriate. Such situations include:

- Irreparable fractures of the glenoid or humeral head
- Recurrent luxation with resulting erosion of the glenoid, rendering surgical stabilization impossible
- Chronic pain associated with severe osteoarthritis.

The decision to undertake arthrodesis should not be taken lightly. The clinical signs of shoulder disease should be severe enough to warrant this intervention. Some degree of mechanical alteration of gait is inevitable and client counselling prior to the surgery is important so that there is a clear understanding of the goals of this surgery.

A craniolateral approach is used followed by preparation for arthrodesis, bone grafting and internal fixation (see Operative Technique 17.9). Plate and screws are generally used for fixation.

Following successful arthrodesis, limb function can be good, presumably through extra movement of the scapula across the thoracic wall and increased movement of the elbow. However, there is limited published information on outcome following scapulohumeral arthrodesis.

References and further reading

Adamiak Z and Szalecki P (2003) Treatment of bicipital tenosynovitis with double tenodesis. *Journal of Small Animal Practice* **44**, 539–540

Bardet JF (1998) Diagnosis of shoulder instability in dogs and cats: a retrospective study. *Journal of the American Animal Hospital Association* **34**, 42–54

Bardet JF (1999) Lesions of the biceps tendon diagnosis and classification. *Veterinary and Comparative Orthopaedics and Traumatology* **12**, 188–195

Bennett D and Campbell JR (1979). Unusual soft tissue orthopaedic problems in the dog. *Journal of Small Animal Practice* **20**, 27–39

Bennett RA (1986) Contracture of the infraspinatus muscle in dogs: a review of 12 cases. *Journal of the American Animal Hospital Association* **22**, 481–487

Boemo CM and Eaton-Wells RD (1995) Medial displacement of the tendon of origin of the biceps brachii muscle in 10 greyhounds. *Journal of Small Animal Practice* **36**, 69–73

Bruce WJ, Spence S and Miller A (1997) Teres minor myopathy as a cause of lameness in a dog. *Journal of Small Animal Practice* **38**, 74–77

Butterworth SJ (2003). The use of methylprednisolone in the management of shoulder lameness in the dog. Abstract from BSAVA Congress 2003. *Journal of Small Animal Practice* **44**, 336

Campbell JR (1968) Shoulder lameness in the dog. *Journal of Small Animal Practice* **9**, 189–198

Clayton Jones DG and Vaughan LC (1970) The surgical treatment of osteochondritis dissecans of the humeral head in dogs. *Journal of Small Animal Practice* **11**, 803–812

Cook JL (2002) Arthroscopic findings and results of radiofrequency treatment of shoulder instability in dogs. *Proceedings of the 12th Annual Symposium of the American College of Veterinary Surgeons, San Diego*

Cook JL (2003) Diagnosis and treatment of shoulder instability in dogs. *Proceedings of the 13th Annual Symposium of the American College of Veterinary Surgeons, Washington DC*

Cook JL, Kenter K and Fox DB (2004) Arthroscopic biceps tenodesis in dogs: technique and results in 6 cases. *Journal of the American Animal Hospital Association* **41**, 121–127

Cook JL, Kenter K and Tomlinson JL (2001) Arthroscopic treatment of shoulder instability using radiofrequency-induced thermal modification. *Proceedings of the 28th Annual Veterinary Orthopedic Society Conference* p. 37

Cook JL, Renfro DC, Tomlinson JL and Sorensen JE (2005a) Measurement of angles of abduction for diagnosis of shoulder instability in dogs using goniometry and digital image analysis. *Veterinary Surgery* **34**, 463–468

Cook JL, Tomlinson JL, Fox DB, Kenter K and Cook CR (2005b) Treatment of dogs diagnosed with medial shoulder instability using radiofrequency-induced thermal capsulorrhaphy. *Veterinary Surgery* **34**, 469–475

Coughlan A and Miller A (1998) *Manual of Small Animal Fracture Repair and Management*. BSAVA Publications, Cheltenham

Danova NA and Muir P (2003) Extracorporeal shock wave therapy for supraspinatus calcifying tendinopathy in two dogs. *Veterinary Record* **152**, 208–209

Deneuche AJ and Viguier E (2002) Reduction and stabilisation of a supraglenoid tuberosity avulsion under arthroscopic guidance in a dog. *Journal of Small Animal Practice* **43**, 308–311

Erdem V and Pead MJ (2000) Haemangiosarcoma of the scapula in three dogs. *Journal of Small Animal Practice* **41**, 461–464

Fitch RB, Breshears L, Staatz A and Kudnig S (2001) Clinical evaluation of prosthetic medial glenohumeral ligament repair in the dog (ten cases). *Veterinary and Comparative Orthopaedics and Traumatology* **14**, 222–228

Flo GL and Middleton D (1990) Mineralisation of the supraspinatus tendon in dogs. *Journal of the American Veterinary Medical Association* **197**, 95–97

Fowler JD, Presnell, KR and Holmberg DL (1988) Scapulohumeral arthrodesis: results in seven dogs. *Journal of the American Animal Hospital Association* **24**, 667–672

Fox SM and Bray JP (1992) Surgical correction for rupture of the transverse humeral ligament in a racing greyhound. *Australian Veterinary Practitioner* **22**, 2–5

Gibbs C, Denny HR and Kelly DF (1984) The radiological features of osteosarcoma of the appendicular skeleton in dogs: a review of 74 cases. *Journal of Small Animal Practice* **25**, 177–192

Gahring DR (1985) A modified caudal approach to the canine shoulder joint. *Journal of the American Animal Hospital Association* **21**, 613–618

Goring RL, Parker RB, Dee L and Eaton-Wells RD (1984) Medial displacement of the tendon of origin of the biceps brachii muscle in the racing greyhound. *Journal of the American Animal Hospital Association* **20**, 933–938

Harari J and Dunning D (1993) Fractures of the scapula in dogs: a retrospective review of 12 cases. *Veterinary and Comparative Orthopaedics and Traumatology* **6**, 105–108

Harvey CE (1974) Forequarter amputation in the dog and cat. *Journal of the American Animal Hospital Association* **10**, 25

Hayashi K and Markel MD (2001) Thermal capsulorrhaphy treatment of shoulder instability – basic science. *Clinical Orthopaedics and Related Research* **390**, 59–72

Holsworth IG, Schulz KS and Ingel K (2002) Cadaveric evaluation of canine arthroscopic bicipital tenotomy. *Veterinary and Comparative Orthopaedics and Traumatology* **15**, 215–222

Hohn RB, Rosen H, Bohning RH Jr and Brown S (1971) Surgical stabilisation of recurrent shoulder luxations. *Veterinary Clinics of North America* **1**, 537–548

Innes JF and Brown G (2004) Rupture of the biceps brachii tendon sheath in two dogs. *Journal of Small Animal Practice* **45**, 25–28

Johnston SA (1993) Articular fractures of the scapula in the dog: a clinical retrospective study of 26 cases. *Journal of the American Animal Hospital Association* **29**, 157–164

Kramer M, Gerwing M, Sheppard C and Schimke E (2001) Ultrasonography for the diagnosis of diseases of the tendon and tendon sheath of the biceps brachii muscle. *Veterinary Surgery* **30**, 64–71

Kriegleder H (1995) Mineralization of the supraspinatus tendon: clinical observations in seven dogs. *Veterinary and Comparative Orthopaedics and Traumatology* **8**, 91–97

Laitinen OM and Flo GL (2000) Mineralisation of the supraspinatus tendon in dogs: long-term follow-up. *Journal of the American Animal Hospital Association* **36**, 262–267

Lincoln JD and Potter K (1984) Tenosynovitis of the biceps brachii tendon in dogs. *Journal of the American Animal Hospital Association* **20**, 385–392

McKee WM and Macias C (2004) Orthopaedic conditions of the shoulder in the dog. *In Practice* **26**, 118–129

McKee WM, May C and Macias C (2002). Infraspinatus bursal ossification in eight dogs (Abstract ESVOT-VOS). *Veterinary and Comparative Orthopaedics and Traumatology* **15**, A24

Meyer-Lindenberg A, Koppler M and Fehr M (2002) Treatment of osteochondrosis dissecans of the shoulder joint in dogs: arthroscopic versus conventional removal. Abstract from BSAVA Congress 2002. *Journal of Small Animal Practice* **43**, 302a

Mitchell RAS and Innes JF (2000) Lateral glenohumeral ligament rupture in three dogs. *Journal of Small Animal Practice* **41**, 511–514

Muir P and Johnson KA (1994) Supraspinatus and biceps brachii tendinopathy in dogs. *Journal of Small Animal Practice* **35**, 239–243

Muir P, Johnson KA and Manley PA (1996) Force-plate analysis of gait before and after surgical excision of calcified lesions of the supraspinatus tendon in two dogs. *Veterinary Record* **139**, 137–139

Olivieri M, Piras A and Vezzoni A (1999) Ununited caudal glenoid ossification center in 5 dogs: arthroscopic diagnosis and treatment (Abstract ECVS). *Veterinary Surgery* **28**, 213–214

O'Neill T and Innes JF (2004) Use of thermal capsulorrhaphy to treat instability of the shoulder joint in a dog. *Journal of Small Animal Practice* **45**, 521–524

Person MW (1986) Arthroscopy of the canine shoulder joint. *Compendium on Continuing Education* **8**, 537–547

Piermattei DL (1993) *An Atlas of Surgical Approaches to the Bones of the Dog and Cat, 3rd edn.* pp. 25–27 and 92–121. WB Saunders, Philadelphia

Puglisi TA (1986) Canine humeral joint instability – part I. *Compendium on Continuing Education for the Practicing Veterinarian* **8**, 593–595

Puglisi TA (1986) Canine humeral joint instability – part II. *Compendium on Continuing Education for the Practicing Veterinarian* **8**, 741–749

Read RA (1994) Successful treatment of congenital shoulder luxation in a dog by closed pinning. *Veterinary and Comparative Orthopaedics and Traumatology* **7**, 170–172

Ringwood PB, Kerwin SC, Hosgood G and Williams J (2001) Medial glenohumeral ligament reconstruction for ex-vivo medial glenohumeral luxation in the dog. *Veterinary and Comparative Orthopaedics and Traumatology* **14**, 196–200

Rivers B, Wallace L and Johnstone GR (1992) Biceps tenosynovitis in the dog: radiographic and sonographic findings. *Veterinary and Comparative Orthopaedics and Traumatology* **5**, 51–57

Rudd RG, Whitehair JG and Margolis JH (1990) Results of management of osteochondritis dissecans of the humeral head in dogs: 44 cases (1982–1987). *Journal of the American Animal Hospital Association* **26**, 173–178

Sharp NJ (1988) Craniolateral approach to the brachial plexus. *Veterinary Surgery* **17**, 18–21

Sharp NJ (1995) Neoplasia of the brachial plexus and associated nerve roots. In: *Manual of Small Animal Neurology, 2nd edn.* ed. SJ Wheeler, pp. 164–166. BSAVA Publications, Cheltenham

Sidaway BK, McLaughlin RM, Elder SH, Boyle CR and Silverman EB (2004) Role of the tendons of the biceps brachii and infraspinatus muscles and the medial glenohumeral ligament in the maintenance of passive shoulder stability in dogs. *American Journal of Veterinary Research* **65**, 1216–1222

Spackman CJA, Caywood DD, Feeney DA and Johnston GR (1984) Thoracic wall and pulmonary trauma in dogs sustaining fractures as a result of motor vehicle accidents. *Journal of the American Veterinary Medical Association* **185**, 975–977

Stobie D, Wallace LJ, Lipowitz AJ, King V and Lund EM (1995) Chronic bicipital tenosynovitis in dogs: 29 cases (1985–1992). *Journal of the American Veterinary Medical Association* **207**, 201–207

Targett MP, Dyce J and Houlton JEF (1993) Tumours involving the nerve sheaths of the forelimb in dogs. *Journal of Small Animal Practice* **34**, 221–225

van Bree HJJ (1992) *Positive Shoulder Arthrography in the Dog: the*

Chapter 17 The shoulder

Application in Osteochondrosis Lesions Compared with other Diagnostic Imaging Techniques [thesis]. Utrecht University Press, Utrecht

Van Ryssen B, van Bree H and Missinne S (1993) Successful arthroscopic treatment of shoulder osteochondrosis in the dog. *Journal of Small Animal Practice* **34**, 521–528

Vasseur PB, Moore D, Brown SA and Eng D (1982) Stability of the canine shoulder joint: an in vitro analysis. *American Journal of Veterinary Research* **43**, 352–355

Vasseur PB, Pool RR and Klein K (1983) Effects of tendon transfer on the canine scapulohumeral joint. *American Journal of Veterinary Research* **44**, 811–815

Vaughan LC (1967) Dislocation of the shoulder joint in the dog and cat. *Journal of Small Animal Practice* **8**, 45–48

Vaughan LC (1979) Muscle and tendon injuries in dogs. *Journal of Small Animal Practice* **20**, 711–736

Vaughan LC and Jones DGC (1968) Osteochondritis dissecans of the head of the humerus in dogs. *Journal of Small Animal Practice* **9**, 283–294

Wall CR and Taylor R (2002) Arthroscopic biceps brachii tenotomy as a treatment for canine bicipital tenosynovitis. *Journal of the American Animal Hospital Association* **38**, 169–175

Chapter 17 The shoulder

OPERATIVE TECHNIQUE 17.1
Craniomedial approach to the shoulder

Positioning
Dorsal recumbency, the limb drawn caudally with a tie and the incision made over the craniomedial aspect of the joint. Placement of a foam wedge between the limb and thoracic wall can aid access to the craniomedial aspect of the shoulder.

Assistant
Desirable but not essential.

Tray extras
Treves self-retaining retractors; Weitlander self-retaining retractors; Gelpi retractors (large and/or small); instruments for placement of any implants required for fixation of a planned greater tubercle osteotomy (Kirschner wires, orthopaedic wire).

Surgical technique
A skin incision is made from a point just medial and caudal to the acromion, passing distally over the craniomedial aspect of the humerus (Figure 17.24a). The fascia along the lateral border of the brachiocephalicus muscle is incised (with or without ligation of the omobrachial vein) to allow retraction of the muscle (Figure 17.24b) and exposure of the superficial pectoral muscle, which is elevated in a similar manner. The biceps brachii muscle and tendon of origin will be exposed (Figure 17.24d) and can be followed proximally to the transverse humeral ligament and then to the scapular tuberosity.

> **PRACTICAL TIP**
> Exposure of the tuberosity can be improved by osteotomy of the greater tubercle (Figure 17.24e), which allows reflection of the supraspinatus muscle, followed by incision of the joint capsule.

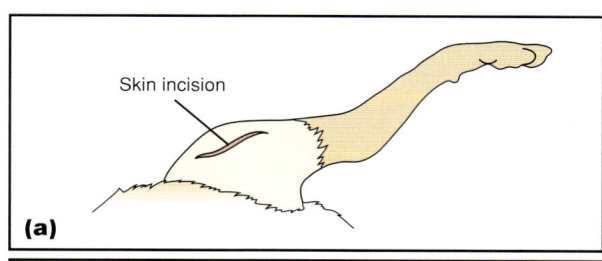

17.24 Craniomedial approach to the shoulder.
(a) With the dog in dorsal recumbency the limb is drawn caudally and the incision made over the craniomedial aspect of the joint. **(b)** The fascia is incised to allow retraction of the brachiocephalicus muscle. **(c)** The superficial and deep pectorals are released from their insertion on the humerus. (continues)

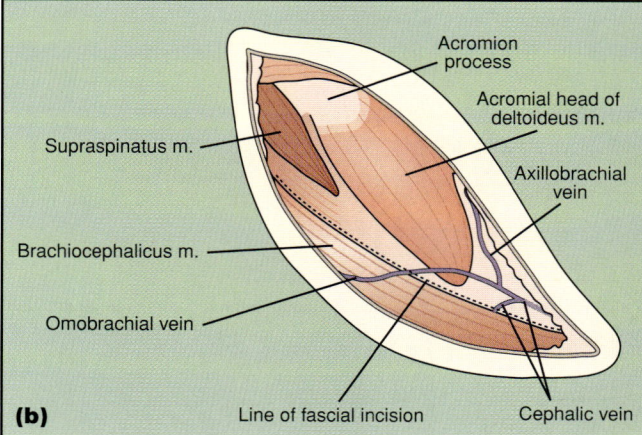

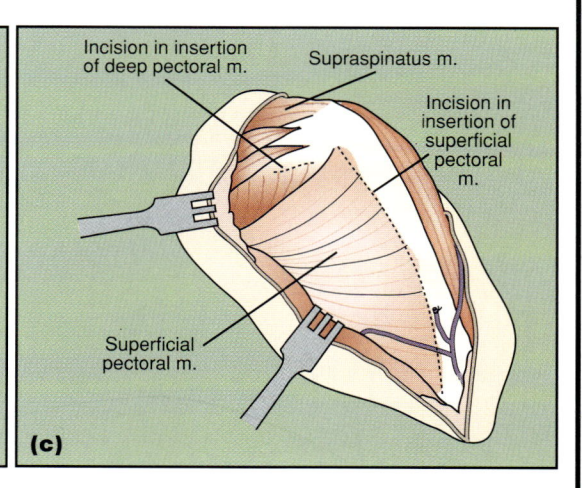

OPERATIVE TECHNIQUE 17.1 *continued*
Craniomedial approach to the shoulder

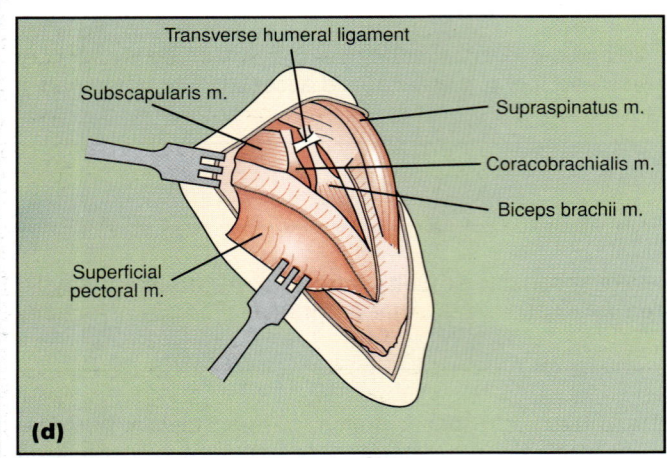

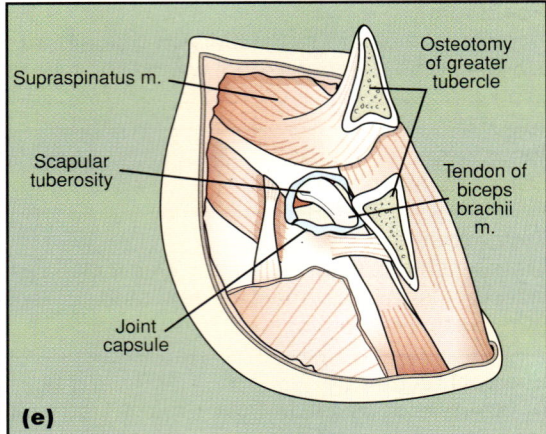

17.24 (continued) **(d)** Retraction of the pectorals exposes the biceps brachii tendon of origin. **(e)** Exposure of the more proximal part of the tendon can be improved by osteotomy of the greater tubercle.

Closure
The greater tubercle must be reattached during closure using crossed Kirschner wires, a lagged bone screw, or pins and a tension band wire. The remaining closure involves reattachment of the deep and then superficial pectoral muscles using absorbable simple continuous or interrupted cruciate sutures.

Postoperative care
See individual procedures. Generally: 4 weeks of rest if no osteotomy has been performed; if osteotomy is performed, rest for 8 weeks and confirm osteotomy healing radiographically.

Complications
See individual procedures.

Chapter 17 The shoulder

OPERATIVE TECHNIQUE 17.2
Craniolateral approach to the shoulder

Positioning
Lateral recumbency with operative limb uppermost. Placement of a foam wedge between the limb and operating table helps support the limb.

Assistant
Desirable but not essential. Of the indications listed, an assistant is possibly most useful for treatment of shoulder luxation.

Tray extras
Treves self-retaining retractors; Weitlander self-retaining retractors; Gelpi retractors (large and/or small).

Surgical technique
A skin incision is made from about a third to half the way up the scapular spine to the distal end of the deltoid tuberosity (Figure 17.25a). The deep fascia is incised over the scapular spine (Figure 17.25b), which releases the insertions of the omotransversarius and trapezius muscles cranially and the origin of the scapular head of

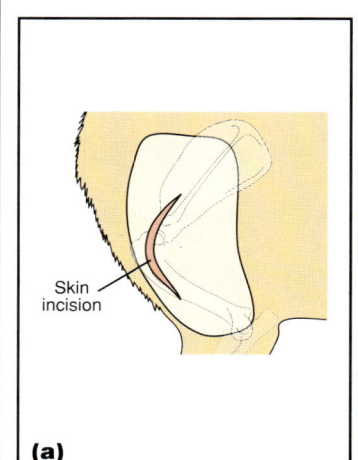

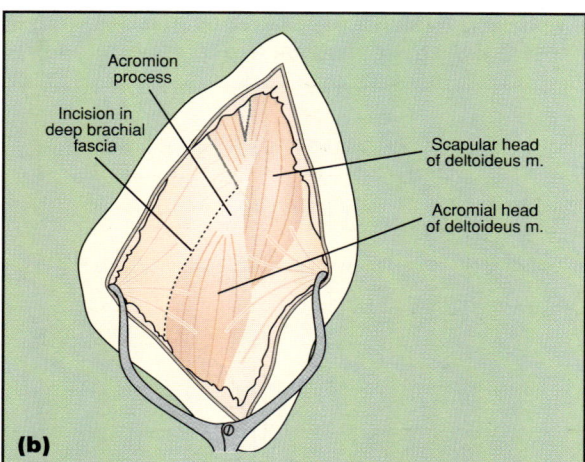

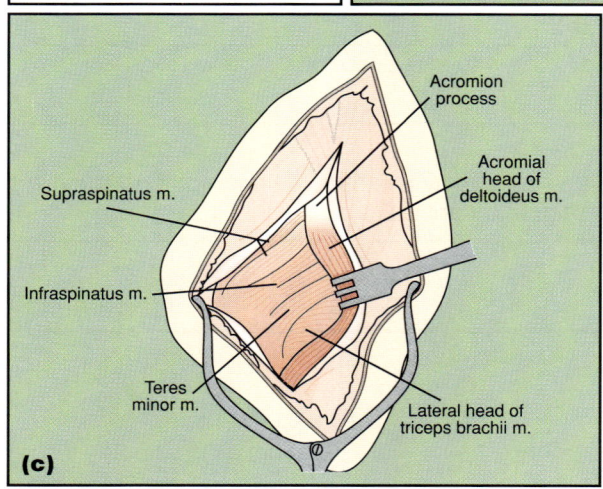

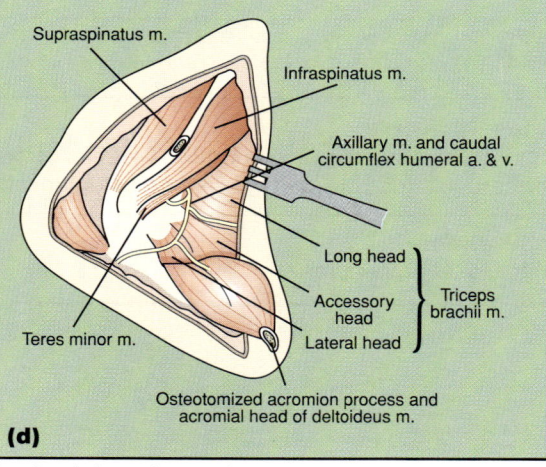

17.25 Craniolateral approach to the shoulder. **(a)** With the dog in lateral recumbency a skin incision is made from midway down the scapular spine to the distal limit of the deltoid tuberosity, passing cranial to the acromion process. **(b)** An incision is made in the deep brachial fascia of a length dictated by which structures are required to be exposed. **(c)** Retraction of the acromial head of the deltoid muscle exposes the insertions of the infraspinatus and teres minor muscles, which can be incised and reflected to expose the lateral glenohumeral ligament and capsule. **(d)** Tenotomy of the acromial head of the deltoid muscle or osteotomy of the acromion process allows reflection of the deltoid for improved exposure of the lateral aspect of the joint.

→

Chapter 17 The shoulder

> **OPERATIVE TECHNIQUE 17.2** *continued*
> **Craniolateral approach to the shoulder**

the deltoid muscle caudally, thus exposing the supraspinatus and infraspinatus muscles. This incision is extended distally, towards the omobrachial vein, to expose the acromial head of the deltoid muscle. Tenotomy of the infraspinatus muscle tendon of insertion improves exposure of the lateral capsule (Figure 17.25d). The scapular neck can now be exposed by elevation of the spinatus muscles.

PRACTICAL TIP
Improved exposure of the scapular neck can be achieved by reflection of the acromial head of the deltoid muscle, either by tenotomy or osteotomy of the acromial process. However, for the indications listed, exposure of the scapular neck can usually be achieved without the need for these additional steps.

Closure
If tenotomy has been performed, repair would require tendon sutures in the acromial head of the deltoid, or, if acromial osteotomy has been performed, reattachment of the acromion is needed, using either Kirschner wires and a tension band or wire sutures (Figure 17.26). The remaining closure involves reattachment of fascia, including insertions of the omotransversarius and trapezius muscles, with simple continuous or interrupted cruciate sutures using an absorbable suture material (e.g. polydioxanone).

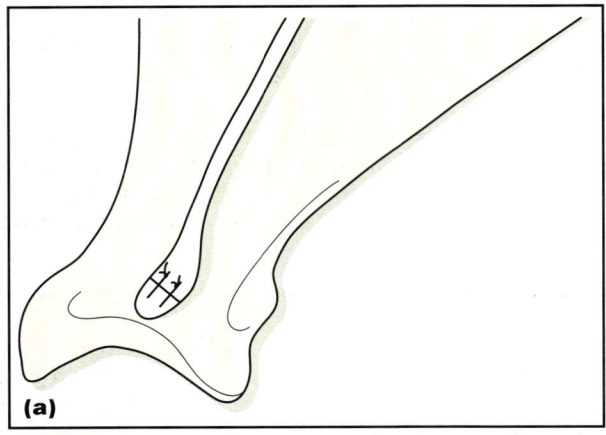

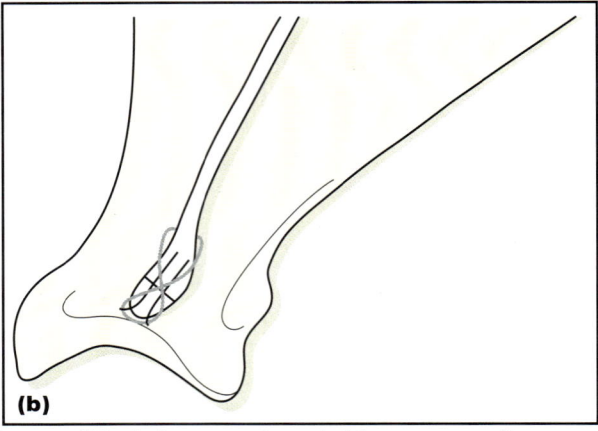

17.26 If an acromion osteotomy has been performed, closure will include re-attachment of the process with **(a)** wire sutures or **(b)** a pin and tension-band technique.

Postoperative care
See individual procedures. Generally: 4 weeks of rest if no osteotomy has been performed; if osteotomy is performed, rest for 8 weeks and confirm osteotomy healing radiographically.

Complications
See individual procedures.

Chapter 17 The shoulder

OPERATIVE TECHNIQUE 17.3
Caudolateral approach to the shoulder

Positioning
Lateral recumbency with operative limb uppermost. Placement of a foam wedge between the limb and operating table helps support the limb.

Assistant
An assistant is valuable in aiding exposure of the caudal humeral head, in particular, since this requires marked internal rotation of the limb. Alternatively, this can be achieved by an unscrubbed assistant manipulating the limb under the surgical drapes.

Tray extras
Treves self-retaining retractors; Weitlander self-retaining retractors; Gelpi retractors (large and/or small).

Surgical technique
There are three variations on this surgical approach. The first two both give satisfactory exposure, but the second is slightly more limited and the third creates a 'deeper' approach requiring retraction of larger muscle masses (although, if no assistant is available, it is often easier to expose an OCD lesion using this approach with the aid of self-retaining retractors alone).

For all, a skin incision is made from halfway along the scapular spine, passing caudal to the acromion and curving distally to and about one third of the way down the humerus (approximately at the distal end of the deltoid tuberosity) (Figure 17.27a). The subcutaneous tissues are dissected to allow identification of the two heads of the deltoid muscle. These are then separated by blunt dissection and retracted (Figure 17.27c).

Variation 1
The teres minor muscle is identified along with a neurovascular bundle just caudal to it (made up of the cephalic vein, muscular branch of the axillary nerve and the caudal circumflex humeral vessels). The muscle is retracted cranially and the nerves and vessels carefully dissected off the joint capsule and then pushed, or retracted, caudally (Figure 17.27d). An incision is made through the joint capsule to expose the caudal humeral head (Figure 17.27e).

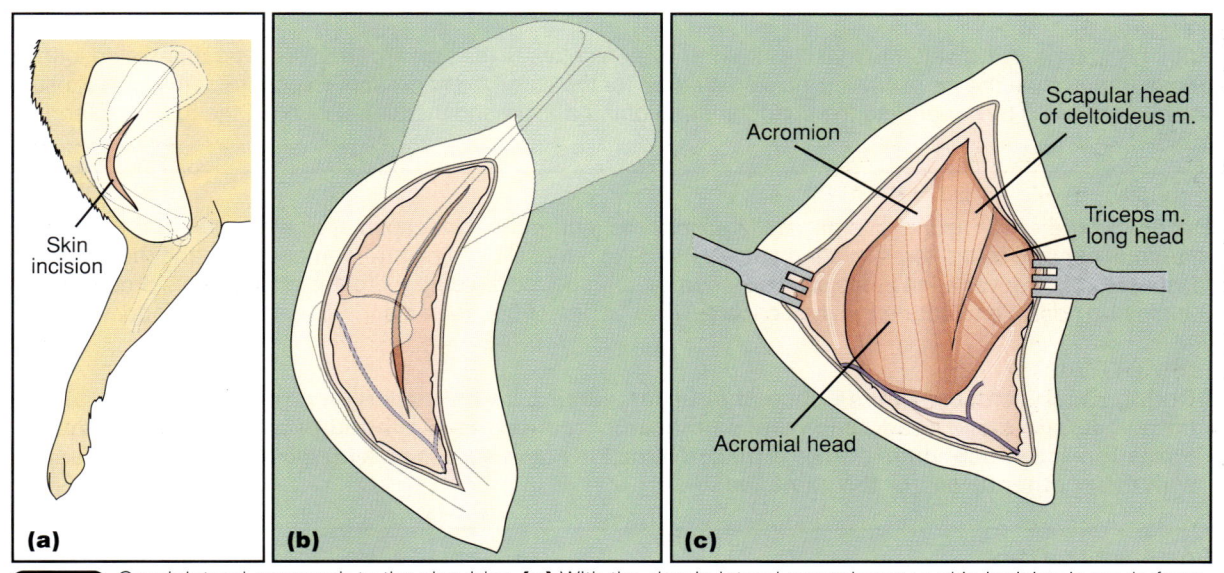

17.27 Caudolateral approach to the shoulder. **(a)** With the dog in lateral recumbency a skin incision is made from midway down the scapular spine to the distal limit of the deltoid tuberosity, passing caudal to the acromion process. **(b)** The fascia overlying the deltoid muscle is incised over the division between the scapular and acromial heads of the muscle which can usually be seen or palpated; the omobrachial vein normally forms the distal limit of this incision, and where the division meets the scapular spine forms the proximal limit. **(c)** Using blunt dissection the two heads of the deltoid muscle are then separated to the same limits as in (b). (continues)

→

235

Chapter 17 The shoulder

OPERATIVE TECHNIQUE 17.3 continued
Caudolateral approach to the shoulder

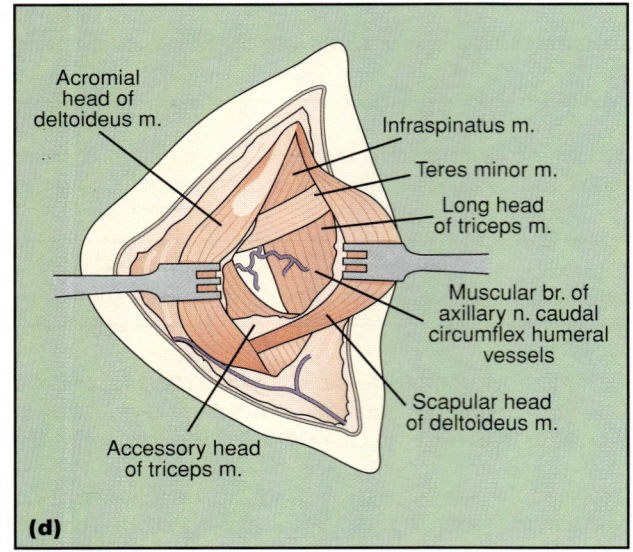

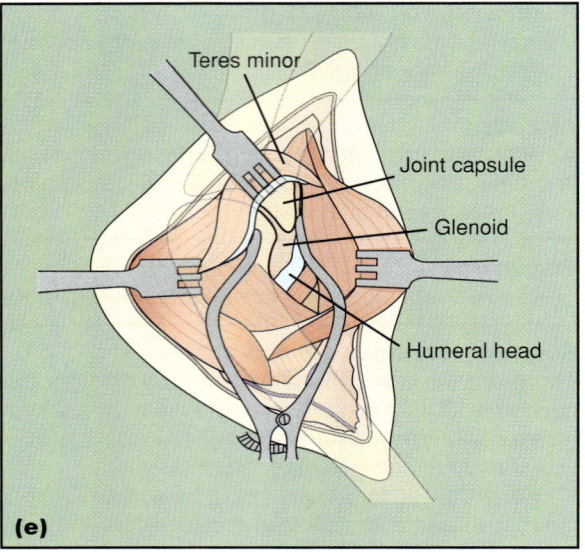

17.27 (continued) **(d)** Cranial retraction of the acromial head and caudal retraction of the scapular head of the deltoid muscle expose the teres minor muscle and the neurovascular complex over the caudal joint capsule. **(e)** Undermining the neurovascular bundle with blunt dissection will allow it to drop away caudally, providing ready access to the caudal joint capsule which is then incised to expose the caudal humeral head.

Variation 2
Having separated the heads of the deltoid, it is possible to gain access to the joint by blunt dissection between the teres minor and infraspinatus muscles (and thus avoid being close to the nerves and vessels mentioned above).

Variation 3
With this approach it is better to make a straight incision between the proximal and distal landmarks described above, rather than the more curved incision created for the standard approach. Exposure of the joint capsule may be achieved by separating the scapular head of the deltoid and the lateral head of the triceps (Gahring, 1985).

Closure
During closure of variation 1 it is generally possible to suture the joint capsule, or at least suture the caudal margin of capsule to the teres minor muscle. The deltoid muscle bellies are then apposed and the overlying fascia sutured. For variation 2, the joint is closed by suturing the teres minor to the infraspinatus. For variation 3 it may be possible to suture the joint capsule. The bellies of the deltoid and triceps are then apposed.

> **PRACTICAL TIP**
> During routine closure of the subcutaneous fat, picking up the underlying fascia with every other throw helps to close dead space and significantly reduce the likelihood of postoperative seroma formation. If a subcuticular suture is placed then it is again best to pick up the subcutaneous tissue with every other throw for the same reason.

Postoperative care
See individual procedures. Generally: 4 weeks of rest.

Complications
Seroma formation can occur but is very uncommon if the practical tip relating to closure is observed. If seen then it is best treated conservatively and will generally resolve slowly; drainage is not recommended because of the risk of introducing infection.

Chapter 17 The shoulder

OPERATIVE TECHNIQUE 17.4
Arthroscopy of the shoulder joint

Positioning and patient preparation
Lateral recumbency with operative limb uppermost. Placement of a foam wedge between the limb and operating table helps support the limb and prevent the shoulder joint space closing.

A square area of hair is clipped, centred on the acromion. Four field drapes are used and are covered by a sterile impervious transparent adhesive disposable drape.

Assistant
Not necessary for diagnostic arthroscopy. Desirable for operative arthroscopy, particularly for right shoulder for the right-handed surgeon (and left shoulder for left-handed surgeon).

Tray extras
Arthroscopy tower with light source, camera unit, monitor; 2.7 mm 30-degree arthroscope with sleeve and blunt obturator (2.4 mm arthroscope in small dogs and cats and 4 mm arthroscope in giant breeds); two 50 mm (2 inch) 20 gauge needles; two 10 ml hypodermic syringes; giving set; sufficient quantity of Hartmann's solution (usually 1 litre); for operative arthroscopy appropriate operative instruments will need to be added, e.g. appropriately sized cannulas, switching stick, range of arthroscopic grasping forceps, arthroscopic probe.

Surgical technique

Lateral portals
A hypodermic needle is placed into the craniolateral aspect of the shoulder joint between the acromion process and the greater tubercle. Synovial fluid is aspirated and 5–10 ml of Hartmann's injected into the joint space. A second hypodermic needle is placed into the joint approximately 1 cm distal to the acromion process (or slightly caudal to this). The needle should pass easily into the joint and move freely. A stab incision is made with a No. 11 blade along the path of this needle to enter the joint space. The sleeve and blunt obturator are then passed along this tissue track as the needle is removed. After the joint is entered, the obturator is removed and the arthroscope inserted. The light source, camera and giving set are attached and the fluid flow commenced.

The joint should be inspected in an orderly fashion, starting cranially and medially and passing caudally. After the medial aspect of the joint has been inspected, the articular surfaces are observed, followed by the craniolateral and caudolateral aspects.

An instrument portal is usually established caudolaterally, initially by placement of a hypodermic needle under arthroscopic guidance. A stab incision along the line of this needle then allows placement of a switching stick over which the cannula is placed. Removal of the switching stick allows placement of operative instruments.

Craniomedial portal (push-through technique)
If a craniomedial portal is required, this can be established using a push-through technique. Using the lateral portal, the arthroscope is pushed against the joint capsule between the subscapularis tendon and the biceps brachii tendon. The sleeve is held in this position as the arthroscope is removed and a switching stick inserted and used to puncture the capsule and push through the soft tissues to exit under the skin craniomedially. An incision over the protruding switching stick allows the stick to be pushed further and the arthroscope sleeve is moved from the lateral position over the stick and guided into the joint craniomedially. This portal allows inspection of the medial gutter and the lateral aspect of the joint.

> **PRACTICAL TIP**
> All portals are interchangeable if necessary.

Closure
Single skin sutures are placed in the portal sites.

Postoperative care
Generally: 48 hours rest following diagnostic arthroscopy. If operative procedures are used, the period of rest is extended as appropriate to each individual procedure.

Complications
Accumulation of subcutaneous fluid can occur during the procedure. This can cause some joint space collapse; it resolves within 48–72 hours.

Chapter 17 The shoulder

OPERATIVE TECHNIQUE 17.5
Arthrotomy for osteochondritis dissecans of the humeral head

Positioning
Lateral recumbency with operative limb uppermost. Placement of a foam wedge between the limb and operating table helps support the limb.

Assistant
- Valuable in aiding exposure of the caudal humeral head, in particular, since this requires marked internal rotation of the limb. Alternatively, this can be achieved by an unscrubbed assistant manipulating the limb under the surgical drapes.
- Desirable to assist with inward rotation of the humeral head which is required to expose the remaining connection of the OCD flap, which is invariably medial.

Tray extras
Treves self-retaining retractors; Weitlander self-retaining retractors; Gelpi retractors (large and/or small); Hohmann retractors (of appropriate size and including blunt-ended variants); bone skid; OCD curette(s); Kirschner wires or small drill bits for forage of any eburnated subchondral bone; forceps designed for arthroscopic surgery (useful because of their size).

Surgical technique
Follow Operative Technique 17.3. Once the OCD lesion is identified, the aim is to remove all the under-run cartilage and any 'joint mice' from the caudal joint pouch. The latter can generally be retrieved by probing the caudal joint pouch with a pair of haemostats. It is advisable to refrain from placing a Hohmann retractor into the joint space until the majority of the flap has been removed, otherwise there is a chance that the retractor will push the flap off the humeral head and into the medial or cranial joint space, from which retrieval can be difficult. It is useful to grasp the flap with forceps, place a curette under it to the point where it is attached and then lever the flap from the surrounding cartilage. The margins of the defect are then inspected to ensure the entire area of under-run cartilage has been removed, leaving sharp edges all around. Granulation tissue within the defect is left in place but any areas of eburnated bone may be foraged with a Kirschner wire or small drill bit to encourage granulation.

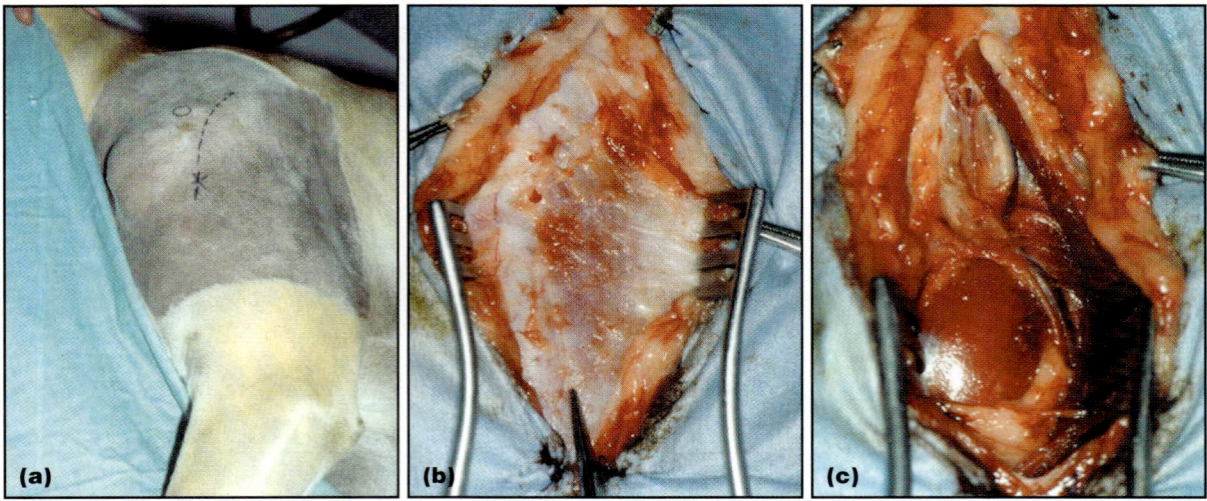

17.28 Surgical treatment of OCD. **(a)** Landmarks for the incision. O marks the acromion. The incision starts about halfway down the scapular spine and ends towards the distal extremity of the deltoid tuberosity. **(b)** Subcutaneous tissue is dissected and retracted to expose the fascia over the deltoid muscle. **(c)** An incision is made through the fascia over the division between the two heads of the muscle and the two are then separated and retracted to expose the teres minor muscle and the neurovascular complex over the caudal joint capsule (compare with Figure 17.27d). (continues)

Chapter 17 The shoulder

OPERATIVE TECHNIQUE 17.5 *continued*
Arthrotomy for osteochondritis dissecans of the humeral head

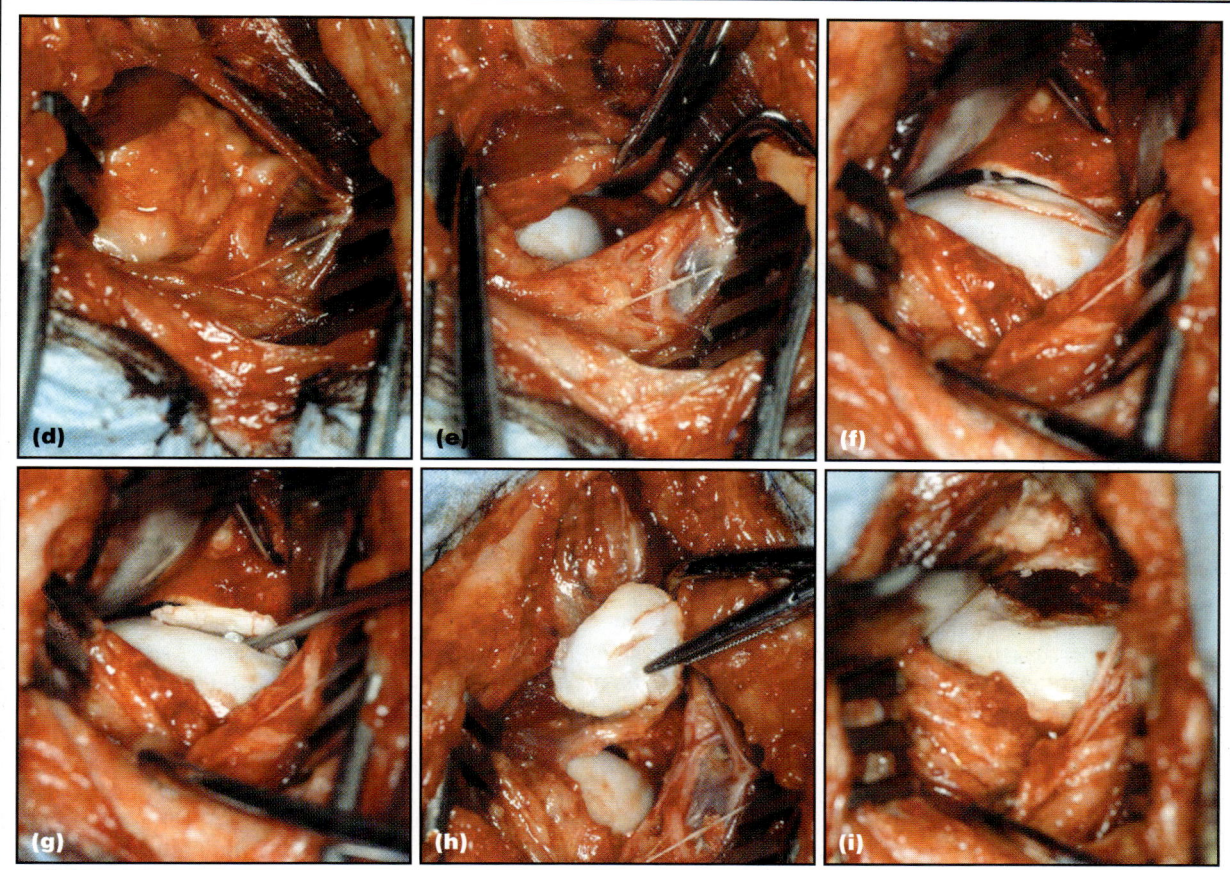

17.28 (continued) **(d)** The muscular branch of the axillary nerve and the caudal circumflex humeral vessels are then dissected from the joint capsule and are carefully retracted caudally (if they do not 'fall away' on their own) whilst the teres minor muscle is retracted cranially. **(e)** The capsule is incised to expose the humeral head (compare with Figure 17.27e). **(f)** Inward rotation of the shoulder is usually required to bring an OCD lesion into view; a Hohmann retractor is in place here for clarity of image but care should be taken to try to remove the cartilage flap first otherwise the retractor may push it off into the medial joint space from where retrieval can prove difficult. **(g)** A probe is used to elevate the cartilage flap and prise it away from its medial attachments, preferably whilst the lateral edge is held firmly with forceps. **(h)** The cartilage flap is removed, preferably in one piece. **(i)** The defect on the humeral head is then examined to ensure that all the margins are clear of detached cartilage, any granulation tissue or fibrocartilage is left on the floor of the defect but any eburnated subchondral bone may be foraged in an attempt to improve vascularization and encourage the formation of fibrocartilage.

Closure
After thorough flushing of the joint with sterile normal saline, closure is achieved as described in Operative Technique 17.3.

Postoperative care
The dog should be restricted to lead exercise and room rest for 6–8 weeks whilst the cartilage defect heals. The distance walked is governed only by what does not make the patient significantly worse (in terms of degree of lameness or stiffness after rest). After that period most cases should be sound and can be returned to normal exercise over the following month.

Complications
- Seroma formation (see Operative Technique 17.3).
- If there is failure to remove completely all the under-run cartilage, lameness may persist and repeat surgery is indicated.

Chapter 17 The shoulder

OPERATIVE TECHNIQUE 17.6
Lateral shoulder stabilization

Positioning
See Operative Technique 17.2.

Assistant
Desirable but not essential.

Tray extras
See Operative Technique 17.2
  Periosteal elevator; drill bits and sleeves of appropriate sizes to create bone tunnels; wire to create loops to facilitate placement of prosthesis through tunnels;

- Bone screws and spiked washers, together with appropriate drill bit, depth gauge, (tap) and screwdriver; or
- Suture screws, together with appropriate drill bit, depth gauge and screwdriver; or
- Tissue anchors, together with the appropriate 'driving' instrumentation.

  Material for the prosthesis, generally non-absorbable and either coated braided polyester (Ethibond, Ethicon) or monofilament nylon (leader line). Crimps and crimping pliers if these are to be used to secure the material.

Surgical technique
Follow Operative Technique 17.2.
  In order to expose the distal end of the scapular spine for anchorage of a lateral prosthesis, osteotomy of the acromion can be performed (Figure 17.29a). However, by separating the two heads of the deltoid muscle it is quite possible to retrieve suture material placed through a tunnel in the scapular spine and then pass it back under the acromial head of the deltoid muscle.
  A cranial to caudal tunnel is drilled through the scapular spine as far distally as possible and the prosthesis anchored proximally by passage through this and back under the acromial head of the deltoid muscle. The distal attachment for the prosthesis is on the lateral aspect of the greater tubercle (Figure 17.29b), either where the ligament insertion can be seen or close to the insertion of the infraspinatus muscle if the remnants of ligament cannot be identified. Fixation of the prosthesis can be achieved by creation of a caudocranial tunnel in the greater tubercle (which can be difficult to execute). Alternatives to this include fixation under a bone screw and spiked washer, through a suture screw or a tissue anchor (Figure 17.29c). When tying or crimping the prosthesis it is important not to overtighten, since this will create abduction of the limb and encourage early failure of the material.

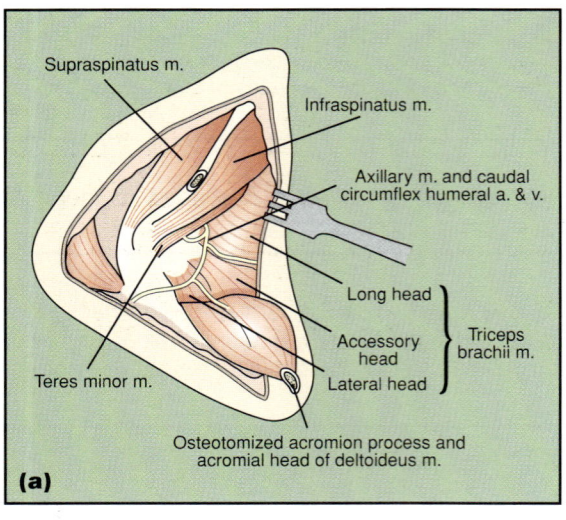

17.29 Lateral stabilization of the shoulder joint. **(a)** The caudal aspect of the scapular spine can be accessed by osteotomy of the acromion process, but separation of the two heads of the deltoid muscle will usually suffice; osteotomy is shown here for clarity. (continues)

Chapter 17 The shoulder

OPERATIVE TECHNIQUE 17.6 continued
Lateral shoulder stabilization

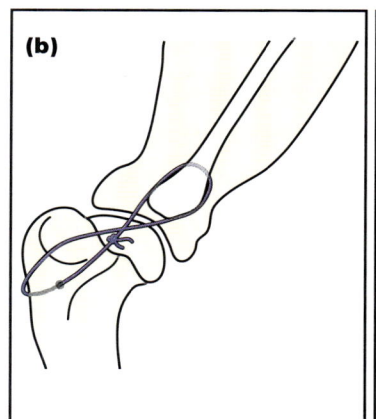

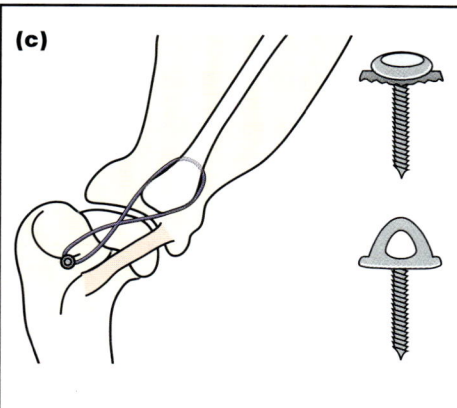

17.29 (continued) **(b)** A lateral prosthesis of braided polyester or monofilament leader line is passed through a tunnel created in the distal scapular spine and a second tunnel drilled in the greater tubercle or **(c)** is anchored around or through an implant (bone screw with spiked washer/suture screw/tissue anchor) placed in the greater tubercle close to the insertion of the teres minor muscle.

PRACTICAL TIP
Placement of a combined lateral and medial prosthesis (Figure 17.30) requires access to the medial aspect of the joint. This can be achieved by retraction of the supraspinatus muscle.

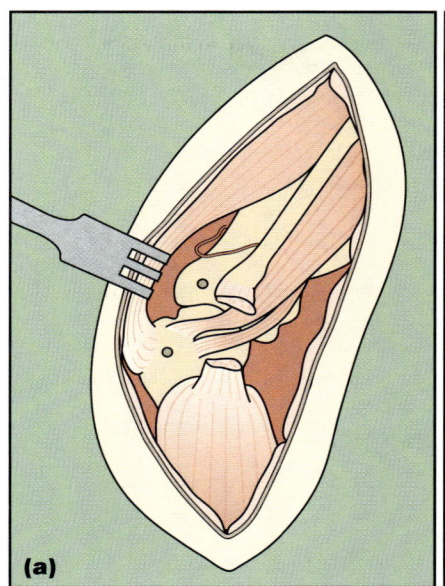

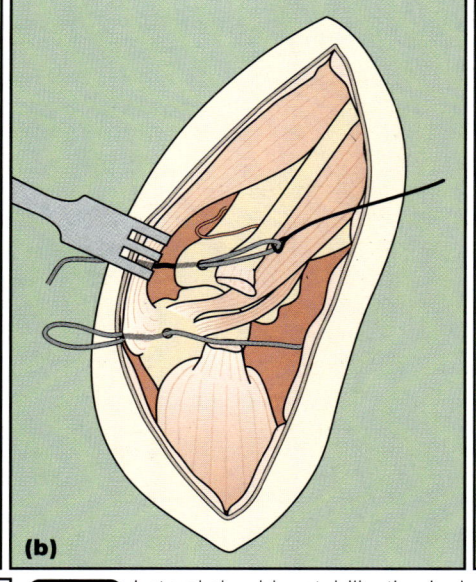

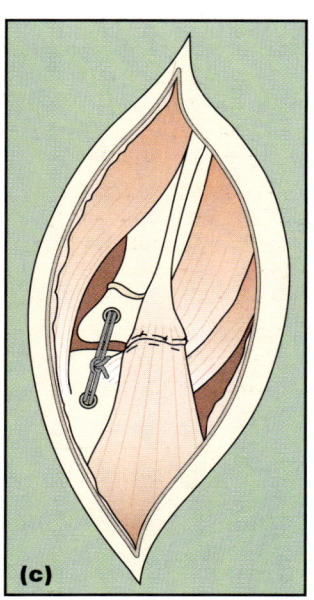

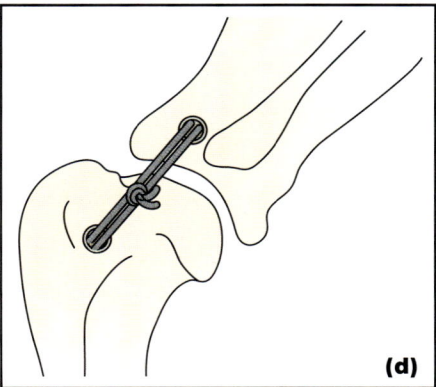

17.30 Lateral shoulder stabilization including modification to combine lateral and medial stabilization. **(a)** The scapular neck and proximal humerus are exposed as shown in Figure 17.25. **(b)** Transverse tunnels are created in the scapular neck and humerus close to the insertion of teres minor. A prosthesis of braided nylon or leader line is passed through these. **(c)** After repair of any available joint capsule, the prosthesis is tightened so the joint is stable but not restricted in range of motion, and tied (or crimped). **(d)** Position of prosthesis.

241

Chapter 17 The shoulder

> **OPERATIVE TECHNIQUE 17.6** *continued*
> **Lateral shoulder stabilization**

Closure
See Operative Technique 17.2.

Postoperative care
Following surgery the dog should be restricted to lead exercise and room rest for 6–8 weeks whilst fibrosis becomes established. The distance walked is governed only by what does not make the patient significantly worse (in terms of degree of lameness or stiffness after rest). After that period most cases should be sound and can be returned to normal exercise over the following month.

Complications
Implant failure is an uncommon complication.

Chapter 17 The shoulder

OPERATIVE TECHNIQUE 17.7
Medial shoulder stabilization

Positioning
See Operative Technique 17.1.

Assistant
Desirable but not essential.

Tray extras
See Operative Technique 17.1; suture screws or tissue anchors, with instrumentation to apply them; crimps and pliers for crimping if these are used to secure the suture; small Hohmann retractors.

Surgical technique
Follow Operative Technique 17.1. The subscapularis muscle is incised and elevated to reveal the medial joint capsule and remnants of the medial glenohumeral ligament. This exposure is aided by placement of small Hohmann retractors behind the scapula and cranially under the supraspinatus muscle (Figure 17.31a). Suture screws or tissue anchors are then placed at the points of origin (two) and insertion (one) of the ligament. Sutures of braided polyester or monofilament nylon are then placed to recreate both components of the ligament (Figure 17.31b). When tying or crimping the prosthesis it is important not to overtighten since this will create adduction of the limb and encourage early failure of the material.

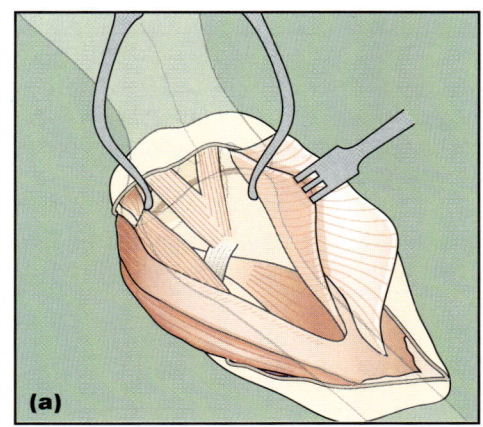

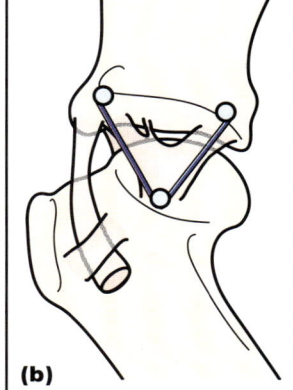

17.31 Medial stabilization of the shoulder joint. **(a)** Incisions are made in the coracobrachialis and subscapularis tendons to expose the joint capsule and glenohumeral ligament. Exposure can be helped by placement of a small Hohmann retractor caudal to the scapula and a second one under the supraspinatus muscle, passing cranial to the scapula. **(b)** Suture screws or tissue anchors are then introduced at the identified points of origin and point of insertion of the medial glenohumeral ligament, and two separate sutures of braided polyester or monofilament leader line are used to replace both the cranial and caudal components of the ligament.

Closure
See Operative Technique 17.1.

Postoperative care
Following surgery the dog should be restricted to room rest for 6–8 weeks. After that, a gradual return to lead exercise is recommended; the distance walked is governed only by what does not make the patient significantly worse (in terms of degree of lameness or stiffness after rest).

Complications
Implant failure is an uncommon complication.

Chapter 17 The shoulder

OPERATIVE TECHNIQUE 17.8
Tenotomy or tenodesis of the biceps brachii tendon of origin

Positioning
See Operative Technique 17.1.

Assistant
Desirable but not essential.

Tray extras
See Operative Technique 17.1.

- Tenotomy: No. 11 scalpel blade
- Tenodesis – there are three methods to fixate the tendon origin:
  - Method 1 – ligament staple of appropriate size (usually 8 or 11 mm) and a means of driving it home (mallet ± staple guide)
  - Method 2 – Bone screw and spiked washer and appropriate drill bit; sleeve; depth gauge; (tap if non-self tapping screw); screw driver
  - Method 3 – Drill bit to create tunnel in greater tubercle; monofilament nylon to aid passage of tendon through tunnel; wire to form loop with which to pull nylon through the tunnel; appropriate suture material to secure tendon to supraspinatus tendon of insertion laterally (non-absorbable monofilament or long-lasting absorbable, e.g. PDS, Ethicon).

Surgical technique
Follow Operative Technique 17.1. Once the biceps tendon has been exposed it can be followed proximally to its point of origin on the scapular tuberosity and released using a scalpel blade. If such a tenotomy is to be accompanied by tenodesis then it may be better to cut the tendon after first securing it to the proximal humerus (only possible with Methods 1 and 2). Tenodesis can be achieved in a number of ways.

Method 1
The simplest technique is to place a ligament staple over the tendon and drive it into the humerus (Figure 17.32a). A tenotomy can then be performed, the tendon folded over the staple and sutured to itself with 3.5 or 3 metric (0 or 2/0 USP) polydioxanone.

Method 2
The biceps tendon can be secured to the humerus with a bone screw and spiked washer (Figure 17.32b).

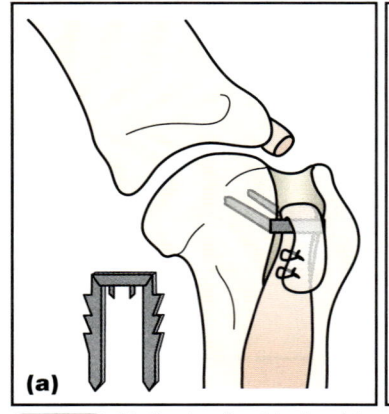

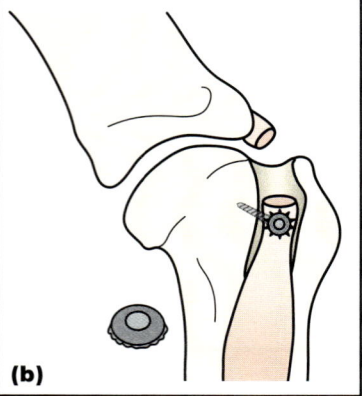

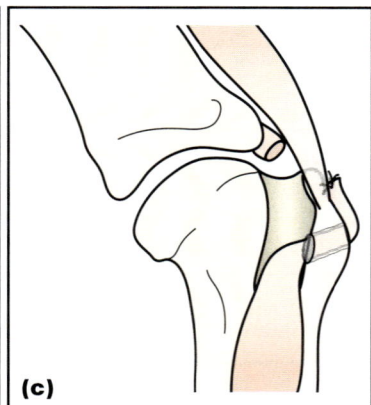

17.32 Methods of achieving biceps tenodesis. **(a)** A ligament staple is used to secure the tendon to the proximal humerus; the tendon is then incised from the scapular tuberosity, folded over the staple and sutured to itself. **(b)** A bone screw and spiked washer are used to secure the tendon to the proximal humerus before or after it is incised from the scapular tuberosity. **(c)** The tendon is incised from the scapular tuberosity, drawn through a tunnel created in the greater tubercle and sutured to the supraspinatus tendon of insertion laterally.

→

OPERATIVE TECHNIQUE 17.8 continued
Tenotomy or tenodesis of the biceps brachii tendon of origin

Method 3
The tendon can be drawn through a transverse tunnel created in the greater tubercle and then sutured to the supraspinatus tendon of insertion laterally (Figure 17.32c).

Method 4
Methods 2 and 3 can be combined (Adamiak and Szalecki, 2003).

WARNING
In all cases it is important that the elbow is held in extension when the tendon is fixed to the humerus, otherwise the joint will have a reduced range of motion postoperatively.

It is quite possible to perform tenodesis without tenotomy of the biceps and some would argue that doing so should help preserve scapulohumeral joint stability whilst, it is hoped, removing the pain from tenosynovitis by stopping movement of the tendon within its sheath. The decision as to whether to perform tenotomy or not is subjective with no scientific study to support one over the other. The authors' current opinion is to perform tenotomy since any tendinitis contributing to the pain might continue if the tendon is not released from its origin.

Closure
See Operative Technique 17.1

Postoperative care
Following surgery the dog should be restricted to lead exercise and room rest for 6–8 weeks whilst the tenodesis becomes established. The distance walked is governed only by what does not make the patient significantly worse (in terms of degree of lameness or stiffness after rest). After that period most cases should be sound and can be returned to normal exercise over the following month.

Complications
Implant failure is an uncommon complication.

Chapter 17 The shoulder

OPERATIVE TECHNIQUE 17.9
Scapulohumeral arthrodesis

Positioning
See Operative Technique 17.2.

Assistant
Desirable but not essential.

Tray extras
Treves self-retaining retractors; Weitlander self-retaining retractors; Gelpi retractors (large and/or small); bone skid; periosteal elevator; oscillating saw; a range of suitable implants for stabilization of the arthrodesis site and reattachment of the greater tubercle/acromion (bone plates, screws, washers, Kirschner wires); the instrumentation that is required to apply those implants (drill, drill bits, sleeves, depth gauge, taps, screwdriver, wire cutters, wire benders, wire twisters – all depending on what implants are being used); plate bending irons/pliers/press for contouring the plate; curette/rongeurs/bone cutters for harvesting cancellous bone from 'off cuts'; a Kirschner wire or Steinmann pin bent to an angle of 105–110 degrees preoperatively as a guide during surgery.

Surgical technique
Follow Operative Technique 17.2. An osteotomy of the greater tubercle is performed to expose the cranial surface of the proximal humerus and the supraspinatus muscle should be elevated proximally to expose at least half of the scapular spine. Tenotomies of the infraspinatus and teres minor tendons of insertion, and tenotomy of the acromial head of the deltoid (or osteotomy of the acromion) are required to expose adequately the lateral aspect of the scapulohumeral joint from cranial to caudal.

The articular surfaces are then removed by making parallel osteotomies across the humeral head and the glenoid, such that when the two surfaces are apposed the angle through the joint is in the order of 105–110 degrees. The surfaces are held in position by placement of a Kirschner wire or, if possible, a lagged bone screw (although the latter is often prevented by the fact that the screw would hamper plate application).

An appropriately sized dynamic compression plate (DCP) is then contoured to fit along the cranial border of the scapular spine and cranial surface of the proximal humerus (Figure 17.33a). This will require quite a marked twist in the plate over the point of the shoulder. Although use of a reconstruction plate would make the contouring much easier, such plates are manufactured in a way that makes them malleable and so much more prone to fatigue failure than comparably sized DCPs. A DCP is also preferable to a round-holed plate as it allows screws to be placed at an angle and still sit properly in the plate hole. Provision should be made to place between five and seven plate screws on each side of the osteotomy. The screws in the scapula are aimed at the base of the scapular spine, since the cross-section of the bone at this point is triangular making adequate purchase more likely. However, it is to be expected that some of these screws will strip the threads in the pilot hole, which is the reason for making provision for more plate screws than are absolutely necessary in the first place. During plate application an attempt is made to place one plate screw in lagged fashion if such an implant was not placed initially. A useful way of achieving this is to place a temporary Kirschner wire to stabilize the osteotomy, such

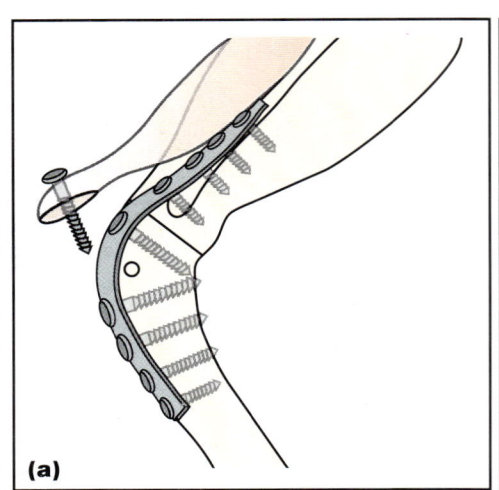

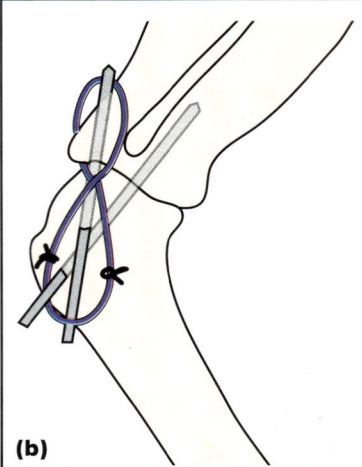

17.33 Scapulohumeral arthrodesis. **(a)** A contoured bone plate is used to stabilize the site in medium and large breeds of dog. The plate is applied to the scapula in such a way as to direct the bone screws into the base of the scapular spine as the triangular cross-section of the scapula at this site will help screw purchase. **(b)** Kirschner wires and a tension-band wire are used to stabilize the site in small dogs and cats.

OPERATIVE TECHNIQUE 17.9 *continued*
Scapulohumeral arthrodesis

that the plate is applied over the Kirschner wire with it protruding through a plate hole. Once plate screws have been secured towards the ends of the plate the Kirschner wire is replaced with a lagged bone screw. If it is not possible to introduce a lagged bone screw then an attempt can be made to compress the site using the plate, if it is a DCP. However, this can prove difficult given the extreme contouring used and the fact that the bone screws in the scapula often show poor purchase. If more than four plate screws are placed into the humerus then it may be advantageous to make the most distal one monocortical to try to reduce any stress riser at the end of the plate. If this is utilized then the pilot hole must not penetrate the transcortex.

> **PRACTICAL TIP**
> In the case of small dogs and cats adequate stability may be achieved by placement of Kirschner wires or small Steinmann pins and a tension-band wire over the cranial aspect of the joint (Figure 17.33b).

Since there is a large surface area of cancellous bone in contact there is no need to augment this site with cancellous bone harvested from elsewhere. However, if any such bone graft can be retrieved from the excised part of the humeral head or glenoid then it can be packed around the osteotomy line.

Closure
Closure involves reattachment of the tendons of the infraspinatus, teres minor and deltoid muscles or reattachment of the acromion with either sutures or Kirschner wires and a tension band wire. The osteotomy of the greater tubercle cannot be repaired because of the presence of the implants, but it can be reattached to the lateral aspect of the proximal humerus using a bone screw and spiked washer. The remainder of the closure is as described in Operative Technique 17.2.

Postoperative care
External support is advantageous until radiographic evidence of fusion becomes apparent, usually by about 6 weeks post surgery. This requires application of either a body cast or a Spica splint. Care should be taken to observe for evidence of excoriation of the skin in the axilla due to rubbing by the cast. Once radiographic fusion is underway, external support can be withdrawn but the patient must remain on lead exercise and room rest for a further 6–8 weeks, at which point it is to be hoped that radiographs will show arthrodesis to be complete with no evidence of implant loosening (Figure 17.34).

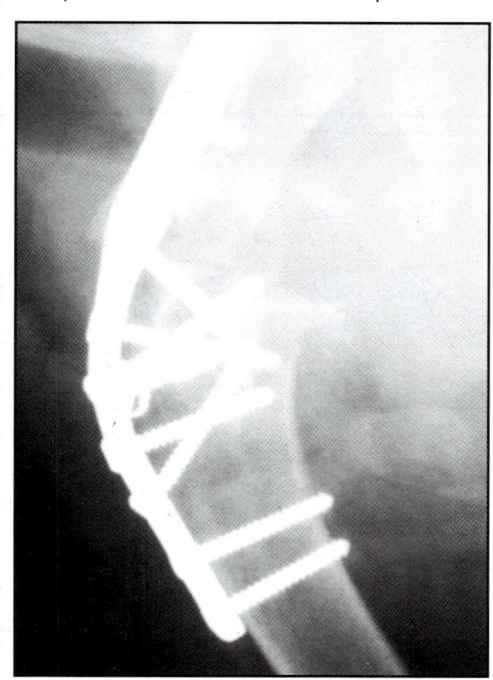

17.34 Mediolateral postoperative radiograph of a 12-year-old Shetland Sheepdog treated for pain from a chronic medial shoulder luxation by arthrodesis.

Chapter 17 The shoulder

OPERATIVE TECHNIQUE 17.9 continued
Scapulohumeral arthrodesis

From that time on, exercise can be gradually returned to normal in line with what the patient is able to accomplish. Because of compensation by movement through the omothoracic junction (Figure 17.35), loss of movement in the scapulohumeral joint causes remarkably little functional disability. A mechanical lameness persists as the limb is circumducted during protraction to avoid dragging the toes. Overall, the functional outcome is usually very good (Fowler *et al.*, 1988).

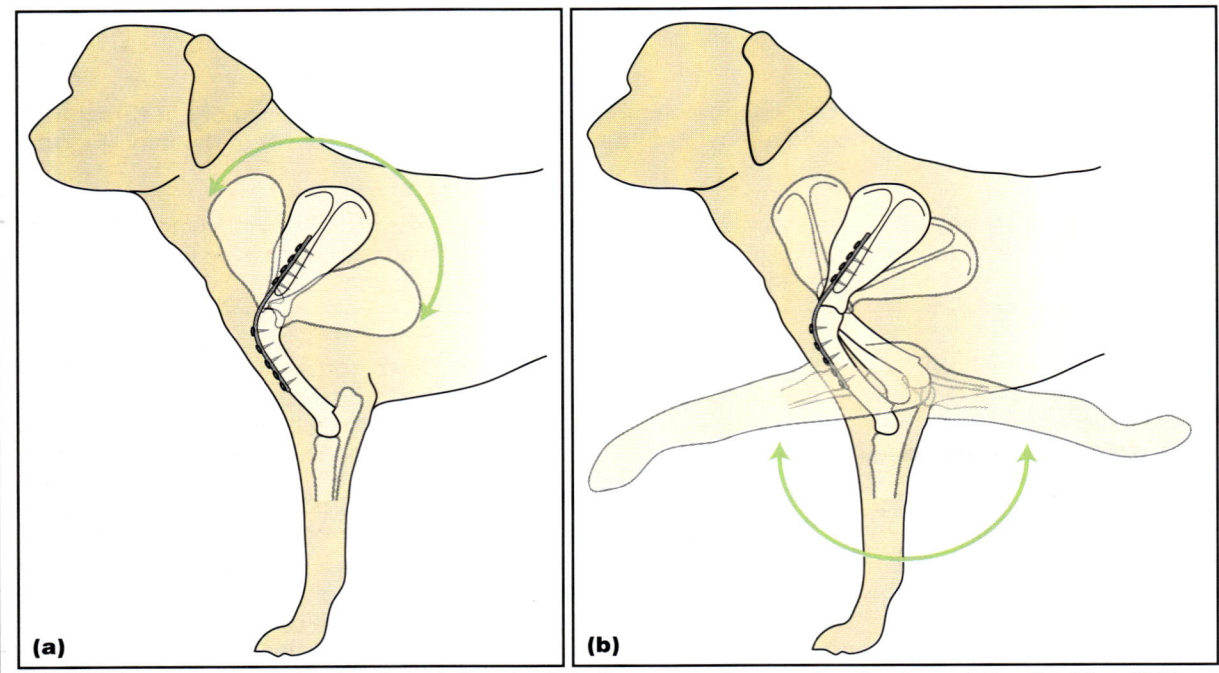

17.35 Mobility through the omothoracic junction **(a)** allows a good range of motion through the distal limb **(b)** to compensate for loss of movement in the scapulohumeral joint.

Complications
Implant failure is an uncommon complication.

18

The elbow

Geoff Robins and John Innes

Introduction

The canine elbow joint is the most common source of non-traumatic thoracic limb lameness in dogs and osteoarthritis of the elbow is becoming more commonly recognized in cats. The architectural complexity of the elbow joint makes it susceptible to subtle incongruence and the early diagnosis of osteoarthritis can be difficult. Although considerable progress has been made in recent years in diagnostic and treatment methods for diseases of the elbow joint, the precise cause and definitive treatment of the developmental conditions of the elbow remain controversial.

Arthroscopy has become an important tool for the diagnosis and treatment of diseases of the elbow. Arthroscopy permits both the full inspection of all articular structures and minimally invasive treatment.

The close association of the three bones that make up the elbow and the fact that it is surrounded by muscles, with vital neurovascular structures on the lateral, cranial and medial aspects, ensure that there is little room for error with any surgical intervention. In practical terms the elbow can be a difficult joint to work on, with few straightforward surgical approaches.

Clinical anatomy

The elbow joint is a stable compound ginglymus, or hinge joint, capable of flexion to about 20 degrees, extension to about 140 degrees and a limited amount of rotation (approximately 60 degrees).

Bony anatomy

The elbow has three articulations: the humeroradial joint; the humeroulnar joint; and the radioulnar joint. A common joint cavity exists for all three articulations. The articular surface of the distal humerus, the humeral condyle, is positioned cranial to the long axis of the shaft and is shaped like an inclined cylinder. It is divided into a small lateral area, the capitulum humeri, which articulates with the radial head, and the larger medially located trochlea humeri, which articulates with the trochlear notch of the ulna. The humeral condyle develops as lateral and medial components that should fuse during development to form the single condyle. The lateral and medial epicondyles are readily palpable surgical landmarks but they are located proximal and caudal to the horizontal axis of the humeral condyle, which is an important consideration when inserting implants to stabilize distal humeral fractures.

The proximal ulna, the olecranon, has three processes on its cranial surface. The largest is the anconeal process, which slopes backwards to the two smaller, unnamed processes that lie side-by-side near the proximal extremity of the ulna. In flexion these two processes function as a trochlear groove for the large triceps tendon, which is attached to the tip of the olecranon. The anconeal process of the ulna articulates with the caudal intercondylar surface of the humerus and fits into the supratrochlear fossa when the joint is fully extended. The proximal ulna does not lie in the midline of the antebrachium. When viewed from behind it has a medial to lateral inclination in a proximal to distal direction and this should be considered when internal fixation devices are inserted down the medullary canal of the ulna. The trochlear notch of the ulna articulates with the trochlea of the humerus. Distal to the trochlear notch are two prominences called the medial and lateral coronoid processes; the medial process is larger and is located more distally than the lateral. The radial head articulates with a curved depression between the two coronoid processes called the radial notch and is held in place by the annular ligament.

Ligaments

The joint is supported by well developed lateral and medial collateral ligaments (Figure 18.1). These arise as single origins on the lateral and medial epicondyles and insert as double radial and ulnar branches. The stability of the elbow is assisted during extension by the presence of the anconeal process within the supratrochlear fossa of the humerus. The annular ligament forms a loop on the cranial aspect of the joint encompassing the radial head, with medial and lateral attachments just distal to the coronoid processes of the ulna.

The lateral collateral ligament originates on the lateral epicondyle and, after blending with the annular ligament, divides distally into two crura. The larger cranial portion inserts on to the radial head, while the thinner caudal part inserts on the ulna. A sesamoid bone is occasionally found between the ligament and the radial head. The smaller and weaker medial collateral ligament originates on the medial

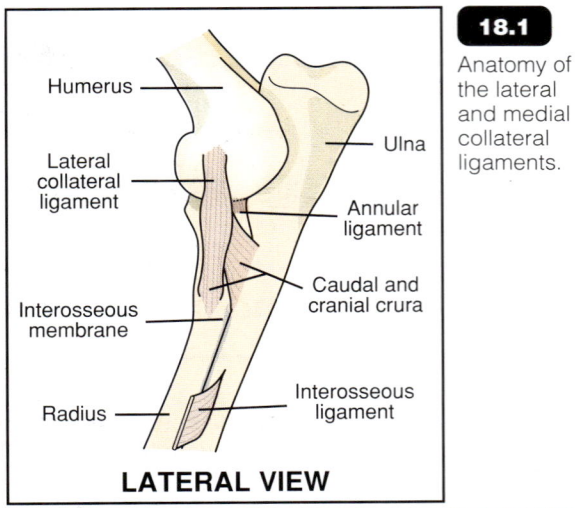

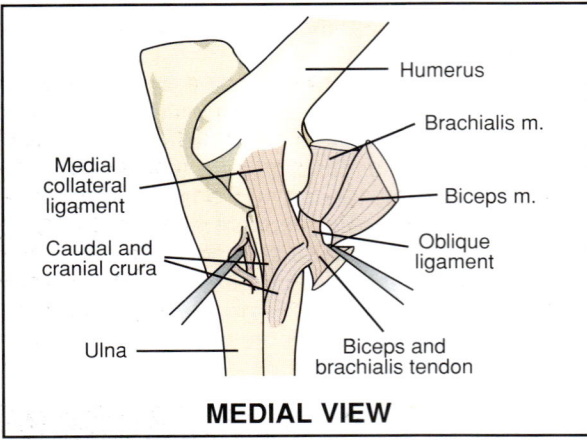

Chapter 18 The elbow

18.1 Anatomy of the lateral and medial collateral ligaments.

LATERAL VIEW
- Humerus
- Lateral collateral ligament
- Interosseous membrane
- Radius
- Ulna
- Annular ligament
- Caudal and cranial crura
- Interosseous ligament

MEDIAL VIEW
- Humerus
- Brachialis m.
- Biceps m.
- Oblique ligament
- Biceps and brachialis tendon
- Medial collateral ligament
- Caudal and cranial crura
- Ulna

epicondyle and also divides into two crura. The weaker cranial part attaches on to the radial head, while the stronger caudal part passes deeply into the interosseous space where it attaches mainly to the ulna, but also to the radius.

Muscles and tendons
The main muscle groups surrounding the elbow joint are the extensors of the elbow caudally (triceps brachii and anconeus), the flexors of the elbow cranially (brachialis, biceps brachii), the carpal and digital extensors laterally and distally, and the carpal and digital flexors medially and distally. The extensor muscles of the carpus and digits originate directly or indirectly from the lateral epicondyle of the humerus. These muscles, in a cranial to caudal direction, are:

- Extensor carpi radialis
- Common digital extensor
- Lateral digital extensor
- Extensor carpi ulnaris.

The supinator muscle lies under the extensor carpi radialis and the lateral collateral ligament lies between the lateral digital extensor and the extensor carpi ulnaris.
Most of the flexor muscles of the carpus and digits originate from the region of the medial epicondyle of the humerus. These muscles, in a cranial to caudal direction, are:

- Flexor carpi radialis
- Deep digital flexor
- Superficial digital flexor
- Flexor carpi ulnaris.

The pronator teres lies cranial to the flexor carpi radialis and the medial collateral ligament lies between these two muscles.

Nerves
The radial nerve courses across the distal third of the lateral aspect of the humerus but is unlikely to be encountered during elbow joint surgery. However, on the medial aspect, the ulnar nerve passes close to the medial epicondylar ridge. In addition, a branch of the median nerve to the flexors of the carpus and digits and a branch of the brachial artery pass distal to the medial aspect of the elbow joint close to the inner surface of the pronator teres muscle; care must be taken during medial approaches to the elbow not to damage this branch. In the cat, the medial epicondyle contains an epicondyloid foramen through which the median nerve travels.

Arthroscopic anatomy of the normal elbow joint
Arthroscopic examination of the elbow joint (see Operative Technique 18.1) is most commonly performed from the medial aspect (Figure 18.2) (Van Ryssen *et al.*, 1992).

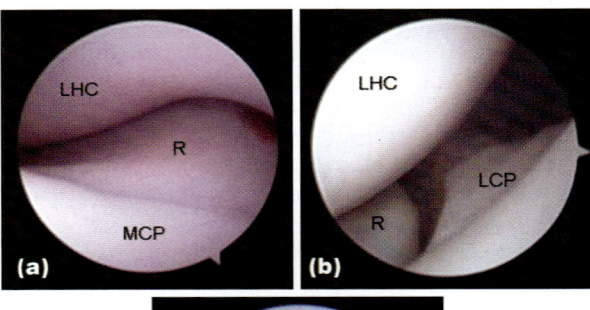

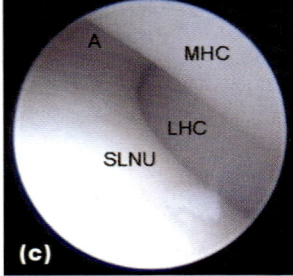

18.2 Arthroscopic appearance of the normal canine elbow joint from the medial portal. **(a)** The light pole is positioned at 9 o'clock to view the radial head, humeral condyle and medial coronoid process. **(b)** The arthroscope is positioned with the light pole at 12 o'clock to view over the 'horizon' of the semilunar notch of the ulna and inspect the lateral compartment of the elbow joint. **(c)** The arthroscope is viewing proximally and caudally, with the light pole positioned at 5 o'clock. (A, anconeus; LCP, lateral coronoid process; LHC, lateral humeral condyle; MCP, medial coronoid process; MHC, medial humeral condyle; R, radial head; SLNU, semilunar notch of ulna).

250

Chapter 18 The elbow

From this approach the following structures can be evaluated:

- Medial side of the anconeal process
- Medial side of the trochlear notch
- Medial and lateral coronoid processes
- Medial, cranial and caudal aspects of the radial head.

More detail on general arthroscopy can be found in Chapter 15.

Surgical approaches to the elbow

Caudolateral approach
The caudolateral approach (see Operative Technique 18.2) is indicated for the following procedures:

- Excision or fixation of un-united anconeal process
- Surgical reduction of elbow luxation.

Medial approach
The medial approach (see Operative Technique 18.3) is indicated for exploration of the medial compartment of the elbow for OCD lesions and fragmentation of the medial coronoid process.

Transolecranon or caudal approach
This approach is usually reserved for those cases where a wide exposure is required, for example for the open reduction and fixation of T and Y fractures of the distal humerus (see *BSAVA Manual of Small Animal Fracture Repair and Management*), although in experienced hands it is possible to repair these fractures via a combined medial and lateral approach. The caudal approach may be achieved via an olecranon osteotomy or tenotomy of the triceps tendon. This approach is illustrated in Operative Technique 18.4.

'Open-book' approach
This approach, first described by Lenehan and Nunamaker (1982), is a modified lateral approach to the elbow through an osteotomy of the ulna below the elbow joint, but above the interosseous ligament (see Operative Technique 18.5). It is indicated for examination of multiple compartments of the elbow and treatment of chronic luxation.

Congenital luxation

This uncommon problem occurs in two distinct forms, sometimes referred to as types 1 and 2. There is some confusion in the literature on the classification of the two types so in this chapter they will be described as humeroulnar luxation and radial head luxation. A third type of congenital elbow luxation has been associated with generalized joint laxity and other congenital skeletal deformities, including ectrodactyly.

Humeroulnar luxation
This type of congenital luxation results in a severe disability, often with complete luxation of the elbow. It is associated with 90 degrees of outward rotation of the proximal ulna, removing the trochlear notch and the anconeal process from effective articulation with the humerus, and displacing the triceps tendon. This results in marked rotation and lateral deviation of the antebrachium, lateral rotation of the paw and marked reduction in elbow extension. The condition is usually recognized at birth or within the first 3 months of life. It can be uni- or bilateral and has its highest incidence in small breeds. Breeds at risk include Yorkshire Terrier, Boston Terrier, Shetland Sheepdog, Miniature Poodle, Pekingese, Miniature Pinscher, Pomeranian, Pug, Cocker Spaniel, English Bulldog and Chihuahua.

Diagnosis
Gait analysis may demonstrate crossing of the thoracic limbs and mild to severe gait abnormality. Physical examination will demonstrate decreased range of motion and palpable lateral displacement of the proximal ulna. Radiographs will demonstrate a varying degree of luxation.

The craniocaudal projection of the elbow may reveal a normal frontal view of the humerus but a lateral view of the proximal ulna, whereas in the lateral projection the situation will be reversed, reflecting the 90-degree rotation of the proximal ulna relative to the distal humerus (Figure 18.3). Other changes that may be present include hypoplasia or aplasia of the anconeal process, trochlear notch, humeral condyle and coronoid processes, plus distortion of the olecranon (Kene *et al.*, 1982).

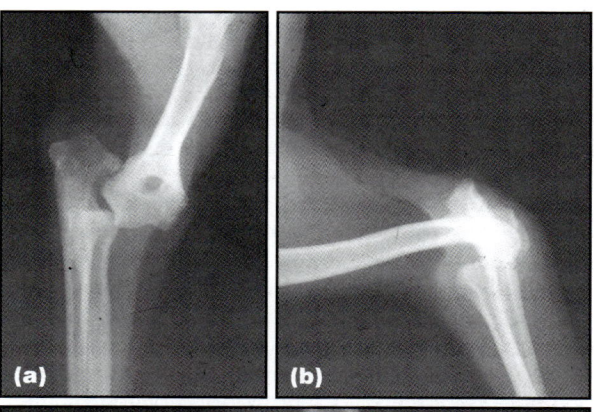

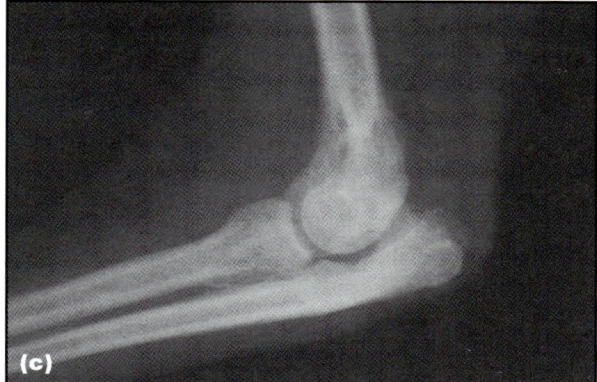

18.3 Congenital humeroulnar luxation: **(a)** craniocaudal view before reduction; note the lateral rotation of the proximal ulna; **(b)** mediolateral view; **(c)** mediolateral view post-reduction. (continues) ▶

Chapter 18 The elbow

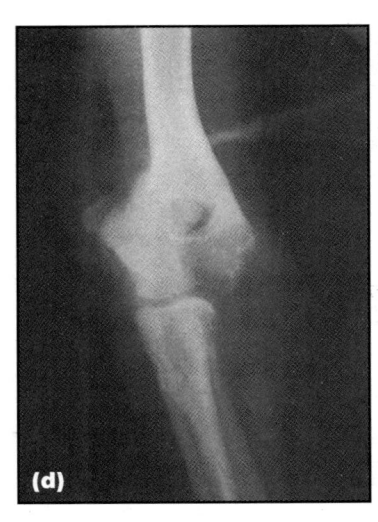

18.3 (continued) Congenital humeroulnar luxation: **(d)** craniocaudal view post-reduction.

Treatment
Conservative or medical management in these cases is generally unrewarding as the disease tends to worsen with skeletal maturation. Treatment by closed reduction should be attempted as soon as possible. If the reduction is unstable, temporary fixation in extension, using transarticular Kirschner wires or a hypodermic needle, should be attempted. The reduction is supported with a padded bandage until the pins are removed after 10–14 days. Relocation of the proximal ulna and stabilization can be achieved by the transcutaneous transverse placement of two small Steinmann pins, one through the condyle of the humerus and the other through the olecranon. Reduction is maintained by placing a tensioned elastic band from the medial aspect of the proximal pin to the lateral aspect of the distal pin. This causes the ulna to be rotated in a caudomedial direction. The caudal aspect of the elbow must be protected by a padded splint to prevent pressure necrosis. The bands and pins are removed after 10–14 days and external support is then continued for about 3 weeks (Milton *et al.*, 1979).

If closed reduction is impossible then open reduction can be attempted, but the results in some cases are poor. This is often the situation with neglected cases and it should be emphasized that surgery may be contraindicated if the animal is able to bear weight and walk on the limb. A number of procedures have been utilized and are tailored to suit the individual's needs. Milton *et al.* (1979) recommended the following procedures: medial capsulorrhaphy; lateral desmotomy; rotational osteotomy of the ulna; transposition of olecranon; fixation of the proximal ulna to the radius; reconstruction of the trochlear notch; and partial anconeal process resection. The joint is usually approached by osteotomy of the olecranon (see Operative Technique 18.4).

Radial head luxation
In this type of luxation the elbow does not luxate completely (the relationship between the humerus and ulna is normal); the proximal radius is displaced in a caudal and lateral direction. In general, the degree of disability is not as severe as with humeroulnar luxation. There is usually only mild limb deviation, but extension is reduced and the elbow is thickened with a marked lateral swelling. There may be caudal bowing of the proximal ulna. Affected animals are usually 4–5 months old at presentation and the following breeds have been identified with this condition: Pekingese, Yorkshire Terrier, Boxer, Bulldog, Rough Collie, Labrador Retriever, Old English Sheepdog, Bullmastiff, Bearded Collie, Bull Terrier and Pomeranian. Significantly, this radial type of congenital luxation is seen more commonly in medium to large-sized dogs than the ulnar type.

Diagnosis
Gait abnormalities may be mild to moderate and the patient may stand with an abducted elbow. The displaced radial head may be visible and palpable lateral to the joint. The radiographic changes seen with this type of elbow luxation (Figure 18.4) are different to the changes seen in the elbow joint following premature closure of the distal ulnar growth plate. The degree of radial head displacement is far greater with the congenital luxation and the proximal radial epiphysis is deformed due to lack of contact between the radial head and the lateral portion of the distal humeral condyle.

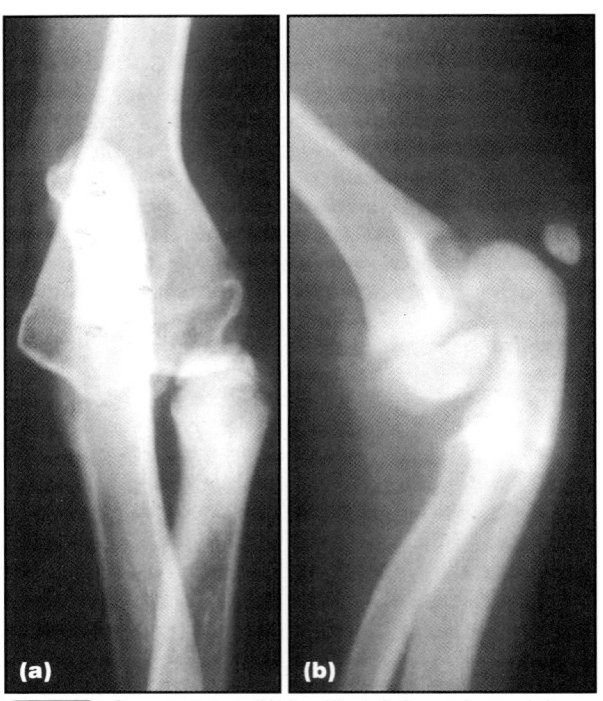

18.4 Congenital radial luxation: **(a)** craniocaudal view; **(b)** mediolateral view. Note the convex shape of the radial head, caused by lack of normal load-bearing forces.

Treatment
Conservative therapy may be the treatment of choice in mild cases although the patient should be monitored closely for progression of luxation. In the early stages, the radial head may be manipulated back into position and retained by tightening the surrounding soft tissues. In most cases an osteotomy of the radius or the ulna may be needed to effect reduction (Milton and Montgomery, 1987); osteotomy of the radius is usually stabilized using a bone plate and screws. Unfortunately,

Chapter 18 The elbow

in long-standing cases the deformity of the articular surface of the proximal radius makes perfect reduction impossible. A single case report records the successful reconstruction of the joint using a fascial strip to reconstruct the annular ligament (Bell–Tawse procedure), in addition to radial osteotomy and temporary transarticular pinning (Spadari *et al.*, 2001). Resection of the radial head can be utilized to salvage the joint if there is intractable pain and lameness, but affected animals often tolerate the displaced radial head quite well and in these cases no treatment is offered.

Traumatic luxation

Traumatic elbow luxation is an uncommon injury due to the intrinsic stability of the elbow joint and is usually seen in animals over 1 year of age. In dogs, the radius and ulna usually luxate in a lateral direction, as the large caudal projection of the medial epicondyle of the humerus prevents medial displacement. Luxation occurs when a lateral force is applied to the distal humerus when the joint is flexed and the antebrachium is twisted. Lateral displacement of the ulna is only possible when the anconeal process is disengaged from the supracondylar fossa and this only occurs when the joint is flexed more than 90 degrees. Rupture of both of the collateral ligaments has been reported in up to 50% of traumatic elbow luxations. In cats, elbow luxation is an uncommon injury; due to differences in the anatomy, however, lateral, medial and cranial luxations can occur.

Diagnosis
Most animals with traumatic elbow luxation are presented with a known history of trauma, usually involving impact with an automobile, although elbow luxations may be seen after falling or dog fighting. The affected animal presents with a characteristic carriage of the limb. The leg is carried in semi-flexion, with the lower limb abducted and supinated. Palpation and manipulation will reveal a painful joint with a limited range of movement, an obvious deformity and a readily palpable trochlear notch. The diagnosis should be confirmed radiographically. Two views should be taken (Figure 18.5), as a lateral projection on its own can be misleading. Radiographs should be carefully examined for evidence of articular fractures. It is important to examine the patient for additional injury, particularly to the chest or spine, due to the cause and location of the injury. Concurrent neurological injury to the affected limb is rare.

Treatment
Relocation of the luxated elbow by closed reduction is usually best undertaken as soon as possible, before an organized intra-articular haematoma makes complete reduction difficult (see Operative Technique 18.6). The collateral ligaments are checked for damage once the successful reduction has been confirmed by palpation and/or radiographs. With the carpus flexed to 90 degrees and the elbow supported in a weightbearing position, the normal amount of lateral rotation of the carpus and paw is limited by the medial collateral ligament to 45 degrees, but may increase to more than 90 degrees if the ligament is stretched or ruptured. Similarly, medial rotation is limited to about 70 degrees by the lateral collateral ligament and damage to it may cause this to increase to 140 degrees or more (Figure 18.6). If the joint is still unstable following relocation, then reconstruction of the damaged collateral ligament is indicated (see Operative Technique 18.7). Open reduction is rarely indicated.

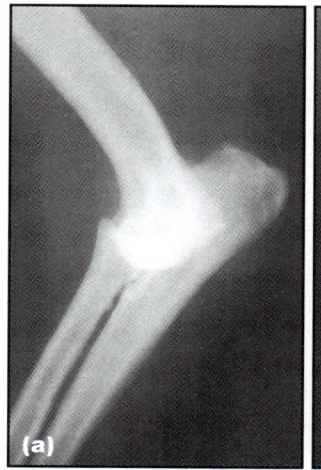

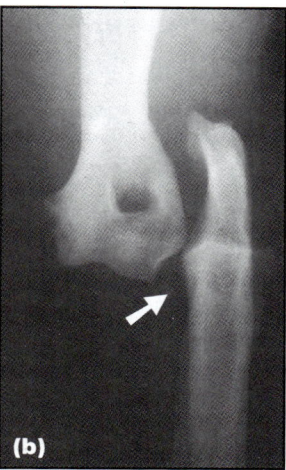

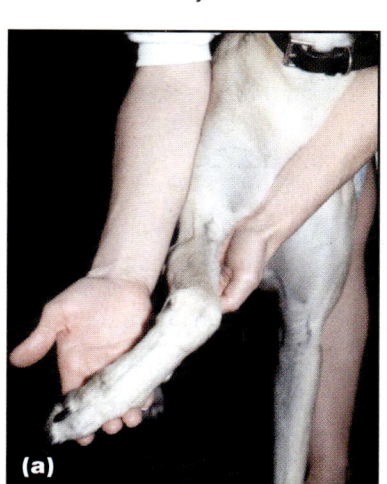

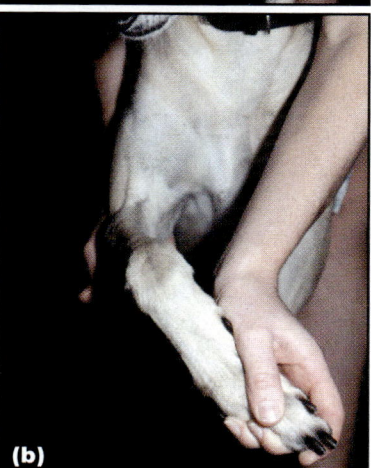

18.5 Traumatic elbow luxation: **(a)** mediolateral view; **(b)** craniocaudal view. Note the small avulsion fracture (arrowed) indicating ligament damage.

18.6 Testing for collateral ligament integrity following closed reduction of a luxated elbow joint. **(a)** Testing medial collateral integrity: with the carpus flexed to 90 degrees and the elbow supported in a weightbearing position, the normal amount of lateral rotation of the carpus and paw is limited by the medial collateral to 45 degrees, but may increase to more than 90 degrees if the ligament is stretched or ruptured. **(b)** Testing lateral collateral integrity: medial rotation is limited to about 70 degrees by the lateral collateral and damage to it may cause this to increase to 140 degrees or more.

Chapter 18 The elbow

Elbow dysplasia

Elbow dysplasia may be strictly defined as the abnormal development of the cubital joint. In dogs numerous disease processes have been included under the term elbow dysplasia; however, three major diseases predominate:

- Un-united anconeal process (UAP)
- Fragmentation of the medial coronoid process (FCP)
- Osteochondritis dissecans (OCD) of the medial portion of the humeral condyle.

Each condition is usually seen in isolation but any combination of the three is possible; having all three conditions at once is unlikely. Other diseases that may be included within elbow dysplasia include joint incongruity, incomplete fusion of the medial epicondyle and idiopathic osteoarthritis of the medial compartment of the elbow joint. Elbow dysplasia has not been reported in cats, although there is ever greater recognition of osteoarthritis of the elbow in cats.

Un-united anconeal process

Aetiology and pathogenesis

Normally the anconeal process develops as part of the ulnar diaphysis, but in certain breeds, such as the German Shepherd Dog, it develops as a separate centre of ossification. This fourth ossification centre appears at about 10–13 weeks of age, and is fused to the ulna by 18–20 weeks.

In certain breeds, such as the Basset Hound, separation is secondary to non-traumatic premature closure of the distal ulnar growth plate. Theoretically, the shortened ulna and the relative lengthening of the radius puts pressure on the trochlea of the humerus, which in turn forces the humerus proximally, exerting sufficient pressure on the anconeal process at a critical stage of its development to result in its separation (Figure 18.7). Theories for UAP in other breeds, particularly the German Shepherd Dog, include its being a form of osteochondrosis, disruption of microcirculation during development, radioulnar incongruity and humeroulnar incongruity (Figure 18.8).

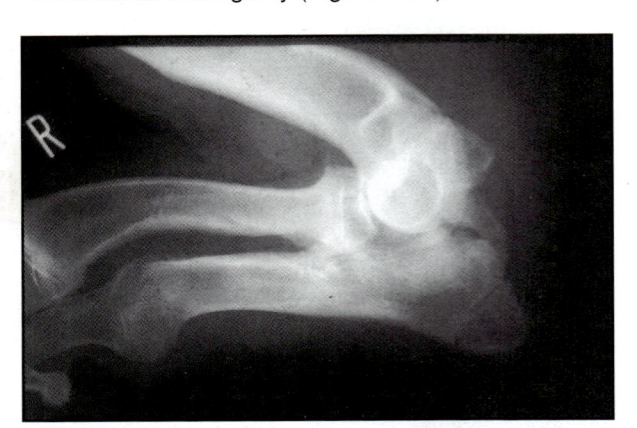

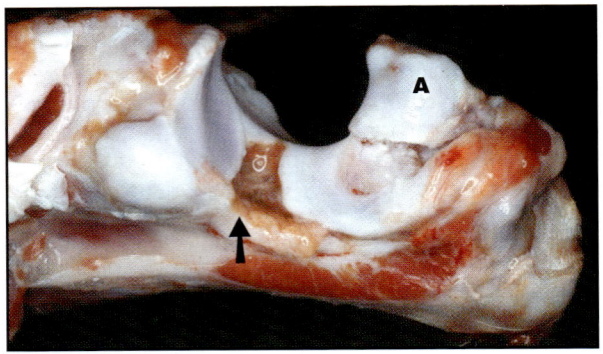

18.8 A post-mortem picture of an un-united anconeal process (A). The synovial fossa (arrowed) is seen as a normal variant in some dogs on the medial aspect of the semilunar notch of the ulna.

The instability and irritation following separation of the anconeal process results in osteoarthritis. The advent of arthroscopic examination of elbows with UAP has revealed a high incidence of associated lesions, particularly FCP (Bardet, 2000). This may account for the poor outcome seen in some cases in the past when these associated lesions went unrecognized. Therefore, arthroscopic examination of an elbow with UAP is indicated to inspect the remainder of the joint.

Diagnosis

The condition can occur in one or both elbows. Affected animals are usually presented with progressive thoracic limb lameness at about 4–5 months of age. Although the condition is seen most frequently in German Shepherd Dogs, it is also seen occasionally in other large-breed dogs, such as the Wolfhound, Rottweiler, St. Bernard and Great Dane. Affected animals may have a strange gait with the elbow abducted. This position may also be adopted when the animal is standing and the foot may be outwardly rotated. Palpation and manipulation of the joint will reveal a thickened joint with a varying amount of synovial fluid effusion. The range of joint movement will be reduced, with pain and sometimes crepitus on full flexion and extension.

The diagnosis is confirmed by taking a fully flexed lateral radiograph of the joint. The flexed view is important so that superimposition of the medial epicondyle on the olecranon can be avoided (Figure 18.9). A clear

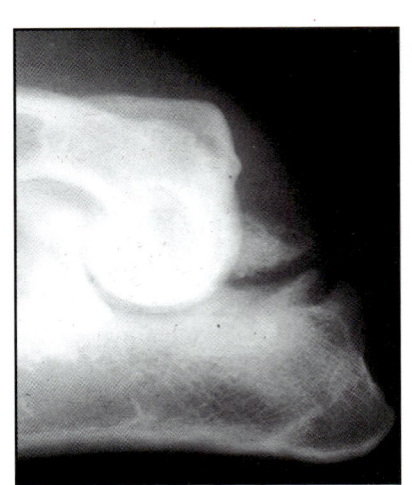

18.7 Mediolateral view of an un-united anconeal process in a Bassett Hound. There is proximal displacement of the anconeal process associated with a relatively short ulna.

18.9 Fully flexed mediolateral view of the elbow of a 5-month-old German Shepherd Dog with UAP. Full flexion of the elbow allows appropriate inspection of the anconeal process.

line of separation below the anconeal process is diagnostic, but in some cases there appears to be only partial separation. A varying amount of osteoarthritis will also be evident. In addition, the congruency of the elbow joint should be assessed from radiographs taken in the normal extended lateral and craniocaudal projections. Shortening of the olecranon has been observed on the affected side (Guthrie, 1989).

Judgment of elbow joint congruity should be done with caution as it is highly subjective and prone to error when evaluating subtle abnormalities (Mason et al., 2002). Invasive surgeries should not be performed to correct incongruity unless it has been diagnosed definitively. Computed tomography (CT) may provide the means to measure joint incongruity objectively. Arthroscopy can be used to confirm the diagnosis but is more useful for evaluation of the remainder of the joint for concurrent abnormalities, such as FCP or OCD.

Treatment and prognosis
Surgical treatment is usually recommended over conservative medical therapy, although there is inadequate clinical evidence to demonstrate categorically the superiority of one technique over another. Occasionally, medical management (see Chapter 7) may be used when surgical treatment is not an option (e.g. very chronic disease, economic constraints). There are a number of choices of surgical treatment for UAP depending on the age and breed of the patient, the presence of incongruity and the relative stability of the anconeal process. However, all dogs develop osteoarthritis with varying amounts of functional impairment following surgery (Guthrie, 1989).

Removing the anconeal process (see Operative Technique 18.8): This was traditionally the treatment of choice but is now reserved for chronic cases. However, following surgery, all these dogs develop osteoarthritic change with varying amounts of functional impairment (Guthrie, 1989) and the possibility of the existence of associated lesions should also be considered (Bardet, 2000).

Osteotomy of the proximal ulna (see Operative Technique 18.9): If subluxation and incongruency of the joint are identified, relief of the intra-articular pressure by osteotomy of the diaphysis of the ulna may result in spontaneous union of the separated anconeal process. Sjöstrom et al. (1995) reported a high level of success with this approach, particularly if the UAP is firmly attached to the underlying ulna. However, Matis (1992) reports that healing may occur with the process in a displaced location which, in turn, results in a distorted trochlear notch.

Combination of internal fixation and ulnar osteotomy (see Operative Technique 18.8): The best results appear to be achieved by combining internal fixation with a lag screw, Kirschner wires, or a combination of a Kirschner wire and a lag screw, with a relieving dynamic osteotomy of the ulna performed via a caudolateral approach (Böhmer et al., 1987; Krotscheck et al., 2000).

Fragmentation of the medial coronoid process

Aetiology and pathogenesis
Currently, FCP of the ulna is the commonest cause of elbow lameness in young, rapidly growing dogs of the large and giant breeds. Although this condition affects many breeds, it is particularly prevalent in Rottweilers, Labrador Retrievers and Bernese Mountain Dogs. Other breeds affected include German Shepherd Dogs, Golden Retrievers, St. Bernards, Chow Chows, Rhodesian Ridgebacks and Newfoundlands. The condition has also been identified in some smaller breeds of dog.

There is no separate centre of ossification for the coronoid processes (Guthrie et al., 1992). Numerous theories have been proposed for the cause of FCP and these include osteochondrosis, radioulnar incongruity and humeroulnar incongruity (Wind, 1986; Wind and Packard, 1986). Histological examination of the affected coronoid region reveals changes more consistent with a fracture than with osteochondrosis. The area(s) involved may be under abnormal loads and forces and, while the exact cause of FCP remains unclear, recent studies have revealed that in a normal elbow there is almost equal loading of the radial head and the medial coronoid process during weightbearing.

FCP has been identified in cases of pathological premature closure of a radial growth plate. In these cases the radioulnar incongruity is usually obvious on radiographs and both the medial and lateral coronoid process may be affected.

In some developmental cases there is evidence of elbow incongruity secondary to asynchronous development of the radius and ulna (radioulnar incongruity), which results in a relative overgrowth of the ulna causing retraction of the radial head from the elbow joint and exposure of the coronoid processes to abnormal shearing forces from the distal humerus.

It is difficult to assess accurately the presence of incongruency between the radial head and the radial notch of the ulna. More accurate assessment can be achieved by centring the X-ray beam on the joint and avoiding extremes of flexion or extension, but judgment of elbow joint congruity should be approached with caution as it is highly subjective and prone to error when evaluating subtle abnormalities (Mason et al., 2002). CT may be used to measure joint incongruity objectively.

Humeroulnar incongruity (Figure 18.10) is the abnormal development of the trochlear notch of the ulna resulting in an arc of curvature with too a small radius to accommodate the humeral trochlea. However, recent studies have demonstrated that a degree of humeroulnar incongruity is normal in both the human and the canine elbow (Preston et al., 2000). Recent studies are focusing on the use of CT for objective measurement of elbow joint incongruity (Holsworth et al., 2003).

Chapter 18 The elbow

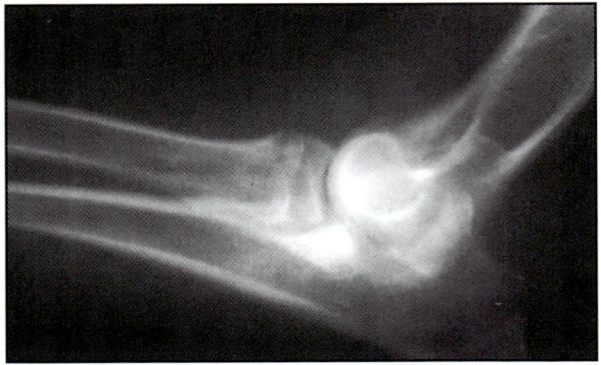

18.10 Short radius syndrome. Mediolateral projection shows incongruity of the humeroulnar joint (note the widening of the proximal humeroulnar joint space and narrowing of the distal humeroulnar joint space). Short radius syndrome can often be associated with FCP.

Pathology

One or more fragments of bone may have fractured from either the inner aspect of the medial coronoid process immediately adjacent to the radial head, or from the apex of the process. The fragment(s) often remain attached to the annular ligament. The fragments may project from the articular surface causing erosion of the adjacent medial humeral condyle (kissing lesion) (Figure 18.11).

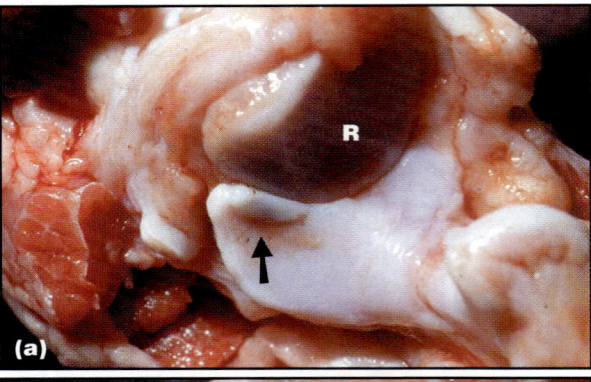

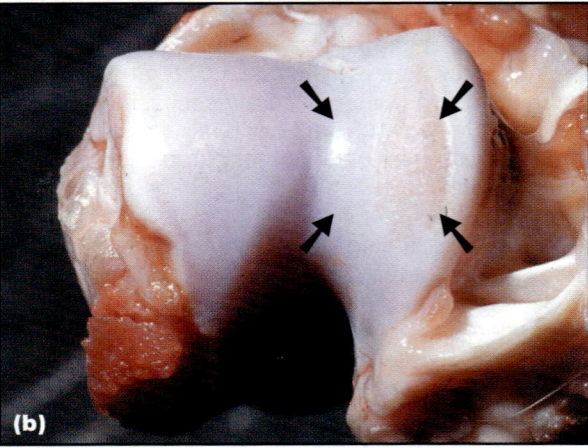

18.11 Post-mortem specimens of the pathology associated with FCP. **(a)** View of the radial (R) and ulnar articular surfaces; a fragment is arrowed. **(b)** View of the humeral articular surface. Note the area of articular cartilage erosion on the medial humeral condyle, a so-called 'kissing' lesion (arrows)

Rarely, the coronoid process may remain attached to the surrounding cartilage; the affected cartilage is thicker and therefore whiter than the normal cartilage, but the underlying bone is fractured. Other lesions that may be identified are chondromalacia and fissures of the coronoid process, erosion of articular cartilage in the trochlear notch and OCD of the medial humeral condyle. The end result is osteoarthritis and the severity depends, in part, on the mobility of the fragments and the presence of other primary lesions such as OCD. Mild cases of FCP are associated with minimal changes to the cartilage of the medial compartment of the elbow joint (medial portion of the coronoid process and medial portion of the humeral condyle). More severe cases may be associated with full thickness (grade IV) cartilage loss of these surfaces. The resulting disease is termed medial compartmental osteoarthritis of the elbow. Similar pathology may occur in the absence of an FCP fragment.

Diagnosis

Clinical signs: The first signs of lameness are usually noticed at about 4–5 months of age but FCP and medial compartmental disease may be diagnosed at any age. The lameness is usually subtle at first, especially if both legs are affected. An early sign may be outward rotation of the pes, with the elbow held close into the body, giving the dog a 'duck-footed' appearance. The lameness is usually worse following rest or heavy exercise. As the condition persists the secondary changes associated with osteoarthritis develop, resulting in a reduced range of flexion and extension. A painful response to manipulation, especially on external rotation and hyperextension, is a consistent finding. In advanced cases there may be crepitus and thickening of the joint, particularly on the lateral side caudal to the humeral epicondyle. The degree of joint fluid effusion varies but is usually not pronounced unless there is a coexisting problem, such as OCD or UAP.

Radiography: The definitive diagnosis of FCP on conventional radiographs poses some problems because the location of the fragment(s) means that there is usually superimposition of other structures. In cases with large fragments, the fragment may be visible on the craniocaudal or the craniolateral–caudomedial oblique projection. If available, CT is an accurate method of assessing congruency as well as imaging the FCP, especially if the software allows three-dimensional reconstructions.

Suspicion of FCP or medial compartmental disease can often be made from the radiographs, based on the evidence of osteophytosis on the radiographs and the elimination of all other known causes of arthritis. However, these changes take some weeks, sometimes months, to develop and therefore they may not be evident on the initial radiographs, especially if the animal has been lame for less than 3–4 weeks. The first evidence of osteoarthritis is usually an increase in bone density (sclerosis) and loss of trabecular pattern in the region of the ulna just caudal to the coronoid process (radial notch) (Figure 18.12). Identification of this radiographic sign can lead to a high suspicion of elbow dysplasia significantly earlier than other radiographic findings.

Chapter 18 The elbow

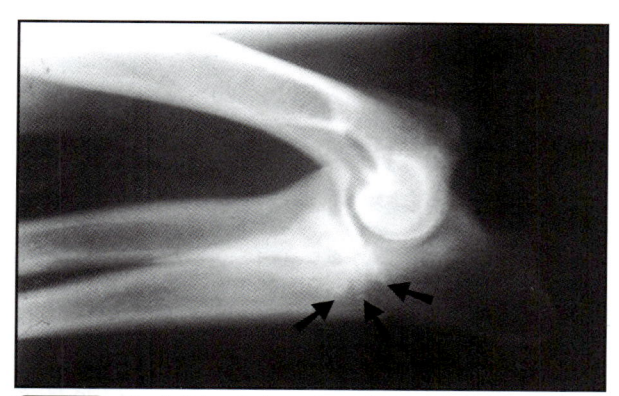

18.12 Mediolateral view of an elbow joint with elbow dysplasia. There is sclerosis in the region of the radial notch (arrowed).

In some dogs this change may be the only radiographic finding for the life of the patient. Later on in the course of the disease, osteophytes may appear on the caudal non-articular proximal surface of the anconeal process. Initially these osteophytes appear as a slight irregularity on the margin of the bone. It is therefore important to take good-quality flexed lateral radiographs and to avoid rotation. If the initial radiographs appear normal and the lameness persists, and advanced imaging or arthroscopy are not available, follow-up radiographs are recommended within 4–8 weeks (Figure 18.13).

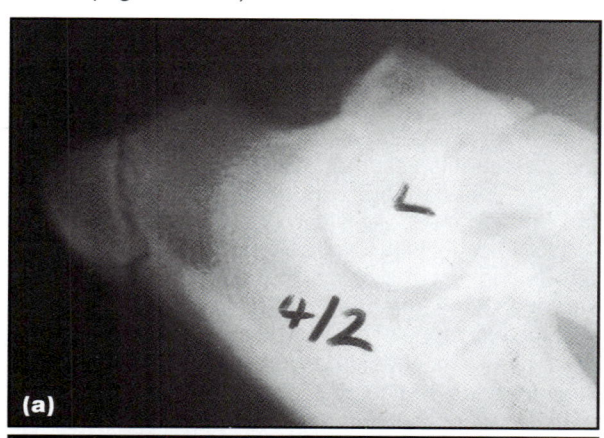

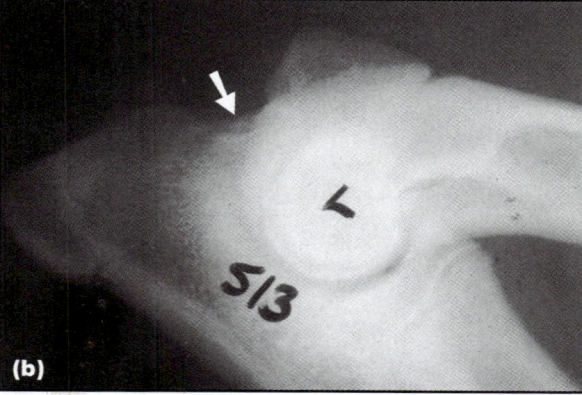

18.13 Two radiographs of the same elbow joint approximately 4 weeks apart. **(a)** The initial radiograph is within normal limits. **(b)** Four weeks later, small osteophytes are present on the proximal border of the anconeal process (arrows) indicating pathology within the elbow joint.

As the condition persists, osteophytes will be found adjacent to the medial coronoid process (seen on the craniocaudal view) and on the cranial aspect of the radial head (seen on the mediolateral view). As well as the flexed lateral radiograph it is recommended that a craniocaudal projection is taken to identify possible OCD lesions and an extended lateral projection to determine the congruency of the joint. Oblique craniocaudal projections are recommended in certain instances as they highlight the caudal and cranial aspects of the joint on the lateral and medial sides, respectively. As previously mentioned, CT may be used for definitive diagnosis of bone fragmentation and is being investigated for use for more accurate, objective analysis of radioulnar incongruity.

Arthroscopy: Definitive diagnosis of the type and severity of elbow dysplasia is obtained through arthroscopy. This technique enables observation of all articular structures of the joint and positive diagnosis of FCP, OCD, UAP and cartilage disease (van Bree and Van Ryssen, 1992) (Figure 18.14). Concomitant cartilage disease is graded on a modified Outterbridge scale (Figure 18.15).

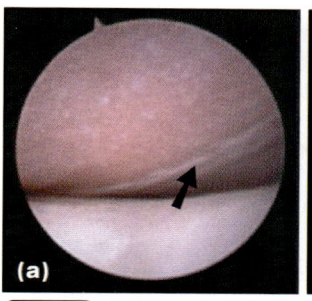

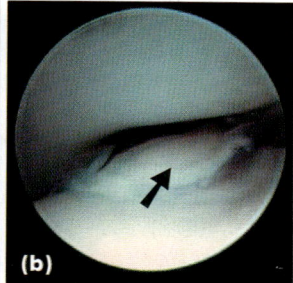

18.14 Arthroscopic views (medial portal) of pathology associated with elbow dysplasia. **(a)** The medial humeral condyle is devoid of articular cartilage with exposure of subchondral bone. Note the clear line of demarcation (arrowed) from the lateral compartment, where there is cartilage that appears grossly healthy. **(b)** A slightly displaced fragment (arrowed) of the medial coronoid process.

Grade	Cartilage disease
0	Normal cartilage
I	Chondromalacia: softening and swelling
II	Fibrillation Superficial fissures: velvet-like appearance Superficial erosion: pitting or cobblestone appearance Lesions do not reach subchondral bone
III	Deep fissures to subchondral bone Deep ulceration not to subchondral bone
IV	Exposure of subchondral bone with or without bone cavitation
V	Eburnated bone

18.15 Modified Outterbridge scale used to grade concomitant cartilage disease in elbow dysplasia.

Chapter 18 The elbow

Other techniques: Nuclear scintigraphy may be helpful in cases of thoracic limb lameness where localization is difficult. Positive scintigraphy will demonstrate increased uptake in the region of the elbow joint. Arthrocentesis and joint fluid analysis are often consistent with low to moderate osteoarthritis and can also be used to help confirm the source of lameness.

Treatment

The management of FCP is controversial. Both medical and surgical techniques may be used for treatment of FCP and medial compartmental disease. Details on medical treatment can be found in Chapter 7. Because of the continued progression of osteoarthritis, regardless of surgical treatment, medical treatment may be necessary in surgically treated cases as well.

Fragment removal: Once positive radiographic evidence of joint disease has been confirmed and all other causes have been eliminated, the medial aspect of the joint should be explored, preferably arthroscopically, and the loose piece(s) of bone and cartilage removed (see Operative Techniques 18.1 and 18.10). It is not clear as yet whether arthroscopy provides a better outcome compared with arthrotomy, but arthroscopy does reduce the morbidity associated with fragment removal. There are some initial data that suggest that arthroscopy may provide a better longer-term outcome (Meyer-Lindenberg *et al.*, 2003). In addition, with practice, arthroscopy is usually quicker. Unfortunately, regardless of surgical treatment, some cases (25–35%) remain lame and most will continue to develop osteoarthritis; owners should be made aware of this before surgery.

Ulnar osteotomy: The concept of ulnar osteotomy for FCP originated in a paper by Bardet and Bureau (1996) who reported on the results of treating older dogs with chronic elbow osteoarthritis with oblique osteotomy of the proximal ulna. Ness (1998) then reported a good clinical outcome when young dogs (less than 10 months old) with FCP were treated by fragment removal and simultaneous transverse proximal ulnar osteotomy (see Operative Techniques 18.9 and 18.10). The procedure has a high postoperative morbidity and remains controversial. The osteotomy may be oblique (caudoproximal to craniodistal) or transverse, and an intramedullary pin may or may not be placed. Complications include significant intra-articular haemorrhage, wound dehiscence, osteomyelitis and delayed or non-union. Typically, the recovery period is 3 months and dogs will remain lame until the osteotomy has healed. A follow-up radiograph at 6–8 weeks provides the clinician with information on osteotomy healing. Proponents of the procedure suggest that the long-term outcome may be improved by improving joint congruity but there are no published data to support this.

Radial lengthening osteotomy is currently being investigated as an alternative means of correcting perceived joint incongruity and decreasing loads on the medial compartment of the joint.

Unfortunately, despite early surgical intervention, some cases remain lame and continue to develop osteoarthritis after surgery; owners should be made aware of this before surgery.

Other surgical options: As medial compartmental disease proceeds and cartilage is lost on the articular surfaces it is likely that the joint collapses towards the medial side. Treatment of severe cartilage loss in the medial compartment is primarily medical; however other surgical options may be considered. Arthroscopy provides the ability to perform topical treatment, including microfracture or abrasion arthroplasty. These techniques are designed to create vascular channels from the underlying bone marrow to the area of cartilage damage. Pluripotential mesenchymal stem cells may then migrate to the region of cartilage disease to aid in healing. While these procedures are simple to perform arthroscopically, their value may be minimal without additional surgery to minimize the destructive forces on the area of diseased cartilage. Additional procedures under development for management of severe medial compartmental disease include corrective osteotomies, resection of the medial coronoid process and joint replacement (see later in this chapter).

Osteochondritis dissecans of the medial condyle of the humerus

Aetiology and pathology

The aetiology and pathogenesis of OCD of the canine elbow joint is poorly understood. Like other OCD lesions, it is thought that the lesion initiates deep within the articular–epiphyseal cartilage complex in the developing joint. Extrapolation from other species suggests that areas of necrosis around the vascular channels in this tissue appear to extend gradually to the joint surface leading to a cartilage flap (Ekmann and Carlson, 1998; Al-Hizab *et al.*, 2002).

OCD occurs with low frequency in Rottweilers and has its highest incidence in Labrador and Golden Retrievers. In common with OCD in other joints, there is a high incidence of bilateral involvement. The lesion is usually found near the outer edge of the central weightbearing region of the articular surface of the medial part of the humeral condyle (Figure 18.16). OCD may be identified in conjunction with FCP and medial compartmental osteoarthritis.

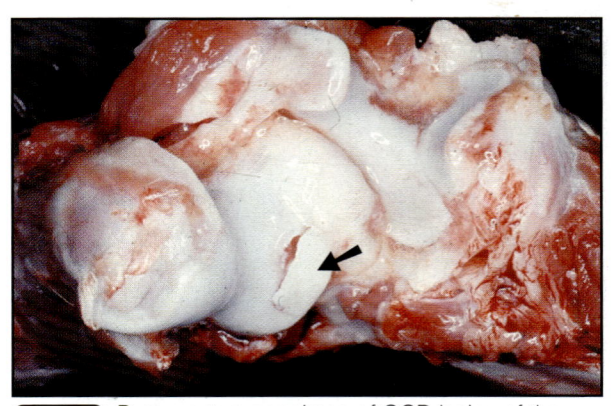

18.16 Post-mortem specimen of OCD lesion of the medial part of the humeral condyle. There is an under-run cartilage flap (arrowed).

Diagnosis
The clinical signs are very similar to FCP. A flexed lateral radiograph will show the presence of osteoarthritis on the anconeal process and a craniocaudal or craniolateral–caudomedial oblique projection will usually reveal a defect in the subchondral bone of the medial part of the humeral condyle (Figure 18.17). Occasionally, ossification of the cartilage flap will make it visible. In long-standing cases, the flap may detach and become lodged in the caudomedial aspect of the joint capsule. It may grow in this location forming a linear osteochondral ossicle, which may only be visible on a craniolateral–caudomedial oblique projection (Robins, 1980). CT is not routinely necessary for diagnosis of OCD although the full extent of the lesion is well defined with this technique.

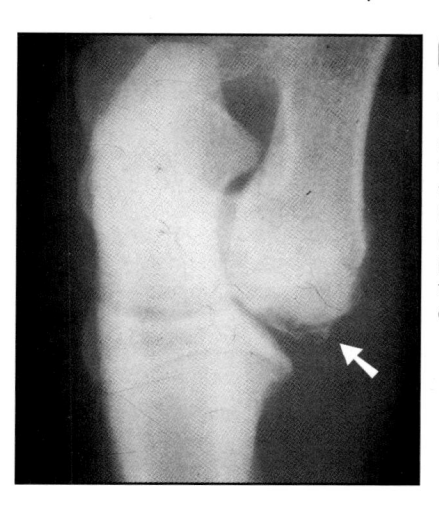

18.17 A 15-degree oblique craniocaudal view of an elbow with a large OCD lesion (arrowed) on the medial part of the humeral condyle.

Diagnosis and treatment of OCD may be performed through arthroscopy (Figure 18.18). This enables thorough evaluation of the joint for other lesions including FCP and additional cartilage disease.

Nuclear scintigraphy may be helpful in cases of thoracic limb lameness where localization is difficult.

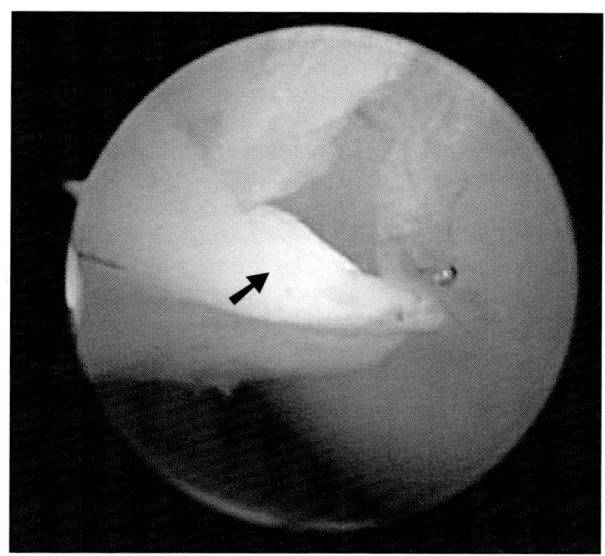

Positive scintigraphy will demonstrate increased uptake in the region of the elbow joint. Arthrocentesis and joint fluid analysis are often consistent with low to moderate osteoarthritis and can also be used to help confirm the source of lameness.

Treatment
Surgical or arthroscopic exploration of the medial aspect of the joint is the treatment of choice (see Operative Techniques 18.1 and 18.10). The cartilage flap is removed and the defect subjected to light curettage. Arthroscopic treatment is preferred because of increased visibility and decreased postoperative morbidity. With early diagnosis and treatment, uncomplicated cases of OCD appear to have a better chance of making a full recovery than cases with FCP.

Incongruity secondary to growth plate damage

Epiphyseal fractures and separation of the growth plates of the radius and ulna are common. The high incidence of growth impairment that occurs following these injuries may result in deviation of the limb and subluxation of the carpal and elbow joints. Further information on these conditions may be found in Chapter 6. This chapter will only consider the consequences for the elbow joint.

Distal radial growth plate closure
This problem is reported to be less common than distal ulnar closure, but in practice it may account for more than 50% of the cases. The cause is generally unknown, but trauma to the distal radial growth plate is the likely cause. Historically, there is a strong correlation between a fall from a height, a transient lameness and then a gradual onset of lameness some weeks later. Symmetrical and asymmetrical growth plate closure occurs with damage to the lateral side of the plate being most common. Proximal radial growth plate closure is very rare.

The most significant clinical aspects of this problem are the pain and lameness that result from retraction of the radial head, subluxation of the elbow and secondary osteoarthritis. In most cases treatment by relocation of the radial head by lengthening the radius, shortening the ulna, or a combination of both will result in a satisfactory clinical result (see Chapter 6). In a series of 35 cases, more than 50% of affected elbows had coronoid pathology secondary to subluxation of the radial head (Robins, 1987) and arthroscopic inspection of the elbow joint prior to corrective surgery is indicated. Because of the reduced humeroulnar joint space, a lateral portal for the elbow joint is useful because the humeroradial joint space is widened. Placement of the arthroscope across the radial head allows inspection of the medial coronoid process. An instrument portal can also be established if fragment removal is required.

Distal ulnar growth plate closure
Subluxation of the elbow joint is frequently encountered with premature closure of the distal ulnar growth plate (Figure 18.19). It is caused either by a relative

18.18 Arthroscopic view of the cartilage flap (arrowed) as seen from a medial portal in a dog with OCD of the medial part of the humeral condyle.

Chapter 18 The elbow

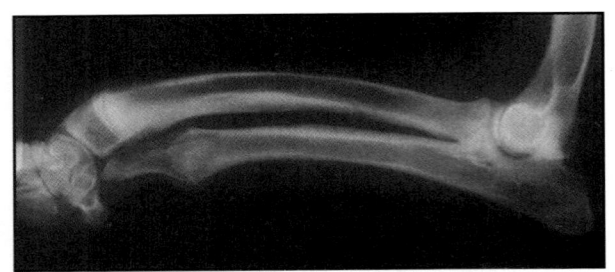

18.19 Closure of the distal ulnar growth plate. Note the bowing of the antebrachium (radius curvus) and the subluxation of the elbow and carpus. At the elbow joint, the humeroradial joint space is narrowed with concomitant narrowing of the proximal portion of the humeroulnar joint space, with widening of the distal humeroulnar joint space.

overgrowth of the radius in a proximal and lateral direction or distal displacement of the proximal ulna. The net effect is for the humeral condyle to be squeezed between the radial head and the anconeal process resulting in subluxation of the joint and osteoarthritis.

Correction of this joint incongruity is best achieved in combination with other procedures to straighten and lengthen the entire antebrachium. In order to maximize leg length it is preferable to lengthen the ulna rather than shorten the radius (see Chapter 6).

Salvage procedures for the elbow joint

Total elbow joint replacement

Prosthetic elbow joint replacement is a new procedure. It is indicated for the treatment of intractably painful elbow joints affected by osteoarthritis. Candidates for this surgery must have exhausted conservative management options and must have severe disease causing an unacceptable compromise in quality of life. The short-term (12 month) success rate of total elbow replacement (TER) is reported as 16 out of 20 (80%) (Conzemius *et al.*, 2003). Reported complications included luxation, infection and fracture of the humeral condyle. Complications requiring removal of the prosthesis may require arthrodesis, amputation or euthanasia.

Biomedtrix released the first canine TER system in late 2004. This cemented system consists of a stemmed humeral component manufactured from cobalt chrome together with a polyethylene radioulnar component (Figure 18.20). Components come in four sizes (extra small, small, medium and large). Implants are sized to the medullary canals of the radius and ulna using the lateral radiograph. The humeral component is chosen to match. If necessary, the humeral component can be downsized by one size relative to the radioulnar component. Following a lateral approach to the elbow involving elevation of the insertion site of the lateral collateral ligament, the elbow is luxated. The collateral ligament must be repaired following surgery and a synostosis between the radius and ulna is also performed to avoid loosening of the radioulnar component.

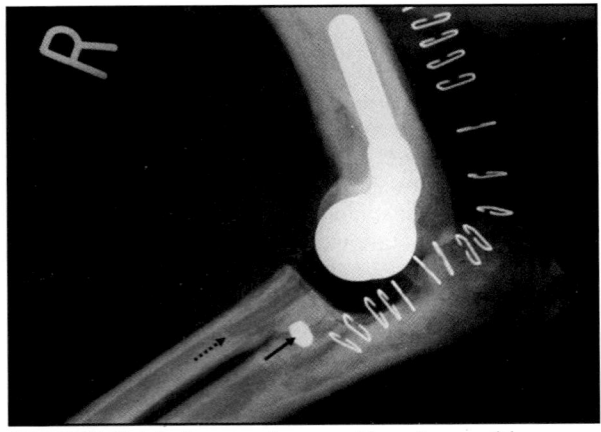

18.20 Total elbow replacement in a 4-year-old Labrador Retriever. The suture anchor (solid arrow) is used for repair of the lateral collateral ligament which is elevated during the surgical approach. The outline of the polyethylene radioulnar component can be seen in the proximal radius (dotted arrow).

Elbow arthrodesis

Arthrodesis of the elbow joint is indicated for the severely and intractably painful elbow joint that cannot be treated with TER, or for a failed TER. The procedure impairs thoracic limb function and causes a moderate to severe mechanical disability. Postoperatively, animals may have difficulty with steps and rough ground. It is therefore a procedure that is indicated for severe conditions of the elbow only, and is best performed by an experienced surgeon.

The joint angle is assessed in the standing patient prior to surgery, but an angle of approximately 110 degrees has been suggested. Bone plate fixation via a caudal, transolecranon approach is the preferred choice in most cases. The olecranon is screwed to the proximal humerus at the end of the procedure, so sufficient allowance must be made for this. The remining proximal ulna is shaped for application of a caudal curved bone plate to the caudal aspect of the humerus and ulna. The joint is approached via a caudolateral approach including transection of the collateral ligament to allow the joint to be hinged open. Articular cartilage is removed and the cavity packed with cancellous bone graft. A bone plate is applied to the caudal humerus and ulna. The plate is bent to 10 degrees more than the desired joint angle to account for bone shape. At least eight cortices (four screws) are purchased proximal and distal to the joint. The most distal humeral screw is placed into the radial head in a lagged fashion and the most proximal ulna screw is lagged into the distal humerus. The olecranon is fixed to the medial epicondyle with a lag screw and an anti-rotational Kirschner wire. A padded dressing is applied for 10–14 days and changed as necessary. Activity should be restricted until arthrodesis is confirmed radiographically (8–10 weeks).

References and further reading

Al-Hizab F, Clegg PD, Thompson CC and Carter SD (2002) Microscopic localization of active gelatinases in equine osteochondritis dissecans (OCD) cartilage. *Osteoarthritis and Cartilage* **10**, 653–661

Bardet JF (2000) Treatment of the ununited anconeal process under arthroscopy in dogs. *Proceedings of the 10th Congress of the European Society of Veterinary Orthopaedics and Traumatology* p.101

Bardet JF and Bureau S (1996) La fragmentation du processus coronoïde chez le chien. *Pratique Medicale et Chirurgicale de l'Animal Companie* **31**, 451–463

Barr ARS and Denny HR (1985) The management of elbow instability caused by premature closure of the distal radial growth plate in dogs. *Journal of Small Animal Practice* **26**, 427–435

Böhmer E, Matis U and Waibl H (1987) Zur operativen Darstellung der Processus anconeus ulnae beim Hund (Modifikation des Zuganges von Chalman und Slocum). *Tierärztliche Praxis* **15**, 425

Clayton-Jones DG and Vaughan LC (1970) Disturbances in the growth of the radius in the dogs. *Journal of Small Animal Practice* **11**, 453–468

Conzemius MG, Aper RL and Corti LB (2003) Short-term outcome after total elbow arthroplasty in dogs with severe, naturally occurring osteoarthritis. *Veterinary Surgery* **32**, 545–552

Ekman S and Carlson CS (1998) The pathophysiology of osteochondrosis. *Veterinary Clinics of North America: Small Animal Practice* **28**, 17–32

Gilson SD, Piermattei DL and Schwarz PD (1989) Treatment of humeroulnar subluxation with dynamic proximal osteotomy. *Veterinary Surgery* **18**, 114–122

Guthrie S (1989) Some radiological and clinical aspects of ununited anconeal process. *Veterinary Record* **124**, 661–662

Guthrie S, Plummer JM and Vaughan LC (1992) Post natal development of the canine elbow joint – a light and electron-microscopic study. *Research in Veterinary Science* **52**, 67–71

Holsworth IG, Wisner E, Scherrer WE, Kass P, Pooya H and Schulz KS (2003) Accuracy of computerized tomographic evaluation of canine radio-ulnar incongruence in vitro. *Proceedings of the 30th Annual Conference of the Veterinary Orthopedic Society, Steamboat Springs, Colorado* p.37

Kene ROC, Lee R and Bennett D (1982) The radiological features of congenital elbow luxation/subluxation in the dog. *Journal of Small Animal Practice* **23**, 621–630

Krotscheck U, Hulse DA, Bahr A, Jerram RM (2000) Ununited anconeal process: lag-screw fixation with proximal ulnar osteotomy. *Veterinary and Comparative Orthopaedics and Traumatology* **13**, 212–216

Lenehan TM and Nunamaker DM (1982) Lateral approach to the canine elbow by proximal ulnar diaphyseal osteotomy. *Journal of the American Veterinary Medical Association* **180(5)**, 523–530

Mason TA and Baker MJ (1978) Surgical management of elbow joint deformity associated with premature growth plate closure in dogs. *Journal of Small Animal Practice* **19(11)**, 639–645

Mason DR, Schulz KS, Samii VF, Fujita Y, Hornof WJ, Herrgesell EJ, Long CD, Morgan JP and Kass PH (2002) Sensitivity of radiographic evaluation of radio-ulnar incongruence in the dog in vitro. *Veterinary Surgery* **31**(2), 125–132

Matis U (1992) Treatment of ununited anconeal process. *Proceedings of the 6th Congress of the European Society of Veterinary Orthopaedics and Traumatology* p.16

Meyer-Lindenberg A (1999) Der isolierte Processus anconaeus: retro- und prospective Untersuchungen zur operative Behandlung. *Tierärztliche Praxis* **27**, 309

Meyer-Lindenberg A, Langhann A, Fehr M and Nolte I (2003) Arthrotomy versus arthroscopy in the treatment of the fragmented medial coronoid process of the ulna (FCP) in 421 dogs. *Veterinary and Comparative Orthopaedics and Traumatology* **16**, 204–210

Milton JL and Montgomery RD (1987) Congenital elbow dislocations. *Veterinary Clinics of North America* **17**, 873–878

Milton JL, Horne RD, Bartels JE and Henderson RA (1979) Congenital elbow luxation in the dog. *Journal of the American Veterinary Medical Association* **175**, 572–582

Ness MG (1998) Treatment of fragmented coronoid process in young dogs by proximal ulnar osteotomy. *Journal of Small Animal Practice* **39**, 15–18

Olsson S-E (l993) Pathophysiology, morphology and clinical signs of osteochondrosis in the dog. In: *Disease Mechanisms in Small Animal Surgery*, ed. MJ Bojrab, pp. 777–796. Lea and Febiger, Philadelphia

Preston CA, Schulz KS, Stover S, Taylor K and Kass P (2000) In vitro determination of contact areas in the normal elbow joint of dogs. *American Journal of Veterinary Research* **61**, 1315–1321

Robins GM (1980) Some aspects of the radiographical examination of the canine elbow joint. *Journal of Small Animal Practice* **21**, 417–428

Robins GM (1987) The management of distal radial growth plate closure. *Australian Veterinary Practitioner* **17**, 143–144

Sjostrom L, Kasstrom H and Kallberg M (1995) Ununited anconeal process in the dog – pathogenesis and treatment by osteotomy of the ulna. *Veterinary and Comparative Orthopaedics and Traumatology* **8**, 170–176

Spadari A, Romagnoli N and Venturini A (2001) A modified Bell–Tawse procedure for surgical correction of congenital elbow luxation in a Dalmatian puppy. *Veterinary Comparative Orthopaedics and Traumatology* **14**, 210–213

van Bree H and Van Ryssen B (1992) Diagnostic and surgical arthroscopy of the lame elbow. *Proceedings of the 6th Congress of the European Society of Orthopaedics and Traumatology* p.14

Van Ryssen B, van Bree H and Simoens P (1992) Elbow arthroscopy in clinically normal dogs. *American Journal of Veterinary Research* **54**, 191–198

Vezzoni A (2000) Dynamic ulnar osteotomies in treating canine elbow dysplasia. *Proceedings of the 6th Congress of the European Society of Veterinary Orthopaedics and Traumatology*, pp.94–98

Wind AP (1986) Elbow incongruity and developmental elbow diseases in the dog. 1. *Journal of the American Animal Hospital Association* **22**, 711–724

Wind AP and Packard ME (1986) Elbow incongruity and developmental elbow diseases in the dog. 2. *Journal of the American Animal Hospital Association* **22**, 725–730

Chapter 18   The elbow

> **OPERATIVE TECHNIQUE 18.1**
> Arthroscopy of the elbow

Indications
Diagnosis of elbow pain and lameness, treatment of FCP, OCD, [UAP] and infective arthritis, synovial biopsy.

Patient positioning and preparation
Unilateral arthroscopy
See Operative Technique 18.2.
Bilateral arthroscopy
Dorsal recumbency with both thoracic limbs abducted. Hair is clipped across the chest to join the medial clips on both limbs.

Tray extras
1.9 mm or 2.4 mm 30-degree foreoblique arthroscope with appropriate sleeve and blunt obturator; 1 litre of lactated Ringer's (Hartmann's) fluid in positive pressure infusor system and sterile giving set; light source; video camera and control box; monitor; image archiving system (e.g. VHS video, digital video, hard drive system); arthroscopy instruments: selection of cannulae, switching stick, hooked probe, 2 mm drilling mill, Smillie knife (mini motorized shaver system).

Surgical approach
Medial portal sites for egress, arthroscope and instruments (Figure 18.21).

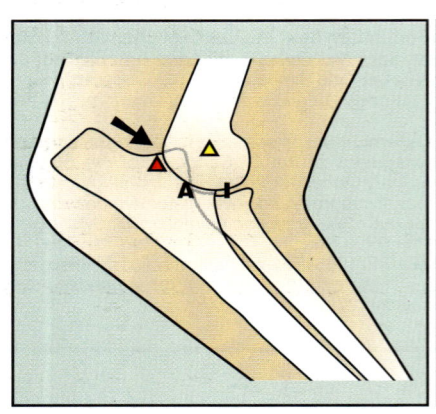

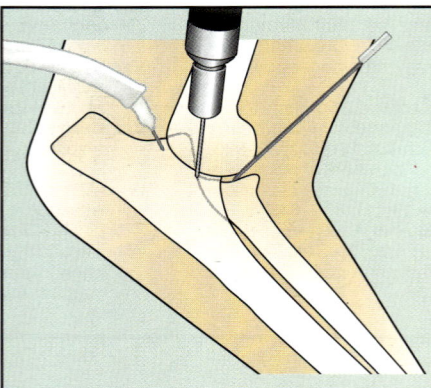

18.21 Portal positions for medial elbow arthroscopy. The arthroscope portal is identified as one point on an equilateral triangle with the medial epicondyle and caudodistal corner of the medial epicondylar ridge forming the other two points. A, arthroscope portal; I, instrument portal; arrow, egress portal; △, medial epicondyle; ▲, caudodistal corner of medial epicondylar ridge.

Surgical technique
A 20 gauge needle is placed caudal to the medial epicondylar ridge and proximal to the anconeal process to puncture the joint caudoproximally. Between 5 ml and 10 ml of Hartmann's is injected to distend the joint (the joint distension should be visible medially). The arthroscope portal is established by using a 20 gauge hypodermic needle to find the medial joint line approximately 1 cm distal and caudal to the medial epicondyle. Easy passage of the needle into the humeroulnar joint space confirms the correct site and fluid should flow easily through this needle. A no. 11 scalpel blade is passed along the line of this needle to the level of the joint. The needle is withdrawn and the arthroscope sleeve with the blunt obturator is passed into the joint. The obturator is removed and the arthroscope inserted. The joint is inspected in a logical fashion with extensive use of the light pole to maximize the view of the arthroscope.

→

Chapter 18 The elbow

OPERATIVE TECHNIQUE 18.1 continued
Arthroscopy of the elbow

Structures inspected are as follows:

1. Anconeal process (light pole at 3 o'clock (L) or 9 o'clock (R))
2. Semilunar notch of the ulna
3. Lateral coronoid process and radial head (the light pole must be at 12 o'clock for this view)
4. Lateral humeral condyle
5. Medial humeral condyle (light pole at 9 o'clock (L) or 3 o'clock (R))
6. Medial coronoid process (light pole at 9 o'clock (L) or 3 o'clock (R))
7. Medial collateral ligament.

Triangulation is achieved by again using a hypodermic needle approximately 1 cm distal and 1 cm cranial to the medial epicondyle. Entry of the needle into the joint is observed through the arthroscope and the optimal angle of the needle is assessed such that it can easily reach the desired region of the joint without undue stress. The portal is established by using a scalpel blade as before and a switching stick is introduced. An appropriately sized cannula is placed over the stick and the stick withdrawn. Instruments are placed through the cannula as appropriate.

Treatment of fragmented coronoid process
Non-displaced fragments are treated by milling using a hand mill (2 mm diameter) or motorized system. Fragments are soft because the bone is necrotic and so hand instruments are usually sufficient. Milling is commenced at the cranial extremity of the fragment to detach the fragment from the annular ligament. Flushing of the joint through the egress cannula encourages cartilage and bone debris to be expelled from the joint through the instrument cannula. Displaced fragments are more challenging. They must first be detached from any soft tissue attachments cranially using a Smillie knife or forceps. Holding smaller fragments in the forceps and twisting the fragment may help to break soft tissue attachments and allow the fragment to be withdrawn. Once the fragment is detached from the soft tissues it may be removed in several pieces with forceps. Larger fragments may jam on the cannula opening and necessitate combined removal of the cannula and forceps.

Treatment of OCD
OCD fragments can usually be easily removed with forceps although larger fragments may require several bite-sized pieces to be removed.

Closure
Single skin sutures are placed in each portal site.

Postoperative care
Protective dressing is placed over portal sites.

Chapter 18 The elbow

OPERATIVE TECHNIQUE 18.2
Caudolateral approach

Positioning
Lateral recumbency, with the affected leg uppermost.

Assistance
Optional, depending on the procedure.

Tray extras
Gelpi-style self-retaining retractors or small stifle distractor; two pairs of Senn hand-held retractors, if working with an assistant.

Surgical technique
A curved skin incision is made behind the caudal edge of the lateral condyle of the humerus centred on the easily palpable lateral epicondylar process (Figure 18.22a). The fascia is divided along the cranial edge of the lateral head of the triceps muscle. Retraction of the fascia will reveal the anconeus muscle, which is then divided across its fibres in its mid section (Figure 18.22b). Alternatively the anconeus muscle can be sharply incised and elevated from its attachment to the lateral epicondylar ridge (Figure 18.22c). Retraction of the muscle with the underlying joint capsule exposes the caudal joint compartment, the lateral condyle of the humerus and the anconeal process.

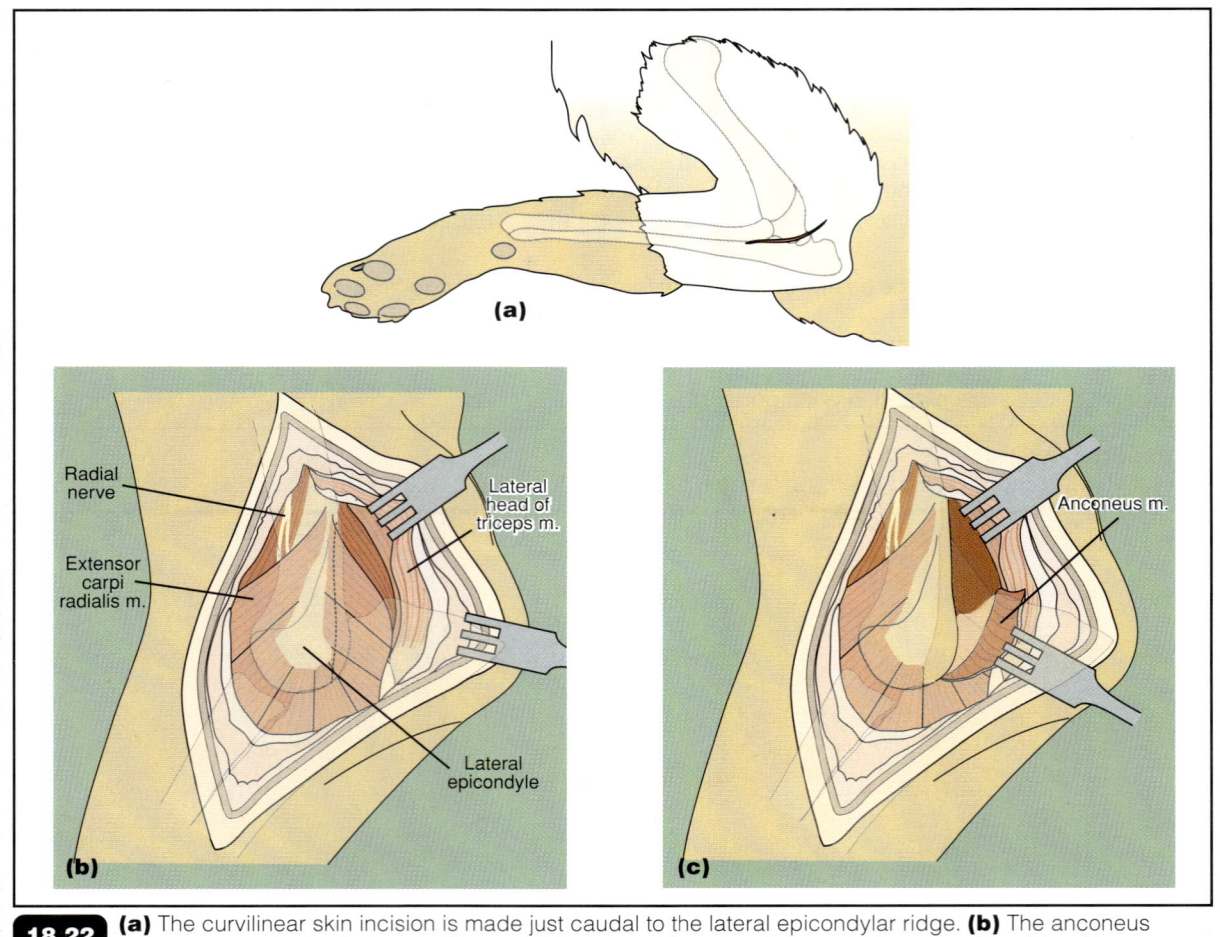

18.22 (a) The curvilinear skin incision is made just caudal to the lateral epicondylar ridge. (b) The anconeus muscle can be incised along its fibres or (c) elevated from its origin on the lateral epicondylar ridge.

Chapter 18 The elbow

OPERATIVE TECHNIQUE 18.2 *continued*
Caudolateral approach

PRACTICAL TIP
Full flexion of the elbow is necessary to explore the anconeal process thoroughly. However, with the joint in this position the surrounding muscles can make visibility difficult. Enough exposure is gained by this approach to remove the anconeal process easily, but if internal fixation is to be conducted then the modified approach (see below) is preferred.

Modified approach
If internal fixation of the separated anconeal process is anticipated, a modification of the caudolateral approach is recommended to provide better access to the anconeal process in the flexed position (Böhmer *et al.*, 1987). The area is exposed by separating between the lateral and long heads of the triceps muscle along a line which is caudal to, but parallel with the humerus. Distally the attachment of the lateral head of the triceps is separated from the olecranon, leaving some the tendon behind to facilitate closure later (Figure 18.23). The anconeus

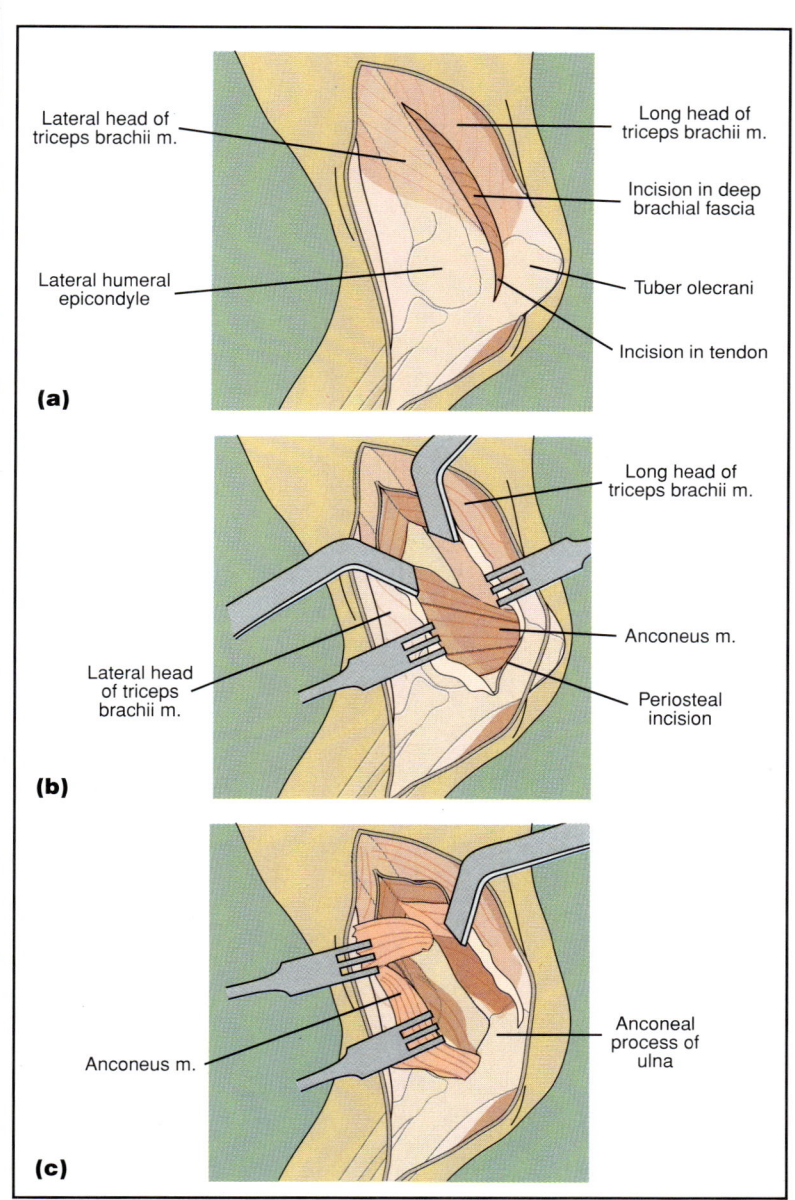

18.23 A modified caudolateral approach to the elbow joint. This approach may be preferred for internal fixation of the anconeal process.

265

Chapter 18 The elbow

> **OPERATIVE TECHNIQUE 18.2** *continued*
> **Caudolateral approach**

muscle is then bluntly dissected from the long head of the triceps muscle. The periosteal insertion of the anconeus muscle is incised on the ulna, the olecranon and the lateral epicondylar crest of the humerus. Retraction of the anconeus muscle cranially and the long head of the triceps caudally achieves superior exposure of the caudal compartment of the elbow joint.

Closure
The joint capsule and the divided anconeus muscle are closed with a simple continuous pattern using absorbable monofilament sutures, followed by the fascia, subcutaneous tissue and skin.

Postoperative care
The joint is protected with a light dressing for 5–7 days. If internal fixation has been performed then more support is provided with a Robert Jones bandage for 2 weeks.

Chapter 18 The elbow

OPERATIVE TECHNIQUE 18.3
Medial approach

Positioning
Lateral recumbency, with the affected leg on the downside. The upper leg is pulled caudally. A small sandbag or folded towel is positioned under the affected elbow to act a fulcrum, which will help with exposure.

Assistant
Essential to help with manipulation of the joint to gain adequate exposure of the interior of the joint through this limited approach.

Tray extras
Gelpi self-retaining retractors or small stifle distractors; Senn hand-held retractors.

Surgical technique
A curved 6–8 cm skin incision is centred over the medial epicondyle (Figure 18.24a). Numerous layers of subcutaneous fascia are divided to expose the medial epicondyle and the flexor muscles of the antebrachium.

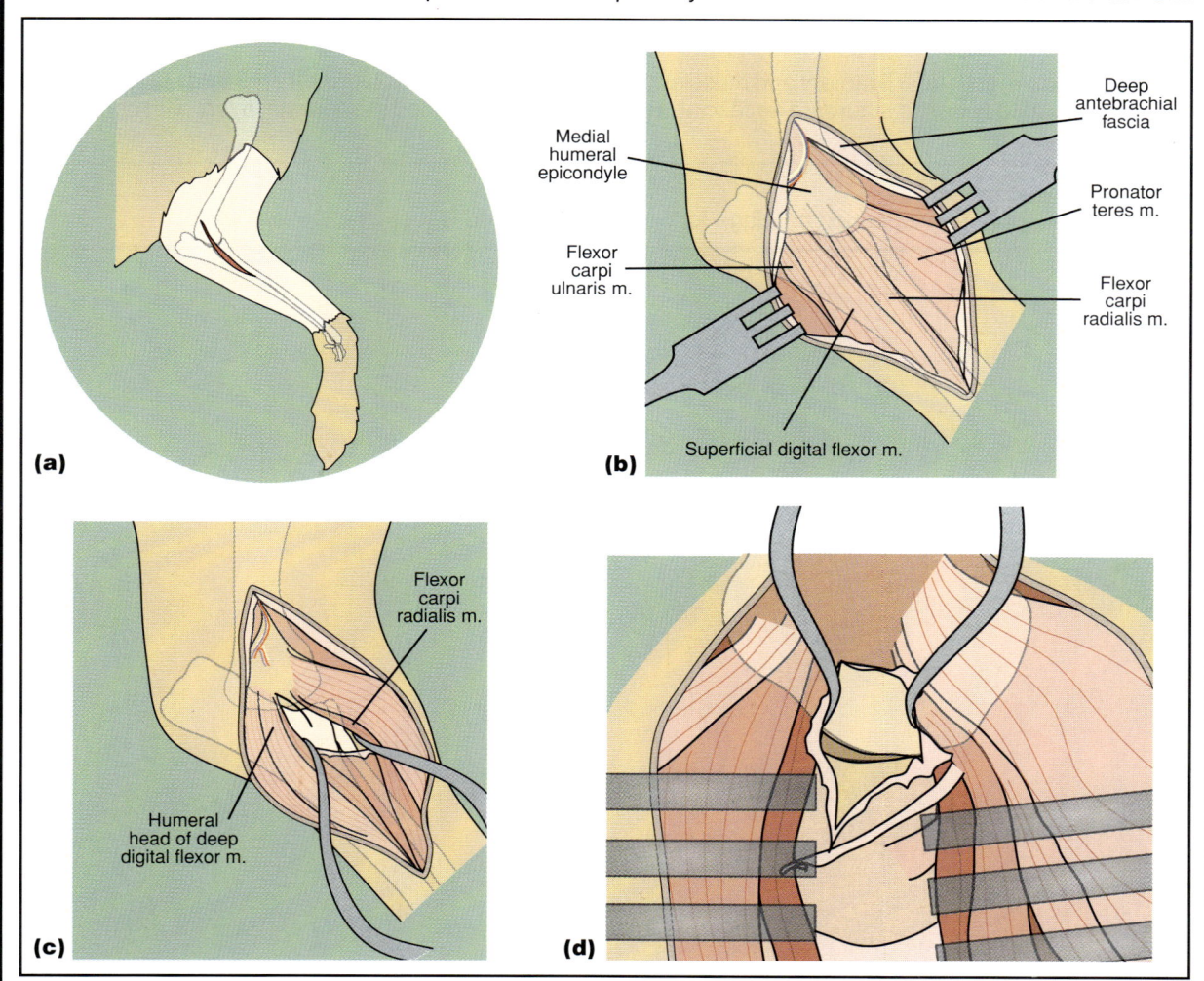

18.24 **(a)** The skin incision is centred over the medial epicondyle and extends proximally and distally for 3–4 cm.
(b) Incision through the underlying fascia and subsequent retraction, exposes the origin of the flexor tendons.
(c) Blunt dissection between the deep digital flexor tendon and the flexor carpi radialis tendon exposes the joint capsule. (An alternative approach is to separate between the flexor carpi radialis and pronator teres tendons.)
(d) The joint capsule is incised. Internal rotation of the elbow joint can aid inspection of the medial coronoid process. If necessary, the caual aspect of the medial collateral ligament can be incised to increase exposure.

→

Chapter 18 The elbow

OPERATIVE TECHNIQUE 18.3 *continued*
Medial approach

> **WARNING**
> The ulnar nerve is located at the proximal end of the incision and care should be taken when the fat in this area is divided. The proximity of the brachial artery and vein and the median nerve to the underside of the pronator teres muscle should be recognized.

Exposure of the joint is achieved by muscle separation, either between the pronator teres and the flexor carpi radialis or between the flexor carpi radialis and the deep digital flexor that lies caudal to it (Figure 18.24c). If more exposure is required the insertions of the relevant muscles can be partially transected.

The joint capsule and, if necessary, the medial collateral ligament are divided parallel with the joint surface (Figure 18.24d). Retraction of the joint capsule will reveal the medial part of the humeral condyle and the outer aspect of the medial coronoid process. Better exposure of the deeper aspects of the joint can be achieved by abduction and pronation of the radius and ulna or alternatively by flexing the carpus and using the sandbag as a fulcrum to lever the joint open. The elbow joint is a close-fitting joint and this approach provides limited but adequate exposure.

Closure
The joint capsule, collateral ligament and muscles are repaired with absorbable sutures. Slight elevation of the limb may facilitate tying the sutures. The fascial layers and skin are closed in separate layers with continuous absorbable sutures.

Postoperative care
The joint is supported in a padded bandage for 5–7 days. Exercise is restricted for 2–3 weeks.

Chapter 18 The elbow

OPERATIVE TECHNIQUE 18.4
Transolecranon or caudal approach

Positioning
Dorsal recumbency with the affected leg supported in extension.

Assistant
Essential.

Tray extras
Equipment for selected method of repair; Kirschner wires and monofilament wire for the tension band fixation of the osteotomy; pin/wire cutters and twisters; Gelpi and Hohmann retractors; sharp-pointed and serrated bone-holding forceps; bone saw; drill.

Surgical technique
A skin incision is made over the caudolateral aspect of the elbow (Figure 18.25a); the fat and fascia are incised and undermined to allow reflection of the skin on both sides of the joint. The fascia along the cranial border of the medial head of the triceps muscle is incised and the ulnar nerve is identified and retracted from the olecranon (Figure 18.25b). The cranial margin of the lateral head of the triceps is also freed from its fascial attachments. The proximal shaft of the ulna is then exposed by separation of the flexor carpi ulnaris medially and the extensor carpi ulnaris laterally. A transverse hole is drilled in the ulna below the elbow joint with a 2 mm drill. A length of heavy-gauge wire is then placed through this hole to be used later as part of the tension band, but at this stage it gives the assistant surgeon something to use to exert traction on the ulna to help in exposure and reduction of the fracture. If a lag screw is to be used to repair the osteotomy then the drill hole should be placed before the osteotomy is performed.

A transverse osteotomy of the olecranon is performed using an oscillating saw or Gigli wire, distal to the insertion of the triceps tendon but proximal to the anconeal process. It is important to identify and protect the ulnar nerve during this part of the procedure. The exposure is completed by reflecting the triceps muscle and

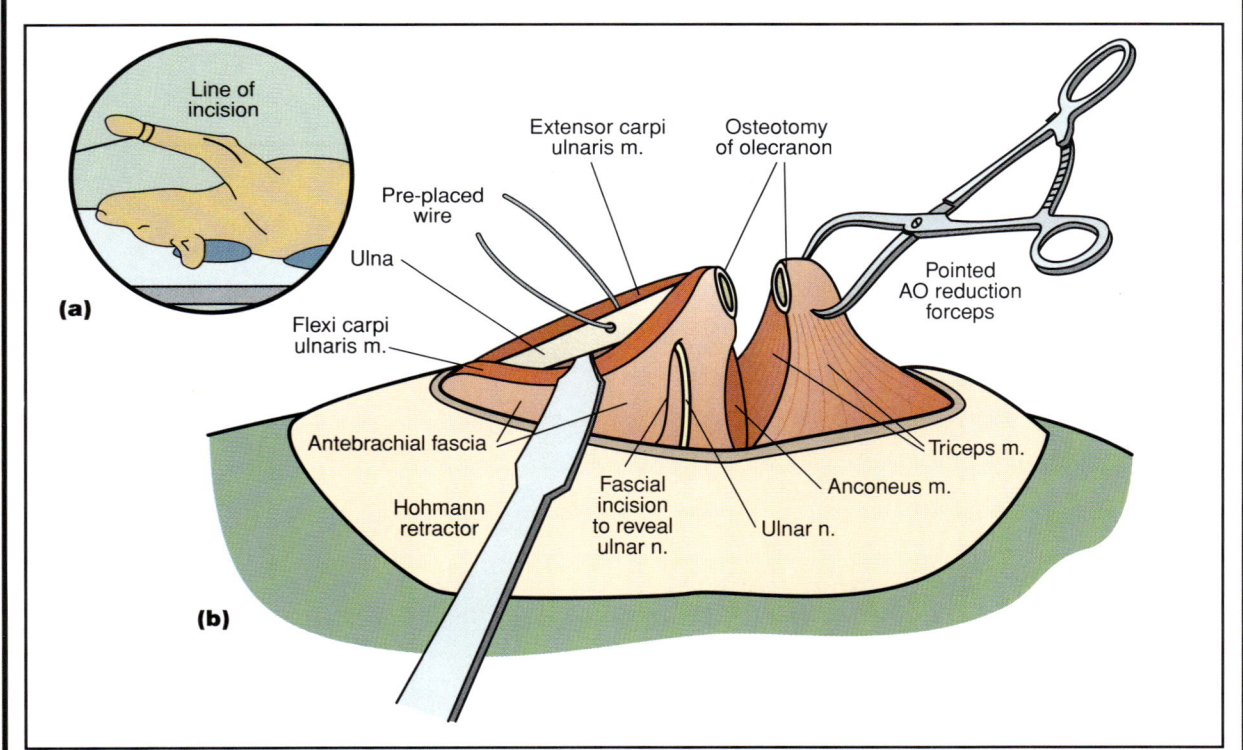

18.25 (a) The skin incision is caudolateral to the elbow joint. (b) The fascia is incised taking care to identify and avoid the ulnar nerve on the medial aspect. The olecranon osteotomy is completed with a Gigli wire and a drill hole inserted in the proximal ulna. A wire is placed through the hole to aid retraction. (continues) →

Chapter 18 The elbow

OPERATIVE TECHNIQUE 18.4 continued
Transolecranon or caudal approach

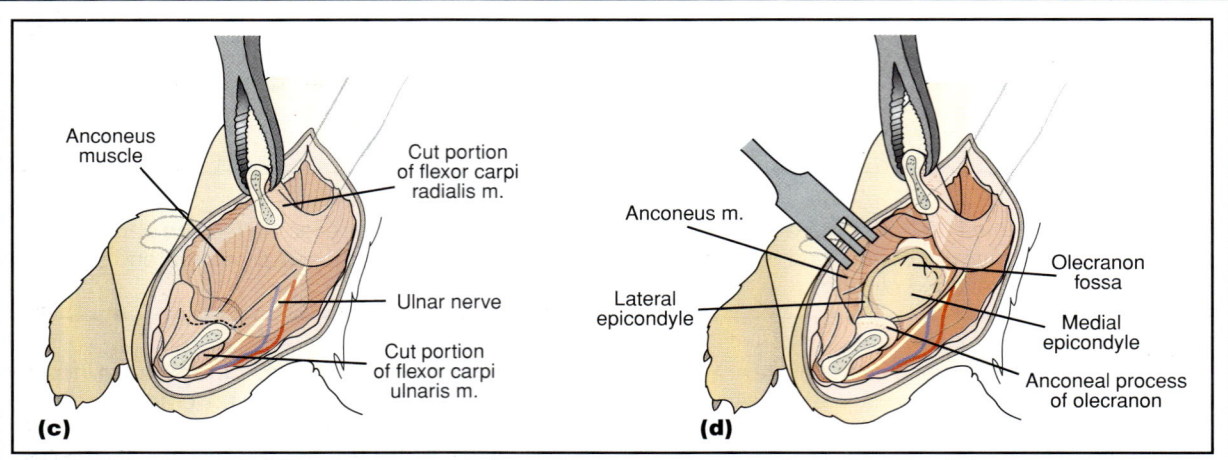

18.25 (continued) **(c)** The olecranon and attached triceps tendon are retracted proximally to expose the anconeus muscle. **(d)** The insertion of the anconeus muscle is incised to expose the caudal joint.

the attached olecranon proximally while the remnants of the anconeus muscle and the joint capsule are reflected from the caudal aspect of the joint (Figures 18.25c,d). Exposure of the fracture is improved by flexion of the joint.

Closure
At closure no attempt is made to reattach the anconeus muscle or the joint capsule. The olecranon is reattached either with a lag screw, supported by a figure-of-eight wire, or with a tension band wire using parallel Kirschner wires. The remaining tissues are closed in layers.

Postoperative care
The leg should be supported for about 7–10 days in a heavily padded bandage.

Chapter 18 The elbow

OPERATIVE TECHNIQUE 18.5
'Open-book' approach

This approach, first described by Lenehan and Nunamaker (1982), is a modified lateral approach to the elbow through an osteotomy of the ulna below the elbow joint, but above the interosseous ligament.

Positioning
Dorsal with limb extended or lateral with the affected leg uppermost.

Assistance
Optional but an advantage for retraction and manipulation.

Tray extras
Self-retaining retractors; Kirschner wires (or a fine intramedullary pin) and orthopaedic wire to repair the osteotomy; pin and wire cutters and twisters.

Surgical technique
A long caudolateral skin incision extends from just proximal to the lateral epicondyle to the level of the mid shaft of the ulna (Figure 18.26a). After subcutaneous dissection, the muscles are elevated from the lateral and medial sides of the ulna by subperiosteal dissection (Figure 18.26b). On the lateral side the anconeus muscle is also

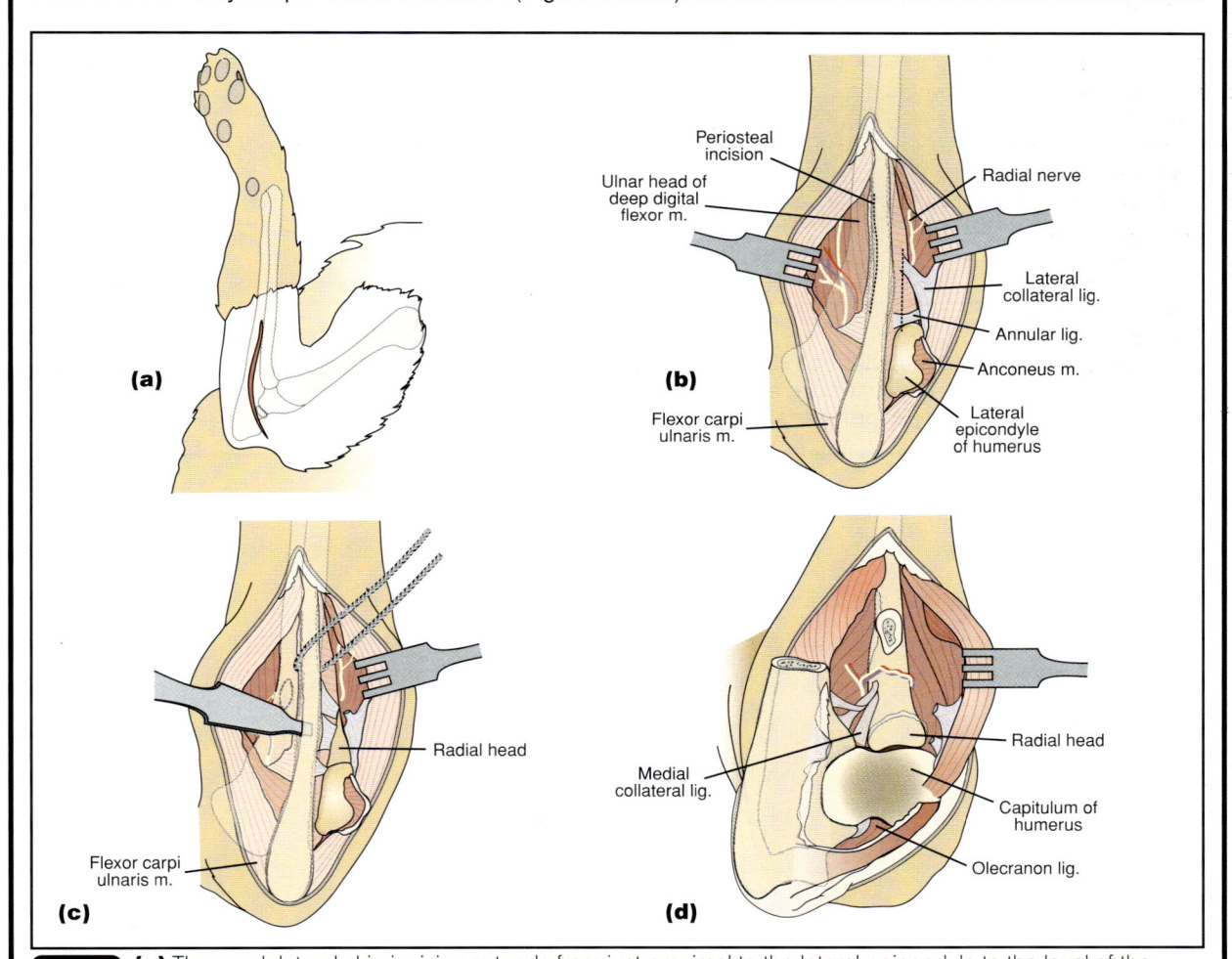

18.26 (a) The caudolateral skin incision extends from just proximal to the lateral epicondyle to the level of the midshaft of the ulna. (b) The muscles are elevated from the lateral and medial sides of the ulna by subperiosteal dissection. (c) The osteotomy is completed with either a Gigli wire (shown) or an oscillating saw. (d) Medial rotation of the proximal ulna exposes the humeral condyle and the radial head.

271

Chapter 18 The elbow

> **OPERATIVE TECHNIQUE 18.5** *continued*
> 'Open-book' approach

divided. The annular ligament is identified below the lateral aspect of the radial head and divided near its attachment to the ulna. The ulna is now osteotomized just proximal to the interosseous ligament using an oscillating saw or Gigli wire (Figure 18.26c). Medial rotation of the proximal ulna exposes the humeral condyle and the radial head (Figure 18.26d) and, with some manipulation, the entire elbow joint can be opened like a book.

Closure
The ulnar osteotomy is stabilized with a Kirschner wire (or fine intramedullary pin) and a tension-band wire (Figure 18.27). The soft tissues are returned to their normal location and held with a series of interrupted sutures placed in the surrounding fascia. No attempt is made to reconstruct the annular ligament.

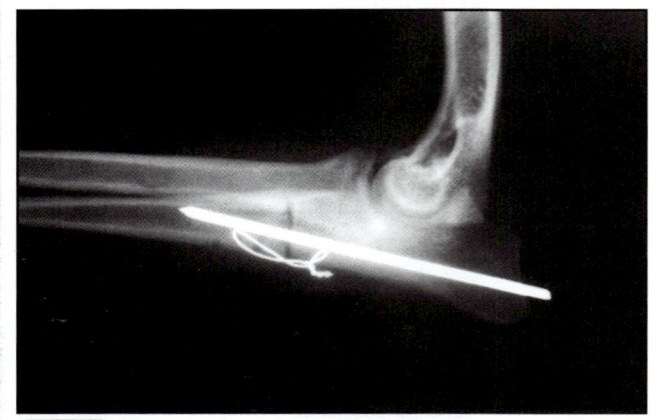

18.27 The osteotomy is repaired with an intramedullary pin and a reinforcing wire.

Postoperative care
A Robert Jones bandage is applied for 10 days and this is followed by restricted exercise for a further 4 weeks. Passive range-of-motion exercises are encouraged. Despite this apparently radical approach, the end result is less traumatic than other approaches where generous exposure is required.

Chapter 18 The elbow

OPERATIVE TECHNIQUE 18.6
Closed reduction of luxations

Positioning
Lateral recumbency with the affected limb uppermost.

Assistance
Depends on the size of the patient. Repeated attempts at closed reduction in a big dog can be very tiring.

Technique
First it is established by palpation and from the radiographs if the elbow is completely luxated (the usual situation) or if the anconeal process is still retained medial to the lateral epicondyle. The elbow is flexed fully and held in this position for a few seconds to fatigue the surrounding muscles. The radial head, the semilunar notch of the ulna and the humeral condyles are identified by palpation.

The elbow is placed in about 110 degrees of flexion. With the carpus flexed to 90 degrees, the antebrachium is rotated inward (pronation) using the metacarpal region as a handle (Figure 18.28a). With the thumb of the opposite hand, the anconeal process is manipulated towards the lateral epicondyle of the humerus. Medial pressure is applied to the olecranon to force the anconeal process medial to the lateral epicondyle. Once this has been achieved the elbow is extended slightly to lock the anconeal process in this position. Now the thumb pressure is changed to the radial head and the amount of antebrachial rotation is increased. Gradual flexion of the elbow and adduction of the antebrachium will force the elbow medially using the anconeal process as a fulcrum (Figure 18.28b). This may be aided by slight abduction of the elbow joint.

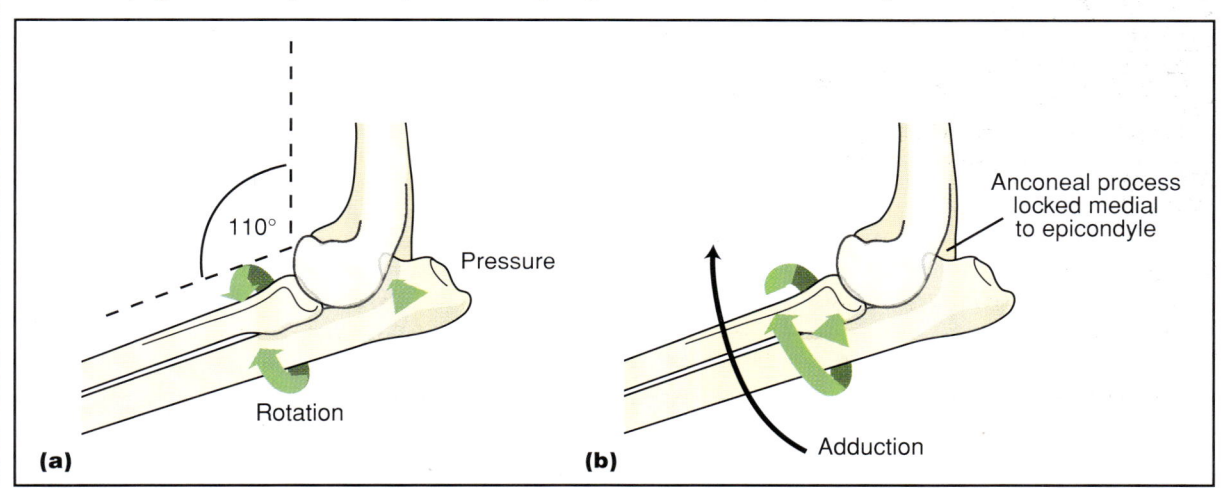

18.28 Closed reduction of elbow luxation. **(a)** The elbow is extended and pressure applied to the lateral aspect of the anconeal process whilst simultaneously internally rotating the elbow joint. **(b)** With the anconeal process engaged, the elbow is slowly extended with simultaneous pressure on the lateral aspect of the radial head.

Successful reduction is usually accompanied by a dramatic return to a normal range of joint motion and restoration of normal anatomical relationships.

The collateral ligaments are then checked for damage once the successful reduction has been confirmed by palpation and/or radiographs (see Operative Technique 18.7).

Post-reduction care
The joint is supported in extension in a Robert Jones bandage for 10 days.

Chapter 18 The elbow

OPERATIVE TECHNIQUE 18.7
Collateral ligament repair

Positioning
Lateral recumbency with the affected limb positioned so that the affected collateral ligament is uppermost. If both medial and lateral sides of the joint are to be approached then it may be easier to have the patient in dorsal recumbency, with the affected limb elevated and extended.

Assistance
Not essential if self-retaining retractors are available.

Tray extras
Self-retaining retractors, such as a small joint distractor or Weitlander; drill with appropriate drill bits; screws; malleable wire, wire cutters and twisters; spiked or plain washers; tissue anchors, if available.

Surgical approach
This will depend on which collateral ligament is to be repaired. The prominent medial and lateral epicondylar processes are convenient landmarks. The lateral or ulnar collateral ligament extends from the lateral epicondyle and divides distally (see Figure 18.1). The cranial portion is attached to the neck of the radius. As it crosses the joint it blends with the annular ligament. The caudal portion attaches to the ulna. The medial or radial collateral ligament extends from the medial epicondyle and divides distally into a weaker cranial part which attaches to the radial tuberosity and a stronger caudal part which attaches mainly to the ulna.

Surgical technique
The affected collateral ligament is exposed by dissection between the overlying muscles and the ends of the ligament are identified. Occasionally primary repair of the ligament may be possible with the use of an appropriate suture (Figure 18.29). However, in most cases no attempt is made to resuture the torn ends as the fibres are too badly damaged. The origin and insertion of collateral ligament are identified and, if available, tissue anchors or self-tapping suture screws are inserted at these points. Malleable monofilament wire, nylon or heavy monofilament absorbable suture is then placed between these anchors using a figure-of-eight pattern (Figure 18.30). Bone screws can be used, but a washer will usually need to be placed under the head of the screw to stop the suture material slipping over the screw as it is tightened. In rare instances when the collateral ligament has been avulsed from the bone it is possible to reattach the ligament using a spiked washer and a bone screw.

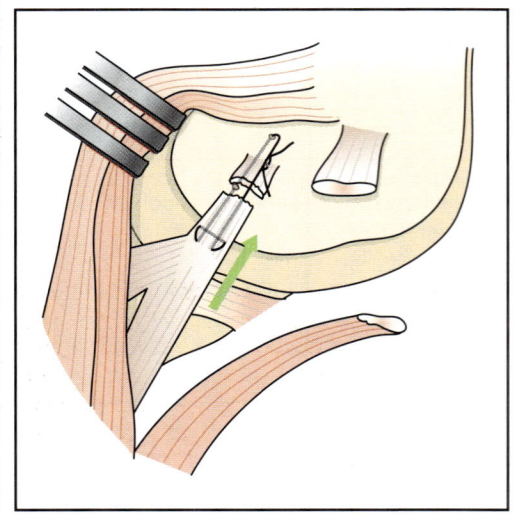

18.29 Repair of a torn lateral collateral ligament with a locking loop suture pattern.

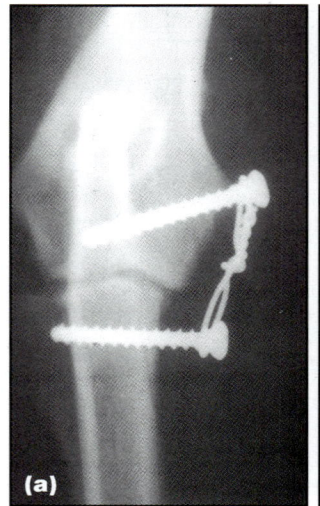

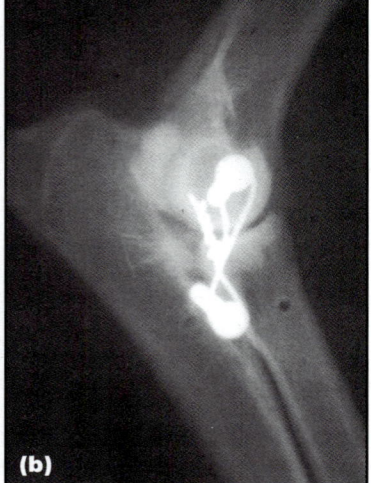

18.30 Repair of a medial collateral ligament with a combination of screws and wire.

Postoperative care
The elbow is immobilized in extension with a Robert Jones bandage for 7–10 days. The implants are usually left *in situ*.

Chapter 18 The elbow

OPERATIVE TECHNIQUE 18.8
Un-united anconeal process

Positioning
Lateral recumbency, affected leg uppermost.

Assistant
Essential if internal fixation is to be undertaken. If removal of the process is the objective then assistance is not necessary if appropriate self-retaining retractors are available.

Tray extras
Self-retaining retractors, such as a small joint distractor or Weitlander; Senn hand-held retractors; oscillating saw; appropriately sized screws and equipment; drill guides and aiming device; small sharp-pointed bone holders; periosteal elevator or osteotome.

Surgical approach
Caudolateral approach (see Operative Technique 18.2). For removal of the anconeal process, the surgeon can use the caudolateral approach, but modify this and incise through the anconeal process. For fragment fixation, a caudolateral approach is used but the origin of the anconeal process is elevated from the lateral epicondylar ridge of the humerus. Full flexion of the joint improves the visualization of the UAP.

Surgical technique

Process removal
The process is removed via a caudolateral approach through the anconeus muscle. A pair of sharp reduction forceps can be used to grasp the process, while its attachments are released with an osteotome (Figure 18.31).

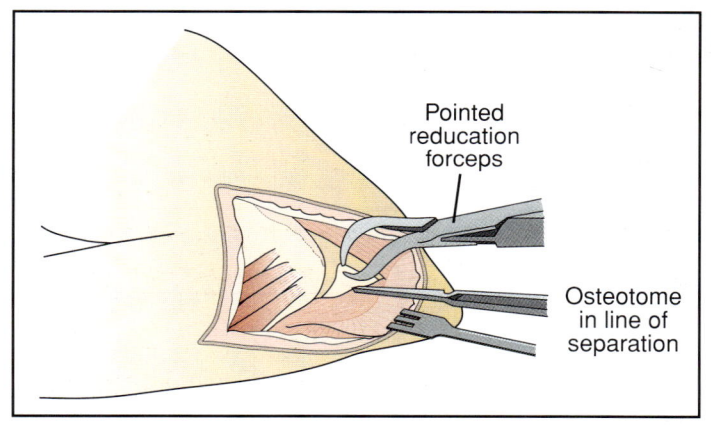

18.31 Removal of an un-united anconeal process.

Elbow exploration and ulnar osteotomy
If subluxation and incongruency of the joint are identified, relief of the intra-articular pressure by osteotomy of the diaphysis of the ulna may result in spontaneous union of the separated anconeal process, especially if exploration of the caudal compartment of the joint reveals that the UAP is firmly attached to the underlying ulna.

A proximal dynamic sliding osteotomy of the ulna is performed. The inclined osteotomy is performed, usually with an oscillating saw, in a proximal to distal, caudal to cranial direction, starting approximately level with the radial head and finishing above the interosseous ligament. The direction of osteotomy and the direction of the pull of the muscles results in lengthening of the ulna and self-stabilization of the fragments with no need for internal fixation. Transverse osteotomies are easier to perform but result in greater patient morbidity (see Operative Technique 18.9).

Internal fixation and ulnar osteotomy
The best results will be achieved by combining internal fixation with Kirschner wires in dogs under 6 months of age or a combination of a Kirschner wire and a lag screw in older individuals performed via a caudolateral approach (see Operative Technique 18.2). Accurate placement of the implants can be difficult as the UAP is quite small. A drill guide can be very helpful in first placing a Kirschner wire. Once the Kirschner wire has been successfully located within the UAP it can be used as a guide for the lag →

OPERATIVE TECHNIQUE 18.8 continued
Un-united anconeal process

screw, which is placed from the caudal surface of the ulna into the anconeal process.

A pressure-relieving dynamic osteotomy of the ulna is also performed with the position and direction of the osteotomy varying according to the breed of the patient and the degree of incongruency. In chondrodystrophic breeds the osteotomy should be performed in the middle or lower third of the ulnar diaphysis because of the high incidence of non-unions when proximal osteotomies are performed in these breeds. In non-chondrodystrophic patients a proximal dynamic sliding osteotomy is performed (Figure 18.32).

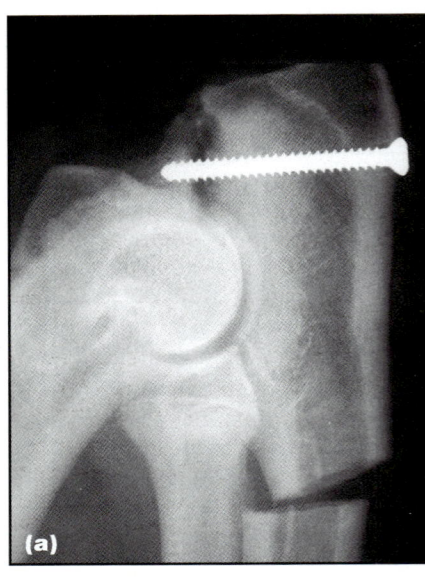

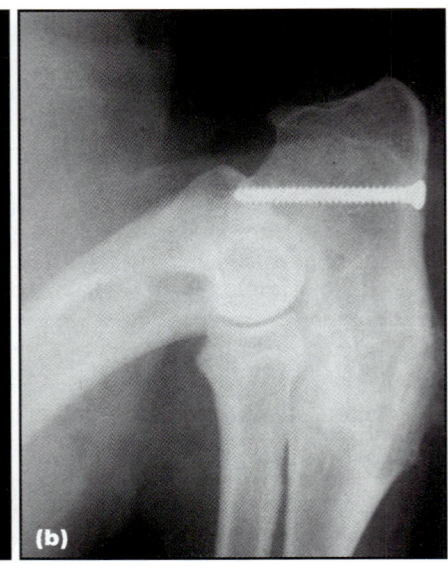

18.32 Fixation of a UAP with a single lag screw combined with a dynamic proximal osteotomy. **(a)** Immediately post-operative view. **(b)** View 12 weeks after operation: there is fusion of the anconeus and union of the osteotomy.

In situations where internal fixation has been performed on the UAP but there is no incongruency, a transverse osteotomy can be performed in the middle or distal portions of the ulnar diaphysis (Meyer-Lindenberg, 1999). This is done to protect the implants from shear stress and potential failure.

Closure
The anconeus muscle is reattached with absorbable sutures.

Postoperative care

- The joint should be immobilized in a padded bandage for about 7 days after surgery to reduce postoperative swelling.
- Following ulnar osteotomy, analgesia may be required for some weeks until healing has occurred.
- Following internal fixation and/or ulnar osteotomy, follow-up radiographs should be taken at 4–8 weeks to check on healing of the anconeus and ulnar osteotomy.

Chapter 18 The elbow

OPERATIVE TECHNIQUE 18.9
Dynamic ulnar osteotomy/ostectomy

Positioning
Lateral recumbency with the affected leg uppermost.

Assistant
Not necessary if appropriate self-retaining retractors are available.

Tray extras
Self-retaining retractors such as a small joint distractor or Weitlander; mini Hohmann retractors or small spoon Hohmann; oscillating saw; rongeurs of various sizes; periosteal elevator.

Surgical approach
A direct incision is made over the caudal aspect of the ulna for a proximal osteotomy or a lateral incision is made for a distal osteotomy. The surrounding muscles are retracted by making a sharp incision through the periosteum, which is then undermined with a periosteal elevator or by dry swab dissection. The retraction is maintained with a combination of self-retaining retractors and Hohmann retractors inserted under the periosteum.

Surgical technique
The position and direction of the osteotomy varies according to the breed of the patient and the degree of incongruency. In chondrodystrophic breeds the osteotomy should be performed in the middle or lower third of the ulnar diaphysis because of the high incidence of non-unions when proximal osteotomies are performed in these breeds.

In patients with incongruency a proximal dynamic sliding osteotomy is indicated (Figure 18.33). The inclined osteotomy is performed, usually with an oscillating saw, in a proximal to distal, caudal to cranial direction, starting approximately level with the radial head and finishing above the interosseous ligament. If an oscillating saw is not available then the cut can be completed by making a series of drill holes along the line of the proposed osteotomy and then cutting along the line of holes with a sharp osteotome.

> **WARNING**
> The ulnar cortical bone is quite thick in this area and prone to split longitudinally when attempts are made to perform the osteotomy with an osteotome.

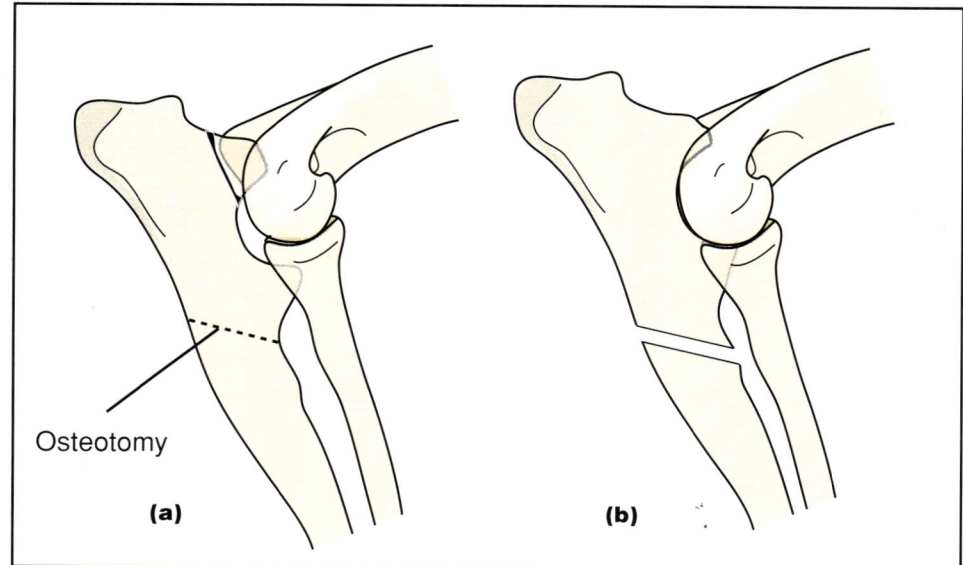

18.33 Dynamic oblique proximal ulnar osteotomy for UAP. **(a)** An oblique osteotomy in this direction allows lengthening of the ulna with some self-stabilization. **(b)** Displacement of the proximal segment of the ulna has restored congruency.

Chapter 18 The elbow

> ## OPERATIVE TECHNIQUE 18.9 continued
> ### Dynamic ulnar osteotomy/ostectomy
>
> The direction of osteotomy and the direction of the pull of the muscles results in lengthening of the ulna and self-stabilization of the fragments. Internal fixation is optional. Transverse osteotomies are easier to perform but result in greater patient morbidity. In young dogs the transverse osteotomy can be performed with a pair of rongeurs.
>
> In young dogs with active growth plates, Vezzoni (2000) recommended performing the osteotomy 2–3 cm above the distal ulnar growth plate, using rongeurs to reduce the possibility of causing damage to the interosseous blood vessels. This causes much less patient morbidity and the elastic interosseous ligament allows for a dynamic shift in the relationship between the radius and the ulna (Figure 18.34).
>
> **18.34** Distal ulnar osteotomy is an alternative in young dogs and causes less postoperative morbidity.
>
> ### Closure
> The periosteum is closed with a simple continuous pattern using a monofilament absorbable suture. The remaining tissues are closed routinely.
>
> ### Postoperative care
> A padded bandage is applied to provide pressure on the soft tissues and to provide support for 10 days. The owners are warned to expect significant swelling at the site of the osteotomy as it heals with a large amount of periosteal callus formation. A prolonged period of lameness will also occur until the bone ends are stable.

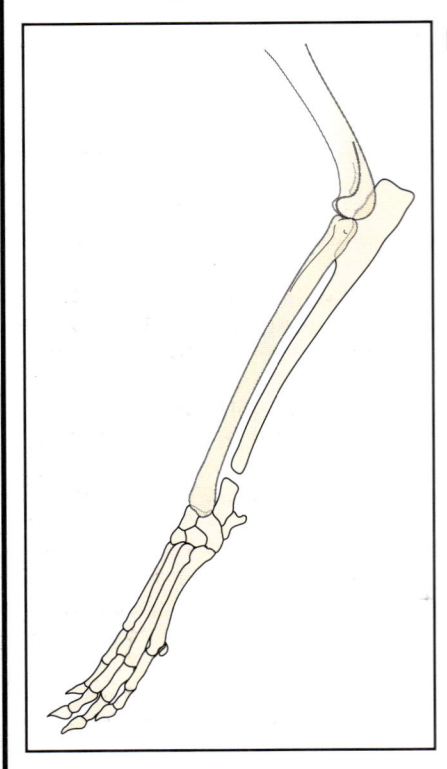

Chapter 18 The elbow

OPERATIVE TECHNIQUE 18.10
Fragmented coronoid process and osteochondritis dissecans

Positioning
Lateral recumbency, with the affected leg on the downside. The upper leg is pulled caudally. A small sandbag or folded towel is positioned under the affected elbow to act a fulcrum, which will help with exposure.

Assistant
Essential to help with manipulation of the joint to gain adequate exposure of the interior of the joint through this limited approach.

Tray extras
Small periosteal elevator or chisel; OCD curette; small Volkman's curette.

Surgical approach
See Operative Technique 18.3.

Surgical technique
The medial aspect of the joint is explored surgically and any loose piece(s) of bone and cartilage are removed. The fragmented piece(s) of the coronoid are removed by elevation of the fragment(s) with a small chisel and transection of the attachments to the annular ligament. All visible articular surfaces are inspected for evidence of erosion and OCD lesions. If erosive and chondromalacic lesions are present then it may be insufficient to just remove the fragmented coronoid. It is recommended either to drill holes in the diseased cartilage and exposed subchondral bone or to remove the surrounding cartilage and 0.5–1 mm of subchondral bone from the medial coronoid process in an attempt to shift the load away from this area on to the humeroradial side of the joint (Olsson, 1993). The joint is flushed with large quantities of sterile saline prior to closure.

Ulnar osteotomy is indicated in cases with incongruency and in cases that have not responded satisfactorily to fragment removal (see Operative Technique 18.9).

Bardet and Bureau (1996) reported on the results of treating selected cases of FCP by performing an oblique osteotomy of the proximal ulna, particularly in cases that had not responded satisfactorily to arthrotomy and fragment removal. The osteotomy is performed below the joint at the junction of the proximal and middle third of the diaphysis. The oblique cut is positioned so that the proximal ulna is allowed to rotate slightly in a proximal and medial direction (Figure 18.35). No attempt is made to stabilize the osteotomy which heals by callus formation in 6–8 weeks. The results revealed a significant clinical improvement in 90% of the 40 joints operated on, but osteoarthritis was progressive in 60% of the joints.

Ness (1998) reported a good clinical outcome when young dogs (less than 10 months old) with FCP were treated by fragment removal and simultaneous transverse proximal ulnar osteotomy, performed with an oscillating saw 2.5 cm distal to the humeroradial joint.

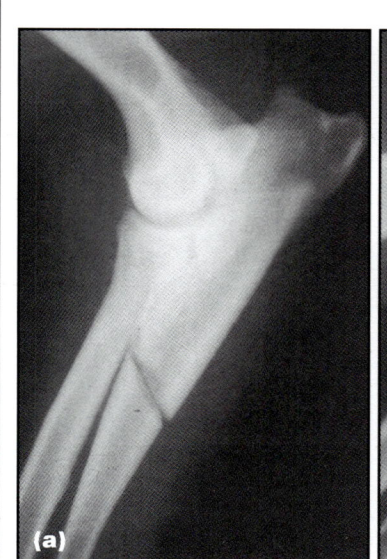

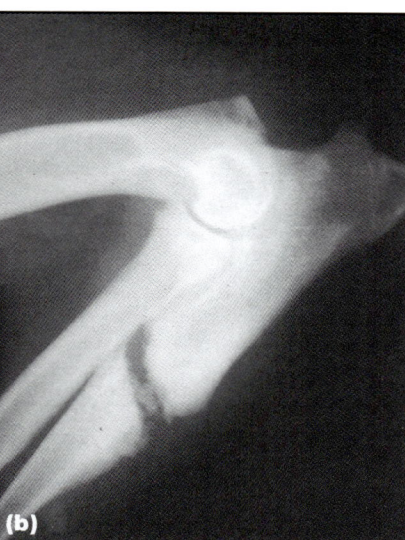

18.35 Lateral radiographs of the elbow of a 1-year-old Rottweiler with fragmentation of the medial coronoid process that had failed to respond satisfactorily to surgical removal of fragments. **(a)** An oblique osteotomy was performed 6 weeks after the initial surgery. The direction of the cut not only releases intra-articular tension but also allows some caudal drift of the proximal ulna. **(b)** After 12 weeks the oteotomy was healing, with periosteal callus, and the dog was sound.

Chapter 18 The elbow

> **OPERATIVE TECHNIQUE 18.10** *continued*
> **Fragmented coronoid process and osteochondritis dissecans**
>
> ---
>
> **Closure**
> See Operative Technique 18.3.
>
> ---
>
> **Postoperative care**
> A pressure bandage is applied for 5–7 days postoperatively. The owners are instructed to restrict the dog's exercise for a further 4 weeks. Swelling of the soft tissues under the incision is an infrequent complication and may be associated with excessive postoperative exercise.

19

The carpus

Mike Guilliard

Anatomy

The carpus is a three-level hinge (ginglymus) joint comprising the antebrachiocarpal joint, the middle carpal joint and the carpometacarpal joint. Approximately 70% of carpal motion is from the antebrachiocarpal joint, 25% from the middle carpal joint and 5% from the carpometacarpal joint. Together with flexion and extension, there is a small amount of lateral angulation placing the medial aspect in tension.

There are seven named carpal bones: in the proximal row are the radial, ulnar and accessory carpal bones; and in the distal row are the first, second, third and fourth carpal bones. In addition there is a small sesamoid bone within the tendon of insertion of the abductor pollicis longus tendon, situated medial to the distal aspect of the radial carpal bone.

The carpus is reliant on ligaments to maintain its stability (Figure 19.1). The main support structures are the strong collateral ligaments, the palmar radiocarpal and ulnocarpal ligaments and fibrocartilage, and the flexor mechanism. The latter comprises the two flexor carpi ulnaris tendons attaching to the free end of the accessory carpal bone (ACB); the ACB acts as a fulcrum with its distal accessoriometacarpal ligaments forming a tension band (Figure 19.2). The ACB articulates with the ulnar carpal bone and the styloid process of the ulna. The palmar process of the radial carpal bone acts as a fulcrum for the palmar support structures of the medial carpus.

During weightbearing there is a small degree of carpal hyperextension, the extent depending on the breed. In the galloping Greyhound the degree of hyperextension has been seen to reach 90 degrees.

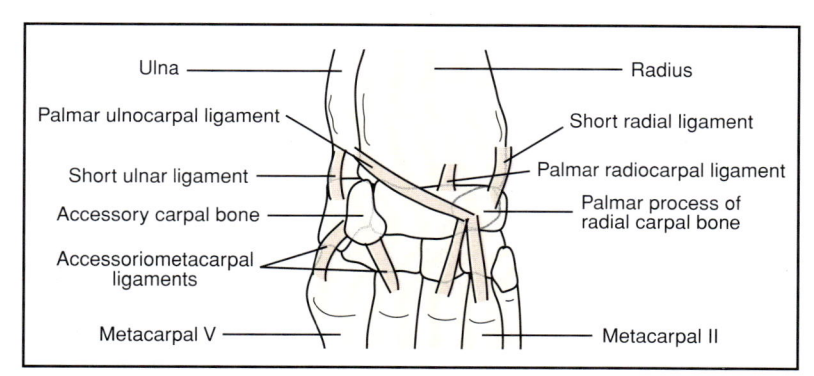

19.1 Ligaments of the palmar aspect of the carpus. The palmar fibrocartilage is not shown.

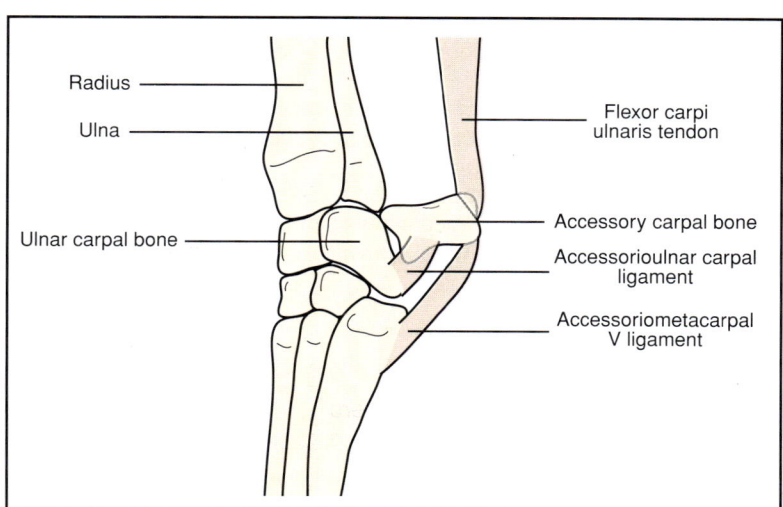

19.2 Diagram of the lateral aspect of the carpus showing the main soft tissue attachments of the accessory carpal bone.

Chapter 19 The carpus

Diagnosis of carpal lameness

The definitive diagnosis of carpal lameness can be a clinical challenge and careful consideration of the signalment, history and clinical findings is required prior to consideration of further diagnostic investigations. The racing Greyhound is particularly prone to carpal injury from the repetitive stresses of galloping around the bends in an anticlockwise direction. Whilst a mild intermittent lameness may be tolerated by the owner of a pet animal, it can be devastating to the career of a racing Greyhound.

Clinical examination

Clinical localization of the injury to the carpus involves careful observation, palpation and manipulation. Gross deformity can arise acutely from trauma, resulting in damage to the supporting soft tissues or fractures and luxations, or more chronically as a result of degenerative changes to the soft tissues leading to ligament laxity, periarticular fibrosis and periarticular new bone deposition. Soft tissue swelling may involve the whole carpus or can be focal, indicating the area of concern. The importance of palpation cannot be overemphasized and is critical in the diagnosis of certain soft tissue injuries. All soft tissue swellings should be palpated for structural deficits, focal pain and firmness.

The carpus should be manipulated to assess the range of normal and abnormal movement. Hyperflexion detects pain and a decreased angle of flexion. Abnormal range of motion is best determined by comparison with the contralateral carpus. The degree of normal flexion is highly variable between individual dogs and can range from full flexion to almost 90 degrees. The forward draw test, in which the metacarpus is moved in a dorsopalmar direction with the distal antebrachium firmly held, will induce a pain response in some carpal injuries. Manipulation also facilitates detection of joint instability and is best performed under general anaesthesia.

Radiography

The standard orthogonal extended views may give sufficient information. Flexed, oblique and stressed views can be useful in particular for the detection of small chip fractures, undisplaced fracture lines and joint instabilities. Contrast arthrography of the antebrachiocarpal joint has not been shown to be helpful.

Advanced imaging

A cadaver study has shown that the major ligaments can be imaged consistently using magnetic resonance imaging (Nordberg and Johnson, 1998) but there is a lack of knowledge concerning its use in the clinical situation. Similarly, although computed tomography would, in theory, have the resolution to provide useful information, its use has not been reported for carpal lameness.

Arthrocentesis

Synoviocentesis will detect inflammatory arthropathies and in traumatic cases will help to determine whether there is involvement of the antebrachiocarpal joint. In the acute injury, normal quantity and appearance of the synovial fluid suggests that the lameness does not involve this joint. Arthrocentesis is a simple procedure with access through the dorsal aspect of the flexed antebrachiocarpal joint. There is no communication between the antebrachiocarpal joint and the middle carpal joint.

Developmental disorders

Flexural deformity of the carpus

This is a not uncommon, marked deformity that is seen in young puppies, between 8 and 12 weeks of age. It can be unilateral or bilateral and presents as a 'knuckling' of the carpus, resulting in a stumbling gait. A growth disparity between the relevant bones and the soft tissues may be the cause. The majority of dogs make a complete recovery within 4 weeks without specific treatment (Vaughan, 1992), although it is wise to ensure that an appropriate balanced diet is being fed and affected puppies should be allowed only moderate exercise. Support bandaging is contraindicated as this will stress-protect and weaken the tissues.

Carpal hyperextension in puppies

This presents as a bilateral excessive degree of carpal hyperextension, which in its extreme form can result in a palmigrade stance. It is most commonly seen in German Shepherd Dogs. Treatment is aimed at increasing muscle tone through controlled exercise. By maturity, carpal posture should have improved considerably. As with flexural deformity, a balanced diet is appropriate and external coaptation is contraindicated. Secondary nutritional hyperparathyroidism can also cause carpal laxity.

Growth plate disorders

Premature closure of the distal radial and ulnar growth plates will produce asynchronous or stunted growth of the radius and ulna. This can lead to clinical problems proximal to the carpus, including bowing of the antebrachium, elbow incongruity and a shortened limb. Carpal valgus may result from premature closure of the distal ulnar growth plate, whilst a varus deformity may occur as a result of distal radial growth plate disturbances.

Unless the angular deformities are successfully treated, secondary degenerative changes are likely to occur. Simple treatment options involve osteotomy or ostectomy of either the radius or ulna to allow independent growth, and distal epiphyseal stapling to counter carpal varus or valgus. These procedures are now becoming superseded by the use of the circular external fixator, which allows accurate correction of angular deformities together with limb lengthening (see also Chapter 6).

Soft tissue injuries of the carpus

Soft tissue injuries can involve the ligaments, tendons, palmar fibrocartilage and joint capsules of the carpus. Clinical signs are usually swelling, varying degrees of lameness and carpal instability.

The dorsal aspect

Sprain of the dorsal radiocarpal ligament
The dorsal radiocarpal ligament runs diagonally from its origin on the proximal rim of the antebrachiocarpal joint (on the distal radial prominence between the middle and lateral dorsal grooves) to insert on the ulnar carpal bone. Sprain of this ligament results in a low-grade chronic lameness and is seen in high-activity dogs and racing Greyhounds (Guilliard, 1997). There is pain on carpal flexion and a characteristic soft tissue swelling is identified along the course of the ligament on the dorsolateral aspect of the carpus. Lateral extended and flexed carpal radiographs are indicated to exclude an avulsion fracture that often involves the origin of the ligament in the Greyhound (Figure 19.3). Treatment is by immobilization of the carpus for 3 weeks in a splinted support bandage and the prognosis is very good. If an avulsion fracture is present the fragment should be surgically removed.

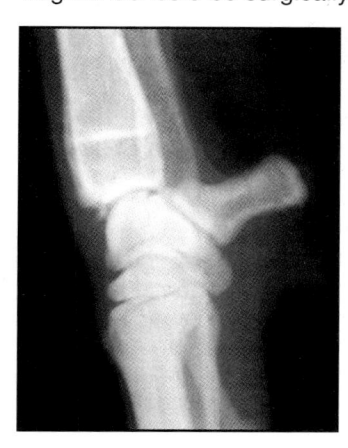

19.3 Lateral view of the extended carpus, showing an avulsion fracture of the origin of the dorsal radiocarpal ligament within the antebrachiocarpal joint.

Injury to the abductor pollicis longus tendon
The tendon of insertion of the abductor pollicis longus muscle, enclosed in a synovial sheath, runs in the most medial sulcus of the dorsal radius, crossing the medial aspect of the carpus to insert medially on the base of metacarpal I. It acts as an abductor and extensor of the first digit and is important for adduction of the carpus. The tendon runs under the straight part of the short radial collateral ligament and the tendon sheath is intimately involved with the ligament. A small sesamoid bone within the tendon can be seen on the medial aspect of the carpus on a dorsopalmar radiograph. A number of separate clinical conditions are seen in this area and the extent of the pathological involvement of the tendon sheath and the short radial ligament is unclear.

Stenosing tenosynovitis of the abductor pollicis longus tendon: This can cause chronic lameness, with pain on carpal hyperflexion. There is a firm swelling on the medial aspect of the antebrachiocarpal joint. In advanced cases, proliferative bone reactions are seen involving the radial sulcus and the tubercle medial to the sulcus. Initial treatment is by local peritendinal injection of 0.5 ml methylprednisolone (40 mg/ml) together with carpal splinting for 3 weeks. If lameness persists, surgical removal of the proliferative soft tissue and bone should be undertaken to free the tendon (Grundmann and Montavon, 2001).

Sprain of the abductor pollicis longus tendon: This is a separate clinical entity and appears as a soft tissue swelling along the distal course of the tendon from the radial rim on the dorsomedial aspect of the carpus. It is seen in the running breeds and is presented as an observation rather than a cause of lameness.

Sprain of the short radial collateral ligament
This condition is seen in the racing Greyhound. There is a marked diffuse swelling over the dorsomedial carpus, with lameness and no instability. A subsequent proliferation of enthesophytes at the origin of the ligament on the medial radial tubercle has been reported. Strict rest with carpal support bandaging for 6 weeks is indicated. After a suitable rehabilitation programme, the prognosis for a return to racing is good (Guilliard and Mayo, 2000a).

Enthesiopathy of the origin of the short radial collateral ligament
Although not generally a cause of lameness, the radiographic abnormalities in this condition can be marked. The origin of the straight part of the short radial collateral ligament is on the unnamed tubercle on the medial aspect of the distal radius. This tubercle can develop an irregular outline and occasionally what appears to be a small avulsion fracture of the origin of the ligament. In a prospective study of 100 Greyhounds there was an incidence of 14% with no effect on racing performance (Guilliard, 1998). The increased size of the tubercle was palpably apparent in many of these cases. It is also seen in other breeds, notably the Labrador Retriever. Similar radiographic findings are seen with stenosing tenosynovitis of the abductor pollicis longus tendon together with dorsal proliferative changes.

Subluxation of the second carpal bone
This is an uncommon cause of carpal lameness in the racing Greyhound. There is a slight diffuse swelling over the dorsal aspect of the second carpal bone with focal pain on digital pressure. The mediolateral radiographic view shows a slight bony protuberance on the dorsal aspect of the middle carpal joint. A definitive diagnosis is made on a palmaromedial dorsolateral oblique view, where the subluxated dorsal articular surface of the second carpal bone is seen (Figure 19.4) (Guilliard, 2001a). The differential diagnosis includes a fracture of the second carpal bone. Surgical reduction with temporary fixation seems to offer a good prognosis (Figures 19.5 and 19.6).

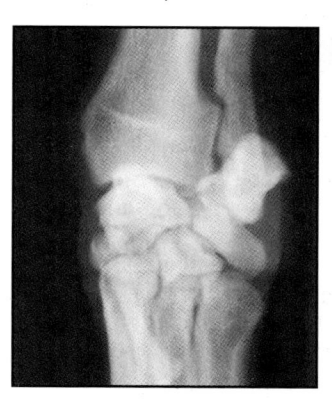

19.4 Palmaromedial dorsolateral oblique view of the carpus, showing subluxation of the proximal articular surface of the second carpal bone.

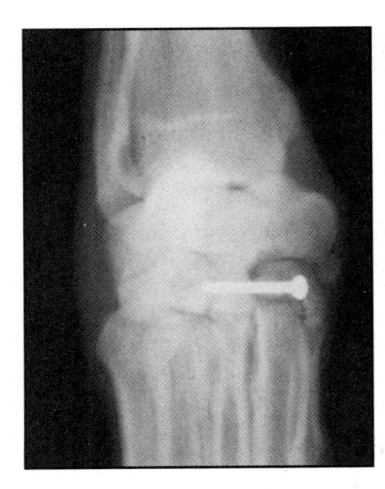

Chapter 19 The carpus

19.5 Second carpal bone subluxation in a racing Greyhound. A positional screw has been placed through the second carpal bone into the third and fourth carpal bones.

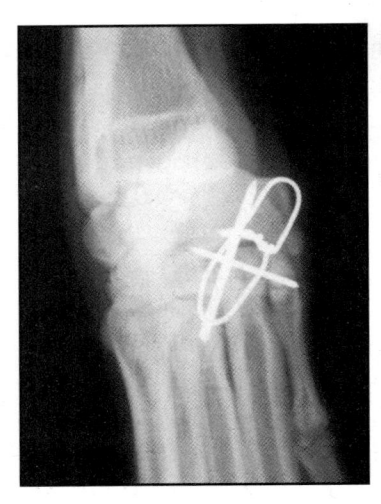

19.6 Second carpal bone subluxation reduced with pins and a tension-band wire.

The palmar aspect

Strain of the flexor carpi ulnaris tendon

The two tendons of the flexor carpi ulnaris muscle insert on the free end of the ACB. The dorsal tendon is the more prone to injury, which presents as an obvious thickening at the tendon insertion. An avulsion fracture from the ACB (type IV) may be present, so radiography is mandatory.

Strain of the flexor carpi ulnaris tendon is a cause of lameness in the racing Greyhound and the severity of the lameness is varied. Dogs can race with this injury but performance is reduced.

Surgical treatment of tendon or bone avulsions is indicated. The avulsed fragment of bone is rarely of a suitable size to be reattached with a lag screw, and surgery should be aimed at apposing the end of the tendon to the bone by suturing it to adjacent soft tissues. Any repair is protected initially by splinting the carpus in 90 degrees of flexion. The degree of flexion is reduced during dressing changes over the subsequent 6 weeks. This splinting technique is also suitable for the treatment of strain injuries without an avulsion. Prognosis for the pet dog is excellent but is more guarded in the performance animal. This condition needs careful differentiation from tears of the palmar fascia.

Tear of the superficial palmar fascia

There is an extensive fascial sheath covering the palmar aspect of the carpus, and in the larger breeds a bursa is present over the free end of the ACB under the fascia. A horizontal tear into the bursa is a common injury in the racing Greyhound, resulting in a low-grade lameness with a discrete swelling (Guilliard and Mayo, 2000b).

Diagnosis is by careful palpation that will differentiate between a thickened flexor carpi ulnaris tendon and a fascial tear, the latter having a characteristic palpable dimple over the tear. Occasionally both injuries may be concurrent. Chronic tears have a thicker fibrous swelling and the dimple is harder to appreciate. Although some of these cases resolve satisfactorily without treatment, suturing of the defect and protecting the repair by supporting the carpus in flexion give a good prognosis for a successful return to racing.

Vertical tears of the palmar fascia can also occur. Again these are easily sutured, but they can be associated with a carpal sprain injury and the prognosis is more guarded.

Carpal sprain injury

Carpal injury is very common in the racing Greyhound and in a high percentage of these dogs a precise diagnosis cannot be made. These cases are given the generic diagnosis of carpal sprain injury and involve grade 1 or 2 sprain injuries to ligamentous structures, with mild to moderate stretching or partial rupture of fibre bundles. No gross instability is present. Typically the presentation is one of mild to moderate lameness after racing. The range of flexion may be reduced and pain is present on hyperflexion. Synoviocentesis shows an increased volume of cytologically non-inflammatory joint fluid that is often serosanguineous. Such cases will often respond well initially to complete rest and appropriate support dressings. The prognosis for a return to the previous racing form is guarded, however, and recurrence is common.

Instabilities and luxations

These are seen acutely as a result of high-energy trauma from road traffic accidents or falls and from high-performance exercise in racing or coursing breeds. Instability and joint subluxation can also occur chronically as a result of degenerative or inflammatory conditions which affect the periarticular soft tissue support structures.

Displacement of the accessory carpal bone

The ACB articulates with the styloid process of the ulna and the ulnar carpal bone. The articulation lies on the lateral palmar aspect of the carpus with the free end of the bone in the midline. The lateral ligaments are on the tension side of the joint. ACB displacement can also be associated with hyperextension injuries.

Two rare conditions have been described (Guilliard, 2001b) involving either complete luxation of the bone, associated with disruption of all the ligaments and joint capsule of the accessoriocarpal joint, or lateral subluxation of the bone where soft tissue support damage is incomplete. In both cases severe lameness results with either gross general swelling of the carpus, in particular over the palmar aspect, or, in the case of subluxation, specifically over the palmarolateral aspect. Radiographic examination confirms luxation on standard orthogonal views but subluxation may be occult and subtle instability is difficult to assess due to significant soft tissue swelling. In such cases soft tissue support damage is confirmed by surgical exploration and damaged tissues are sutured and the carpus supported in flexion. The prognosis for cases of ACB subluxation is good. In cases of complete luxation, salvage pancarpal arthrodesis (see Operative Technique 19.1) is indicated, with the redundant ACB being discarded.

In the cat, the main articulation of the ACB is with the ulna, and subluxation can be a cause of chronic carpal lameness. A lateral subluxation of the articular end of the ACB can be detected on careful palpation. Comparison with the contralateral carpus is helpful. As is the case in the dog, this condition can be difficult to confirm radiographically. A lateral arthrotomy allows accurate reduction, and fixation is achieved by placing cross pins, one through the lateral ACB into the ulna, and the other down the length of the bone into the ulnar carpal bone (Figure 19.7).

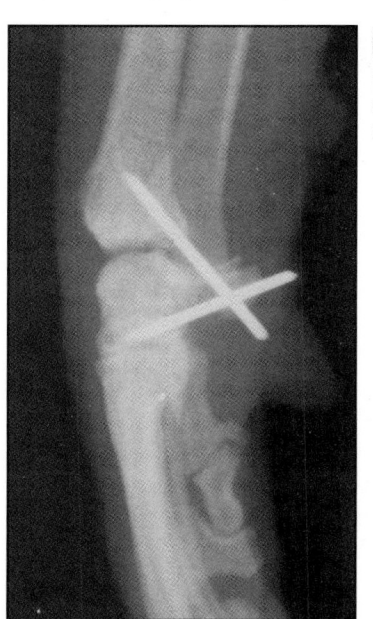

19.7 Reduction of ACB subluxation in a cat, using cross pins.

19.8 Stressed dorsopalmar radiograph of the carpus of a Pekingese, showing subluxation of the medial aspect of the antebrachiocarpal joint due to rupture of the short radial collateral ligaments. A small avulsion fracture is also present.

Stability is restored by prosthetic ligament replacement or primary repair, although this is particularly difficult with the short ligament. Bone tunnels are drilled in the medial prominence of the radial carpal bone and in the distomedial radius. Permanent (either nylon, wire or braided polyester) suture material is passed through the tunnels in such a manner as to simulate the course of both the long and short parts of the medial support.

Injuries to the lateral ligaments are less common and less serious because they are subject to less distractive (tensile) forces. Nonetheless, these injuries result in carpal instability, and surgical repair, using either ligament repair, augmentation or replacement (Figure 19.9), is indicated.

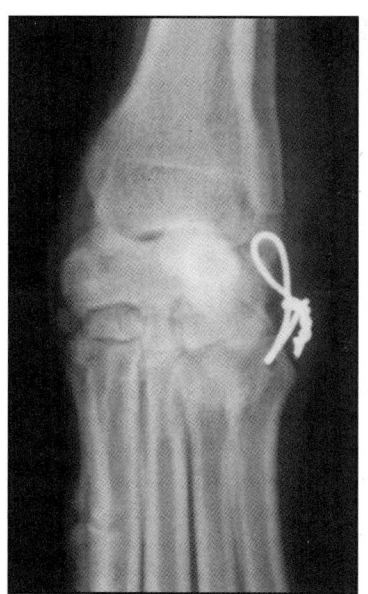

19.9 Repair of ruptured lateral carpal support structures using a tension-band wire.

Radial (medial) collateral ligament rupture

The medial radial collateral ligament comprises two components: the straight (long) ligament and the oblique (short) ligament. The straight ligament is in tension during extension; the oblique ligament is in tension during flexion. Rupture of these ligaments results in a carpal valgus, with a medial dorsopalmar instability and severe lameness. Diagnosis is by stressed radiography (Figure 19.8). An avulsion fracture of the styloid process of the radius may also be present.

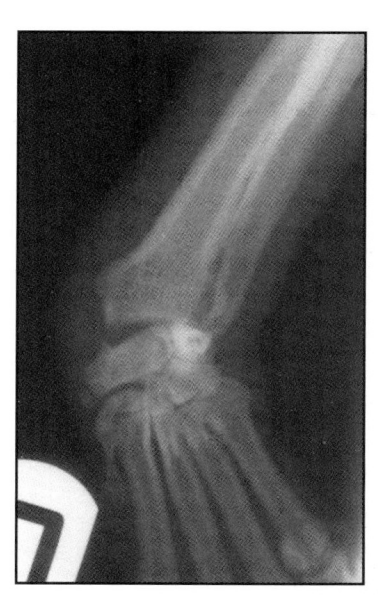

Middle carpal luxation and subluxation

Complete disruption of the middle carpal joint is unusual. Partial carpal arthrodesis is indicated (see Operative Technique 19.2). Subluxation, with medial instability, is much more common. Dorsomedial

Chapter 19 The carpus

ligamentous disruption between the radial carpal and second carpal bone (and occasionally between the second carpal and the base of metacarpal II), results in a valgus deformity of the foot. Dorsomedial stability is restored through ligament replacement within tunnels through the palmaromedial process of the radiocarpal bone and the base of metacarpal II. Care must be taken to identify coexistent hyperextension, associated with damage to the palmaromedial ligaments and fibrocartilage, necessitating pancarpal arthrodesis.

Radial carpal bone luxation

This is an uncommon injury of both the dog and cat. The radial carpal bone rotates on its medial axis with the lateral aspect of the bone moving in a palmar and then dorsal direction to lie behind the carpus; the ligamentous attachments of the palmar process remain intact. Diagnosis is from orthogonal radiographs where an obvious defect is seen in the medial carpus (Miller *et al.*, 1990). Treatment involves reduction and fixation with a pin or screw into the ulnar carpal bone. The medial ligaments are also reconstructed (Figure 19.10). Prognosis is good in the pet dog.

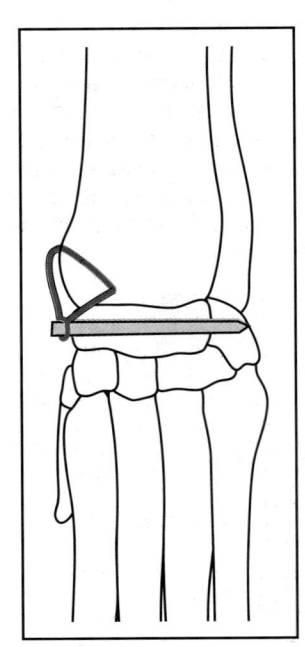

19.10 Luxation of the radial carpal bone repaired with a pin and prosthetic short radial ligaments.

Carpal hyperextension injuries

Carpal hyperextension is usually the result of a fall or road traffic accident causing rupture of the palmar carpal ligaments and fibrocartilage. Concomitant fractures of the carpal bones may also be present. The dog will present with a dropped carpus or palmigrade stance. It is also seen as a bilateral degenerative condition, notably in Rough Collies, and as a sequel to inflammatory polyarthropathy.

The level and degree of instability are assessed during clinical examination and confirmed by stressed, lateral radiographic views. Instability may be identified at the antebrachiocarpal joint, the middle carpal joint, the carpometacarpal joints or a combination of these.

In addition to obvious hyperextension, proximal tilting of the ACB, associated with failure of the two accessoriometacarpal ligaments, may be noted. There may also be proximal elevation of the palmar part of the ulnar carpal bone with increased joint width between the ulnar carpal bone and the fifth metacarpal bone. Chip fractures along the dorsal margin of the distal row of carpal bones due to impingement forces have been identified (Johnson, 1998) and the bases of the metacarpal bones appear to overlap the distal row of carpal bones on a stressed lateral film.

Treatment for traumatic cases using external support inevitably fails as subsequent weightbearing on the limb causes stretching or breakdown of the healing tissues. Partial or complete carpal arthrodesis (see Operative Techniques 19.1 and 19.2), depending on the level of instability, carries a good prognosis; the majority of dogs gain almost full limb function within 4 months. Partial carpal arthrodesis involves the fusion of the middle carpal and carpometacarpal joints. Pancarpal arthrodesis also includes fusion of the antebrachiocarpal joint.

Carpal luxation

This is a rare injury in dogs, sustained during high-performance pursuit activities such as coursing, presumably from stumbling at high speed on rough terrain. The carpus luxates caudally to lie behind the radius and ulna. The diagnosis is made by radiography (Figure 19.11). There may be a concomitant distal ulnar fracture. Reduction is easily achieved and carpal extension gives reasonable stability as the collateral ligaments are usually still intact. External coaptation is indicated for 3–4 weeks. If articular cartilage damage is present, together with bilateral instability associated with collateral support disruption, elective pancarpal arthrodesis (see Operative Technique 19.1) should be considered.

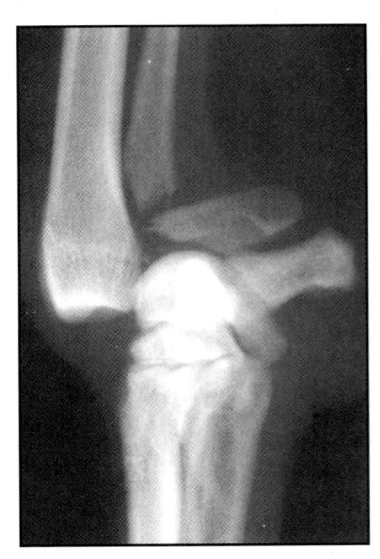

19.11 Lateral radiographic view of a carpal luxation with a fracture of the distal ulna in a Lurcher. The collateral ligaments were intact. This was treated by the insertion of an intramedullary pin in the ulna and by holding the joint in normal congruency for 3 weeks with cross pins. The dog made a full recovery.

The distal ulnar fracture, if present, is repaired with an intramedullary pin, and the reduced carpus is held in extension by two transarticular cross pins for 3 weeks (Figure 19.12).

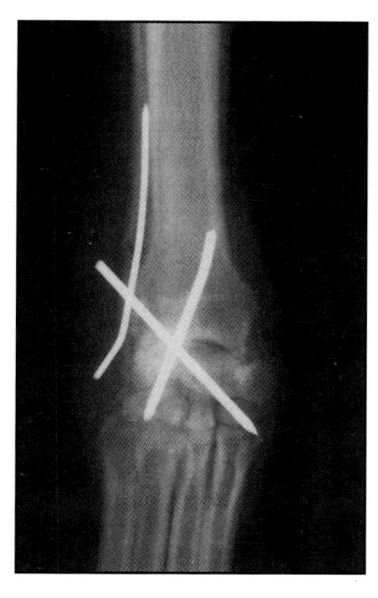

Chapter 19 The carpus

19.12 Carpal luxation repaired with temporary cross pins and an intramedullary pin in the ulna. The dog became sound and could work again.

though not too aggressive, debridement and copious wound lavage are indicated. The open or partially closed wound is then managed appropriately (see *BSAVA Manual of Canine and Feline Wound Management and Reconstruction*) to encourage a healthy granulating bed initially which is subsequently epithielialized. Re-establishment of the medial support using surgical implants is not usually necessary in cases treated with temporary (4–6 weeks) external transarticular fixation. Prognosis varies according to the extent of articular damage and resultant joint instability. Early or delayed pancarpal arthrodesis (see Operative Technique 19.1) can usefully salvage those cases where tissue loss is such that poor function is anticipated or where chronic lameness and pain persist.

Shear injuries

Shear injuries occur when the tissues are abraded by traction over a rough surface, resulting in a considerable loss of the soft tissues and bone. The medial aspect of the carpus is usually affected. The extent of the injury is determined by clinical and radiographic examination and by careful surgical debridement with the removal of all foreign material, non-viable soft tissues and bone.

Stability is achieved using a transarticular external fixator allowing access to the wound for appropriate dressing management (Figure 19.13). Meticulous,

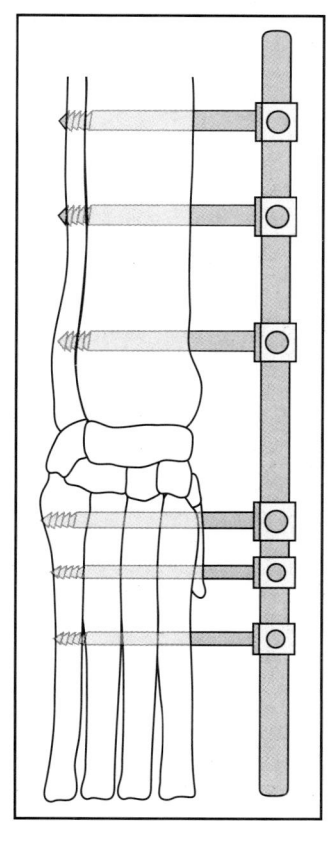

Fractures

Fractures involving the carpus are covered in detail within the *BSAVA Manual of Small Animal Fracture Repair and Management*. Carpal fractures are usually associated with either high-impact trauma, in which case lameness is severe, or high-performance injury. They can be associated with instability either due to loss of bony buttress support to surrounding carpal bones or through avulsion of ligamentous support structures. In the racing Greyhound, fractures are often more subtle with minimal lameness and are a result of repetitive stressing of bone that is undergoing reparative remodelling in response to performance loads. Small articular avulsion fractures, in the absence of instability can be a cause of chronic low-grade lameness, in which case the fragments are removed (Figure 19.14).

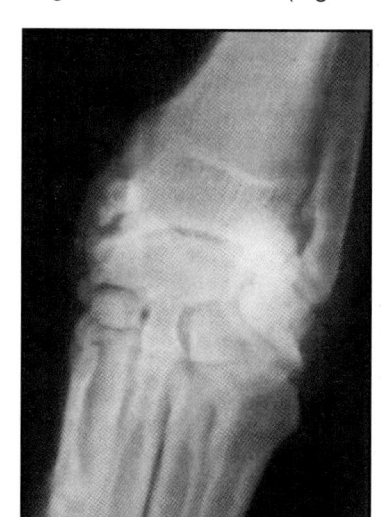

19.13 Carpal shear injury supported by an external skeletal fixator placed medially.

19.14 A large fragment of bone is seen on the medial aspect of the antebrachiocarpal joint in a cross-breed dog. This caused a chronic mild lameness which resolved after fragment removal. The fragment was thought to have avulsed from the palmar process of the radial carpal bone at the insertion of the short radial collateral ligament.

References and further reading

Boemo CM (1993) Chip fractures of the dorsal carpus in the racing greyhound: 38 cases. *Australian Veterinary Practitioner* **23**, 39–147

Grundmann S and Montavon PM (2001) Stenosing tenosynovitis of the abductor pollicis longus muscle in dogs. *Veterinary Comparative Orthopaedics and Traumatology* **14**, 95–100

Guilliard MJ (1997) Dorsal radiocarpal ligament sprain causing intermittent lameness in high activity dogs. *Journal of Small Animal Practice* **38**, 463–466

Chapter 19   The carpus

Guilliard MJ (1998) Enthesiopathy of the short radial collateral ligaments in racing greyhounds. *Journal of Small Animal Practice* **39**, 227–230

Guilliard MJ (2001a) Subluxation/luxation of the second carpal bone in two racing greyhounds and a Staffordshire bull terrier. *Journal of Small Animal Practice* **42**, 356–359

Guilliard MJ (2001b) Accessory carpal bone displacement in two dogs. *Journal of Small Animal Practice* **42**, 603–606

Guilliard MJ and Mayo AK (2000a) Sprain of the short radial collateral ligament in a racing greyhound. *Journal of Small Animal Practice* **41**, 169–171

Guilliard MJ and Mayo AK (2000b) Tears of the superficial palmar fascia in five racing greyhounds and a labrador retriever. *Journal of Small Animal Practice* **41**, 218–220

Johnson KA (1987) Accessory carpal bone fractures in the racing greyhound. *Veterinary Surgery* **16**, 60–64

Johnson KA, Piermattei DL, Davis PE and Bellenger CR (1988) Characteristics of accessory carpal bone fractures in 50 racing greyhounds. *Veterinary and Comparative Orthopaedics and Traumatology* **2**, 104–107

Johnson KA (1998) Carpal injuries. In: *Canine Sports Medicine and Surgery*, ed. MS Bloomberg, JF Dee and RA Taylor, pp.100–119. WB Saunders, Philadelphia

Li A, Bennett D, Gibbs C *et al.* (2000) Radial carpal bone fractures in 15 dogs. *Journal of Small Animal Practice* **41**, 74–79

Miller A, Carmichael S, Anderson TJ and Brown I (1990) Luxation of the radial carpal bone in four dogs. *Journal of Small Animal Practice* **31**, 148–154

Nordberg CC and Johnson KA (1998) Magnetic resonance imaging of normal canine carpal ligaments. *Veterinary Radiology and Ultrasound* **39**, 128–136

Vaughan LC (1992) Flexural deformity of the carpus in puppies. *Journal of Small Animal Practice* **33**, 381–384

Chapter 19 The carpus

OPERATIVE TECHNIQUE 19.1
Pancarpal arthrodesis

Positioning
Lateral recumbency, affected limb uppermost, clipped and prepared beyond the shoulder. Placement of a foam wedge under the shoulder on the opposite limb to elevate the ipsilateral shoulder is of assistance. Alternatively, dorsal recumbency with operative limb pulled caudally.

Assistant
Essential.

Tray extras
Gelpi self-retaining retractors; powered surgical tools for burring (cartilage debridement) and drilling; trephine or pin for access to cancellous bone harvest site; curette or scoop; plating set.

Surgical technique
A dorsal midline approach is made, from the distal third of the radius to the distal third of the metacarpal region (Figure 19.15a). Antebrachiocarpal and middle carpal and carpometacarpal joints are opened and any excess capsular soft tissue removed. The articular surfaces are debrided of all cartilage. The tendons of the extensor carpi radialis on the proximal parts of metacarpals II and III are cut at their insertion. Cancellous bone is harvested from the ipsilateral proximal humerus and packed into the joint spaces at all levels (Figure 19.15d). A minimum seven-hole pancarpal arthrodesis (PCA) compression plate (or DCP) is centred on the radial carpal bone and the mid body of metacarpal III and applied in compression over the carpus to fix the joint in approximately 10 degrees of extension (Figure 19.15e).

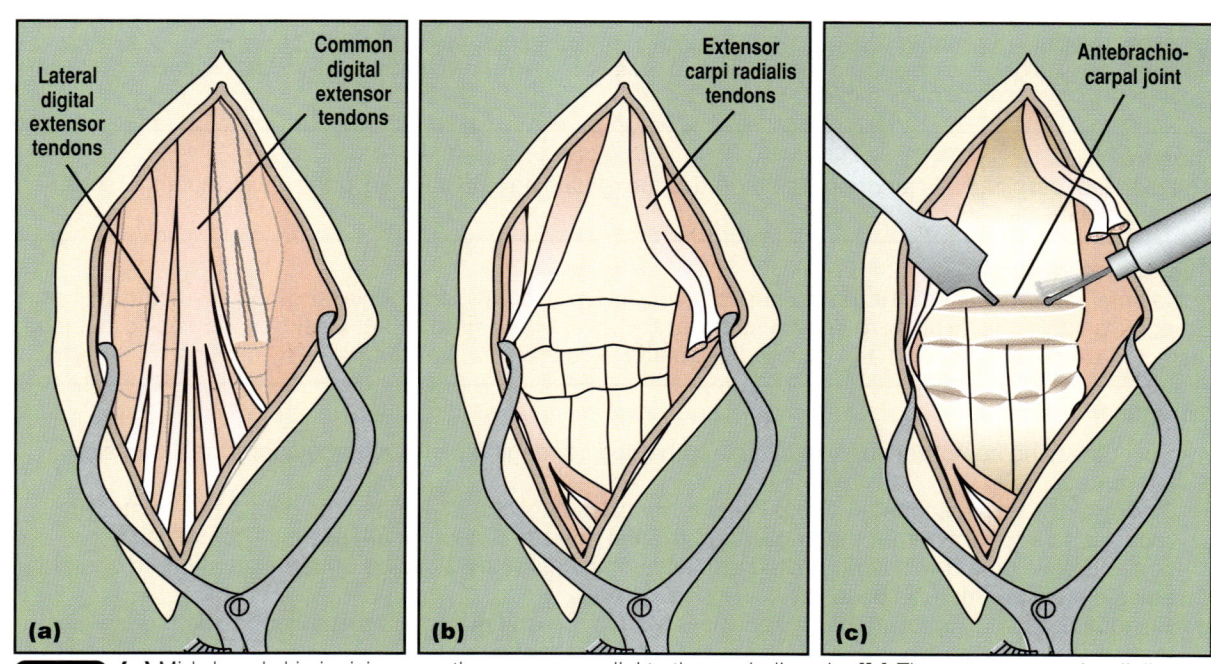

19.15 (a) Mid-dorsal skin incision over the carpus parallel to the cephalic vein. (b) The extensor carpi radialis tendons are sectioned and the common digital extensor tendon is retracted. (c) Following fibrous capsular excision, the joints are meticulously debrided of articular cartilage. (continues) ▶

Chapter 19 The carpus

OPERATIVE TECHNIQUE 19.1 continued
Pancarpal arthrodesis

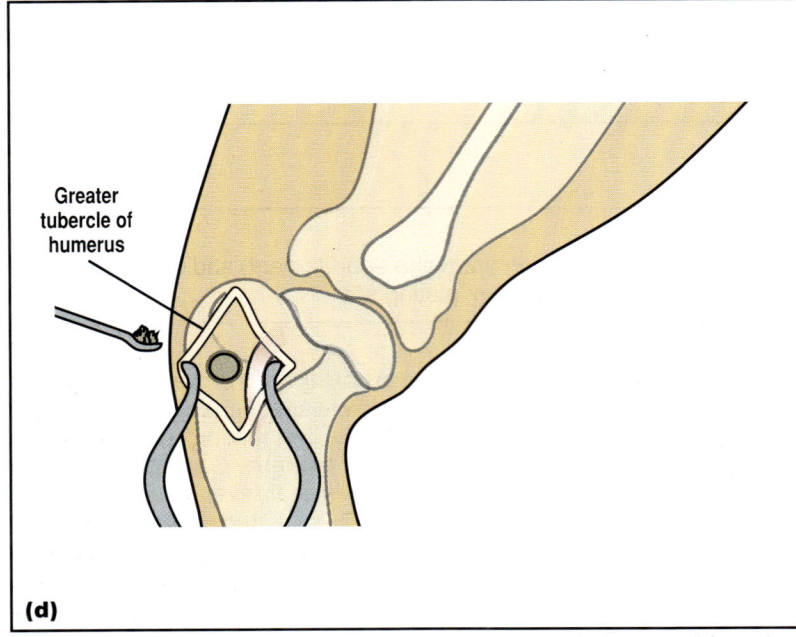

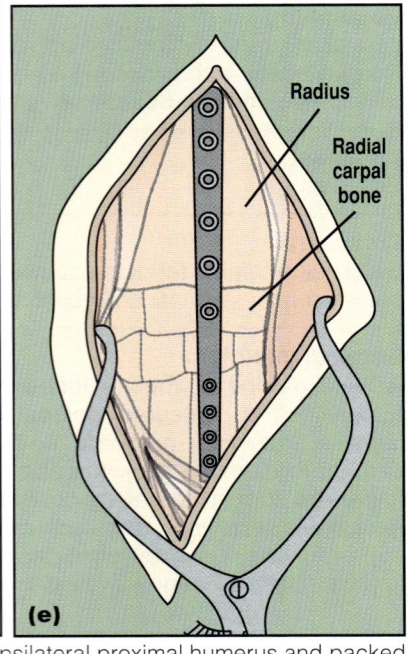

19.15 (continued) **(d)** Autogenous cancellous bone is harvested from the ipsilateral proximal humerus and packed into the debrided joint spaces. **(e)** A hybrid plate is applied in compression, centred on metacarpal III, the radial carpal bone and the distal radius.

Closure
The extensor carpi radialis tendons are sutured to the remaining joint capsule, and subcutaneous tissues and skin are closed routinely.

Postoperative care
A short moulded palmar splint is maintained for 4 weeks. Exercise is short, regular and lead-restricted until early signs of radiographic fusion are seen, usually at 8–12 weeks. A further 6–8 weeks of increasing but lead-restricted exercise is advised and radiographic union is complete at between 4 and 6 months.

Complications
- Splint/dressing complications – avoidable with good bandaging technique and appropriate dressing aftercare.
- Fracture or pain associated with the implant site on metacarpal III – use of the hybrid PCA plate with reduced screw diameter for the metacarpal fixation holes and appropriate exercise control in postoperative period will usually avoid problems. Implant removal can be undertaken after radiographic union if pain or lameness persists.
- Residual instability or failure of arthrodesis is usually a result of poor cartilage debridement or surgical immobilization or inadequate postoperative exercise management.

Chapter 19 The carpus

OPERATIVE TECHNIQUE 19.2
Partial carpal arthrodesis

Positioning
Lateral recumbency, affected limb uppermost, clipped and prepared beyond the shoulder. Placement of a foam wedge under the shoulder on the opposite limb to elevate the ipsilateral shoulder is of assistance. Alternatively, dorsal recumbency with operative limb pulled caudally.

Assistant
Essential.

Tray extras
Gelpi self-retaining retractors; powered surgical tools for burring (cartilage debridement) and drilling; trephine or pin for access to cancellous bone harvest site; curette or scoop; plating set.

Surgical technique
A dorsal midline approach is made, as for Operative Technique 19.1, but the incision starts immediately proximal to the antebrachiocarpal joint. Care is taken to preserve the extensor carpi radialis tendon insertions, and the tendon inserting on the base of metacarpal III may require suturing to II if a T plate is used. Middle carpal and carpometacarpal joints are opened and debrided of cartilage. Cancellous autograft is packed into joint spaces. A T plate is applied, centred on metacarpal III, ensuring that there is no interference with the antebrachiocarpal joint. Alternatively, in small dogs and cats two cross pins may be inserted diagonally from the bases of metacarpal bones II and V into the radial and ulnar carpal bones on the opposite side from the pin insertion site. Axial arthrodesis wires may also be used, inserted into linear slots in the distal metacarpals and passed proximally to transfix the carpometacarpal joint and the middle carpal joint without penetrating the antebrachiocarpal joint.

Closure
Routine subcutis and skin closure.

Postoperative care
A short moulded palmar splint is maintained for 4 weeks. Exercise is short, regular and lead-restricted until early signs of radiographic fusion are seen, usually at 8–12 weeks. A further 6–8 weeks of increasing but lead-restricted exercise is advised and radiographic union is complete at between 4 and 6 months.

Complications
- Interference from implants on the antebrachiocarpal joint.
- Failure to identify early or mild instability in the antebrachiocarpal joint may lead to subsequent degenerative change and hyperextension, necessitating pancarpal arthrodesis.

20

The distal limb

Richard Eaton-Wells

Introduction

The anatomy of the metacarpophalangeal, metatarsophalangeal, proximal interphalangeal and distal interphalangeal joints in the dog and cat are similar in both the thoracic and pelvic limbs. This chapter will use terminology for the thoracic limb, unless otherwise stated.

Surgical anatomy

Detailed anatomy of the canine and feline digits can be found in standard veterinary anatomy texts. The weightbearing digits are numbered II to V, from an axial to an abaxial direction. Each digit has the following joints:

- metacarpophalangeal joint (MCPJ)
- proximal interphalangeal joint (PIPJ)
- distal interphalangeal joint (DIPJ).

Metacarpophalangeal joint

The two central digits, metacarpals III and IV, are longer than II and V, their sagittal ridges are better defined, and the two articular surfaces for the palmar sesamoids are more equal in size and shape. The medial and lateral metacarpals, digits II and V, diverge distally and palmarly, their articular condyles are less well defined, and their sagittal ridges do not equally divide the articular area. The distal metacarpals form a dorsally convex arcade.

> **The distal divergence of the medial and lateral metacarpals results in the deep flexor tendons of digits III and IV being placed centrally behind sesamoids III to VI, respectively, while the flexor tendon in digits II and V is eccentrically placed, resulting in more pressure being applied to sesamoids II and VII (Figure 20.1).**

A pair of sesamoid bones is located on the palmar surface of each MCPJ in each of the weightbearing digits; the sesamoid bones are numbered I to VIII axially to abaxially. Each pair of sesamoids is embedded within the tendon of insertion of the interosseous muscle on the respective digit. They articulate primarily with the palmar aspect of the metacarpal head and, secondarily, with the first phalanx. Each pair of sesamoids is joined by a thick fibrous band, the intersesamoidean ligament, which forms a groove in which the superficial and deep digital flexor tendons run.

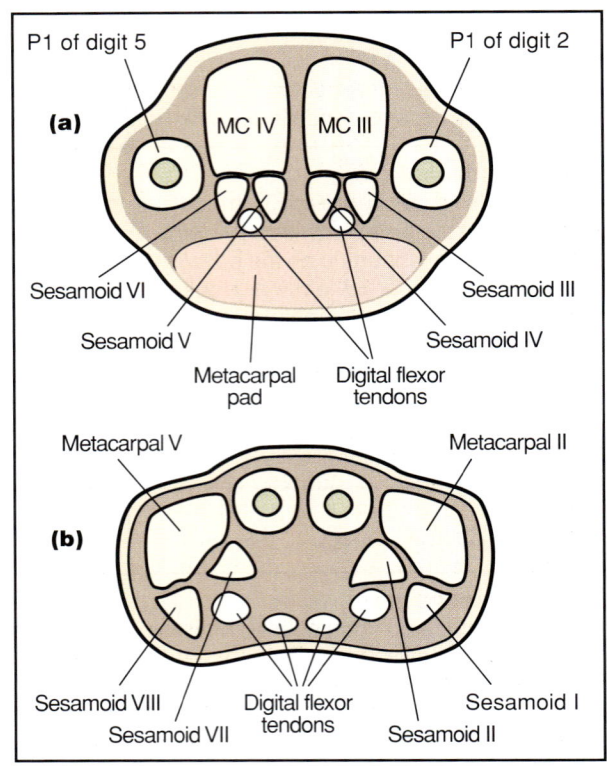

20.1 Metacarpal anatomy. **(a)** Cross-section through the metacarpus at the level of the axial sesamoid bones. **(b)** Cross-section through the metacarpus at the level of the abaxial sesamoid bones. (Reproduced from the *BSAVA Manual of Small Animal Fracture Repair and Management*.)

The shape of the sesamoid bones varies: I and VIII are shorter and have a wider base than III, IV, V and VI. II and VII are also shorter and almost pear-shaped. All sesamoids are supported on the palmar aspect of the metacarpal head by the sagittal ridge and multiple ligaments. There is also an extension of the interosseous muscle tendon, which runs dorsally and attaches to the common digital extensor tendon in the distal third of the first phalanx.

The four weightbearing MCPJs are compound saddle joints supported by a pair of medial and lateral collateral ligaments that arise from the distal end of the metacarpal bone and fan out to attach to the lateral or medial aspect of the first phalanx. The intersesamoidean ligament consists of short transverse fibres which join the two sesamoids together. The lateral and medial collateral sesamoidean ligaments form two parts, with the proximal ligament passing dorsally to attach just caudal to the MCP collateral ligament. The more distal component crosses the joint and attaches to the tubercle on the caudomedial or caudolateral aspect of the first phalanx. A pair of cruciate ligaments extends from the base of each sesamoid, crosses the MCP joint diagonally and attaches to the respective tubercles on the first phalanx. Covering the cruciate ligaments, the distal sesamoidean ligament is made up of a broad flat band, which attaches the distal end of the sesamoids to the first phalanx.

A small dorsal sesamoid is incorporated within the common digital flexor tendon as it crosses the dorsal aspect of the joint. It is held in place by: the common digital extensor tendon dorsally; delicate fibres attached to extensions from the interosseous muscles; and the joint capsule medially and laterally. The joint capsule encases these structures and the joint is supported by the medial and lateral collateral ligaments. These arise from the distal end of the metacarpus and pass distally to attach to the palmar aspect of the proximal end of the first phalanx.

The first digit or 'dew claw' is a rudimentary structure with a shortened metacarpal bone and phalanges. The distal end, or head, is enlarged laterally, with a single sesamoid located on the ventral aspect of the MCPJ.

Interphalangeal joints

Each PIPJ consists of the convex head of the first phalanx articulating with the proximal fossa of the second phalanx. These two surfaces are enclosed in a joint capsule, which has considerable inherent strength. This joint capsule is thickened dorsally and is closely adherent to the extensor tendon. There is a small dorsal sesamoid embedded within this dorsal thickening. The joint capsule is also thickened ventrally and involves the insertion of the superficial digital flexor. There is also a medial and a lateral collateral ligament; these attach to the dorsal distal surface of the proximal phalanx and fan out as they extend distopalmarly to attach to the palmar aspect of the proximal end of the distal phalanx. These collateral ligaments have a vertical orientation in the normal weightbearing position and are relatively lax until the toe is extended. The joint capsule provides significant stability when the joint is flexed.

The DIPJ comprises the distal end of P2, the proximal end of P3, the joint capsule, the insertion of the deep digital flexor tendon and the collateral ligaments. These ligaments are thin fan-shaped structures on the medial and lateral aspect of the joint.

Clinical examination

The use and breed of the animal being examined is an important piece of information. Digital injuries are more common in racing and working dogs. However, failure to examine fully the extremities of all lame dogs will result in injuries being missed. It is also important to ascertain if the animal is currently, or has recently been, taking any anti-inflammatory agent or nutraceutical that could mask a mild lameness.

Due to the minimal soft tissue coverage of the area, careful observation and palpation will often lead to a correct diagnosis. Swellings of individual digits, differences between the left and right side and uneven digital pad wear should alert the clinician to the possibility of disease. Obvious congenital disorders should also be noted, although they may not be of clinical significance. The distal limb is easily palpated and most injuries should be diagnosed on physical examination and confirmed radiographically (see later).

If the area is painful or the animal resents palpation, local anaesthesia is an easy and useful technique as an aid to diagnosis. There are paired nerves that run on the dorsal and palmar (plantar) aspects on the medial and lateral side of each digit. Sufficient local anaesthetic, approximately 0.5 ml per side, is infused to deaden the area, thus allowing a more complete examination. The use of local anaesthesia to 'block' a toe can result in an altered gait in some dogs. Cats may be observed loose in the examination room, but it is often difficult to persuade them to walk normally.

The start of the lameness examination should involve the careful observation of the animal's extremities at rest. This can provide clues to causes of lameness, such as the 'bunched' toes associated with injuries to the gastrocnemius muscle or its tendon (Figure 20.2). The animal should then be examined at a slow and a fast walk. This part of the examination is best performed outside, where the dog has a normal and familiar surface to walk on, allowing the presence and extent of any lameness to be assessed. Dog trainers and breeders are very adept at disguising lameness with upward pressure on the lead, so a loose lead must be emphasized. Examinations of gait inside or on slippery surfaces will often result in the dog changing gait to suit the surface, thus making small changes in gait more difficult to detect. The length of both the cranial and caudal phases of the stride should be assessed, as should any evidence that the animal is 'scuffing' its toenails. This may be by noted by hearing the nails catch on the ground. Careful questioning of the owner with regard to the extent of the lameness, or what makes it better or worse, is also an essential part of the history-taking. The presence of a lameness that is more pronounced on uneven surfaces, such as pebbles, may indicate a phalangeal or pad problem.

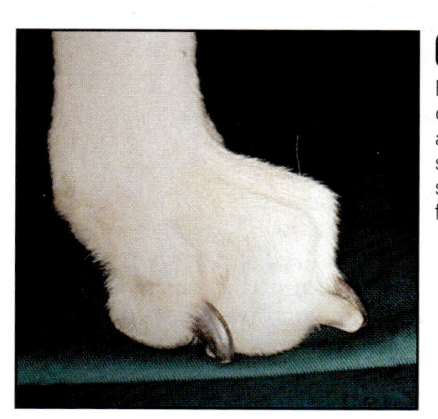

20.2 Flexion of the digits due to apparent shortening of the superficial digital flexor tendon.

Chapter 20 The distal limb

It is important to be methodical when examining the extremities. The examination can be performed from proximal to distal or *vice versa*. The author's preference is to start at the toenails and pads and work proximally. This chapter will therefore be presented in that order. It is also a good idea to examine the non-lame leg first. This allows the clinician to get a feel for what is normal in the particular animal and allows the patient time to become accustomed to digital examination. Conditions affecting the feet are summarized in Figure 20.3.

Pads and webbing
Cuts and lacerations
Excessive or uneven wear
Puncture wounds
Foreign bodies, with or without tenosynovitis
Corns
Blisters
Viral papillomas
Sand ulcers
Split webbing, full or partial
Ingrown toe nails
Interdigital cysts
Toenails
Torn toenails/'quick'
Infections/paronychia
Ungual crest fractures
Third phalanx
Intra-articular fractures
Deep digital flexor tendon avulsions
Infections
Tumours
Osteomyelitis
Distal interphalangeal joint
Collateral ligament injuries/open wounds
Intra-articular fractures
Septic arthritis
First and second phalanges
Fractures: simple, comminuted, open, Salter–Harris
Collateral ligament avulsions
Osteomyelitis: bacterial, fungal
Tumours: soft tissue, osteogenic
Proximal interphalangeal joint
Collateral ligament injuries: unilateral, bilateral, with or without gross luxation
Luxation of the dorsal sesamoid
Immune-mediated arthropathy
Osteoarthritis
Septic arthritis

20.3 Conditions affecting the feet.

Pads and webbing

Pad lacerations should be noted, as should uneven wear, comparing both individual digits and different feet. Excessive wear may be initially recognized by the loss of the normal roughened pad surface. In more extreme cases, there may be both a smoothed pad and loss of pigment in its weightbearing surface. The animal will often have a history of lameness when walked on small stones or rough ground, but is sound when walked on smooth or soft surfaces, such as concrete or grass. Pads that are excessively worn are prone to puncture wounds from sharp objects or pieces of glass. Most glass is radiolucent and is therefore difficult to detect radiographically. Glass is also rarely still present when the dog is presented for examination, but the resultant deficit allows other objects such as dirt and grains of sand to lodge within the pad (Figure 20.4a). If puncture wounds involve the deep digital flexor tendon, a chronic tenosynovitis may develop. This results in a mild lameness and may be detected by palpation of the flexor tendon on the palmar (plantar) aspect of the phalanges with the digits in extension. Acute tenosynovitis is more painful on palpation and the animal is often three-legged lame. Puncture wounds that are not treated adequately may result in a corn developing (Figure 20.4b).

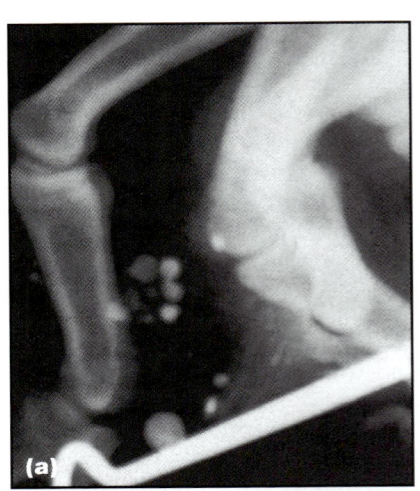

20.4 (a) Sand within the pad and palmar soft tissues after a penetrating pad injury. (b) Corn developed following inadequate treatment of a penetrating pad injury.

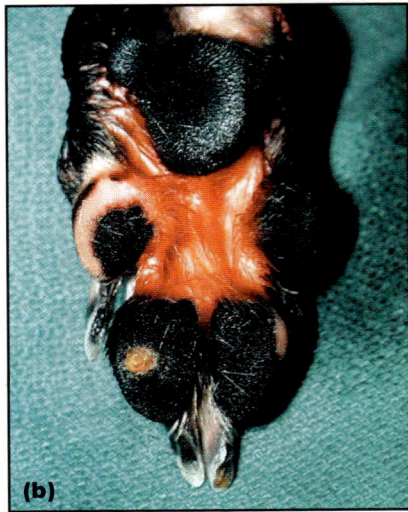

The webbing between the individual toes should be assessed. Palpation of the leading edge of the webbing will reveal the normal thickened palmar (plantar) component. It is important to re-appose this accurately when webbing lacerations are repaired. Full-thickness splits in the dorsal and ventral components of the webbing are obvious, not least because of the amount of haemorrhage that accompanies them. Isolated

Chapter 20 The distal limb

lacerations to either the dorsal or ventral surface of the webbing are more easily missed. The presence of viral warts or papillomas (Figure 20.5) should be noted. These are very painful and a common cause of lameness in young Greyhounds. The presence of small areas of cutaneous ulceration or 'sand ulcers' should also be noted. Dogs with long hair between their toes often suffer from accumulations of mud, dirt, snow and ice, which act as a foreign body, causing pain and irritation to the palmar (plantar) aspect of the foot. The presence of other foreign bodies, such as burrs, should be noted. The presence of swellings, with or without a discharging sinus, in the interdigital area may be indicative of interdigital cysts or draining tracts from foreign bodies such as grass seeds.

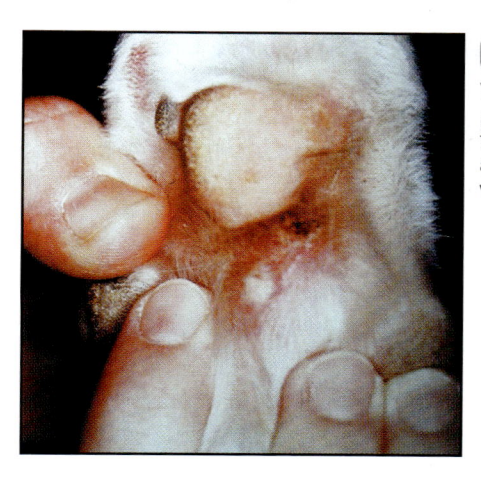

20.5 Viral papilloma in the palmar aspect of the webbing.

The metacarpal/tarsal pad should also be checked for shape and consistency. Dogs with a chronic foot problem often have a slightly smaller and harder pad when compared to the contralateral limb. Excessive wear, or problems such as blisters from running on hot dry ground, should also be noted. The dew claw, if present, should be checked, as excessive length of the toenail will result in injury to the pad.

Digits
Congenital disorders, such as the absence of individual toes or the presence of more than the normal complement, should be noted (see Chapter 6).

Toenails
The toenails should be examined individually, particular care being taken to note the length and colour of the nail and the level of the vascular core. The examination should include the length and continuity of the hairs which protect the 'quick'. Damage or loss of these hairs may be indicative of early neurological dysfunction. Loss of these hairs in the racing Greyhound predisposes the toe to abrasive injuries by small particles such as sand and resultant paronychia. The toenail bed should also be checked for tumours and ulcerative conditions.

Other toenail injuries include trauma, such as a torn nail cuticle and fractures. Splitting of the nail and the resulting lifting of the dorsal cuticle can be subtle and easily missed. The position of the toenail should be noted, as injuries to the deep digital flexor will result in a 'knocked-up' toe (Figure 20.6).

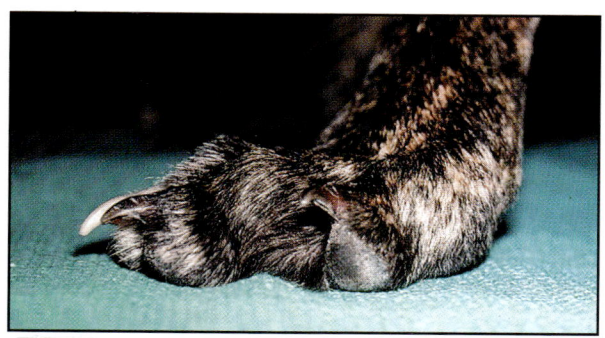

20.6 Rupture of the deep digital flexor tendon causing a 'knocked-up' toe.

Scuffing of the dorsal aspect of the toenails may be an indication of neurological disease. Excessively short toenails will expose the sensitive core, resulting in lameness on uneven or rough ground. This may result from contracted flexor tendons, insufficient extensor activity, or nails that have been cut too short. Rubbing injuries can occur over adjacent digits. These will vary from some loss of hair to a full-thickness skin abrasion.

The nail length should be noted. Excessively long nails are prone to splits in the cuticle, fractures around the ungual crest and interphalangeal collateral ligament injuries. The length of the nail on the dew claw should also be noted. This is often missed when nails are trimmed, resulting in an ingrowing nail. The integrity of the nail itself should be assessed, and any splitting or swelling should be observed.

The vascularity should also be assessed: blueness or discoloration of a clear nail may be an indication of impaired vascularity or of infection.

These conditions are less obvious in dark nails, so the clinician must rely on palpation. In cases where compromise to the blood supply is suspected, trimming the nail back to the vascular core is an easy method of assessing vascularity. Pain on pressure to the nail may indicate a fracture or infection. The nail beds should be assessed for signs of infection, erosions or tumours. Fracture of the distal phalanx can involve the nail, the ungual crest or the base. The latter may have an intra-articular component and can be detected on palpation by the presence of pain and swelling. However, in cases where there is no crepitus, they can be difficult to differentiate from distal interphalangeal injuries without radiography.

In dogs that have undergone phalangeal amputation, a number of complications are recognized. If the dog has only had a toenail removed, all the germinal layer of the ungual crest must be removed or there will be partial regrowth of the nail. This will initially present as a mild lameness, while palpation will reveal a sore point over the amputation site. Later in the course of the disease, the nail regrowth will break out through the skin, resulting in a painful draining wound.

Third phalanx
Problems involving the third phalanx include: injuries to the toenail, ungual crest, articular surface and insertion of the deep digital flexor; infections; tumours; and trauma, such as degloving injuries.

Chapter 20 The distal limb

Removal of the third phalanx by disarticulation of the joint must be accompanied by complete removal of the articular cartilage on the distal end of the second phalanx. Failure to do this may result in chondromalacia. This is detected on palpation by 'mushrooming' of the distal articular surface and pain on palpation.

Distal interphalangeal joint
The medial and lateral collateral ligaments of the DIPJ should be tested with the joint extended and the ligaments under tension; testing in flexion will result in false positive results. DIPJ luxations in the racing Greyhound are often accompanied by rupture of the overlying skin. These present as a profusely bleeding injury. They may also present with the distal end of the second phalanx protruding through the skin. They should be reduced immediately to limit vascular compromise to the area and poor healing.

First and second phalanges
Both the first and second phalanges can be palpated along their entire length. Pain, crepitus, periosteal thickening or soft tissue changes should be noted. Fractures close to the proximal or distal joint may be difficult to differentiate from collateral ligament injuries. Fractures of the second phalanx in the racing Greyhound may be open. It is important to recognize this, and assess the extent of the periosteal damage present, as the prognosis for successful fracture repair and return to racing is guarded when extensive periosteal damage has occurred. Soft tissue changes should also be noted.

Proximal interphalangeal joint
Physical examination should reveal any pain and/or swelling. A joint effusion may also be noted. As with the DIPJ, the collateral ligaments must be tested with the toe in extension, due to the degree of joint laxity in flexion. The joint should be fully extended and pressure applied to the tendon of insertion of the superficial digital flexor to check for partial avulsions or tenosynovitis. Complete rupture or avulsion of the superficial digital flexor will result in a 'dropped' toe (Figure 20.7). The stability of the dorsal sesamoid should also be checked. Gross luxation of the joint can also occur with the proximal end of the second phalanx lying behind the distal end of the first.

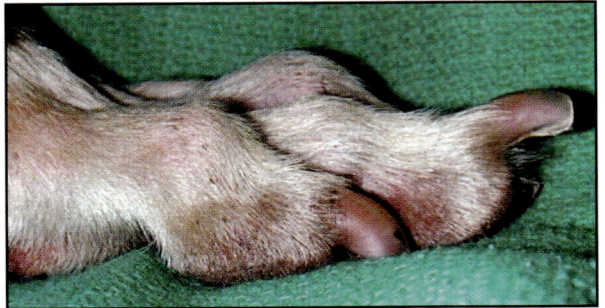

20.7 Rupture of the superficial digital flexor tendon causing a 'dropped' toe.

> **PRACTICAL TIPS**
> - Any dog that has suffered a collateral ligament injury and is clinically lame should be assessed radiographically, because of the high incidence of intra-articular and avulsion fractures associated with these injuries.
> - Dogs, particularly the racing Greyhound, that have had a cast fitted incorporating the foot often have pain on extension of the PIPJ after exercise for some 6–8 weeks after the cast is removed. For this reason, casts applied to Greyhounds should end in the distal third of the metatarsal area.

Swelling around the PIPJ, often associated with the distal end of the first and the proximal end of the second phalanx, on either a single or multiple joints, is suggestive of an immune-mediated polyarthropathy.

Metacarpophalangeal joint
All the MCPJs should be assessed visually for swelling on the dorsal aspect; if present, it should be noted whether this involves either a single or multiple digits. The digits should be flexed and extended, The MCPJ should flex to 90 degrees, though it is normal for some dogs to have less flexion than this in a single or multiple digits. Therefore, it is the presence of pain in a joint with loss of flexion that is significant. Simple loss of flexion of the MCPJ or MTPJ is not indicative of disease. Arthrocentesis and cytology of these joints may be helpful if an immune-mediated disease is suspected.

The joint should be pain-free and stable in flexion, extension, rotation and when stressed mediolaterally. Assessment of the collateral ligaments in digits III and IV is more difficult because of the adjacent digit. The palmar aspect of the distal metacarpal bone and its associated sesamoids should be palpated for pain, swelling and crepitus. The dorsal sesamoid should also be checked for soft tissue swelling, joint effusion, instability or pain.

First digit
It should be remembered that fractures and luxations can occur in the first digit (dew claw), so it is essential that it should be included when examining the extremities.

Radiographic examination
High-quality radiographs are essential for viewing the extremities. The use of the correct exposure, high-detail screens or single emulsion mammography film, and good dark room technique are necessary to achieve this. Multiple views may also be required, due to the overlapping nature of the bones and the subtle injuries that occur. The presence of Mach lines on metacarpal/tarsal radiographs is a normal phenomenon and should not be mistaken for fractures.

> **PRACTICAL TIP**
> A bright light and magnifier are essential for proper interpretation of radiographs of the digits. When reviewing these radiographs, variation in the contrast settings is recommended.

Chapter 20 The distal limb

Preoperative and surgical considerations

General principles of articular surgery are covered in Chapter 12. The foot, however, is particularly difficult to prepare for aseptic surgery. The pads and nails should be scrubbed with a soft brush. The interdigital area should also receive extra attention. If a long procedure is expected, soaking the foot in alcoholic chlorhexidine is recommended. Where possible, the nails should be excluded from the surgery site, either by draping or with adhesive drapes. Because of the minimal soft tissue, surgical incisions are usually directly over the area of interest. Careful soft tissue dissection is necessary to prevent damage to the nerves, vessels and tendons. The use of a tourniquet will render the surgical field bloodless but in unskilled hands may lead to more soft tissue damage.

Metacarpophalangeal luxations

MCP luxations may be single or multiple. Due to the arrangement of the various sesamoidean ligaments, however, an injury to a single ligament is unlikely; therefore these injuries are, by definition, complex. Radiographic examination is necessary to rule out intra-articular avulsion fractures associated with the collateral ligaments or fractures of the sesamoids (Figure 20.8). The prognosis for return to function is good although MCP luxations carry a guarded prognosis for return to successful competitive racing.

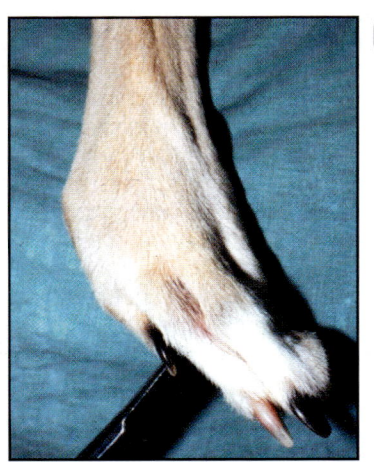

20.8 Multiple metacarpophalangeal luxations with associated sesamoid displacement, resulting in a valgus deformity of the foot.

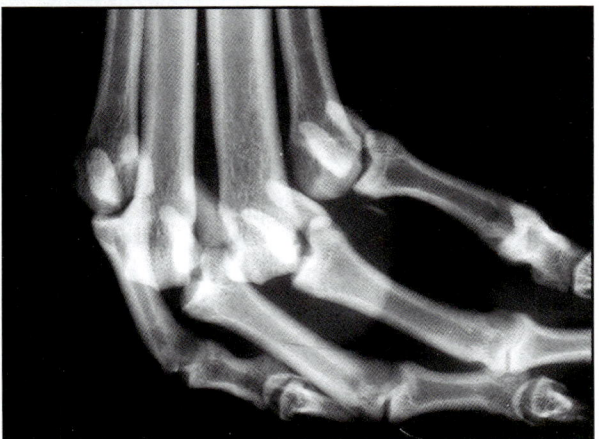

Acute MCPJ luxation

Temporary immobilization with a padded bandage may be necessary in some cases to reduce the swelling and pain. The use of external coaptation as a primary method of repair will result in increased morbidity and loss of joint function. Moreover, it does not provide rotational stability. This loss of rotational stability is the main reason for poor performance if a dog is returned to racing.

Primary repair or reattachment of the collateral ligaments may be possible (see Operative Technique 20.1. Failure of the primary surgical repair is common due to lack of sufficient rotational support, while maintaining good flexion and extension during the postoperative period. Various dressing modalities have been adopted to address this rotational instability problem, but none is particularly successful. Complications include infection, suture failure and significant loss of range of motion.

> **WARNING**
> The likelihood of multiple sesamoid ligament failures with injury to this joint is high and the recognition of the extent of the injury is difficult. This can make adequate treatment difficult.

Chronic MCPJ disease

Chronic instability or osteoarthritis may be treated by sesamoidectomy, excision arthroplasty of the head of the proximal phalanx, arthrodesis of the MCPJ, or digital amputation at the distal metacarpal level.

Arthrodesis

Arthrodesis (see Operative Technique 20.2) of single or multiple MCPJs is an effective salvage procedure for chronic or debilitating osteoarthritis. The normal angle of arthrodesis will be between 100 and 120 degrees. Arthrodesis may cause a slight change in gait but should be well tolerated by a pet. Complications include implant failure and pressure sores from the cast. Chronic lameness after arthrodesis surgery is usually an indication of either infection or the development of a non–union.

Digital amputation

The osteotomy should be bevelled to reduce the incidence of postoperative complications. The prognosis for amputation at the distal metacarpal level varies with the end use of the dog. Single amputations are well tolerated in all breeds; amputations of up to three digits may be tolerated in smaller breeds. Amputation of either digits II or V may not result in loss of performance; however, amputation of either digit III or IV or more than one digit will result in some loss of performance in the racing Greyhound.

> **WARNING**
> In the racing Greyhound it is important not to amputate too high either metacarpal V in the left limb, or metacarpal II in the right limb. If this happens, the adjacent digit will have to undergo significant adaptive hypertrophy to withstand the stresses associated with running around turns. This will certainly result in a period of lameness after a run and occasionally results in a stress fracture.

Chapter 20 The distal limb

Sesamoid disease

The pathogenesis of the various forms of sesamoid disease is poorly understood.

Acute fractures

These usually occur in racing, working or very active pets during periods of excessive activity. They can affect any sesamoid, although II and VII are most commonly affected. The dog is acutely lame and there is swelling of the affected digit with pain and loss of flexion. Diagnostics and treatment are detailed in the *BSAVA Manual of Small Animal Fracture Management and Repair*.

Bipartite or tripartite sesamoids

Bipartite or tripartite sesamoids are a well recognized condition and have been reported in several breeds, particularly the racing Greyhound, Rottweiler and other giant breeds. Sesamoids II and VII are most commonly, but not exclusively, affected. The condition is usually clinically silent and the abnormalities are an incidental finding on radiography. In one survey, 27% of racing Greyhounds were affected (Eaton-Wells, unpublished data). In this series, there was no evidence to suggest a traumatic aetiology, although the method of rearing young Greyhounds, allowing free exercise in large paddocks, may have subjected the sesamoids to chronic trauma. There may be some swelling of the affected digit with loss of flexion, but no pain on palpation. No treatment is necessary.

Sesamoid disease of young dogs

In some breeds, the Rottweiler and Australian Cattle Dog in particular, there is a readily recognized syndrome of chronic pain associated with the MCPJs of all digits. The dogs are presented with either an acute, or acute superimposed on a chronic, thoracic limb lameness. There is a shortened caudal phase of the stride when the dog is gaited and the lameness is worse when walking on 'stony' surfaces. Clinically there are varying degrees of decreased range of motion and there is effusion in the affected joints. Subclinical cases can often be detected by holding the MCPJs flexed for a couple of minutes and then allowing the dog to walk, when there is an obvious lameness which decreases or disappears after a few steps.

The pathogenesis and likely aetiology of 'young dog sesamoid disease' is still unclear, though suggested factors include osteochondrosis, degeneration, trauma and vascular compromise. Multiple authors have reported varying incidences of subclinical sesamoid changes (Read *et al.*, 1992; Robins and Read, 1993; Mathews *et al.*, 2001). The clinical incidence of sesamoid disease is recognized to be more common in large breeds such as the Rottweiler, but smaller breeds such as the Australian Cattle Dog, Australian Kelpie and the Staffordshire Bull Terrier also have a high incidence of both clinical and subclinical disease (Robins and Read, 1993).

The occurrence of clinical signs of sesamoiditis in breeds that also have a high incidence of osteochondral disease has led to the hypothesis that osteochondrosis could be a contributing factor. However, this was not supported histopathologically. It has also been reported that diseased sesamoid bones show various stages of fracture repair, that there are extensive areas of bone necrosis associated with this healing process, and that the extent of the necrosis appears to be inversely correlated to the stage of fracture repair (Robins and Read, 1993). In dogs with a history of acute onset of disease there was evidence of cartilage regeneration and extensive areas of bone necrosis. This is supported by the radiographic appearance of osteoporotic sesamoids during the acute phase of the disease. In cases with a more chronic history, the histological picture was one of extensive fibrous callus formation with cartilage proliferation and osteoclastic activity in the adjacent bone. The authors concluded that vascular compromise was part of the aetiology of this disease, but they were unable to establish whether trauma to the vasculature and subsequent avascular necrosis caused the bone to weaken and fracture, or whether a primary fracture resulted in vascular compromise. Subsequent work demonstrated abundant but variable blood supply (Cake and Read, 1995b).

Radiographs are necessary to confirm the presence of sesamoid abnormalities. Care should be taken in chronic cases, and it may be advisable to assess both left and right feet for the presence of subclinical abnormalities. Evidence of sesamoid changes on physical examination, such as palmar swelling and loss of flexion of the MCPJ or MTPJ without pain or discomfort, are more likely to indicate the presence of single or multiple bi- or tripartite sesamoids. These can be readily identified radiographically by their smooth rounded edges, indicating a chronic process. Radiographs should always be taken of both feet to check for multiple digit involvement.

Young dogs with chronic sesamoid disease will usually have varying degrees of joint effusion. This effusion is particularly noticeable on the dorsal aspect of the joint. Cytology of these joints shows varying degrees of lymphocytic/plasmacytic cellularity and there is pain on flexion. Radiographs of these MCPJs may reveal some or all of the following changes: enlarged sesamoids; partial or gross lysis; multiple fragments contained within the enlarged sesamoid; and early signs of osteoarthritis.

Treatment of both young dogs and those with chronic sesamoid disease should initially be conservative, using non-steroidal anti-inflammatory drugs (NSAIDs). Other possible treatments include nutraceuticals and the many physiotherapy modalities available (e.g. ultrasound, laser or magnetic field therapy). Intra-articular or systemic use of corticosteroids has also produced excellent results in cases that have become refractory to NSAIDs.

Other

The author has noted another MCPJ dysfunction that has not been adequately researched. These dogs, both young and old, are significantly lame. There is pain on flexion of the MCPJ, with or without loss of flexion. The joint capsule is thickened dorsally and there is a small amount of joint effusion. Radiographs do not reveal any significant abnormalities. Cytology of the joint fluid reveals mainly mononuclear cells. Synovial biopsy reveals a lymphocytic, plasmacytic synovitis. These are probably part of an immune-mediated process (see Chapter 7). Treatment involves NSAIDs and local or systemic corticosteroids. In some dogs that were refractory to medical treatment, and in which a cosmetic result was important or the owner was reluctant to agree to amputation, the use of gold beads implanted on either side of the joint has provided excellent results.

Surgical treatment

Sesamoid disease that does not respond to conservative treatment may be treated by surgical excision of the affected bone (see Operative Technique 20.3), removal of both sesamoids, or arthrodesis. Complications of sesamoidectomy include adhesions, resulting in pain on extension of the digit.

Proximal interphalangeal luxations

Luxation or subluxations of the PIPJ may involve single or multiple joints, with varying degrees of ligament failure. The injuries may involve the dorsal sesamoid, the collateral ligaments, the joint capsule or the insertion of the superficial digital flexor, either singularly or in various combinations. Luxations of the dorsal sesamoid will merely result in disruption of the joint capsule, and the degree of pain and dysfunction is usually minimal. This minor injury will cause weakening of the joint's inherent stability and may lead to failure of a collateral ligament. Luxations of a single collateral ligament are usually associated with swelling around the affected joint, and the toe may be luxated manually without discomfort to the dog. Those joints that are painful should be radiographed to check for small fractures or avulsed ligaments. Collateral ligament injuries may be associated with small avulsion fractures; the prognosis for full return to function, if these fractures are not treated, is reduced if the problem is not addressed at the time of initial injury.

Avulsion of the superficial digital flexor tendon from the proximal palmar aspect of the phalanx will result in a 'dropped' toe (see Figure 20.7). In all but show dogs, this is of little consequence. However, in the show animal it may be necessary to re-attach the tendon with either a spiked washer or a wire suture.

Disruption or avulsion of one or both collateral ligaments, luxation of the dorsal sesamoid in the tendon of the common digital extensor tendon, and avulsion injuries associated with the insertion of the superficial digital flexor tendon should be detected on physical examination. All these injuries may be repaired surgically.

Treatment of PIPJ injuries

All digital injuries should be treated with ice packs/baths as soon as possible after the injury to reduce the amount of soft tissue swelling. Minor sprains of the collateral ligaments, the joint capsule and the flexor or extensor tendons should be treated conservatively. There are many treatment modalities, such as massage, ultrasound, laser and magnetic field therapy. The use of blistering agents by lay personnel is still quite common and should be discouraged.

Disruption of one side of the dorsal sesamoid support should be sutured, as this is often a precursor to full collateral ligament injury. If both the medial and lateral support to the dorsal sesamoid is injured or there is disruption of the tendon distally, the sesamoid should be removed.

Disruption of the medial or lateral collateral ligaments should be treated surgically (see Operative Technique 20.4). Complications of this procedure include an inability of the joint to extend fully, due to placing the sutures in the wrong place or overtightening them, and suture failure or pull out allowing the joint to reluxate.

Joints that have suffered injury to both collateral ligaments should also be repaired surgically. This may be achieved by repair or reconstruction of both the medial and lateral collaterals. If this repair is less than ideal, a transarticular Kirschner wire, with the toe approximately 70% extended, is used to provide temporary stability while the ligaments heal. The foot is supported for approximately 2–3 weeks, when the Kirschner wire is removed. This technique allows the digit to stabilize with only minimal loss of function and no pain when the dog is at full stride.

> **PRACTICAL TIP**
> In the racing Greyhound, PIP collateral ligament repair in digits II and V should be protected by either cutting the toenail short or amputation at the ungual crest. The loss of the toenail reduces the incidence of further injury during the healing and return to racing phase.

Where surgical stabilization has failed or the joint has been severely damaged, an interdigital arthrodesis may be performed (see Operative Technique 20.5).

Distal interphalangeal joint injuries

Traumatic luxation

Physical examination will reveal loss of stability in extension, with varying degrees of pain and swelling. A dog may also be presented with gross displacement of the joint; remarkably, this does not appear to be unduly painful and the joint is readily replaced. In fact, the toe may luxate totally on physical examination. Traumatic luxation of the DIPJ in the racing Greyhound may result in the distal end of the second phalanx being forced through the skin. On presentation, there is usually only a small laceration over the joint which bleeds profusely; occasionally, the bone will be protruding though the skin. These small lacerations should always be considered to be grade 1 open collateral ligament injuries until proved otherwise. Radiographs will reveal any fractures or ligamentous avulsions. Surgical exploration directly over the ruptured ligament will reveal whether the joint is salvageable.

The ligament and associated soft tissues may be reconstructed and the toenail amputated (see Operative Technique 20.6). Failure to remove all the ungual crest and associated germinal cells will result in regrowth of part of the nail, causing lameness and dysfunction. Removal of the extensor process may result in the remnants of the third phalanx being retracted palmarly by the flexor tendon, exposing the articular surface of the second digit to trauma. This often results in a chondromalacia/chondritis causing chronic pain in the racing dog.

If the joint is not salvageable, amputation of the joint including the distal end of the second phalanx will be necessary. In the racing Greyhound, repair of the ligament and toenail amputation will allow the dog to return to racing in approximately 4–6 weeks. Digital amputation, however, will require approximately 10–12 weeks before the dog is returned to racing. This loss of racing time should always be considered when treating Greyhound toe injuries. Gross disruption of the DIPJ should be treated by amputation. This is fine for pet dogs, but primary repair should always be attempted in racing dogs.

Failure of the deep digital flexor tendon ('knocked up' toe)

This appears to present as two separate entities: the acute sprain/rupture associated with athletic dogs; and the apparent weakening of the tendon seen in older dogs. Complete rupture, as seen in athletic dogs, results in the dog apparently experiencing marginal pain for a few days; the pain then disappears and the dog returns to normal. In those cases where the tendon has not completely ruptured, it may be necessary to exercise the dog while it is given an anti-inflammatory agent to ensure that the tendon does rupture. This often provides a more rapid resolution of the problem. Care should also be taken when examining dogs which spend a lot of time inside on slippery surfaces as they appear to develop 'flat feet' which are totally pain-free. Treatment involves conservative treatment with NSAIDs.

References and further reading

Cake MA and Read RA (1995a) Canine and human sesamoid disease. *Veterinary Comparative Orthopaedics and Traumatology* **8**, 70–75

Cake MA and Read RA (1995b) The blood supply to the canine palmar metacarpal sesamoid bones. *Veterinary Comparative Orthopaedics and Traumatology* **8**, 76–81

Eaton-Wells RD (1989) Prognosis for return to racing following surgical repair of musculoskeletal injury. In: *Greyhound Medicine and Surgery, Proceedings 122 of the Post Graduate Committee in Veterinary Science*, University of Sydney

Hudson LC and Hamilton WP (1993) *Atlas of Feline Anatomy for Veterinarians.* WB Saunders, Philadelphia

Mathews KG, PD Koblik, JG Whitehair *et al.* (2001) Fragmented palmar metacarpo-phalangeal sesamoids in dogs: a long-term evaluation. *Veterinary Comparative Orthopaedics and Traumatology* **14**, 7–14

Piermattei D and Johnson K (2004) *An Atlas of Surgical Approaches to the Bones and Joints of the Dog and Cat.* WB Saunders, Philadelphia

Read RA, AP Black, SJ Armstrong *et al.* (1992) Incidence and clinical significance of sesamoid disease in Rottweilers. *Veterinary Record* **130**, 533–535

Robins GM and Read RA (1993) Diseases of the sesamoid bones. In: *Disease Mechanisms in Small Animal Surgery, 2nd edn.*, ed. MJ Bojrab, pp. 1094–1101. Lea & Febiger, Philadelphia

Rochat MC and Mann FA (1998) Metatarsophalangeal arthrodesis in three dogs. *Journal of the American Veterinary Medical Association* **34**, 158–163

Van Ee RT and Blass CE (1989) Arthrodesis of the metatarsophalangeal joints in a dog. *Journal of the American Veterinary Medical Association* **194**, 82

Chapter 20 The distal limb

OPERATIVE TECHNIQUE 20.1
Surgical repair of MCPJ collateral ligaments

Patient preparation
Surgical clip from the carpus to the distal phalanges. Suitable surgical scrub. Clear adhesive surgical drapes allow for better visualization of the extremities.

Positioning
Lateral recumbency with the affected ligament uppermost.

Assistant
Optional. Useful for retraction of the various distal metacarpals to provide better access.

Tray extras
Mini self-retaining retractors; 1.5/2.0mm implant set; orthopaedic wire kit plus Kirschner wires if reattachment is to be attempted; power drill.

Surgical approach
The surgical approach is made directly over the damaged ligament where possible, for example over the medial or lateral collateral ligament of digits II and V, respectively. The approach to other collaterals is hampered to a greater or lesser degree by the adjacent digit and the approach has to be altered accordingly. The approach to the lateral aspect of digit III and the medial aspect of digit IV is also more difficult due to the proximity and position of the adjacent metacarpal head.

Surgical technique
Sharp dissection is employed to expose the area. Avulsed ligaments with a bone fragment attached can be replaced and maintained with either a small pin and tension-band wire, or a mini-screw. The avulsed fragment is often too small for the screw to be placed in a lag fashion, so it must therefore be placed as a positional screw (Figure 20.9). Ligament ruptures should be supplemented with one or two sutures of a suitable absorbable material, such as 1 metric (4/0) polyglyconate.

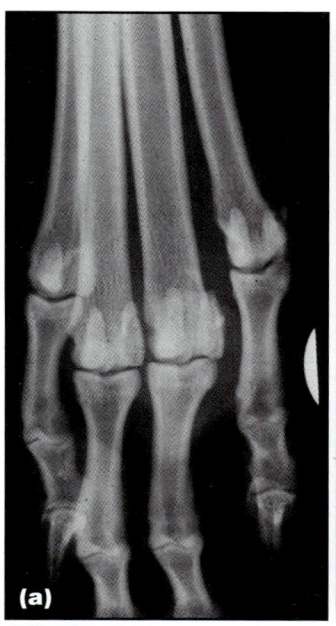

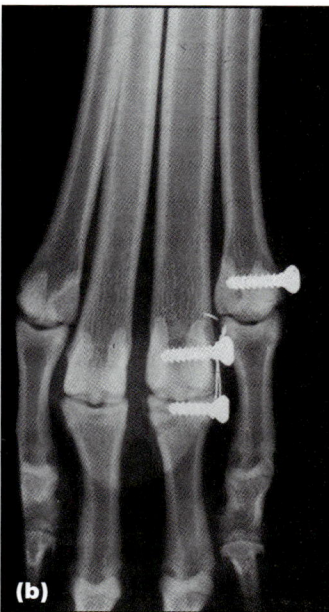

20.9 **(a)** Luxation of fourth and fifth metacarpophalangeal joints. **(b)** MCPJ 4 has been repaired with two screws and a loop of wire. MCPJ 5 has been repaired with a single screw placed through the origin and augmented with a suture anchored in the ligament and secured to the screw.

Closure
Subcutaneous tissue and skin are apposed with 1.5 metric (4/0) absorbable material.

Postoperative care
Light dressing, changed as necessary, for 2–3 weeks. Leash exercise or confinement to a small yard during this time, followed by gradual increasing exercise levels over the next month, prior to allowing free exercise.

Chapter 20 The distal limb

OPERATIVE TECHNIQUE 20.2
Arthrodesis of the MCPJ

Positioning and preparation
Dorsal recumbency with shoulder clipped for harvesting a bone graft.

Assistant
Required to assist and maintain limb in the appropriate position.

Tray extras
Suitable small implants, plates and screws; bone curette; small retractors; Jacobs chuck; small Kirschner wires to maintain bone position while plate applied.

Surgical approach
A dorsal approach is made with retraction of the extensor tendons to expose the joint.

Surgical technique
The articular cartilage is removed with a curette or high-speed burr; the former maintains better integrity of the joint surfaces. The subchondral bone should be foraged with a 1.1 mm drill bit. The joint space is packed with cancellous bone, with the MCPJ at approximately 110 degrees, and a suitable plate placed under compression (Figure 20.10).

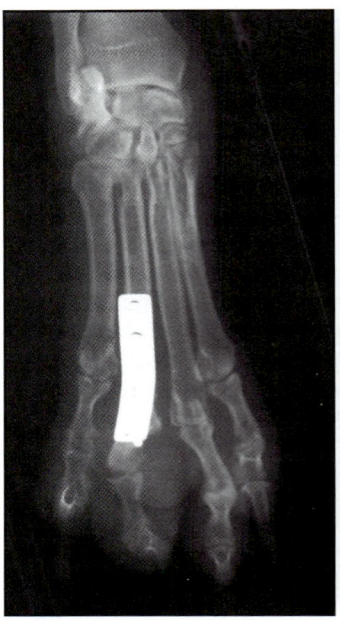

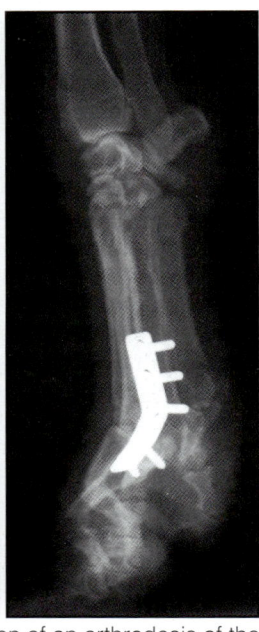

20.10 Dorsal plate stabilization of an arthrodesis of the fourth metacarpophalangeal joint. The dog had a painful arthritic joint that was unresponsive to medical management. (Courtesy of SJ Langley-Hobbs)

Closure
Subcutaneous tissue is closed over the plate with a suitable small monofilament absorbable material. The skin is closed in a routine manner.

Postoperative care
Light dressing for 24 hours followed by a light cast, placed with the foot in a weightbearing position, for 3 weeks. The cast is then split and the caudal half replaced for a further 3 weeks, when follow-up radiographs are taken to assess healing.

Chapter 20 The distal limb

OPERATIVE TECHNIQUE 20.3
Sesamoidectomy

Patient preparation
Clip the entire foot and soak in alcoholic hibitane.

> **WARNING**
> **It is advisable to leave the hairs associated with nails in racing Greyhounds to help protect the nailbed and prevent paronychia.**

Positioning
Thoracic limb: lateral or dorsal recumbency as suits the surgeon.
Pelvic limb: sternal recumbency with the affected limb extended caudally.

Assistant
Useful for limb positioning and retraction.

Tray extras
Either small self-retaining or hand-held retractors; no. 11 scalpel blade for dissecting out the sesamoid.

Surgical approach
A palmaro (plantaro) lateral or medial approach may be used for sesamoids II and VIII. A palmar (plantar) approach directly over the MCPJ concerned is used for the remainder. Care should be taken to avoid the metacarpal/tarsal pad.

Surgical technique
The annular ligament is incised and the flexor tendons identified and retracted to expose the sesamoids within the interosseous muscle (Figure 20.11a,b). A no. 11 scalpel blade is used to dissect out the damaged sesamoid (Figure 20.12). Good haemostasis is essential. The surgical site is flushed, the flexor tendons replaced and annular ligament reapposed with a suitable absorbable suture material.

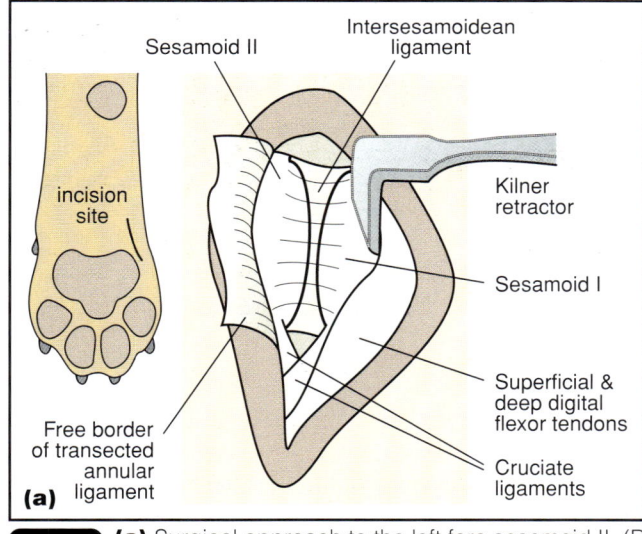

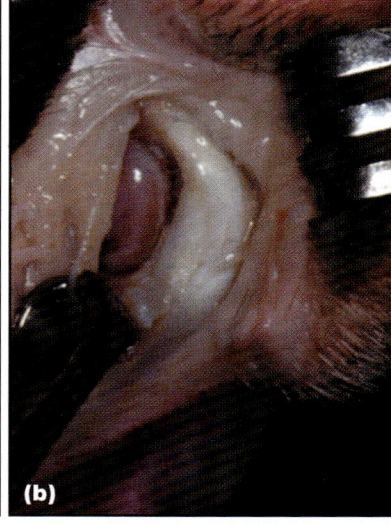

20.11 (a) Surgical approach to the left fore sesamoid II. (Reproduced from the *BSAVA Manual of Small Animal Fracture Repair and Management*.) (b) Surgical approach to palmar sesamoid VII. (Courtesy of JEF Houlton)

OPERATIVE TECHNIQUE 20.3 continued
Sesamoidectomy

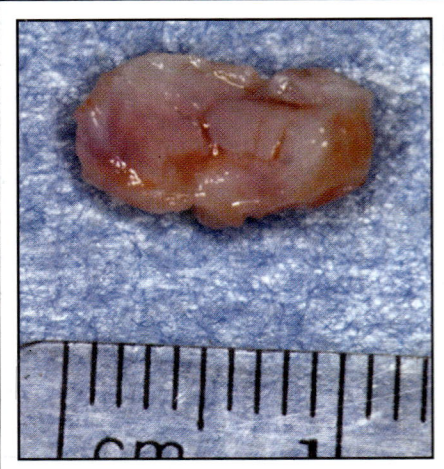

20.12 Excised fractured sesamoid. (Courtesy of JEF Houlton)

Closure
The tendon sheath and annular ligament are closed with several sutures of a suitable small monofilament absorbable material. Subcutaneous and skin closure is routine.

Postoperative care
The foot should be supported with a light dressing for 5–7 days and the dog's exercise levels restricted for 3–4 weeks. Thereafter, exercise is returned to normal over the next 3 weeks. The use of NSAIDs will aid in a smooth recovery to full function. Postoperative physiotherapy in the form of ultrasound or laser acupuncture helps to decrease any loss of mobility.

OPERATIVE TECHNIQUE 20.4
PIPJ collateral ligament repair

Patient preparation
The foot is clipped and prepared for surgery. A soft brush is used to clean the nails and pads; the rest of the foot is prepared routinely. In racing dogs the hairs around the nailbeds should be preserved to reduce the incidence of paronychia resulting from the abrasive action of soil/sand particles. The foot may be soaked in alcoholic hibitane.

Positioning
The dog is placed in lateral recumbency with the affected collateral ligament uppermost. The foot is draped in a normal manner. A surgical self-adhesive drape may be applied.

Assistant
Useful to distract the digits.

Tray extras
Mini self-retaining or hand-held retractors.

Surgical approach
An incision is made directly over the collateral ligament, remembering that it runs in a proximodorsal to palmaro(plantaro)distal direction (Figure 20.13).

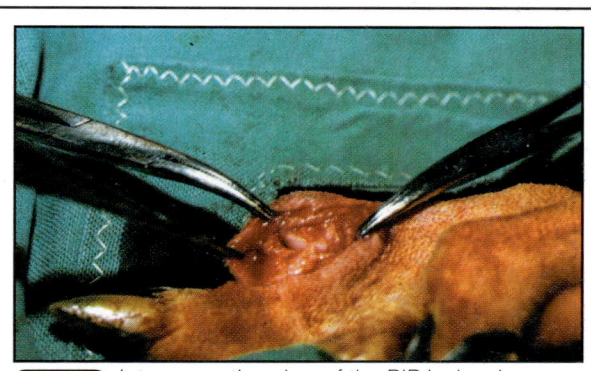

20.13 Intra-operative view of the PIPJ, showing rupture of a collateral ligament.

Surgical technique
Two or three pulley sutures of 1.5 metric (4/0) monofilament absorbable suture material are placed in the appropriate direction and tightened carefully (Figure 20.14). It is important to remember that the toe must be able to extend fully postoperatively; otherwise the dog will become lame after exercise. The knots in the collateral ligament repair are carefully covered with subcutaneous tissue as, in thin-skinned dogs such as the racing Greyhound, suture ends may perforate the skin when the dog is placed back into work. To reduce the stress on the repair, and hence reduce the incidence of recurrence when racing and sporting dogs are returned to full activity, the author prefers to cut back the nail to the level of the pad. Haemostasis is achieved with either a styptic pencil or soap.

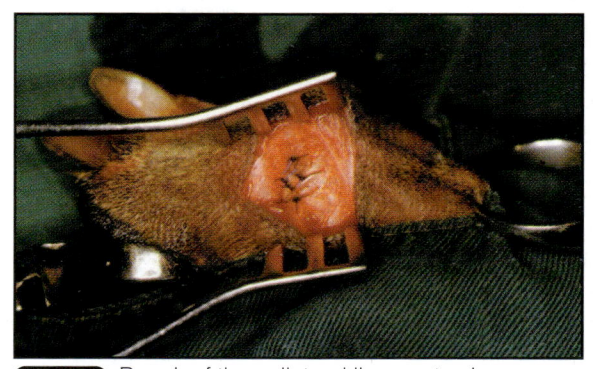

20.14 Repair of the collateral ligament using multiple sutures of 1.5 metric (4/0) absorbable monofilament material.

Closure
Routine.

Postoperative care
The toe should be supported for 2–3 weeks and the dressing changed as necessary. Greyhounds may be exercised on a walking machine from 10 days post repair; other dogs should be confined to leash exercise only for 3–4 weeks.

Chapter 20   The distal limb

OPERATIVE TECHNIQUE 20.5
Arthrodesis of the PIPJ

Patient preparation
Routine preparation of the PIPJ area is carried out. If considering a cancellous bone graft, an appropriate area, such as the proximal humerus, should also be clipped and cleaned.

Positioning
Dorsal or lateral recumbency at the surgeon's preference.

Assistant
Preferred but not essential. Useful to distract the apposing digits.

Tray extras
Suitable small implants, plates and screws; bone curette; small retractors; Jacobs chuck; small Kirschner wires to maintain bone position while plate applied.

Surgical approach
A dorsolateral or dorsomedial approach is used, directly over the affected joint.

Surgical technique
The extensor tendon and dorsal sesamoid are reflected and the joint prepared for arthrodesis. The articular cartilage is removed from each surface, care being taken to maintain the joint alignment and hence the inherent stability. Several 1.1 mm forage holes are drilled into the subchondral bone of the joint surfaces. The interphalangeal space may be packed with cancellous bone collected from the proximal humerus. A small maxillofacial plate, mini-plate or pin and tension band (Figure 20.15) is applied on the dorsal aspect.
In larger breed dogs, an oblique fingerplate may be applied on the lateral or medial aspect of the joint. For a show dog, the toe should be arthrodesed in almost a normal standing position. In racing and sporting dogs, the arthrodesis should be performed with the toe in a semi-extended position to allow for extension of the digit when galloping.

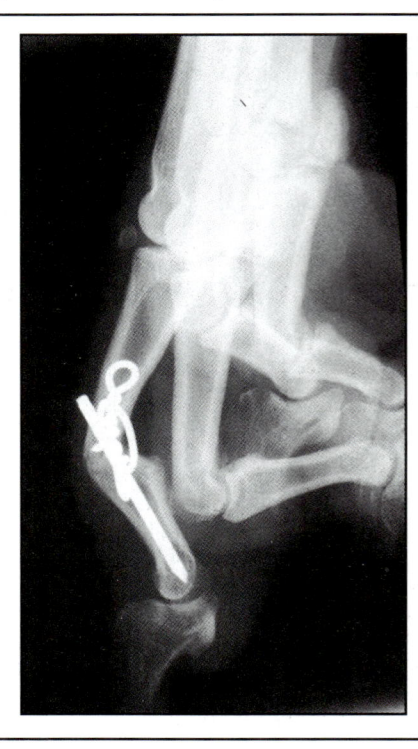

20.15 Pin and tension band arthrodesis of the PIPJ 3 months after surgery.

Closure
Where possible the soft tissues should be closed over the plate. The skin is closed routinely.

Postoperative care
The foot should be supported in a padded dressing until any swelling subsides and then placed in a walking cast for 3–4 weeks. This should then be split, the healing assessed radiographically, and the back half of the splint applied for another 3 weeks. The dog should be confined to exercise on a lead during this time.

Chapter 20 The distal limb

OPERATIVE TECHNIQUE 20.6
DIPJ collateral ligament repair

Patient preparation
The foot is clipped and prepared for surgery. A soft brush is used to clean the nails and pads; the rest of the foot is prepared routinely. The foot may be soaked in alcoholic hibitane.

Positioning
Lateral recumbency with affected ligament uppermost.

Assistant
Not necessary.

Tray extras
Mini self-retaining retractors; curved bone cutters; fine-nosed bone rongeurs.

Surgical approach
An incision is made directly over the ruptured collateral ligament. Careful dissection will reveal the fan-shaped structure of the ligament (Figure 20.16a).

Surgical technique
Two or three pulley sutures of 1.5 metric (4/0) monofilament absorbable material are placed to reconstruct the ligament (Figure 20.16b). The subcutaneous tissue and skin are closed routinely. An inverted Y incision is made around the nail base, extending proximally on the dorsal aspect towards the PIPJ. Careful dissection around the third phalanx down to the ungual crest will expose the germinal tissues. Care is taken not to damage the extensor or flexor process or the joint capsule. The nail is cut short with curved bone cutters (Figure 20.16c) and the ungual crest plus all germinal cells removed with the fine rongeurs (Figure 20.16d).

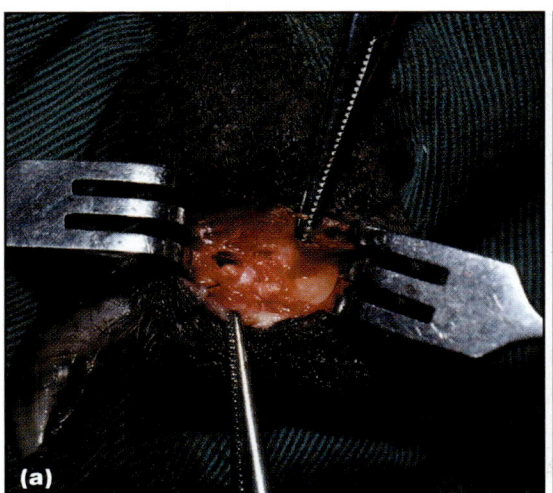

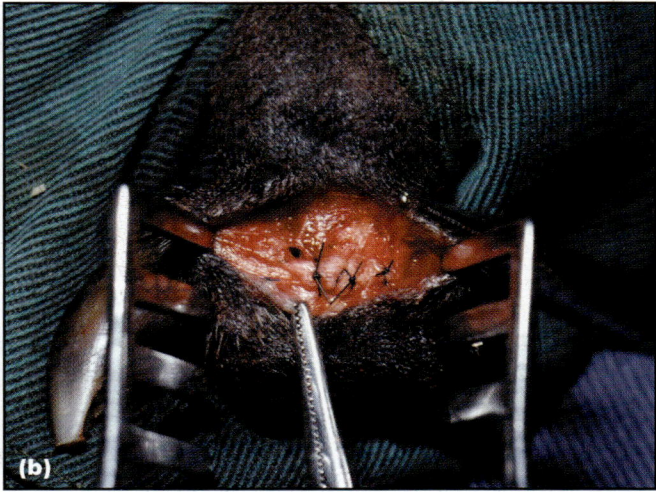

20.16 **(a)** Surgical view of the DIPJ, showing rupture of a collateral ligament. **(b)** Multiple 1.5 metric (4/0) monofilament absorbable sutures used to repair the ligament. (continues)

Chapter 20 The distal limb

> **OPERATIVE TECHNIQUE 20.6** *continued*
> **DIPJ collateral ligament repair** 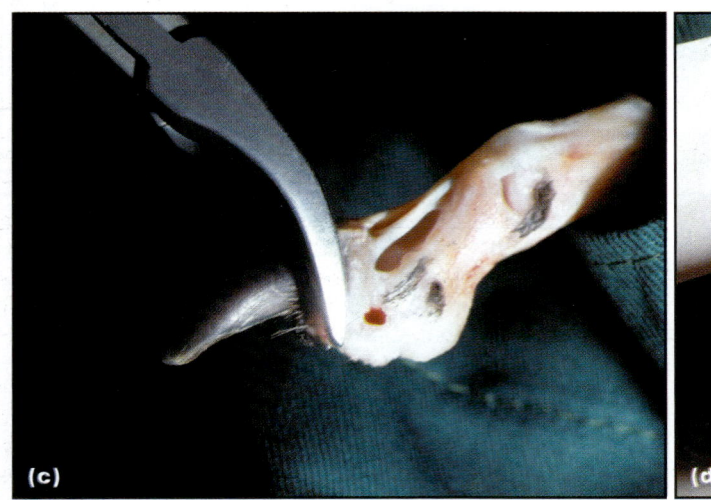
>
> **20.16** (continued) **(c)** Gross specimen illustrating the use of bone cutters to remove the nail as close to the ungual crest as possible. **(d)** Surgical view illustrating the use of small bone rongeurs to remove any remaining ungual crest and ALL the germinal layers.
>
> **Closure**
> The subcutaneous tissue and skin are closed routinely.
>
> **Postoperative care**
> The toes are supported with a light dressing for 10–14 days, and the dog is restricted to leash exercise only for 3 weeks.

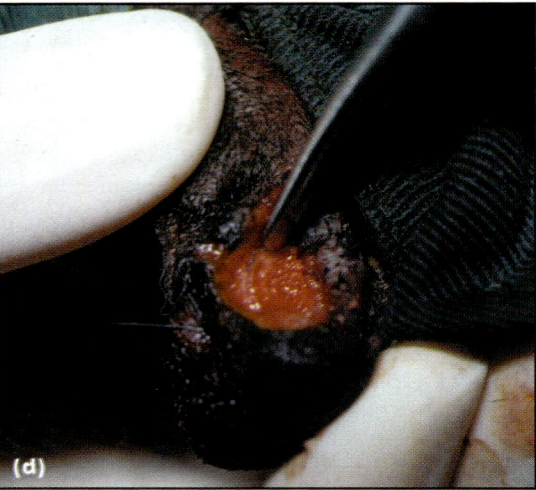

21

The hip

Carlos Macias, James L. Cook and John Innes

Introduction

This chapter deals with a number of developmental and acquired surgical conditions of the hip, excluding fractures. The reader is directed to *The BSAVA Manual of Small Animal Fracture Repair and Management* for information on specific fracture management.

Clinical and surgical anatomy

The hip, or coxofemoral joint, is a diarthrodial (ball and socket) joint, in which the head of the femur resides in the acetabulum of the pelvis. The surface area and the radius of curvature of the articular acetabular surface closely match the articular surface of the femoral head. The acetabulum is further deepened by the labrum, or acetabular lip, a band of fibrocartilage that extends from the acetabular rim dorsally. Ventrally, this structure extends across the acetabular notch as a free ligament, known as the transverse acetabular ligament. The acetabulum is divided into two parts, the articular cartilage (lunate surface) which covers approximately two-thirds of the whole surface, situated dorsomedially, and the acetabular fossa, situated ventromedially from where the teres ligament (also known as the round ligament or ligament of the head of the femur) originates. In normal animals, the femoral head and neck are inclined to the femoral diaphysis by an angle of 130–145 degrees and also anteverted by 12–40 degrees.

The hip joint is a highly constrained joint. The joint is stabilized primarily by the intra-articular teres ligament and the joint capsule. Secondary stabilizers include the acetabular labrum, the gluteal muscles and the hip joint adductors and abductors (iliopsoas, gemelli, quadriceps and internal and external obturator muscles).

The blood supply to the femoral head and neck is potentially from two sources:

- The intraosseous (metaphyseal system) supply, which courses up the femoral neck and, in mature animals only, crosses the physeal scar into the femoral head
- The epiphyseal system, which enters through the joint capsule via the cranial and caudal circumflex femoral arteries.

This arrangement leaves the femoral head in a precarious position in the immature animal because any injury to the epiphyseal system can lead to ischaemic injury to the femoral head. For example, luxation of the hip in an immature dog may tear the capsule and hence the epiphyseal blood supply. The consequence can be ischaemic necrosis. In the cat, there is an additional supply to the femoral head through the teres ligament.

The main muscle groups around the hip are the gluteals (cranial and dorsal), the internal obturator and gemelli (caudal), the biceps femoris (caudal), the vastus lateralis (laterally) and the pectineus ventrally. The ischiatic (sciatic) nerve courses dorsal and caudal to the joint and often needs to be identified and protected during surgery, especially when drilling the acetabulum or making a caudal approach to the joint.

Examination of the hip

Palpation and manipulation

Examination of the hip should commence with gentle palpation of the surrounding musculature. Particular attention should be given to the gluteal muscles, as a degree of atrophy is likely to be noted in the majority of chronic conditions affecting the hip. Palpation of the iliac wing, greater trochanter and ischiatic table will be useful to determine the relative position of the femoral head, especially in cases where a coxofemoral luxation is suspected.

The coxofemoral joint should be manipulated to assess the range of motion and the presence or absence of crepitus. This is usually performed with the animal in a standing position, although in animals with bilateral orthopaedic conditions it may be preferable to perform this manipulation in lateral recumbency. In normal dogs, the range of motion when evaluating flexion and extension is approximately 160 degrees. Dogs with painful conditions of the hip may not allow thorough manipulation. In dogs with chronic hip disease, periarticular fibrosis may limit the range of movement, particularly when attempting hip extension.

It is important to assess the degree of hip laxity, especially when hip dysplasia is suspected. Specific tests allow an evaluation of the degree of laxity: the Ortolani, Barlow and Barden tests. These can be attempted in the conscious animal but they can be painful and therefore may be best performed with the dog heavily sedated or under general anaesthesia. Hip laxity should be evaluated in conjunction with clinical data to avoid over-interpretation.

Chapter 21 The hip

Ortolani test
This is the most widely performed manoeuvre for the detection of hip instability in the young dog. It can be performed with the dog in lateral or dorsal recumbency. With the dog in lateral recumbency, the stifle is grasped with one hand while the other hand is placed on the dorsal aspect of the pelvis to stabilize it. Firm pressure is applied from the stifle in a dorsal direction in an attempt to subluxate the joint. Whilst maintaining this pressure, the limb is gently abducted until a click or 'clunk' is detected (positive Ortolani sign) (Chalman and Butler, 1985). This 'clunk' represents the relocation of the femoral head within the acetabulum. In animals with a positive Ortolani sign, the angle between the limb and the table (when testing in lateral recumbency) at which relocation of the femoral head occurs is termed the reduction angle (Figure 21.1). If the limb is now adducted, whilst dorsal pressure is maintained, re-luxation of the hip will occur. The angle between the limb and the table when re-luxation occurs is termed the re-luxation or subluxation angle.

The Ortolani test can also be used somewhat subjectively to assess the integrity of the dorsal acetabular rim. If the dorsal acetabular rim is intact, the femoral head falls abruptly into the acetabulum; in dogs with a poor acetabular rim the femoral head slides back. The presence of crepitus is suggestive of the existence of osteoarthritic changes. The Ortolani sign is usually absent in dogs with advanced osteoarthritis because pathological changes reduce the sensation of subluxation and reduction.

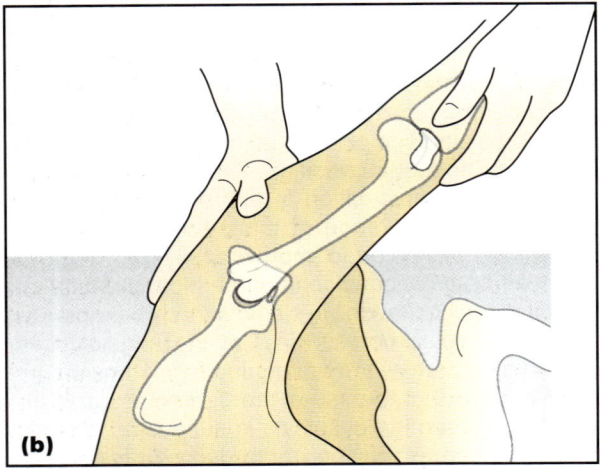

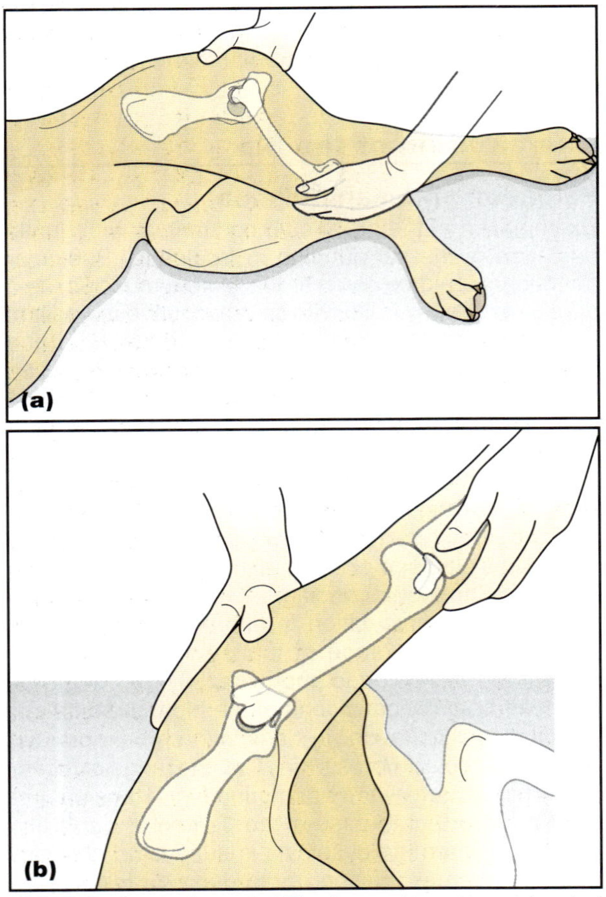

Barlow test
The Barlow test is defined as the detection of femoral head dorsal subluxation. It is essentially the first half of the Ortolani test (Barlow, 1962).

Barden test
Also known as the hip lift test, this is performed with the animal in lateral recumbency. The thigh is grasped firmly whilst standing behind the dog and an attempt is made to lift the limb laterally. It is useful to position the other hand over the region of the greater trochanter in order to detect the lateral displacement. When the greater trochanter can be displaced laterally >0.5 cm the test result is considered to be positive (Barden and Hardwick, 1968).

Arthrocentesis
See Chapter 3.

Radiography
The standard projection for evaluating the hip joint is the ventrodorsal (VD) view, with the pelvic limbs extended caudally (Figure 21.2). Padding material is usually placed between both femurs to aid positioning and it is important to avoid rotation of the pelvis. Ideally, the femurs should be parallel to each other and to the table. The patellas should be centred within the trochlear sulci (femoral grooves) to indicate proper positioning and this is achieved by adducting the femurs and internally rotating the stifles; tape or rope ties can be used to hold the femurs in place.

Additional views include the VD flexed view ('frog-legged view') and the lateral view. The flexed view is particularly useful for the evaluation of acetabular infilling as part of the presurgical evaluation of young dogs with hip dysplasia (if a triple pelvic osteotomy is being considered) and in the diagnosis of slipped capital femoral epiphysis. Further details on imaging the hip joint are provided in the *BSAVA Manual of Canine and Feline Musculoskeletal Imaging*.

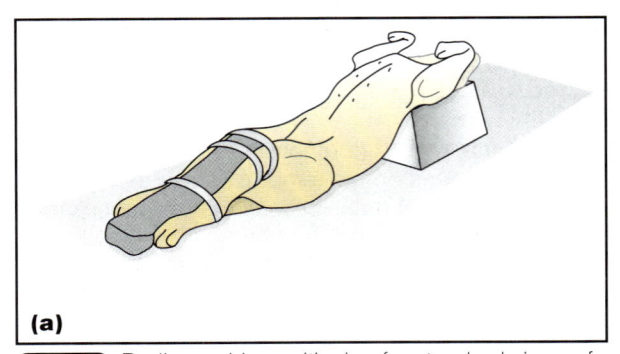

21.1 Ortolani test. **(a)** The femoral head is subluxated by displacing the femur in a proximal direction, with the femur parallel to the table, whilst the dog is in lateral recumbency. **(b)** The femur is then abducted so that the femoral head is relocated within the acetabulum. The angle between the femur and the table at which relocation occurs is termed the angle of reduction.

21.2 Radiographic positioning for standard views of the hip. **(a)** Extended VD view of the pelvis; note the use of padding and tape in order to keep the femurs parallel to each other. (continues)

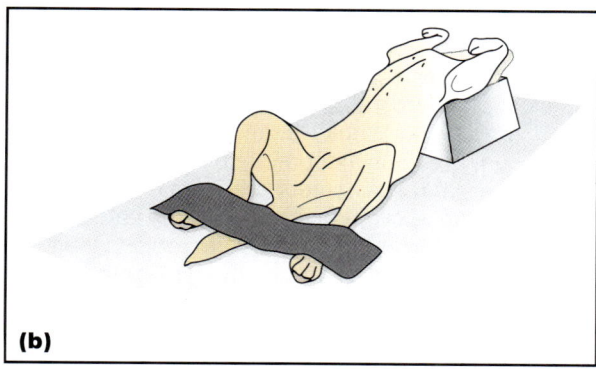

21.2 (continued) Radiographic positioning for standard views of the hip. **(b)** Flexed VD view of the pelvis.

Arthroscopy

Arthroscopy of the hip joint in dogs can provide important information regarding diagnosis, treatment options, and prognosis (see Operative Technique 21.1). Arthroscopic procedures that can readily be performed in the hip joint of dogs include:

- Exploratory/diagnostic arthroscopy
- Articular cartilage grading/assessment for selection of candidates for triple pelvic osteotomy
- Biopsy
- Debridement/wash-out for septic or degenerative arthritis.

Surgical approaches

Craniodorsal approach

The craniodorsal approach (see Operative Technique 21.2) provides good exposure. Indications for this approach include:

- Craniodorsal luxations (transarticular pinning)
- Denervation
- Femoral head and neck excision arthroplasty
- Total hip arthroplasty.

Variations include partial or complete deep gluteal tenotomy.

Dorsal approach

This approach (see Operative Technique 21.3) is advised when extensive exposure of the acetabulum is required. Indications for this approach include:

- Craniodorsal luxations (capsulorrhaphy)
- Acetabular fractures (see *BSAVA Manual of Small Animal Fracture Repair and Management*).

Variations on this approach include the option of gluteal tenotomy rather than trochanteric osteotomy. The trochanteric osteotomy can be repaired with a lag screw or a combination of Kirschner wires and tension-band wire.

Caudal approach

The caudal approach (see Operative Technique 21.4) is indicated for craniodorsal luxations (hip toggle).

Ventral approach

A ventral approach is rarely indicated because of the limited exposure it affords. It can be used for femoral head and neck excision.

Hip dysplasia and osteoarthritis

Hip dysplasia is an inherited developmental disease of the hip joint, characterized by hip laxity and the development of osteoarthritis (Lust *et al.*, 1985; Smith *et al.*, 1995). Hip dysplasia is a very common disease that usually affects both hips. Hip dysplasia is not, however, a devastating disease, with many dogs and cats showing minimal or no clinical signs (Barr *et al.*, 1987). Hip dysplasia affects all breeds of dog, although the prevalence is higher in the large and giant breeds. In cats, there is a higher prevalence in the Maine Coon, Persian, Devon Rex and Himalayan, although the condition is not usually symptomatic. There is no sex predisposition.

Aetiopathogenesis

Laxity of the hip joint is a constant feature of hip dysplasia. A direct correlation between passive laxity and the development of osteoarthritis has been demonstrated (Smith *et al.*, 1995).

The mechanism of inheritance is consistent with a polygenic trait (the phenotypic expression is influenced by genetic and non-genetic factors), with variable estimates of heritability ranging from 0.2–0.6, depending on the population studied. Non-genetic factors that may play a role in the expression of the disease include body size, growth rate, nutrition, exercise and muscle mass.

Dogs with a genetic predisposition to hip dysplasia are grossly normal at birth. During development, there is a loss of congruency between the articular surfaces of the acetabulum and the femoral head. This incongruency leads to the development of osteoarthritis. In particular, in the first 2 months of life, there is stretching of the teres ligament, loss of definition of the dorsal acetabular rim, and subluxation of the femoral head. Further stretching of the joint capsule and progressive subluxation lead to further remodelling of the acetabular rim, articular cartilage degeneration and femoral head remodelling. Acetabular infilling, femoral head remodelling and thickening of the femoral neck all progress, becoming radiographically evident in dogs from 5 months of age onwards. With time, the acetabulum becomes shallower and the femoral head also becomes misshapen. Eventually a gradual thickening of the joint capsule leads to an increase in joint stability.

Pain in the initial stages is thought to be the result of stretching of the joint capsule and the development of microfractures in the dorsal acetabular rim because of the abnormal femoral head loading. Surrounding muscle development is usually delayed because of poor limb use and pain, further contributing to the lack of support during the first 9 months of life. With time, pain due to capsular stretching subsides and there is a gradual increase in stability afforded by the intra- and periarticular changes, mainly because of the increased thickening of the joint capsule. A gradual increase in muscle mass usually follows and contributes to an increase in joint stability.

Chapter 21 The hip

By the time dogs reach skeletal maturity (approximately 12–18 months of age), the hip is usually stable because of capsular thickening, increased muscle mass and bone remodelling. Despite the loss of range of motion, many dogs develop adequate function, especially if not destined for intense work.

From this point on, the osteoarthritic changes usually progress slowly, influenced by the weight of the dog and exercise regimen (Kealy *et al.*, 1997).

Clinical signs and physical examination

The clinical signs associated with hip dysplasia typically have a bimodal age distribution. Although clinical signs can appear at any age, many dogs under 1 year that are affected with hip dysplasia present with clinical signs related to hip instability and secondary synovitis. Older dogs present with clinical signs related to hip osteoarthritis. Because of the high prevalence amongst dogs, hip dysplasia tends to be overdiagnosed in both immature and older dogs.

> **WARNING**
> **The clinician should be very aware of other possible differential diagnoses (Figure 21.3) when evaluating dogs with pelvic limb lameness, even if there are clear radiographic signs of hip dysplasia.**

Differential diagnoses in the young dog
Patellar luxation
Cranial cruciate ligament disease
Hock and stifle osteochondrosis
Legg–Calvé–Perthes disease
Septic arthritis
Spinal disorders
Myasthenia gravis
Myopathies

Differential diagnoses in the mature dog
Cranial cruciate ligament disease
Patellar luxation
Degenerative lumbosacral stenosis
Other spinal disorders
Achilles tendinopathy
Septic arthritis

21.3 Differential diagnoses for hip dysplasia.

Young dogs

Typical clinical signs in the young dog affected with hip dysplasia (4–10 months of age) include some, or all, of the following:

- Variable degree of pelvic limb lameness
- Swaying of the pelvis when walking
- 'Bunny-hopping' gait at faster speeds
- Weakness of the pelvic limbs
- Reluctance to exercise
- Inability to jump
- Inactivity stiffness.

Sudden-onset lameness is rare but can be associated with microfractures of the dorsal acetabular rim or with complete dislocation of the femoral head in cases of severe coxofemoral instability. Owners sometimes detect an audible 'clunk'. Examination of the pelvic limbs usually reveals a degree of gluteal muscle atrophy. The greater trochanters are usually very prominent and hip instability can sometimes be palpated if a hand is placed over the trochanteric region when the animal is walking. Pain can usually be detected, especially if hip extension is attempted. Manipulation of the hip usually reveals instability and, in many cases, a positive Ortolani sign can be detected.

> **WARNING**
> **Care should be taken when attempting the Ortolani manoeuvre in the conscious dog because this can be very painful.**

Palpation of the hip to evaluate instability should be performed with the animal under heavy sedation or general anaesthesia.

Adult dogs

Dogs over 12 months of age with hip osteoarthritis usually present with more vague clinical signs including some or all of the following:

- Difficulty rising
- Pelvic limb inactivity stiffness (often worse after exercise)
- Exercise intolerance
- Difficulty jumping
- Behavioural changes (e.g. aggression when hindquarters touched)
- Sudden-onset lameness (uncommon).

A reduction in the range of hip extension is usually noted, and crepitus (normally non-painful) can be detected on manipulation of the hip. Muscle atrophy is usually mild. Pain on hip extension may be a feature, although hip extension can also exacerbate lumbar or lumbosacral pain. Abduction of the hip may help differentiate hip dysplasia from degenerative lumbosacral stenosis.

> **WARNING**
> **Sudden-onset lameness is very rare in dogs over 12 months of age with hip osteoarthritis, and other differentials need to be considered.**

Diagnostic imaging

Radiography

Radiography is the standard method for the diagnosis of hip dysplasia. The VD extended view remains the accepted position and is adequate for the diagnosis of hip dysplasia in symptomatic dogs. Proper positioning is paramount to avoid pelvic rotation (see above). The radiograph should be assessed for evidence of joint laxity (percentage of femoral head coverage within the limits of the dorsal acetabular rim or degree of subluxation, medial joint space widening, Norberg–Olsson angle) (Figure 21.4) and for signs of osteoarthritis,

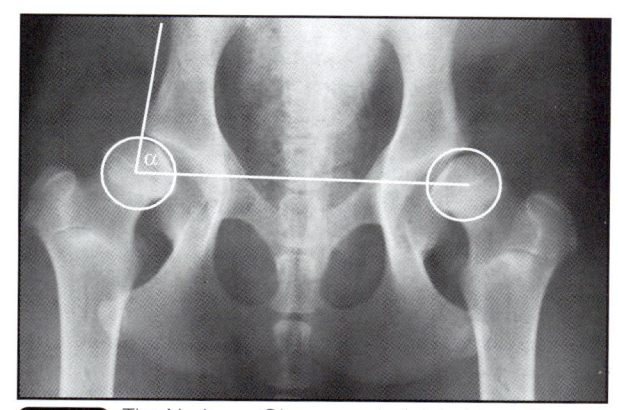

Chapter 21 The hip

21.4 The Norberg–Olsson angle (alpha) is defined by a line connecting the centres of the femoral heads and a second line from the centres of the femoral heads to the effective cranial acetabular rims. Angles smaller than 105 degrees are considered abnormal.

such as: changes in the shape of the dorsal acetabular edge; new bone formation in the acetabular fossa, on the cranial and caudal acetabular edges, and femoral head and neck; and degree of remodelling of the femoral head and neck.

In the young dog, secondary changes can be minimal, and therefore the diagnosis of hip dysplasia is based solely on the degree of femoral head subluxation (Figure 21.5). This is usually measured as the percentage of femoral head that is covered within the limits of the acetabulum. The hips are considered dysplastic if the centre of the femoral head is lateral to the dorsal acetabular rim (less than 50% of femoral head coverage within the limits of the acetabulum). Mildly affected animals may appear normal or have a minimal degree of apparent laxity when evaluating the extended VD projection due to self-tightening of the joint capsule (wind-up mechanism) (Adams *et al.*, 2000). Interpretation of the radiographic features should be made in combination with the history, clinical signs and the results of the physical examination in order to obtain an accurate diagnosis.

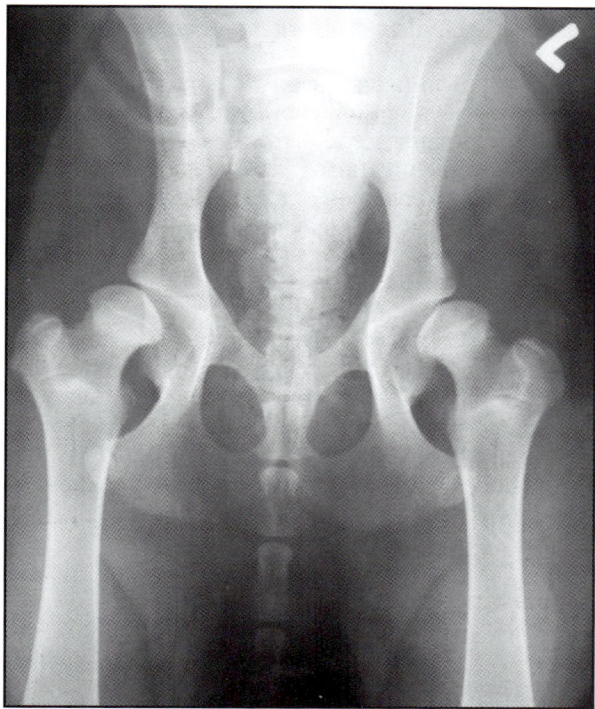

The severity of secondary changes is very variable in dogs with hip dysplasia/osteoarthritis, from a very faint osteophyte in the area of joint capsule attachment to the femoral neck (Morgan's line or caudolateral curvilinear osteophyte) to severe remodelling of the femoral head, femoral neck and acetabulum and marked osteophytosis (Figure 21.6).

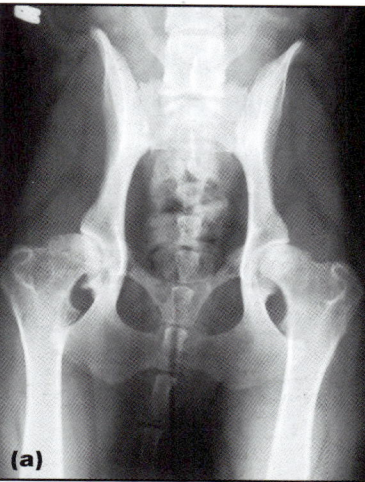

21.5 VD extended radiograph of a 7-month-old Newfoundland with severe hip dysplasia. There is lateral displacement of the femoral heads and poor acetabular coverage. There are minimal secondary changes, although there is a degree of femoral head remodelling.

21.6 VD extended radiographs of two dogs with moderate **(a)** and severe **(b, detail)** osteoarthritic changes secondary to hip dysplasia. Note: thickening of the femoral neck; more triangular femoral head shape; acetabular infilling; and osteophyte formation on the femoral neck and cranial and caudal aspects of the acetabulum.

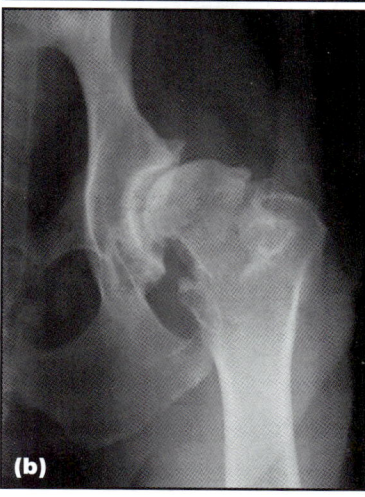

WARNING
There is poor correlation between the severity of radiographic changes and the clinical signs. Many dogs show radiographic features of hip dysplasia but no clinical signs.

Ultrasonography
Ultrasonography can be used in the early detection of dogs with mild to moderate hip dysplasia but is not reliable compared with radiographic methods that evaluate passive hip laxity (Adams *et al.*, 2000).

Chapter 21 The hip

Early detection and screening methods
Due to the high prevalence of hip dysplasia in dogs, several screening/breeding control programmes have been devised based on radiographic evaluation methods. Any reduction in the prevalence of a genetic disease requires early and accurate detection of affected animals so that selective breeding can be adopted.

BVA/KC and OFA schemes
In the UK, the British Veterinary Association/Kennel Club (BVA/KC) scoring scheme is based on the standard VD extended radiograph. It measures radiographic evidence of hip subluxation (laxity) and secondary osteoarthritic changes in dogs with a minimum age of 12 months. Nine parameters are scored on a scale from 0–6 (except the caudal acetabular edge, 0–5). Higher scores indicate a greater degree of radiographic abnormality. The results of both hips are added together to obtain a total hip score value (maximum value 106). Breeding from dogs with scores significantly lower than the breed mean score is recommended in order to reduce the prevalence of the disease. Although the scheme has shortcomings (see below), the introduction of rolling 5-year breed mean scores will provide breeders with additional information (Figure 21.7).

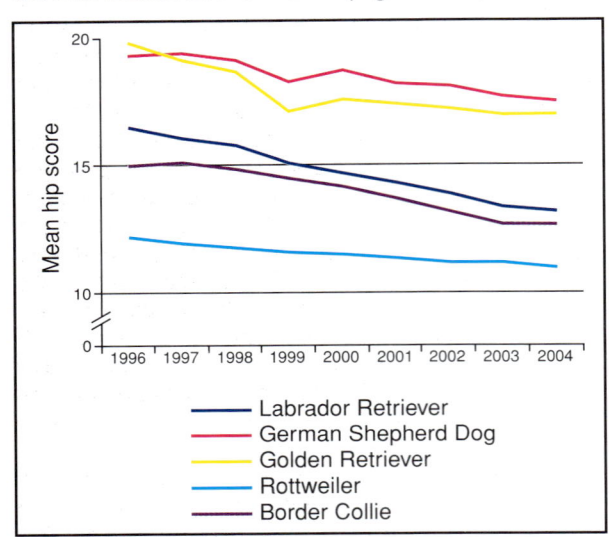

21.7 Rolling 5-year breed mean hip scores for the five breeds most frequently submitted to the BVA/KC Scheme between 1996 and 2004.

In the USA, the Orthopedic Foundation for Animals (OFA) also uses the VD hip-extended projection to evaluate hips but dogs must be at least 24 months of age. The phenotypic evaluation of hips done by the OFA falls into seven different categories. Those categories are normal ('excellent', 'good', 'fair'), 'borderline' and dysplastic ('mild', 'moderate', 'severe'). Three independent radiologists classify the hip into one of the seven phenotypes above, with the final hip grade decided by the consensus grade. The hip grades of excellent, good and fair are within normal limits and are given OFA numbers. This information is accepted by the American Kennel Club (AKC) on dogs with permanent identification (tattoo, microchip) and is in the public domain. Radiographs of borderline, mild, moderate and severely dysplastic hip grades are reviewed by the OFA radiologist and a radiographic report is generated documenting the abnormal radiographic findings. Unless the owner has chosen the open database, dysplastic hip grades are not in the public domain.

The shortcoming of screening methods based on the standard VD extended radiograph – because of their inability adequately to identify laxity, and the poor correlation between the genotype and the development of secondary changes – has been highlighted by Smith *et al.* (1990, 1993, 1995) and, more recently, by Wood and Lakhani (2003). Nevertheless, other countries around the world operate similar systems and readers are advised to consult country-specific information.

Methods based on hip laxity
A high correlation between hip joint laxity and the development of secondary changes has been shown in several studies, despite significant breed differences (Smith *et al.*, 1993, 1995). The accurate assessment of hip laxity requires stress radiographs, which are obtained if the femoral head is forcefully pushed out of the acetabulum prior to taking the radiograph. Stress radiographs are required in order to identify mildly affected dogs that may be otherwise considered normal based on standard VD extended views (because of the wind-up mechanism described previously). Several methods, such as the distraction index method 'Penn-Hip method' (Smith *et al.*, 1990), the dorsolateral hip subluxation score method (Farese *et al.*, 1998) and the stress radiographic method proposed by Fluckiger *et al.* (1999) have been shown to be more reliable for the early screening of dogs with hip dysplasia than is the standard extended VD view.

The advantage of the Penn-Hip screening method (based on accurate and repeatable determination of hip laxity) has been highlighted (Smith *et al.*, 1995; Kapatkin *et al.*, 2002). The incorporation of such screening methods in the UK is unlikely, however, until a method is devised that does not require manual restraint while obtaining the radiograph, bearing in mind that UK Ionising Radiation Regulations prohibit the routine use of manual restraint for small animal radiography.

Management options
The aims of any treatment are: to alleviate pain; to maintain or improve limb function; and, whenever possible, to reduce the progression of osteoarthritis. The decision as to whether conservative or surgical management is indicated should be made on an individual basis, based on severity of clinical signs, age, patient behaviour and potential use, as well as owners' considerations (e.g. ability to provide adequate postoperative care and financial constraints).

Conservative management
Conservative management is indicated in all dogs with mild clinical signs, regardless of age, and it should always be considered as the first line of treatment, even for severely affected cases. Conservative management can produce very satisfactory long-term results regardless of the severity of the initial clinical signs. In a long-term study of conservatively managed dogs with moderate to severe clinical and radiographic signs of hip

dysplasia, 76% of dogs showed minimal or no gait abnormalities despite the radiographic progression of secondary osteoarthritic changes (Barr *et al.*, 1987).

> **The majority of dogs with hip dysplasia can be successfully treated with conservative management, regardless of the initial severity and of the progression of radiographic features.**

In the young dog with unstable painful hips, the objective is to reduce the level of pain whilst improving hip stability. The severity of clinical signs will usually decrease as hip stability increases (due to the development of periarticular fibrosis and improved muscle mass). In the adult dog with hip dysplasia and secondary osteoarthritis, the objective is to control the osteoarthritis-related clinical signs to a level that is acceptable to the dog and owner.

Conservative management can be broadly divided into three aspects: weight regulation and dietary management; exercise regimen; and use of therapeutic agents. These three aspects should be considered simultaneously for a successful outcome to be achieved.

Dietary management: The importance of dietary control cannot be overemphasized. Overnutrition has been shown to increase the phenotypic expression of canine hip dysplasia. In a study of dogs predisposed to canine hip dysplasia, growing dogs fed on a restricted diet were 50% less likely to show radiographic evidence of osteoarthritis at 2 years of age than dogs fed *ad libitum* (Kealy *et al.*, 1992). In addition, in an 8-year follow-up study of dogs predisposed to hip dysplasia, dogs fed on a restricted diet had less progression of secondary osteoarthritic changes than dogs fed *ad libitum* (Kealy *et al.*, 1997).

Young dogs predisposed to canine hip dysplasia or young dogs with symptomatic hip dysplasia will benefit if the food intake is limited so that they develop as lean dogs. Several strategies have been proposed such as reducing the food intake (by limiting the size of the portions as well as limiting the time available for feeding) or switching the diet from growth formulas to adult preparations once 80% of the final growth has been reached. Ensuring lean body development will require close monitoring and critical appraisal of body condition as well as client education. Weight control alone was shown to be beneficial in reducing lameness in the adult dog with established osteoarthritis secondary to hip dysplasia (Impellizeri *et al.*, 2000) and may be the only change required in many dogs with mild clinical signs. The caloric intake should be balanced by the metabolic requirements of the patient and this can be achieved by a combination of reducing the food intake and increasing the level of exercise if tolerated.

Exercise regimen: While exercise is probably best kept to a minimum in the acute painful stages, because it may exacerbate clinical signs, it can be used to improve long-term function. The beneficial effects of exercise in the management of osteoarthritis are well recognized. Exercise improves range of motion, stimulates cartilage metabolism, and strengthens muscles and ligaments, leading to an increase in joint stability and a reduction in pain scores. Whilst high-impact exercise (such as chasing balls, jumping and any other form of vigorous activity) is probably best avoided, low-impact exercise, such as controlled lead walks and swimming, is usually of benefit.

Exercise should be tailored according to the individual and the stage of the disease. In the young dog, a fairly intense and gradually progressive regimen of controlled exercise, including swimming, is recommended so that the developing muscles surrounding the hip can contribute towards an increase in stability. A gradual increase in exercise should be considered based on the clinical response. In the adult dog with established osteoarthritis, exercise should be directed towards maintaining mobility at acceptable levels (for the dog and owner) without exacerbating presenting clinical signs. Exercise on a little and often basis is usually better than prolonged sessions, and this can be gradually increased and modified according to the clinical stages of the disease.

Therapeutic agents: The use of pharmacological substances in the treatment of canine hip dysplasia is well established. The aim should be to use drugs to control pain and therefore improve limb function, as well as to improve the dog's overall quality of life. Non-steroidal anti-inflammatory drugs (NSAIDs) are the mainstays of pharmacological therapy. There is little information regarding the best treatment protocol and most treatment regimens rely on the clinician's individual experience with regard to which drug to use and duration of treatment. In the acute phases of the disease, both in the young and in the adult dog, it may be preferable to consider a prolonged course of medication (3–4 weeks initially). The overall situation should be monitored closely and further recommendations should be made according to the clinical response. Some dogs will require prolonged, almost continuous therapy, whilst other dogs will require intermittent therapy, depending on the severity of clinical signs and exercise regimen.

The use of nutraceuticals remains controversial; additional, more objective data will be required before recommending these products on a general basis. For more information on the use of pharmacological and nutritional agents, see Chapter 7.

Surgical management

Surgical techniques for hip dysplasia can be divided into preventive, palliative and salvage procedures. Each technique has its reported indications, complications, advantages and disadvantages. The surgeon must help the owner make informed decisions regarding treatment of each individual.

Juvenile pubic symphysiodesis (JPS) (Operative Technique 21.5): This is a recently reported innovative technique for preventing canine hip dysplasia (Mathews *et al.*, 1996; Swainson *et al.*, 2000; Dueland *et al.*, 2001; Patricelli *et al.*, 2001, 2002). The technique is designed to use alteration of the natural development of the pelvis to attain acetabular rotation (ventroversion; Figure 21.8) similar to that accomplished via triple pelvic osteotomy

Chapter 21 The hip

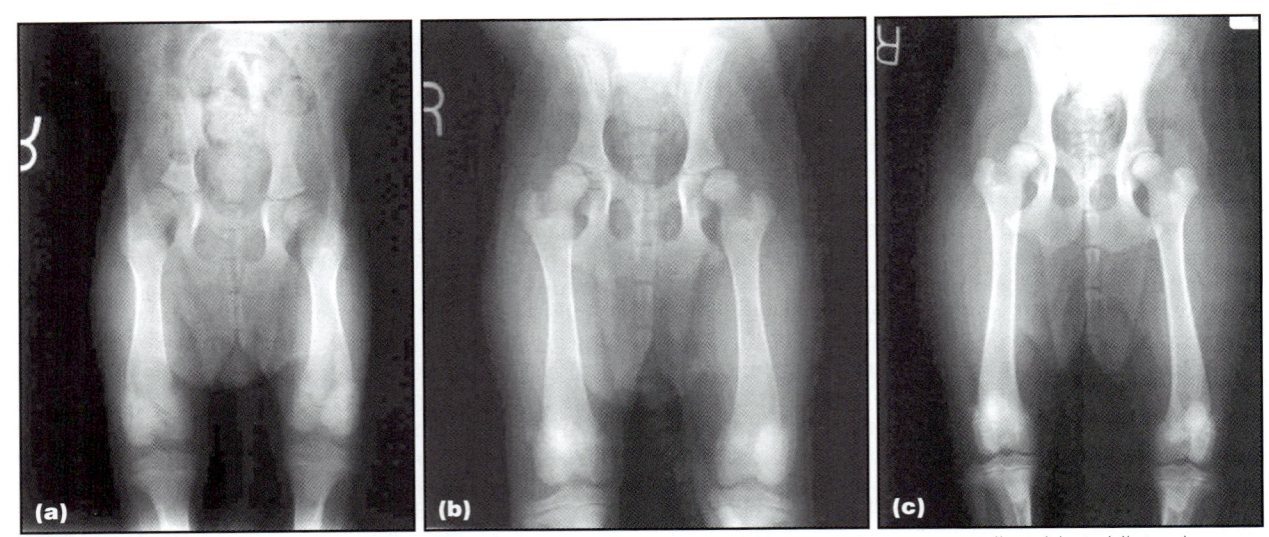

21.8 (a) VD radiographic view of the pelvis of a 15-week-old dog with severe lameness attributable to bilateral coxofemoral joint laxity. (b) The same dog at 19 weeks of age, 4 weeks after JPS was performed. (c) The same dog at 32 weeks of age, 17 weeks after JPS was performed.

(see below). The pubic symphysis is insulted using electrosurgery or staples early in the dog's development (3–5 months of age) so that it ceases to participate in endochondral ossification for pelvic growth. This focal disturbance of growth results in relatively less growth of the ventral pelvis, which results in bilateral acetabular ventroversion and allows for increased femoral head coverage. Because the technique needs to be performed in very young puppies, early evaluation of hip status is critical. Currently, this involves testing for hip laxity at 14–16 weeks of age and deciding on the need for surgery based on the estimated risk of the development of hip dysplasia. Clearly, this is somewhat controversial. Nevertheless, this technique has the advantages of being minimally invasive, resulting in bilateral acetabular rotation, and can be performed in conjunction with a neutering procedure. Early results of this technique in dogs have been very promising (Dueland *et al.*, 2001; Patricelli *et al.*, 2002). Complications include loss of pelvic canal diameter, potential for thermal damage to adjacent tissues and skin, and incisional oedema.

> **WARNING**
> Juvenile pubic symphysiodesis changes a dog's phenotype without changing its genotype. In the authors' opinion, concurrent or subsequent neutering of the dog must be mandatory.

Triple pelvic osteotomy (TPO) (Operative Technique 21.6): If the biomechanical imbalance in a dysplastic hip is corrected early in the progression of canine hip dysplasia, the hip can return to normal function. TPO is designed for this purpose. Ideally, correction takes place prior to skeletal maturity and before secondary changes occur. The goals of TPO are correction of femoral head subluxation and restoration of the hip's weightbearing surface area (Figure 21.9). The procedure is still somewhat controversial but the current consensus is that the ideal candidate is a young dog (<10 months) with clinical signs attributable to hip dysplasia, radiographic subluxation and no secondary osteoarthritic changes. The procedure involves performing osteotomies in the pubis, ischium and ilium to allow axial rotation of the acetabulum, providing increased dorsal acetabular coverage and weightbearing surface area. The ilial osteotomy is then stabilized using a bone plate that maintains the desired degree of rotation (Figure 21.9c). The most appropriate degree of acetabular rotation has been reported to be 20 degrees. Recent studies have shown that no advantage in femoral head coverage, weightbearing surface area or clinical outcome is gained with higher degrees of rotation (Dejardin *et al.*, 1998; Tomlinson *et al.*, 2002).

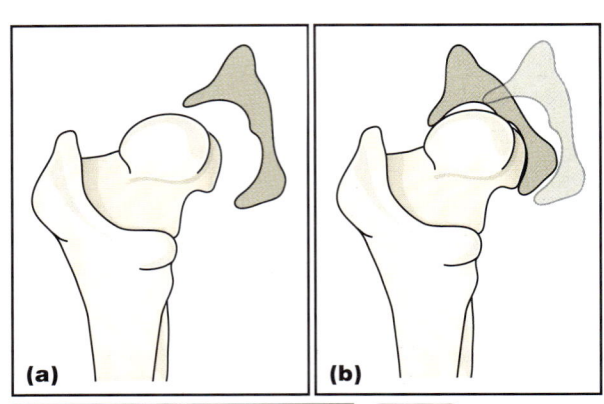

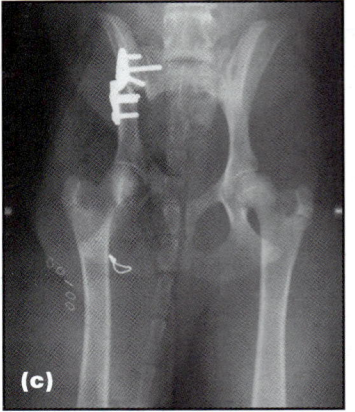

21.9 Laxity and subluxation of the coxofemoral joint prior to **(a)** and after **(b)** TPO. **(c)** VD radiographic view of the pelvis of a dog in which TPO has been performed.

316

Postoperative management involves exercise restriction until there is radiographic evidence of healing of the ilial osteotomy; there is then a gradual return to normal function. TPO can be performed in the contralateral hip 2–6 weeks after the first surgery if surgical selection criteria are still fulfilled. Concurrent bilateral TPO has been advocated by some authors (Borostyankoi *et al.*, 2003). Complications associated with TPO include narrowing of the pelvic canal, constipation, urethral injury, over-rotation of the acetabulum (resulting in limited femoral extension and abduction), implant failure, infection, sciatic nerve palsy, persistent incongruity, and failure to retard the progression of osteoarthritis. Long-term success, as determined by normal weightbearing and limb function, reportedly ranges from 72 to 92% of cases.

Denervation: Denervation of the hip joint capsule has been described as a surgical procedure aimed at palliation of pain. The technique has been performed alone or in conjunction with pectineal and/or iliopsoas releasing procedures (Montavon, 1998; Kinzel *et al.*, 2002). Denervation is accomplished through a craniolateral approach to the hip joint and then, using a periosteal elevator, removing the periosteum of the craniolateral edge of the acetabulum to disrupt the innervation of the cranial gluteal and sciatic nerve components (Kinzel *et al.*, 2002), and/or to disrupt the innervation of the obturator and femoral nerve components by elevating the capsule ventrally (Montavon, 1998). Subjective improvement in lameness after denervation has been reported in approximately 92% of cases in a large clinical study (Kinzel *et al.*, 2002).

Other palliative procedures: Numerous surgical procedures have been advocated for palliative treatment of hip dysplasia including biocompatible osteoconductive polymer (BOP) shelf arthroplasty, intertrochanteric osteotomy, femoral neck lengthening, dorsal acetabular rim arthroplasty (DARthroplasty) and others. Very limited success, if any, using these procedures has been reported in the literature. The authors do not currently advocate the use of these techniques.

Femoral head and neck excision (FHNE) arthroplasty (Operative Technique 21.7): This is a salvage procedure. Joint pain is reduced because only a fibrous pseudojoint exists. The pseudojoint is less biomechanically stable than a normal hip joint and range of motion is reduced. FHNE can be performed at nearly any stage in the progression of hip dysplasia. Most surgeons wait until secondary osteoarthritic changes and the associated pain are persistent. However, severe muscle atrophy may result in a less favourable outcome (Berzon *et al.*, 1980). To attain an optimal level of function after FHNE, the surgical candidate should weigh <18–20 kg (Duff and Campbell, 1977; Gendreau, 1977); because most dogs treated for hip dysplasia are >20 kg, FHNE may result in lower levels of function than other surgical procedures, but the goal of pain relief should still be reached.

FHNE is accomplished through a craniolateral approach to the hip joint. The osteotomy should be performed using an oscillating saw or sharp osteotome. The cut extends from the medial aspect of the greater trochanter to a point immediately proximal to the lesser trochanter. Irregularities at the osteotomy site should be smoothed with rongeurs or a bone rasp. Complete removal of the head and neck is vital to success. Various interpositional muscle flaps have been described for use in promoting fibrous tissue formation within the joint space but no long-term benefit from their use has been reported (Duff and Campbell, 1977; Mann *et al.*, 1987; Prostredney *et al.*, 1991).

Postoperative management involves a rapid return to exercise (first 3–5 days) to promote formation of the fibrous pseudojoint while maintaining muscle mass and range of motion. Physiotherapy involving active and passive range-of-motion exercises should be initiated 2–3 days after surgery. Success rates, as determined by slight or intermittent lameness, reportedly range from 60 to 83% (Duff and Campbell, 1977; Gendreau, 1977; Berzon *et al.*, 1980). Complications include shortening of the limb, abnormal limb motion, muscle atrophy, varying degrees of lameness, patellar luxation and compromised joint function. Pain can persist if excision is inadequate.

Total hip arthroplasty (THA) (Operative Techniques 21.8 and 21.9): This is a salvage procedure that can effectively provide pain relief and high-level function in dogs with hip dysplasia. THA is indicated in dogs that are persistently clinically affected with osteoarthritis resulting from hip dysplasia and are non-responsive to conservative measures. The candidate should be skeletally mature, have pain and/or lameness attributable to the hip, and weigh at least 10–12 kg to accept the prostheses. Contraindications include infection, neurological disease that affects the hindlimbs, and some systemic diseases. Concurrent orthopaedic disease will necessitate careful patient evaluation and may preclude the procedure. THA can be done bilaterally with at least 2–3 months between surgeries. Unilateral THA, however, reportedly results in acceptable function in up to 80% of dogs with bilateral hip dysplasia (Olmstead *et al.*, 1983).

Currently, the most commonly used system is a cemented THA system comprising a high-density polyethylene acetabular component and cobalt chromium femoral heads and endoprostheses (e.g. Biomedtrix CFX). However, other cemented (e.g. Bardet, New Generation Devices) and non-cemented systems (e.g. Biomedtrix BFX) are commercially available and are being used increasingly throughout the world. While there are theoretical advantages for both cemented and non-cemented systems, the relative indications and advantages and disadvantages of each system have not been clearly defined in veterinary medicine. It is important to note that both cemented and non-cemented THAs are technically challenging and unforgiving procedures that can have severe complications and result in unacceptable morbidity.

WARNING
Whilst the techniques for THA are described in this Manual (see Operative Techniques 21.8 and 21.9), the authors caution that THA should only be performed by experienced surgeons with appropriate training, resources and equipment.

Chapter 21 The hip

Postoperative management is vital to a successful outcome. For the first week after surgery, activity is restricted to lead walking with support of the hindlimbs. Activity restriction should continue for the first month, with a gradual return to function 10–12 weeks after surgery. THA is reported to have a 91–95.2% success rate (Budsberg *et al.*, 1996; Marcellin-Little *et al.*, 1999; Skurla *et al.*, 2000). Complication rates vary widely and decrease with increased surgical experience. Complications include luxation, osteomyelitis, aseptic component loosening, femoral fractures, implant failure and sciatic neuropraxia (Olmstead, 1995; Edwards *et al.*, 1997; Marcellin-Little *et al.*, 1999; Schulz, 2000; Skurla *et al.*, 2000). In the light of the excellent results and minimal complications associated with THA, expense and availability are considered the major determinants in clients' decisions.

Postoperative rehabilitation: Postoperative rehabilitation is extremely important following hip surgery of any type. Optimal protocols vary depending on procedure, patient size and intended function (see Chapter 16).

Avascular necrosis of the femoral head (Legg–Calvé–Perthes disease)

Avascular or ischaemic necrosis of the femoral head was independently and simultaneously described in humans in 1910 by the three authors after whom this disease is named. Legg–Calvé–Perthes disease is a developmental avascular necrosis of the femoral head that occurs in juvenile small dogs, particularly the terrier breeds. Commonly affected breeds include the Miniature Poodle and West Highland White, Cairn, Manchester and Yorkshire Terriers (Ljunggren, 1967; Lee and Fry, 1969; Piek *et al.*, 1996). Both sexes are affected equally and the condition is usually unilateral. A multifactorial inheritance pattern consistent with an autosomal recessive gene with high heritability has been demonstrated in the Manchester (Vasseur *et al.*, 1989) and West Highland White Terriers (Robinson, 1992) and has been suggested in other breeds (Robinson, 1992).

Aetiopathogenesis

Despite the evidence to support a genetic basis, the exact cause of the disease is unknown. The vascular supply to the femoral head is derived from epiphyseal vessels that enter the epiphysis along the borders of the joint capsule. A temporary vascular compromise, rather than permanent vascular destruction, is suspected. Histological changes can be divided into three stages. The initial necrotic stage is followed by a partial attempt to repair the necrotic bone by a process of bone resorption/bone formation known as 'creeping substitution'. This results in local failure to provide support to the subchondral bone and the subsequent articular cartilage collapse. The loss of normal articular congruency rapidly leads to development of secondary osteoarthritis.

Clinical signs

Affected dogs usually become lame when they are between 4 and 11 months of age. Sudden-onset lameness may be reported but animals present more commonly with a history of progressive lameness of 1–2 months' duration. Intermittent non-weightbearing lameness is often noted on visual inspection. Manipulation of the hip almost inevitably results in a marked pain response, especially when extension or abduction are attempted. A reduction in the range of motion and crepitus is often noted, especially in more chronic cases where there is established periarticular fibrosis. Varying degrees of gluteal muscle atrophy resulting in a prominent greater trochanter may also be detected.

Diagnosis

The presumptive diagnosis should be confirmed following radiographic examination. A VD extended view of the pelvis is usually sufficient. Initial radiographic signs include areas of reduced radiodensity within the femoral head and neck, and a widened, often irregular, joint space. Deformity of the epiphysis resulting in a grossly abnormal femoral head, sclerosis and thickening of the femoral neck, as well as marked joint incongruency, are noted in more advanced cases (Figure 21.10). These changes are almost pathognomonic. Femoral neck fractures, acetabular remodelling, flattening of the femoral head and periarticular new bone formation can be detected in more chronic cases.

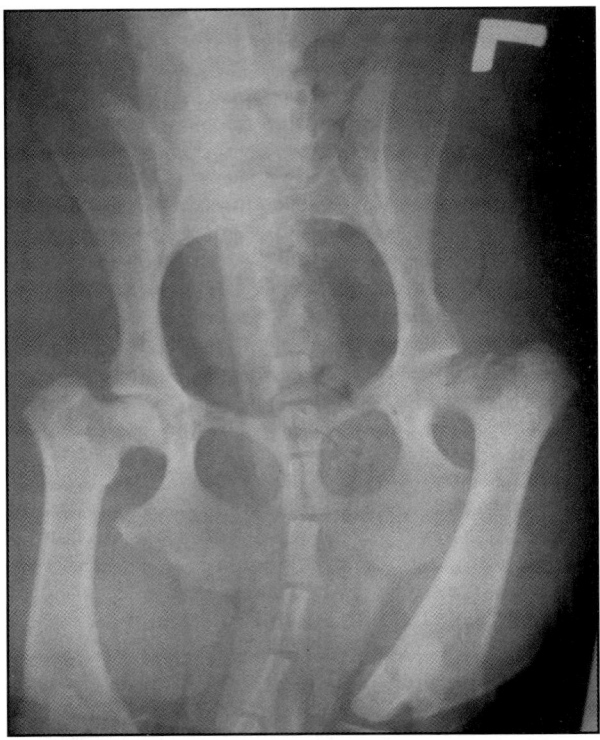

21.10 VD extended radiograph of a 10-month-old West Highland White Terrier with unilateral Legg–Calvé–Perthes disease. The femoral head is collapsed and the articular surface is irregular.

Management

Conservative management is an option for dogs with very mild lameness and minimal radiographic changes, and can result in an excellent functional outcome. Strict rest and the use of analgesics may allow a successful repair and the preservation of joint integrity.

Surgical management with an FHNE arthroplasty (see Operative Technique 21.7) is recommended as the treatment of choice in dogs with marked lameness and advanced radiographic changes, or in dogs that fail to respond to conservative treatment within the first 4 weeks (Piek et al., 1996). The result of the surgery is influenced by the postoperative rehabilitation. Early, active limb use should be encouraged with the use of appropriate analgesia, active physiotherapy techniques and swimming. The prognosis for return to normal function is good to excellent with adequate surgical technique and if an adequate postoperative regimen is followed. Intermittent lameness may be a feature in dogs treated conservatively. Affected animals should not be used for breeding.

Feline metaphyseal osteopathy

It appears that cats may be more likely to have avascular necrosis of the femoral neck, rather than the femoral head. This disorder, termed femoral neck metaphyseal osteopathy, has been reported to occur in male cats less than 2 years of age (Queen et al., 1998). The disease has been characterized clinically by a subtle lameness, which acutely progresses to a severe lameness. Radiographically, radiolucency and loss of definition in the proximal femoral metaphysis are noted. The problem can be unilateral or bilateral. FHNE arthroplasty (see Operative Technique 21.7) was reported to be successful in resolving the lameness in all cases in one study (Queen et al., 1998). Successful non-surgical management of this disorder has not been reported to the authors' knowledge.

Epiphysiolysis

Epiphysiolysis is an idiopathic condition of the hip joint that has been reported in cats and dogs (Dupuis et al., 1997; Craig, 2001; Burke, 2003). The syndrome is defined as separation of the proximal femoral epiphysis that is not associated with trauma. In cats, the problem may be associated with gender (males), obesity and breed (Siamese) (Craig, 2001; Burke, 2003). Both cases reported in dogs were in male Shetland Sheepdogs that were affected bilaterally (Dupuis et al., 1997). Diagnosis is based on clinically localized hip lameness and radiographic evidence of slipped capital physis, with focal osteopenia and femoral neck sclerosis. Histologically, the physis is open, with evidence of chondrodysplasia, osteoclastic resorption and/or fibrous tissue proliferation.

Surgical management is recommended in the majority of clinically affected cases. Surgical repair using Kirschner wires has been proposed for immature animals if there are minimal changes within the femoral neck and surgical reduction is possible (Moores et al., 2004). It may not be possible to identify the line of separation, and surgical stabilization may have to be performed 'blindly', especially in dogs with minimal displacement of the epiphysis. In the majority of cases, however, secondary changes preclude the use of such techniques and therefore surgical options are limited to salvage techniques, such as total hip replacement (see Operative Techniques 21.8 and 21.9) (if the animal is mature enough to allow for this) or FHNE arthroplasty (see Operative Technique 21.7).

Conservative management may allow spontaneous healing in minimally displaced cases; while this may lead to the development of secondary osteoarthritis, it may be an option for dogs with very mild clinical signs, with the option of performing a total hip replacement at a later date if the secondary osteoarthritis leads to a significant clinical problem.

Coxofemoral luxation

Luxation of the coxofemoral joint is the most common luxation in dogs and cats (Johnston et al., 1994), accounting for 39–90% of all luxations reported. Luxation of the hip requires a traumatic incident in the majority of cases. Road traffic accidents are the most common cause, although falls and a variety of other incidents such as slipping, twisting of the limb and playing with other dogs have also been reported (Basher et al., 1986). Affected animals are usually over 1 year of age, as the force that would cause a luxation in the mature animal is more likely to cause a fracture of the proximal femoral physis in the skeletally immature animal. 'Spontaneous', non-traumatic luxations can occur in dogs with hip dysplasia and marked joint laxity with or without secondary osteoarthritic changes (Trostel et al., 2000). Bilateral luxations are uncommon.

Luxation of the femoral head in a craniodorsal direction represents approximately 90% of all luxations, although in some instances the femoral head is dislocated in a caudodorsal or in a ventral direction. Ventral luxations are thought to be more painful due to direct compression of the obturator nerve as the femoral head rests within the obturator foramen.

Clinical signs and examination

Affected animals are presented with a variable degree of lameness, from moderate to non-weightbearing. Dogs with a craniodorsal luxation will usually present with the stifle externally rotated. The greater trochanter is quite prominent and there is an increased distance between the ischiatic tuberosity and the greater trochanter. The limb appears shorter when extended caudally. Pain and crepitus may be detected if manipulation of the hip is performed. Manipulation of the hip may not be possible in dogs with severe pain. A 'thumb' displacement test has been described in order to establish the presence of a luxation. A thumb firmly placed in the soft tissue depression caudal to the greater trochanter will be displaced in the intact hip when outward rotation of the femur is performed and will not be displaced in the case of a coxofemoral luxation.

Dogs with a caudodorsal luxation will show a gentle internal rotation of the stifle. The limb appears slightly longer and the distance between the greater trochanter and the ischiatic tuberosity will be reduced. In dogs with a ventral luxation, the greater trochanter is difficult to locate and the limb is held in slight abduction. Dogs with bilateral luxations will not be able to stand and the appearance may mimic that of spinal conditions, such as intervertebral disc disease.

Chapter 21 The hip

Diagnosis

VD and lateral radiographs of the pelvis should be obtained prior to attempting reduction, to evaluate the direction of the luxation and the possibility of avulsion fractures of the teres ligament as well as to assess other possible concomitant fractures within the pelvis (including acetabular fractures), as these are likely to compromise hip stability (Figure 21.11). In addition, the presence of secondary changes consistent with pre-existing osteoarthritis should be evaluated. Careful assessment will be required to detect small bone fragments within the acetabulum in cases of avulsion fractures of the teres ligament.

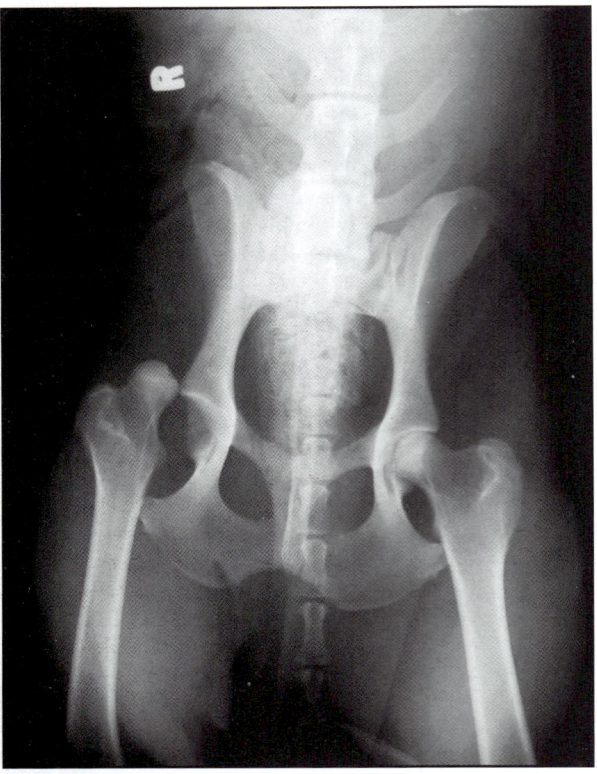

21.11 VD radiograph of the pelvis, showing a right craniodorsal coxofemoral luxation secondary to an avulsion of the teres ligament. Two small fragments within the acetabulum are present and abnormal femoral head morphology is evident.

Treatment

The choice of treatment depends on the presence of pre-existing disease, duration of the luxation and other complicating factors, such as concomitant orthopaedic injuries. Management options can be divided into:

- Closed reduction with or without augmented stabilization using an Ehmer sling; ischial–ilial pin or an external skeletal fixator
- Open reduction and stabilization techniques, such as capsulorrhaphy, ilial–femoral suture, transarticular pinning, hip toggle, anchored extracapsular technique with or without distal transposition of the greater trochanter, TPO
- Salvage options, such as FHNE arthroplasty and total hip replacement.

The majority (90%) of traumatic luxations of the hip joint are craniodorsal in direction. As such, the majority of surgical techniques that have been developed are aimed at this type of luxation. There are many reported techniques for hip luxation and the techniques discussed in this chapter are those that are considered most popular and have been used with success by the authors.

Closed reduction and conservative management

Closed reduction is often possible with recent traumatic luxations. Reduction is best performed as soon as possible after injury, once the patient is stabilized. If a luxation has been present for longer than 7–10 days, closed reduction is unlikely to be successful. Closed manipulation should be performed under general anaesthesia.

Craniodorsal luxation: Closed reduction of a craniodorsal luxation is accomplished with the patient in lateral recumbency with the injured limb uppermost. The animal's hindquarters are secured to the table with a rope tie. Traction on the femur and manipulation of the femoral head will counteract muscle contraction. The leg is then extended, adducted and externally rotated with continued traction to lift the femoral head over the dorsal rim of the acetabulum and reduce the hip. Once reduced, the hip is manipulated and checked for range of motion and stability.

> **PRACTICAL TIP**
> **Radiography should be undertaken to document the reduction.**

If the dog's conformation and temperament allow, an Ehmer sling (Figure 21.12) may be applied for 10–14 days and a conservative management protocol followed. The majority of craniodorsal luxations can be treated in this way, although this approach may fail. Reasons for failure include interposed soft tissue between the femoral head and acetabulum, and hip dysplasia.

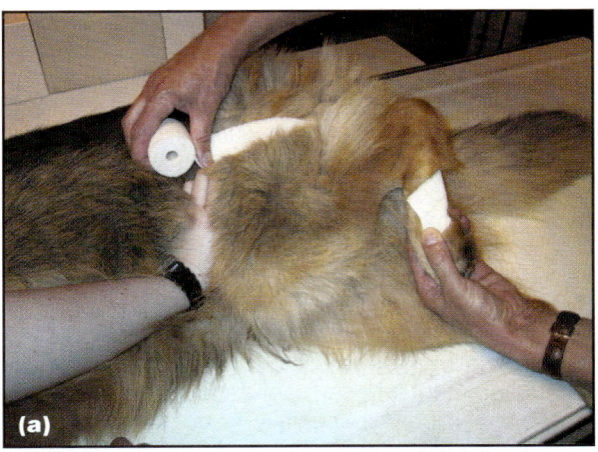

21.12 Application of an Ehmer sling. **(a)** Adhesive dressing material is placed caudal to the metatarsus and passed medial to the tarsus to cross the crus caudocranially. (continues) ▶

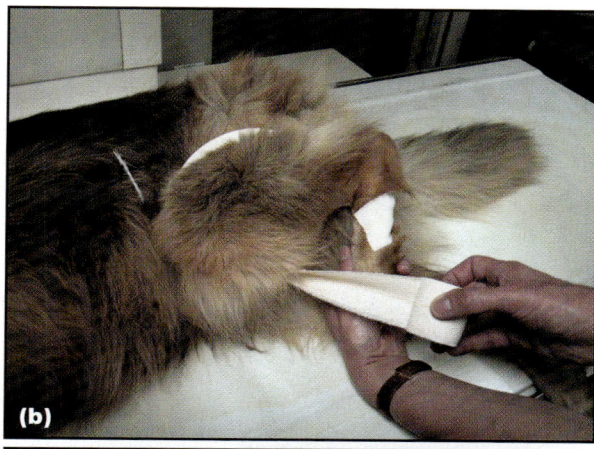

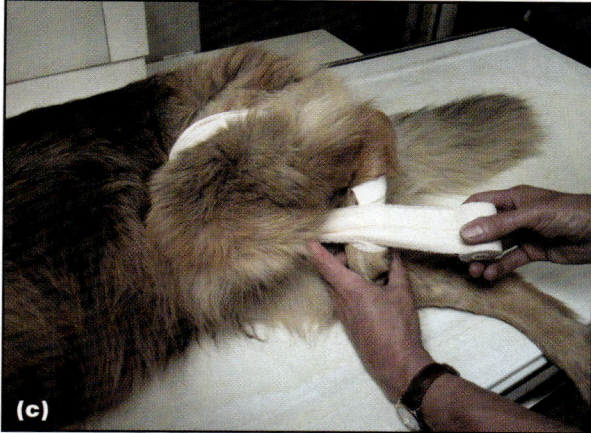

Chapter 21 The hip

Preoperative assessment of the pelvis and hip is extremely important prior to surgical treatment of a luxation. Key points to consider are:

- The direction of luxation
- Other pelvic injuries that may influence the choice of technique
- The presence and severity of any hip dysplasia; a dysplastic hip may be more inherently likely to reluxate and this may influence the choice of technique. Some surgeons will consider TPO or THA in such circumstances, but this may depend on other factors such as age, history and economics
- The presence of any avulsion or chip fractures of the femoral head
- The age of the patient. Skeletally immature dogs that suffer luxation are at risk of ischaemic necrosis of the femoral head if the capsular blood supply has been compromised.

Three techniques commonly employed for craniodorsal luxation are: capsulorrhaphy (prosthetic capsule); transarticular pinning; and the hip toggle. Although there are published reports of each of these techniques, there are few comparative data to suggest which is superior (Evers *et al.*, 1997) and choice is made on the basis of the surgeon's preference and familiarity with the technique.

Capsulorrhaphy (Operative Technique 21.10): This involves placement of horizontal mattress sutures across the craniodorsal aspect of the joint to limit excursion of the femoral head. The sutures are anchored on the dorsal acetabulum at 10 o'clock and 1 o'clock for the left hip and 11 o'clock and 2 o'clock for the right hip. Implants suitable for anchorage of the sutures include suture anchors or a combination of bone screw and spiked washer (see Chapter 14). Suture anchors have the advantage of a low profile and ease of insertion. The dorsal approach is usually used for capsulorrhaphy and thus this technique requires a more involved surgical approach and greater operative time. However, if applied correctly, it has few complications.

Transarticular pinning (Operative Technique 21.11): This involves temporary placement of a Kirschner wire or Steinmann pin across the joint space, travelling up the femoral neck, exiting the femoral head at the fovea capitis and entering the acetabulum at the acetabular fossa. As the femoral head is luxated, the pin can be introduced retrograde from the fovea capitis down the femoral neck to exit the lateral aspect of the proximal femur and then normograde through the acetabulum after femoral head relocation. The pin is left in place for 3–4 weeks and then removed. The pin can be applied through a craniodorsal approach and the procedure is relatively simple, but complications can occur (pin breakage, migration, femoral neck fracture) (Bennett and Duff, 1980; Hunt and Henry, 1985; Julier-Franz *et al.*, 2002). A disadvantage is the necessity for a second minor surgery to remove the pin.

21.12 (continued) Application of an Ehmer sling. **(b)** The bandage is passed medial to the stifle. **(c)** The bandage is passed lateral to the metatarsus to meet the start of the dressing. This process is repeated several times and finally, the whole limb can be wrapped to encase the Ehmer sling.

Other luxations:

- Cranioventral luxations are usually manipulated to the craniodorsal position and reduced as described above
- Ventral luxations are reduced by leverage on the femur by placing a sandbag between the thighs and using this to lever the femoral head back into the acetabulum.
- Caudal luxations can usually be manipulated back to the acetabulum although open reduction may be necessary; soft hobbles fashioned from self-adherent non-adhesive wrap (e.g. Vetwrap) can be used to prevent abduction in the 7–10 days following reduction.

Open reduction and surgical management
Surgical management is indicated when:

- Closed reduction is not possible
- The patient has a temperament or conformation (e.g. chondrodystrophoid, well muscled) that makes use of an Ehmer sling difficult or inadvisable
- The hip is unstable following closed reduction
- There is recurrent luxation after failed conservative treatment.

321

Chapter 21 The hip

Hip toggle (Operative Technique 21.12): The toggle technique is used to create a prosthetic teres ligament. The toggle pin anchors a suture behind a drill hole in the acetabular fossa and this suture then passes through a drill hole in the femoral head, along the femoral neck and is tied laterally with the use of a transverse drill hole to lock one of the suture strands. The hip toggle can be performed through a caudal approach. Since the internal obturator and gemelli muscles are often torn because of the craniodorsal luxation, this is relatively simple. Closed fluoroscopically guided toggling has also been reported in dogs (Serdy *et al.*, 1999).

A toggle pin can be fashioned from a twisted 0.9 mm Kirschner wire (Piermattei, 1965), or a toggle rod can be fashioned from a 3.2 mm Steinmann pin (Flynn *et al.*, 1994). It also possible to purchase dedicated implants with inserters. Mechanical testing failed to show significant advantage of pin or rod (Baltzer *et al.*, 2001). The suture used to create the prosthetic ligament can vary. Mechanical testing (cyclic) indicated that woven polyester had the longest fatigue life and may be a preferred material (Baltzer *et al.*, 2001) although the risk of persistent infection with multifilament sutures may be greater (Varma *et al.*, 1974, 1981); high-breaking-strain monofilament nylon is an alternative suture material.

Prognosis
The prognosis following hip luxation is usually good, although Evers *et al.* (1997) reported that 6 of 23 dogs were lame at a minimum of 8 months follow-up. Development or progression of osteoarthritis in the affected hip is also apparently quite common.

von Willebrand's heterotopic osteochondrofibrosis

von Willebrand's heterotopic osteochondrofibrosis is an uncommon cause of lameness. It has been described predominantly in the Dobermann, although it has also been reported in the German Shepherd Dog and the St Bernard (Layton and Ferguson, 1987; Dueland *et al.*, 1990; Janssens *et al.*,1993). Affected animals are presented with a chronic progressive moderate to severe pelvic limb lameness of insidious onset. Muscle atrophy is usually a feature. The range of hip extension is reduced and pain is usually detected on manipulation of the hip. A palpable mass is sometimes detected caudal and dorsal to the greater trochanter.

The disease is characterized by the development of a soft tissue mass (later calcified) involving the muscles caudal to the hip (mainly gemelli and internal and external obturator muscles). It is thought that minor trauma or spontaneous bleeding leads to focal myopathy. Chondro-osseous tissue is formed following initial fibrosis. Affected animals should test positive for von Willebrand's disease.

The diagnosis may prove challenging in the early stages as there are no radiographic abnormalities. With time, a mild periosteal reaction can usually be detected affecting the ischium and proximal femur. A calcified mass of variable size may be present in the more chronic cases (Figure 21.13b). MRI may be useful to obtain an early diagnosis prior to the development of bony changes.

Surgical resection of the mass to allow restoration of the hip range of movement should be considered in cases that fail to respond to conservative treatment. The use of corticosteroids following surgery has been suggested although information is anecdotal. The owner should be warned of the possibility of recurrence.

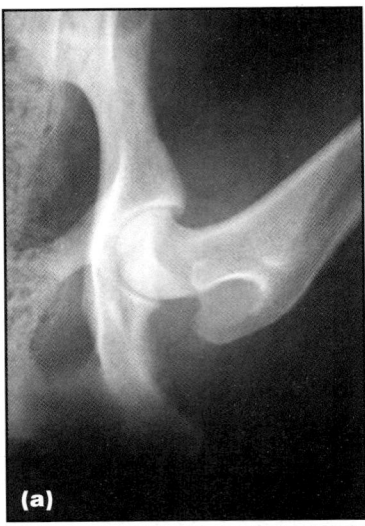

21.13 (a) VD flexed view of the pelvis of a 4-year-old Dobermann with early signs of von Willebrand's heterotopic osteochondrofibrosis. Note the irregular outline of the lateral aspect of the ischium. **(b)** Mediolateral view of a 6-year-old Dobermann with marked mineralization of the soft tissues caudal and distal to the region of the hip.

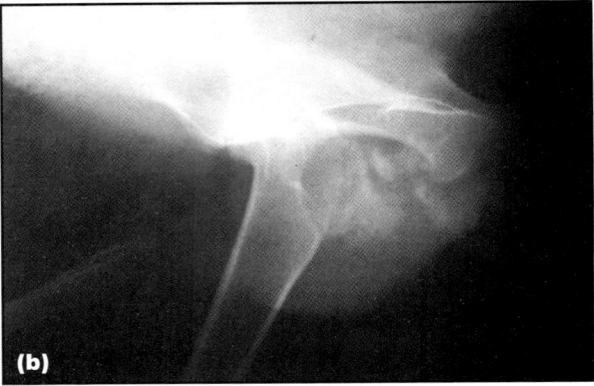

References and further reading

Adams WM, Dueland RT, Daniels R, Fialkowski JP and Nordheim EV (2000) Comparison of two palpation, four radiographic and three ultrasound methods for early detection of mild to moderate canine hip dysplasia. *Veterinary Radiology and Ultrasound* **41**, 484–490

Baltzer WI, Schulz KS, Stover SM, Taylor KT and Kass PH (2001) Biomechanical analysis of suture anchors and suture materials used for toggle pin stabilization of hip joint luxation in dogs. *American Journal of Veterinary Research* **62**, 721–728

Barden JW and Hardwick H (1968) New observations on the diagnosis and cause of hip dysplasia. *Veterinary Medicine Small Animal Clinic* **63**, 238

Barlow TG (1962) Early diagnosis and treatment of congenital dislocation of the hip. *British Journal of Bone and Joint Surgery* **44**, 292

Barr ARS, Denny HR and Gibbs C (1987) Clinical hip dysplasia in dogs: the long term results of conservative management. *Journal of Small Animal Practice* **28**, 243–252

Basher AWP, Walter MC and Newton CD (1986) Coxofemoral luxation in the dog and cat. *Veterinary Surgery* **15(5)**, 356–362

Bennett D and Duff SR (1980) Transarticular pinning as a treatment for hip luxation in the dog and cat. *Journal of Small Animal Practice* **21**, 373–379

Berzon JL, Howard PE, Covell SJ *et al.* (1980) A retrospective study of the efficacy of femoral head and neck excision in 94 dogs and cats. *Veterinary Surgery* **9**, 88–92

Biery DN (2006) The hip joint and pelvis. In: *BSAVA Manual of Canine and Feline Musculoskeletal Imaging*, ed. F Barr and R Kirberger, pp. 119–134. BSAVA Publications, Gloucester

Borostyankoi F, Rooks RL, Kobluk CN, Reed AL and Littledike ET (2003) Results of single-session bilateral triple pelvic osteotomy with an eight-hole iliac bone plate in dogs: 95 cases (1996–1999). *Journal of the American Veterinary Medical Association* **222**, 54–59

Budsberg SC, Chambers JN, Lue SL, Foutz TL and Reece L (1996) Prospective evaluation of ground reaction forces in dogs undergoing unilateral total hip replacement. *American Journal of Veterinary Research* **57**, 1781–1785

Burke J (2003) Physeal dysplasia with slipped capital femoral epiphysis in a cat. *Canadian Veterinary Journal* **44**, 238–239

Chalman JA and Butler HC (1985) Coxofemoral joint laxity and the Ortolani sign. *Journal of the American Animal Hospital Association* **21**, 671

Craig LE (2001) Physeal dysplasia with slipped capital femoral epiphysis in 13 cats. *Veterinary Pathology* **38**, 92–97

Cook JL, Tomlinson JL and Constantinescu GM (1996) Pathophysiology, diagnosis, and treatment of canine hip dysplasia. *Compendium on Continuing Education for the Practicing Veterinarian* **18**, 853–867

Dejardin LM, Perry RL and Arnoczky SP (1998) The effect of triple pelvic osteotomy on the articular contact area of the hip joint in dysplastic dogs: an in vitro experimental study. *Veterinary Surgery* **27**, 194–202

Dueland RT, Adams WM, Fialkowski JP, Patricelli AJ, Mathews KG and Nordheim EV (2001) Effects of pubic symphysiodesis in dysplastic puppies. *Veterinary Surgery* **30**, 210–217

Dueland RT, Wagner SD and Parker RB (1990) von Willebrand heterotopic osteochondrofibrosis in Doberman pinschers: five cases (1980-1987). *Journal of the American Veterinary Medical Association* **197**, 383–388

Duff R and Campbell JR (1977) Long-term results of excision arthroplasty of the canine hip. *Veterinary Record* **101**, 181–184

Dupuis J, Breton L and Drolet R (1997) Bilateral epiphysiolysis of the femoral heads in two dogs. *Journal of the American Veterinary Medical Association* **210**, 1162–1165

Edwards MR, Egger EL and Schwarz PD (1997) Aseptic loosening of the femoral implant after cemented total hip arthroplasty in dogs: 11 cases in 10 dogs (1991–1995). *Journal of the American Veterinary Medical Association* **211**, 580–586

Evers P, Johnston GR, Wallace LJ, Lipowitz AJ and King VL (1997) Long-term results of treatment of traumatic coxofemoral joint dislocation in dogs: 64 cases (1973–1992). *Journal of the American Veterinary Medical Association* **210**, 59–64

Farese JP, Todhunter RJ, Lust G, Williams AJ and Dykes NL (1998) Dorsolateral subluxation of hip joints in dogs measured in a weight-bearing position with radiography and computed tomography. *Veterinary Surgery* **27**, 393–405

Fluckiger MA, Friedrich GA and Binder H (1999) A radiographic stress technique for evaluation of coxofemoral joint laxity in dogs. *Veterinary Surgery* **28**, 1–9

Flynn MF, Edmiston DN, Roe SC, Richardson DC, Deyoung DJ and Abrams CF (1994) Biomechanical evaluation of a toggle pin technique for management of coxofemoral luxation. *Veterinary Surgery* **23**, 311–321

Gendreau C (1977) Excision of the femoral head and neck: the long-term results of 35 operations. *Journal of the American Animal Hospital Association* **13**, 605–608

Hunt CA and Henry WB (1985) Transarticular pinning for repair of hip dislocation in the dog – a retrospective study of 40 cases. *Journal of the American Veterinary Medical Association* **187**, 828–833

Impellizeri JA, Tetrick MA and Muir P (2000) Effect of weight reduction on clinical signs of lameness in dogs with hip osteoarthritis. *Journal of the American Veterinary Medical Association* **216**, 1089–1091

Janssens LAA, Ramon FA, De Schepper AMA and Van Bree H (1993) A case of degenerative myopathy of the obturator externus muscle in a dog. *Veterinary and Comparative Orthopaedics and Traumatology* **6**, 66–69

Johnston JA, Austin C and Breuer CJ (1994) Incidence of canine appendicular musculoskeletal disorders in 126 veterinary teaching hospitals from 1980 through 1989. *Veterinary and Comparative Orthopaedics and Traumatology* **7**, 56–59

Julier-Franz A, Kramer M, Schleicher S, Gerwing M, Schimke E and Tacke S (2002) The surgical treatment of the coxofemoral luxation with a transarticular pin in dogs and cats. *Kleintierpraxis* **47**, 221–230

Kapatkin AS, Mayhew PD and Smith GK (2002) Genetic control of canine hip dysplasia. *Compendium of Veterinary Education* **24**, 681–689

Kealy RD, Lawler DF, Ballam JM, Lust G, Smith GK, Biery DN and Olsson SE (1997) Five-year longitudinal study on limited food consumption and development of osteoarthritis in coxofemoral joints of dogs. *Journal of the American Veterinary Medical Association* **210(2)**, 222–225

Kealy RD, Olsson SE, Monti KL, Lawler DF, Biery DN, Helms RW, Lust G and Smith GK (1992) Effects of limited food consumption on the incidence of hip dysplasia in growing dogs. *Journal of the American Veterinary Medical Association* **201(6)**, 857–863

Keller GG, Reed AL, Lattimer JC and Corley EA (1999) Hip dysplasia: a feline population study. *Veterinary Radiology and Ultrasound* **40**, 460–464

Kinzel S, Hein S, von Scheven C and Kupper W (2002) 10 years' experience with denervation of the hip joint capsule for treatment of canine hip joint dysplasia and arthrosis. [article in German]. *Berliner und Münchener Tierarztliche Wochenschrift* **115**, 53–56

LaFond E, Breur GJ and Austin CC (2002) Breed susceptibility for developmental orthopaedic diseases in dogs. *Journal of the American Animal Hospital Association* **38**, 467–477

Layton CE and Ferguson HR (1987) Lameness associated with coxofemoral soft tissue masses in six dogs. *Veterinary Surgery* **16**, 21–24

Lee R and Fry PD (1969) Some observations in the occurrence of Legg-Calvé-Perthes disease (coxa plana) in the dog, and an evaluation of excision arthroplasty as a method of treatment. *Journal of Small Animal Practice* **10**, 309

Ljunggren GL (1967) Legg-Perthes in the dog. *Acta Orthopaedica Scandinavica* **95**, 1

Lussier B, Lanthier T and Martineau-Doize B (1994) Evaluation of biocompatible osteoconductive polymer shelf arthroplasty for the surgical correction of hip dysplasia in normal dogs. *Canadian Journal of Veterinary Research* **58**, 173–180

Lust G, Rendano VT and Summers BA (1985) Canine hip dysplasia: concepts and diagnosis. *Journal of the American Veterinary Medical Association* **187(6)**, 638–640

Mann FA, Tangner CH, Wagner-Mann C et al. (1987) A comparison of standard femoral head and neck excision and femoral head and neck excision using a biceps femoris muscle flap in the dog. *Veterinary Surgery* **16**, 223–230

Marcellin-Little DJ, DeYoung BA, Doyens DH and DeYoung DJ (1999) Canine uncemented porous-coated anatomic total hip arthroplasty: results of a long-term prospective evaluation of 50 consecutive cases. *Veterinary Surgery* **28**, 10–20

Mathews KG, Stover SM and Kass PH (1996) Effect of pubic symphysiodesis on acetabular rotation and pelvic development in guinea pigs. *American Journal of Veterinary Research* **57**, 427–433

Montavon PM (1998) Alternatives in the treatment of coxarthrosis in dogs: pectineomyectomy, tenotomy of the iliopsoas and neurectomy of the joint capsule (PIN) as a symptomatic treatment for coxarthrosis. *Proceedings of the 4th FECAVA/SCIVAC Congress 1998*, pp.303–304

Moores AP, Owen MR, Fews D, Coe RJ, Brown PJ and Butterworth SJ (2004) Slipped capital femoral epiphysis in dogs. *Journal of Small Animal Practice* **45**, 602–608

Olmstead ML (1995) Canine cemented total hip replacements: state of the art. *Journal of Small Animal Practice* **36**, 395–399

Olmstead ML, Hohn RB and Turner TM (1983) A five-year study of 221 total hip replacements in the dog. *Journal of the American Veterinary Medical Association* **183**, 191–194

Patricelli AJ, Dueland RT, Adams WM, Fialkowski JP, Linn KA and Nordheim EV (2002) Juvenile pubic symphysiodesis in dysplastic puppies at 15 and 20 weeks of age. *Veterinary Surgery* **31**, 435–444

Patricelli AJ, Dueland RT, Lu Y, Fialkowski JP and Mathews KG (2001) Canine pubic symphysiodesis: investigation of electrocautery dose response by histologic examination and temperature measurement. *Veterinary Surgery* **30**, 261–268

Piek CJ, Hazewinkel HA, Wolvekamp WT, Nap RC and Mey BP (1996) Long-term follow-up of avascular necrosis of the femoral head in the dog. *Journal of Small Animal Practice* **37(1)**, 12–18

Piermattei D (1965) Fabrication of an improved toggle pin. *Veterinary Medicine and Small Animal Clinician* **60**, 384–389

Prostredney JM, Toombs JP and Van Sickle DC (1991) Effect of two muscle sling techniques on early morbidity after femoral head and neck excision in dogs. *Veterinary Surgery* **20**, 298–305

Queen J, Bennett D, Carmichael S, Gibson N, Li A, Payne-Johnson CE and Kelly DF (1998) Femoral neck metaphyseal osteopathy in the cat. *Veterinary Record* **142**, 159–162

Rettenmeier JL, Keller GG, Lattimer JC, Corley EA and Ellersieck MR (2002) Prevalence of canine hip dysplasia in a veterinary teaching hospital population. *Veterinary Radiology and Ultrasound* **43**, 313–318

Robinson R (1992) Legg-Calvé-Perthes disease in dogs: genetic aetiology. *Journal of Small Animal Practice* **33**, 275

Schulz KS (2000) Application of arthroplasty principles to canine cemented total hip replacement. *Veterinary Surgery* **29**, 578–593

Chapter 21 The hip

Serdy MG, Schulz KS, Hornof W, Koehler C, Chiu D and Vasseur PB (1999) Closed toggle pinning for canine traumatic coxofemoral luxation. *Veterinary and Comparative Orthopaedics and Traumatology* **12**, 6–14

Skurla CT, Egger EL, Schwarz PD and James SP (2000) Owner assessment of the outcome of total hip arthroplasty in dogs. *Journal of the American Veterinary Medical Association* **217**, 1010–1012

Smith GK, Biery DN and Gregor TP (1990) New concepts of coxofemoral joint stability and the development of a clinical stress-radiographic method for quantitating hip joint laxity in the dog. *Journal of the American Veterinary Medical Association* **96(1)**, 59–70

Smith GK, Gregor TP, Rhodes WH, and Biery DN (1993) Coxofemoral joint laxity from distraction radiography and its contemporaneous and prospective correlation with laxity, subjective score, and evidence of degenerative joint disease from conventional hip-extended radiography in dogs *American Journal of Veterinary Research* **54**, 1021–1042

Smith GK, Popovitch CA, Gregor TP and Shofer FS (1995) Evaluation of risk factors for degenerative joint disease associated with hip dysplasia in dogs. *Journal of the American Veterinary Medical Association* **206**, 642–647

Swainson SW, Conzemius MG, Riedesel EA, Smith GK and Riley CB (2000) Effect of pubic symphysiodesis on pelvic development in the skeletally immature greyhound. *Veterinary Surgery* **29**, 178–190

Trostel CD, Peck JN and deHaan JJ (2000) Spontaneous bilateral coxofemoral luxation in four dogs. *Journal of the American Animal Hospital Association* **36**, 268–276

Tomlinson JL and Cook JL (2002) Effects of degree of acetabular rotation after triple pelvic osteotomy on the position of the femoral head in relationship to the acetabulum. *Veterinary Surgery* **31**, 398–403

Varma S, Ferguson HL, Breen H and Lumb WV (1974) Comparison of 7 suture materials in infected wounds – experimental study. *Journal of Surgical Research* **17**, 165–170

Varma S, Johnson LW, Ferguson HL and Lumb WV (1981) Tissue reaction to suture materials in infected surgical wounds – a histopathologic evaluation. *American Journal of Veterinary Research* **42**, 563–570

Vasseur PB, Foley P, Stevenson S and Heitter D (1989) Mode of inheritance of Perthes' disease in Manchester terriers. *Clinical Orthopaedics* **244**, 281–292

Wood JLN and Lakhani KH (2003) Hip dysplasia in Labrador retrievers: the effects of age at scoring. *Veterinary Record* **152(2)**, 37–40

Wood JL, Lakhani KH and Henley WE (2004) An epidemiological approach to prevention and control of three common heritable diseases in canine pedigree breeds in the United Kingdom. *Veterinary Journal* **68**, 14–27

OPERATIVE TECHNIQUE 21.1
Hip arthroscopy

Positioning
Lateral recumbency, affected limb uppermost.

Assistant
Not essential.

Tray extras
1.9 mm, 2.4 mm or 2.7 mm 30-degree foreoblique arthroscope with appropriate sleeve and blunt obturator; 1 litre lactated Ringer's (Hartmann's) fluid in positive-pressure infusor system and sterile giving set; light source; video camera and control box; monitor; image archiving system (e.g. VHS video, digital video, hard drive system); arthroscopy instruments: selection of cannulae, switching stick, hooked probe, biopsy forceps.

Surgical technique

> **WARNING**
> The hip joint is especially prone to iatrogenic damage to the articular cartilage during arthroscopic portal placement. Extreme care should be taken to distract the joint and use blunt obturators when establishing portals.

An 18–20 gauge spinal needle is placed at 12 o'clock just proximal to the greater trochanter. An assistant applies traction to the limb to aid insertion of this needle. Once the joint is penetrated, synovial fluid is aspirated to confirm the intra-articular location. 5–10 ml of Hartmann's is instilled to distend the joint. A no. 11 scalpel blade is used to make an entry site for the arthroscope sleeve. A sharp trocar is used to insert the sleeve through the soft tissues but it is replaced with a blunt obturator prior to capsular penetration. Once the capsule is penetrated, the obturator is removed and the arthroscope inserted. An egress portal is established at 5 o'clock (right hip) or 7 o'clock (left hip). If required, an instrument portal can be established at 2 o'clock (right hip; Figure 21.14) and 10 o'clock (left hip). The portals may be interchanged using switching sticks if necessary.

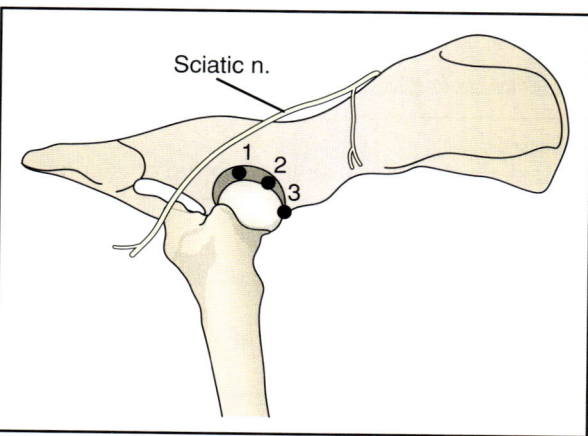

21.14 Position of portals for hip arthroscopy. 1: Arthroscope portal. 2: Instrument portal. 3: Egress portal.

> **PRACTICAL TIP**
> Distal traction placed on the limb by an assistant during needle and portal placement is very helpful in gaining access to the joint while avoiding iatrogenic damage to articular structures.

Complete exploration of the joint can be performed by moving the arthroscope and changing the direction of view with the 30-degree foreoblique 'scope. It is sensible to explore the hip joint (Figure 21.15) in a logical order, such as:

- Acetabulum (articular cartilage, acetabular fossa, ligament of the femoral head, joint capsule, transacetabular ligament, labrum)
- Femoral head articular cartilage.

Chapter 21 The hip

> # OPERATIVE TECHNIQUE 21.1 continued
> ## Hip arthroscopy
>
> **21.15** Arthroscopic images of the canine coxofemoral joint. **(a)** Normal coxofemoral joint, showing the acetabulum (a), acetabular fossa (af), teres ligament (tl) and femoral head (fh). **(b)** Full-thickness articular cartilage loss on the femoral head and pathology of the teres ligament and acetabular fossa. **(c)** Complete rupture of the teres ligament. **(d)** The acetabular labrum, with mild fibrillation, the acetabulum and the femoral head. **(e)** Partial tearing of the teres ligament.
>
> | **Closure** |
> |---|
> | The skin is closed with simple interrupted sutures. |
>
> | **Postoperative care** |
> |---|
> | Rest for 7 days. |
>
> | **Complications** |
> |---|
> | None reported, but iatrogenic injury to the sciatic nerve is theoretically possible if portals are placed too far caudally. |

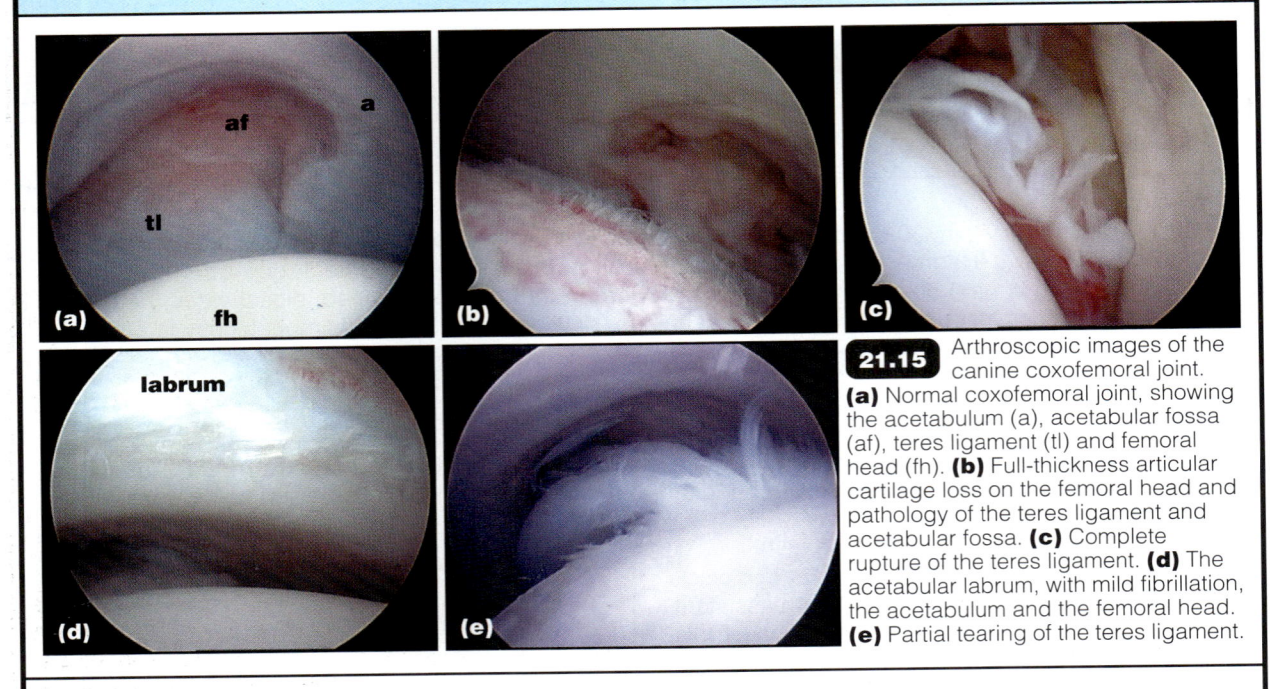

OPERATIVE TECHNIQUE 21.2
Craniodorsal approach to hip

Positioning
Lateral recumbency. A rope tie is used to anchor the patient to the table if intraoperative traction is required (e.g. in hip luxation). A vacuum bed is used if accurate pelvic positioning is necessary (e.g. total hip arthroplasty).

Assistant
Preferred but depends on indication for surgery.

Tray extras
Senn retractors; right-angled Gelpi retractors; large and small Weitlander retractors (or Myerding retractors if assistance available); periosteal elevator; Hohmann retractors.

Surgical technique
The skin incision is centred just cranial to the greater trochanter and can angle cranially or caudally at the proximal end. The incision passes distally and is aimed towards the patella to extend one-third of the length of the femur.

> **PRACTICAL TIP**
> For most procedures, the incision curves cranially at the proximal end but for total hip arthroplasty, it curves caudally to assist preparation of the femur.

The subcutaneous fascia and fat are dissected to reveal the superficial fascia lata. This is incised along the cranial margin of the biceps femoris muscle (Figure 21.16a). Retraction of the biceps femoris allows incision of the deep leaf of the fascia lata, thus freeing the insertion of the tensor fasciae latae muscle. This fascial incision extends proximally along the septum between the tensor muscle and the cranial margin of the superficial gluteal muscle.

> **PRACTICAL TIP**
> The incision in the fascia lata must extend distally for the entire length of the skin incision; otherwise exposure of the hip will be limited.

The fascia lata is retracted cranially and the biceps caudally to allow identification of the middle and deep gluteal tendons of insertion. The vastus lateralis is also identified laterally and the rectus femoris muscle medially. The deep gluteal tendon is separated by blunt dissection from the middle gluteal; it can be readily identified by its silvery tendinous appearance. Retraction of the middle gluteal allows an L-shaped tenotomy incision to be made in the deep gluteal tendon (Figure 21.16b). A stay suture is placed in the freed tendon and the tendon retracted. The joint capsule lies immediately beneath and the small articularis coxae muscle may be visible on the lateral aspect of the capsule.

The capsule is incised along the line of the femoral neck and the incision is extended to the origin of the vastus lateralis on the femoral neck and lesser trochanter. A periosteal elevator is used to elevate the origin of the vastus lateralis. The femoral head can be inspected by placement of intra-articular Hohmann retractors around the femoral neck (Figure 21.16c). External rotation of the hip, by holding the stifle, can also aid inspection.

→

Chapter 21 The hip

OPERATIVE TECHNIQUE 21.2 continued
Craniodorsal approach to hip

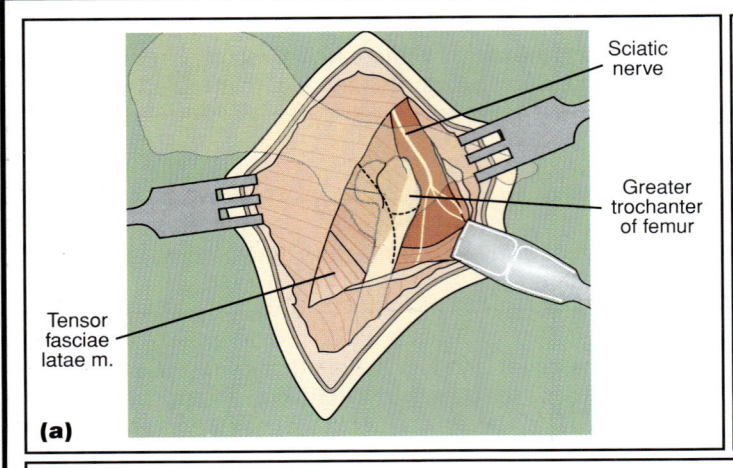

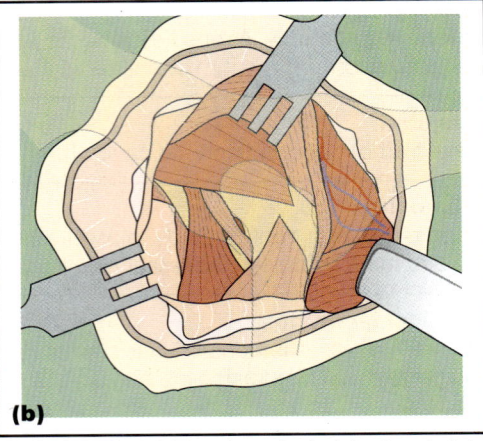

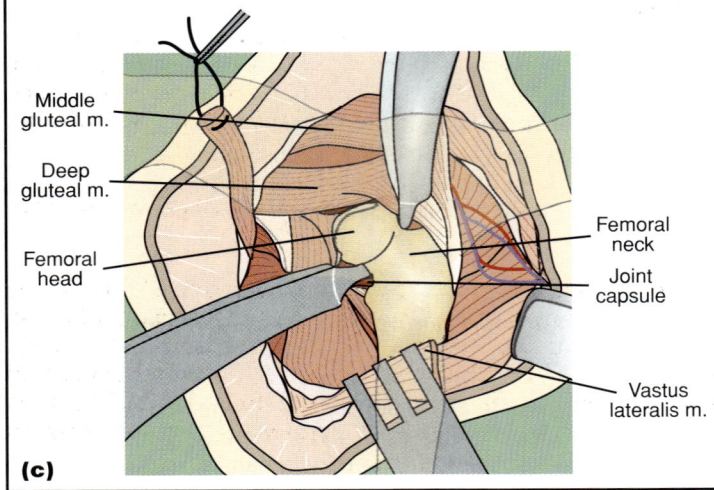

21.16 **(a)** The deep leaf of the fascia lata is incised and the incision curves cranioproximally between the superficial gluteal muscle and the tensor fasciae latae muscle. **(b)** The middle gluteal muscle is retracted using Myerding retractors and this exposes the tendon of insertion of the deep gluteal muscle. This silvery tendon is easily identified. An L-shaped tenotomy is made in the deep gluteal tendon to expose the joint capsule beneath (a stay suture in the transected tendon is useful for retraction). **(c)** The joint capsule is incised parallel to the neck of the femur. If necessary, the origin of the vastus lateralis is elevated from the periosteum of the lateral femur. External rotation of the limb allows inspection of the femoral head.

Closure
The joint capsule is repaired if possible as this will aid stability of the hip. The deep gluteal tenotomy is repaired with a three-loop pulley suture. The vastus lateralis muscle is then sutured to the deep gluteal tendon. The tensor fasciae latae muscle is repaired with continuous sutures and these extend to the superficial gluteal muscle proximally. The superficial fascia is closed to the cranial aspect of the biceps muscle in a similar fashion.

Postoperative care
See individual procedures. Generally: 4 weeks rest is sufficient, but this may be extended.

Complications
See individual procedures.

Chapter 21 The hip

OPERATIVE TECHNIQUE 21.3
Dorsal approach to the hip

Positioning
Lateral recumbency. A rope tie is used to anchor patient to the table if intra-operative traction is required (e.g. hip luxation).

Assistant
Preferred.

Tray extras
Senn retractors; right-angled Gelpi retractors; large and small Weitlander retractors (or Myerding retractors if assistance available); periosteal elevator; Hohmann retractors.

For trochanteric osteotomy and repair: oscillating saw (or osteotome and mallet, or Gigli wire); drill; Kirschner wires; orthopaedic wire; wire twisters; pin bender; pin/wire cutters. A lagged bone screw can be used instead of Kirschner wires and figure-of-eight tension band and appropriate instrumentation (drill bits, depth gauge, tap) will be required if that option is chosen.

Surgical technique
The skin incision is made as in Operative Technique 21.2.

The subcutaneous fascia and fat are dissected to reveal the superficial fascia lata. This is incised along the cranial margin of the biceps femoris muscle. Retraction of the biceps femoris allows incision of the deep leaf of the fascia lata, thus freeing the insertion of the tensor fasciae latae muscle. This fascial incision extends proximally along the septum between the tensor muscle and the cranial margin of the superficial gluteal muscle.

> **PRACTICAL TIP**
> The incision in the fascia lata must extend distally for the entire length of the skin incision; otherwise exposure of the hip will be limited.

The fascia lata is retracted cranially and the biceps caudally to allow identification of the sciatic nerve (see Figure 21.16a). The tendon of insertion of the superficial gluteal muscle is incised close to the third trochanter, leaving sufficient tissue to allow repair. Retraction of the superficial gluteal dorsally allows identification of the middle and deep gluteal tendons of insertion. The trochanteric osteotomy is started just proximal to the third trochanter and the angle of the cut is at 45 degrees to the long axis of the femur (Figure 21.17a,b). The cut is made with an oscillating saw, an osteotome or a Gigli wire. The middle and deep gluteal muscles are retracted proximally and the joint capsule is incised (Figure 21.17c).

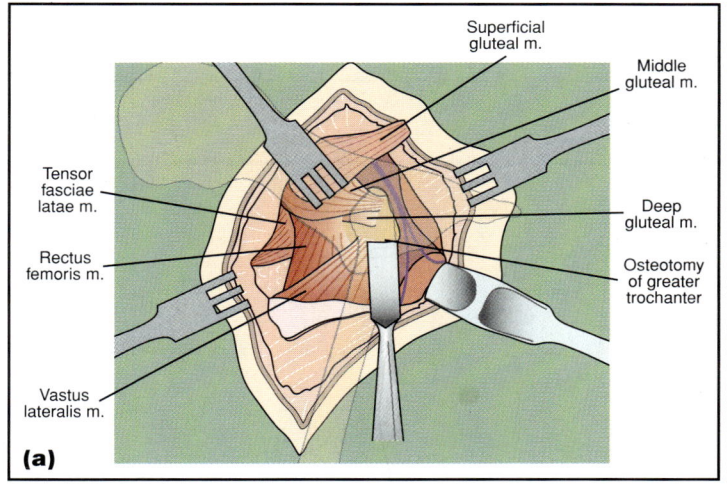

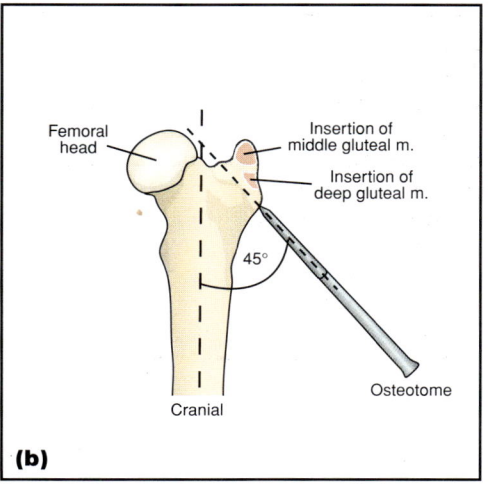

21.17 (a,b) A 45-degree osteotomy of the greater trochanter is performed. Care is taken to ensure sufficient bone stock in the proximal fragment and also to avoid the osteotomy being too distal. (continues)

329

Chapter 21 The hip

OPERATIVE TECHNIQUE 21.3 *continued*
Dorsal approach to the hip

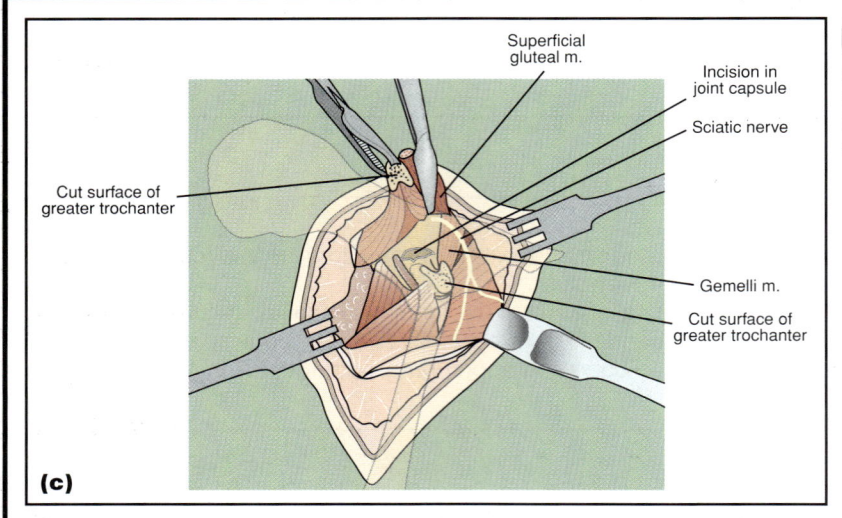

21.17 (continued) **(c)** The middle and deep gluteal muscles are retracted proximally with the osteotomized bone. The joint capsule is exposed and incised as appropriate.

(c)

> **PRACTICAL TIP**
> If an osteotome or oscillating saw is being used, a curved mosquito forceps should be placed under the middle and deep gluteal tendons to act as a target for the osteotomy cut.

Variation
An alternative to trochanteric osteotomy is tenotomy of the middle and deep gluteal tendons. Retraction of the middle and deep gluteals in a dorsal direction exposes the joint capsule. A circumferential joint capsule incision can be made in skeletally mature animals but should be avoided in immature animals.

Closure
The joint capsule is closed with cruciate mattress sutures if possible. The trochanteric osteotomy is repaired using Kirschner wires and a figure-of-eight tension band wire technique. A lagged bone screw provides an alternative. The insertion of the superficial gluteal is repaired with interrupted sutures. The tensor fasciae latae muscle is repaired with continuous sutures and these extend into the superficial gluteal muscle proximally. The superficial fascia is closed to the cranial aspect of the biceps muscle in a similar fashion.

Postoperative care
See individual procedures. A minimum of 8 weeks strict rest is required.

Complications
See individual procedures.

OPERATIVE TECHNIQUE 21.4
Caudal approach to the hip

Positioning
Lateral recumbency. A rope tie is used to anchor patient to the table if intraoperative traction is required (e.g. hip luxation).

Assistant
Not essential.

Tray extras
Senn retractors; right-angled Gelpi retractors; large and small Weitlander retractors (or Myerding retractors if assistance available); Hohmann retractor.

Surgical technique

> **WARNING**
> The sciatic nerve must be identified and protected throughout this approach. The gemelli and internal obturator tendons can be used to retract and protect the nerve.

The incision is centred just caudal to the greater trochanter and extends in a proximodistal direction with the distal extremity at one-third the length of the femur. The superficial fascia is incised at the cranial edge of the biceps muscle. The insertion of the superficial gluteal is cut near the third trochanter and this incision continues in to the deep fascia lata, to free the insertion of the tensor fasciae latae muscle (see Figure 21.16a). Caudal retraction of the biceps allows identification of the sciatic nerve, which should be protected throughout the procedure.

Internal rotation of the femur exposes the combined tendon of insertion of the internal obturator and gemelli muscles; this tendon is cut close to its insertion in the trochanteric fossa (Figure 21.18a). A stay suture is placed in this tendon and the tendon retracted caudodorsally, simultaneously protecting the sciatic nerve (Figure 21.18b). If necessary, the caudal part of the insertion of the deep gluteal is incised to further expose the dorsal aspect of the joint. A Hohmann retractor placed ventral to the femoral neck will aid retraction of caudal musculature. The joint capsule is incised.

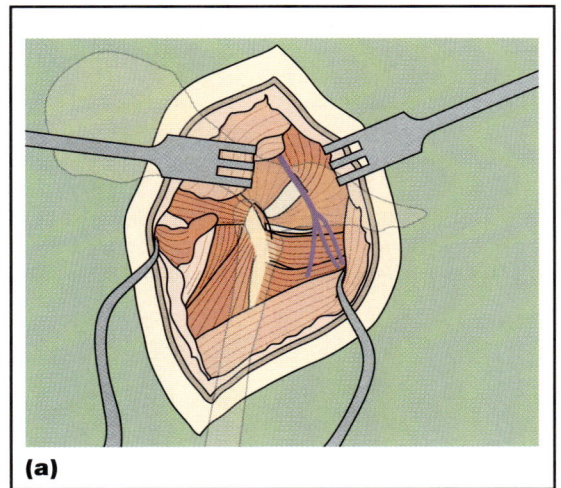

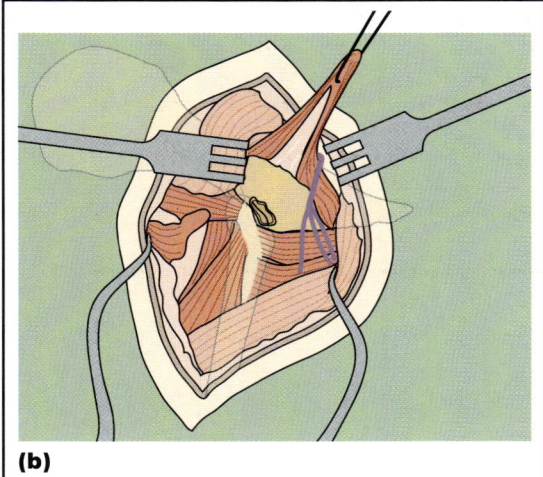

21.18 **(a)** The hip is rotated internally and the biceps femoris muscle is retracted caudally. The sciatic nerve is identified and protected. The tendons of insertion of the internal obturator and gemelli are identified and transected with a scalpel (if there has been traumatic craniodorsal hip luxation, these may already be ruptured). **(b)** Stay sutures in the transected tendons assist retraction dorsally to expose the joint capsule beneath; the retracted tendons also protect the sciatic nerve.

Chapter 21 The hip

OPERATIVE TECHNIQUE 21.4 continued
Caudal approach to the hip

Closure
A Bunnell–Mayer suture is placed in the internal obturator and gemelli tendon and this is sutured to the deep and middle gluteal tendons. The insertion of the superficial gluteal is repaired with interrupted sutures. The tensor fasciae latae muscle is repaired with continuous sutures and these extend into the superficial gluteal muscle proximally. The superficial fascia is closed to the cranial aspect of the biceps muscle in a similar fashion.

Postoperative care
See individual procedures. Generally: 4 weeks' rest are needed but this may be extended.

Complications
Sciatic nerve injury is possible, but this should be avoided if the nerve is protected during surgery.
　See individual procedures.

Chapter 21 The hip

OPERATIVE TECHNIQUE 21.5
Pubic symphysiodesis

Positioning
Dorsal recumbency at end of table, with hindlimbs abducted.

Assistant
No.

Tray extras
Weitlander or Gelpi retractors, large-gauge needle; electrosurgery tip.

Surgical technique
In bitches the skin is incised on the ventral midline over the pubic symphysis, which can be readily palpated. In male dogs a peripreputial incision is made and the penis retracted to one side to allow access to the ventral midline over the pubic symphysis.

Sharp dissection on the ventral midline (Figure 21.19a,b) is used to expose the cartilage and bone and symphysis. Minimal elevation of the origin of the adductor muscles may be necessary. The surgeon reaches one hand under the surgical drapes and palpates per rectum to accomplish retraction of the urethra away from the midline (Figure 21.19c) with simultaneous palpation of the dorsal aspect of the pubic symphysis. With the opposite hand, the electrosurgery needle tip is inserted into the cartilage at the cranial aspect of the pubic symphysis. The needle is inserted from ventral to dorsal until the tip of the needle can be palpated using the finger within the rectum. The needle is then retracted so that the tip lies completely within the symphyseal cartilage. In general, electrosurgery is applied at 40 W in coagulation mode for 10–15 seconds. The process is repeated every 2–3 mm along the symphysis for approximately two-thirds of its length (Figure 21.19d). Prediction equation analysis can be used to plan electrosurgery doses for each case (Patricelli, 2001).

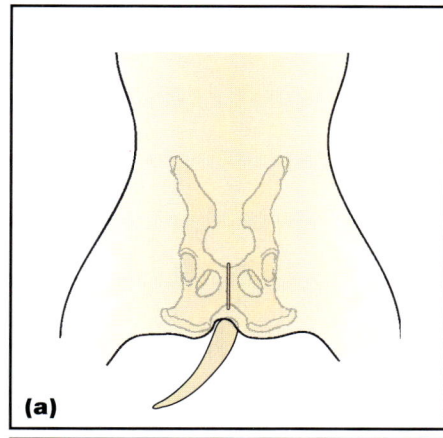

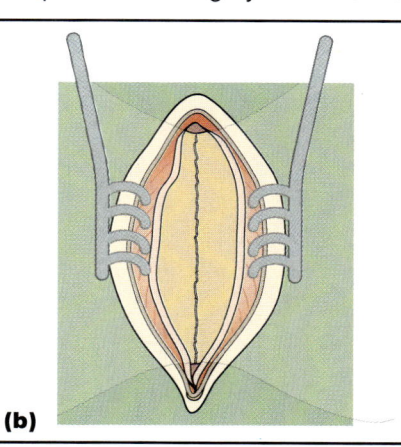

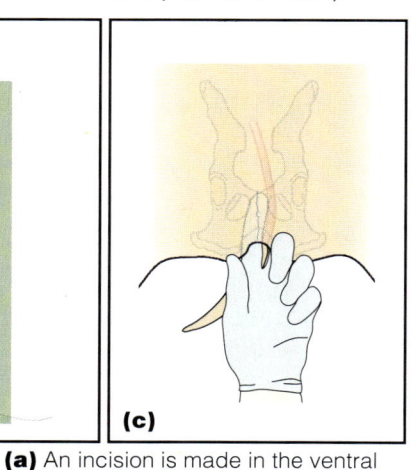

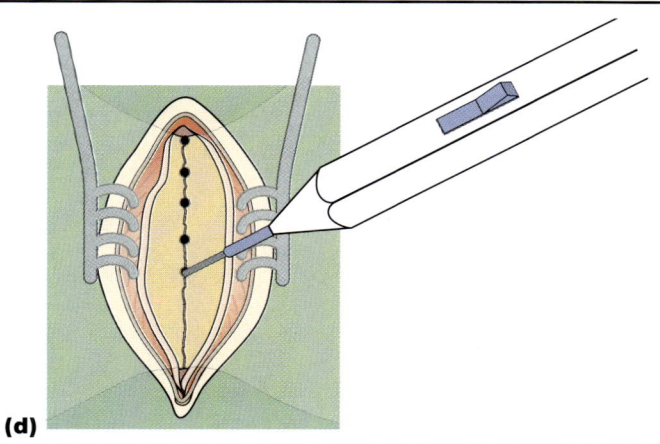

21.19 (a) An incision is made in the ventral midline. (b) The linea alba and subpelvic tendon are incised in the midline. (c) Palpation per rectum to achieve urethral retraction. (d) The electrosurgery probe is inserted into the cartilage of the symphysis at set intervals and for set times.

333

Chapter 21 The hip

OPERATIVE TECHNIQUE 21.5 continued
Pubic symphysiodesis

Closure
After re-establishing aseptic technique, routine closure of subcutaneous tissue and skin is performed.

Postoperative care
Routine incision care and suture removal are performed.

Complications
Skin burns may result on the dorsum if electrosurgery is not grounded well. There is potential for thermal damage to adjacent tissues, such as the urethra.

Chapter 21 The hip

OPERATIVE TECHNIQUE 21.6
Triple pelvic osteotomy

Positioning
Lateral recumbency with the affected limb up.

Assistant
Yes.

Tray extras
Periosteal elevator; Hohmann retractors; Meyerding retractors; bone-holding forceps; sagittal saw (or Gigli wire); drill; bone plates; screws; plating equipment; orthopaedic wire; wire twisters.

Surgical technique

Pubic osteotomy
The affected limb is abducted and extended to allow for palpation of the pectineus muscle. An incision is made over the origin of the pectineus muscle and blunt dissection is performed to allow isolation and transection of the muscle at its origin (Figure 21.20). The pubic ramus is then exposed using a periosteal elevator. The ramus is isolated by placing Hohmann retractors cranial and caudal to the bone. Two osteotomies are performed in the pubic ramus to allow removal of a 3–8 mm section of bone at the level of the pubic eminence. Haemostasis is ensured and the incision is closed. The limb is then returned to a normal resting (adducted, neutral) position.

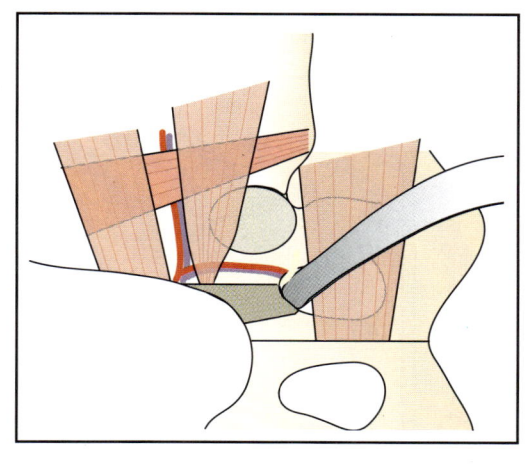

21.20 An incision is made over the origin of the pectineus muscle. Blunt dissection is performed to allow isolation and transection of the muscle at its origin. The pubic ramus is then exposed and isolated by placing Hohmann retractors cranially and caudally. Two osteotomies are made in the pubic ramus to allow removal of a 3–8 mm section of bone at the level of the pubic eminence.

Ischial osteotomy
An incision is made over the midpoint of the ischial tuberosity from dorsal to ventral. Sharp dissection and retraction of the subcutaneous tissues is performed to allow exposure of the ischial tuberosity. Sharp dissection is continued down to the bone for the entire length of the ischial tuberosity to allow initial elevation of the dorsal and ventral periosteum. A periosteal elevator is then used to continue subperiosteal elevation of the dorsal and ventral tissues on the ischial table so that Hohmann retractors can be placed subperiosteally into the obturator foramen from both the dorsal and ventral aspects of the ischial table. With the tissues retracted, a sagittal saw or Gigli wire is used to make a single osteotomy from the approximate midpoint of the ischial tuberosity to the caudolateral aspect of the obturator foramen (Figure 21.21). Holes are created in the tuberosity on either side of the osteotomy, at least 5–8 mm from the cut edge, and orthopaedic wire is placed in hemicerclage fashion. The wire is left loose and the incision is protected until the ilial osteotomy is completed and stabilized.

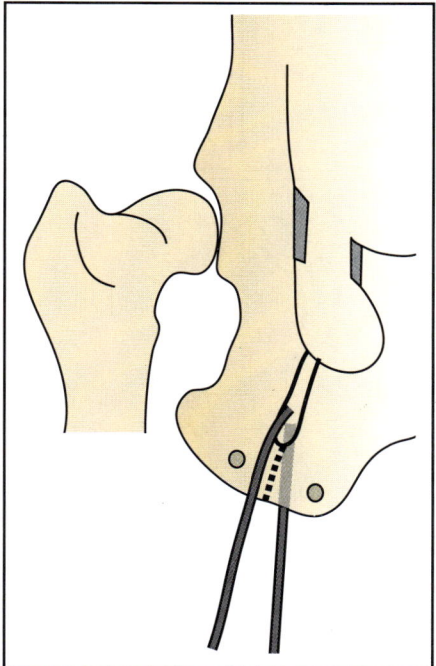

21.21 A Gigli wire may be used for osteotomy.

→

335

Chapter 21   The hip

OPERATIVE TECHNIQUE 21.6 continued
Triple pelvic osteotomy

Ilial osteotomy
The body and wing of the ilium are exposed through a gluteal roll-up approach (Figure 21.22). Meyerding retractors are used to retract the gluteal muscles. A periosteal elevator is used to elevate the musculature on the ventral aspect of the ilial body to allow the surgeon to place a finger on the medial side of the ilium to palpate the location of the sacrum and the sciatic nerve. The intended line for osteotomy of the ilial body is marked such that it is immediately caudal to the sacrum and orientated approximately 10 degrees from perpendicular to the axis of the ilial body. Osteotomy of the ilial body is then completed using a sagittal saw with extreme care given to protecting the subjacent sciatic nerve. A bone-holding forceps is placed on the ilial body caudal to the osteotomy site for rotating the acetabular segment. The ilial osteotomy is then stabilized using a bone plate that maintains the desired degree of rotation. The most appropriate degree of acetabular rotation has been reported to be 20 degrees (Dejardin *et al.*, 1998; Tomlinson and Cook, 2002). The author recommends that one or more screws in the ilial segment proximal to the osteotomy engage the sacral body.

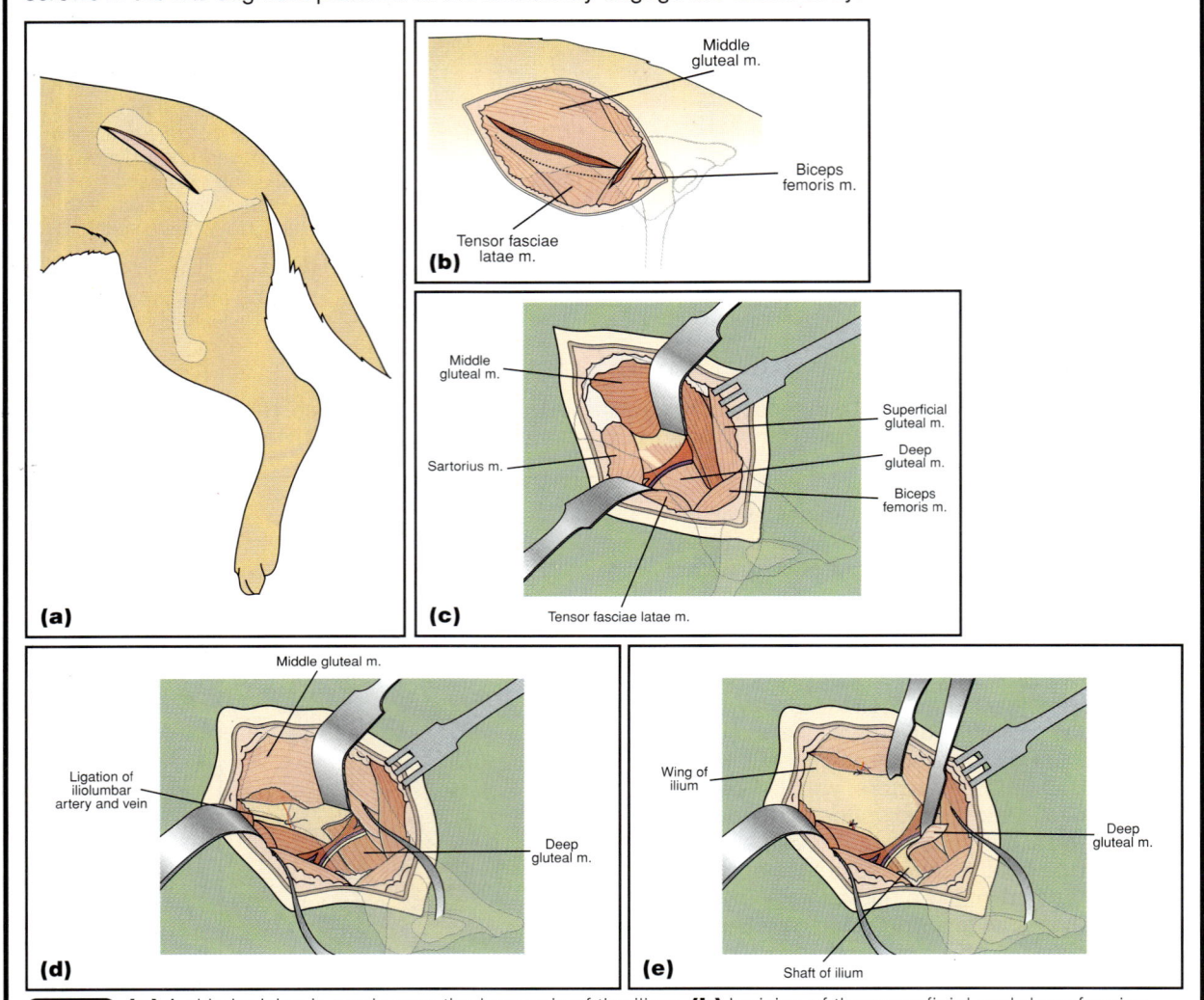

21.22 **(a)** A skin incision is made over the long axis of the ilium. **(b)** Incision of the superficial and deep fascias allows exposure of the intermuscular septum between the tensor fasciae latae and the middle gluteal muscles. **(c)** Dissection along this plane allows retraction of the middle gluteal to expose the deep gluteal muscle. **(d)** An incision in the origin of the middle gluteal muscle allows elevation of the muscle from the ilium. **(e)** Myerding retractors are used to retract the gluteal muscles. A periosteal elevator is used to elevate the musculature on the ventral aspect of the ilial body to allow the surgeon to place a finger on the medial side of the ilium and palpate the location of the sacrum.

→

336

OPERATIVE TECHNIQUE 21.6 continued
Triple pelvic osteotomy

The ischial hemicerclage wire is then tightened and both incisions are closed routinely. The procedure can be performed bilaterally at the same setting.

Closure
Fascia, subcutaneous tissues and skin are apposed routinely.

Postoperative care
Restricted activity (cage rest and leash walking) is necessary for 6 weeks. If appropriate, the procedure can be performed on the contralateral side 3–4 weeks after the first surgery.

Complications
Narrowing of the pelvic canal; constipation; urethral injury; over-rotation of the acetabulum (resulting in limited femoral extension and abduction); implant failure or loosening; infection; sciatic nerve palsy; persistent incongruity; failure to retard the progression of osteoarthritis.

Chapter 21 The hip

OPERATIVE TECHNIQUE 21.7
Femoral head and neck excision arthroplasty

Positioning
Lateral recumbency with the affected limb uppermost.

Assistant
Yes.

Tray extras
Meyerding retractors; sagittal saw or sharp osteotome and mallet; rongeurs; bone rasp.

Surgical technique
After a craniolateral approach to the hip joint, the joint capsule is incised and the femoral head and neck are exposed. The hip joint is luxated and the femur is externally rotated so that the cranial surface of the femoral head and neck are pointed laterally. The osteotomy is then performed using an oscillating saw or sharp osteotome. The osteotomy extends from the medial aspect of the greater trochanter to a point immediately proximal to the lesser trochanter (Figure 21.23). The femoral head and neck are removed and irregularities at the osteotomy site are removed with rongeurs or a bone rasp. The limb should be returned to a neutral position and the hip joint should be put through all functional ranges of motion to ensure that no bony impingement or contact remains. The surgical wound is lavaged and closed routinely.

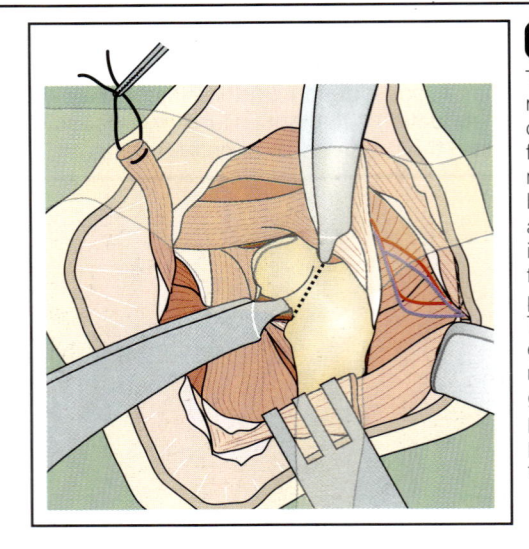

21.23
The femur is externally rotated so that the cranial surfaces of the femoral head and neck are pointed laterally (the surgeon's assistant can hold the ipsilateral stifle such that the patella is pointing to the ceiling). The osteotomy extends from the medial aspect of the greater trochanter to a point immediately proximal to the lesser trochanter.

Closure
The authors recommend precise apposition of the joint capsule using absorbable suture. Fascia, subcutaneous tissues and skin are apposed routinely.

Postoperative care
Postoperative management involves a rapid return to exercise (first 3–5 days) to promote formation of the fibrous pseudojoint while maintaining muscle mass and range of motion. Physiotherapy involving active and passive range-of-motion exercises should be initiated 2–3 days after surgery.

Complications
Shortening of the limb; abnormal limb motion; muscle atrophy; varying degrees of lameness; patellar luxation; compromised joint function; pain (if excision is inadequate).

Chapter 21 The hip

OPERATIVE TECHNIQUE 21.8
Cemented total hip arthroplasty

WARNING
Clinicians should not attempt these surgeries without first receiving practical training in their execution.

The details of the procedure described apply to the use of the Biomedtrix CFX cemented total hip implant. For other implants, follow the manufacturer's recommendations.

Templating
Implant sizes are estimated on radiographs using the proprietary template; because the radiographic magnification may vary slightly from that allowed for in the template, the final implant size is decided at surgery. The acetabular template is placed such that the medial edge is against the medial cortex of the acetabulum (Figure 21.24a); the largest size of cup that will fit within the acetabulum is chosen. The femoral component is sized such that a 1–2 mm cement mantle will be left at all cortices in the diaphysis seen on the VD view (Figure 21.24b) and also on the lateral view (not shown).

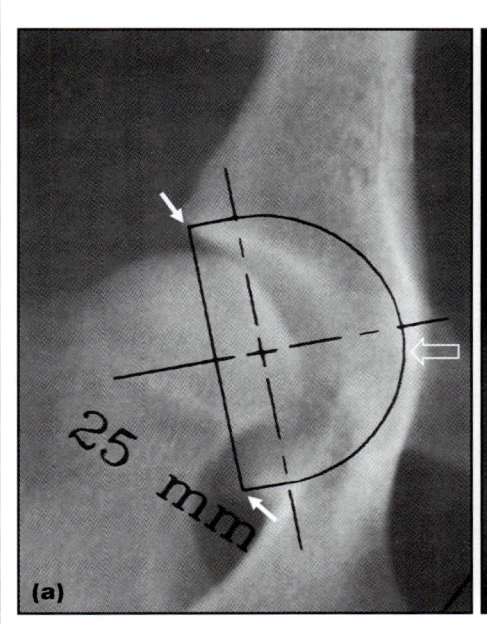

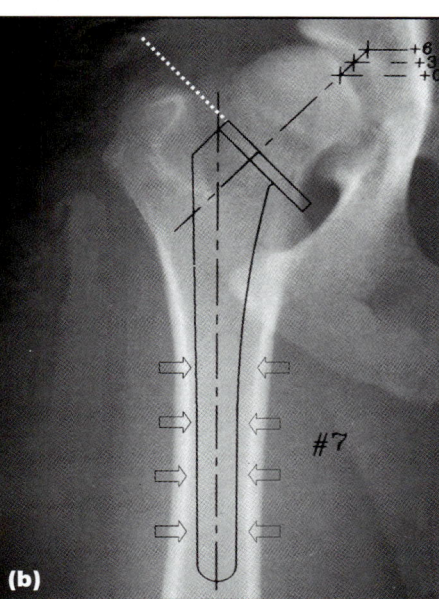

21.24 Templating. **(a)** The acetabular template should 'touch' the medial cortex (open arrow) and be within the limits of the acetabulum (closed arrows). **(b)** The proximal border of the femoral stem template should be aligned with the proximal border of the greater trochanter (dotted line) and the stem should allow for 1–2 mm of cement mantle (open arrows).

Positioning
Lateral recumbency with the affected limb uppermost. Use the Biomedtrix positioning board with columns to align the pelvis in relation to the floor. It is essential for accurate cup placement that the pelvis is aligned with the transaxial plane at 90 degrees to the floor.

Assistant
Essential; a four-person surgical team is ideal, including one person working the instrument trolley. Less assistance leads to less efficiency and longer surgical time.

Tray extras
Biomedtrix CFX total hip arthroplasty instrumentation system; sagittal saw; high-torque drill; Meyerding retractors; curettes; rongeurs; AO reduction forceps; large blunt-tip Hohmann retractor.

→

Chapter 21 The hip

OPERATIVE TECHNIQUE 21.8 continued
Cemented total hip arthroplasty

Surgical technique
After a craniolateral approach to the hip joint with partial tenotomy of the deep gluteal tendon, the joint capsule is incised and the femoral head and neck are exposed. The hip joint is luxated and the femur is externally rotated so that the cranial surface of the femoral head and neck are pointing laterally. The femoral osteotomy is then performed at the desired level along the surface of the cut template (Figure 21.25a) using an oscillating saw. The femoral head and portion of the femoral neck are removed.

The acetabulum is exposed and soft tissue debris is removed. The acetabulum is then reamed with the appropriately sized reamer (Figure 21.25b). Channels are created in the ilium and dorsal acetabular rim using a combination of a drill (same size as the templated femoral component) and Volkmann's curette (Figure 21.25c).

A trial acetabular prosthesis is placed to ensure appropriate fit, positioning and bone coverage. The appropriate acetabular cup is then cemented into place using dough-type polymethylmethacrylate (containing cefazolin or gentamicin) and positioned using the acetabular prosthesis positioning device (Figure 21.25d,e).

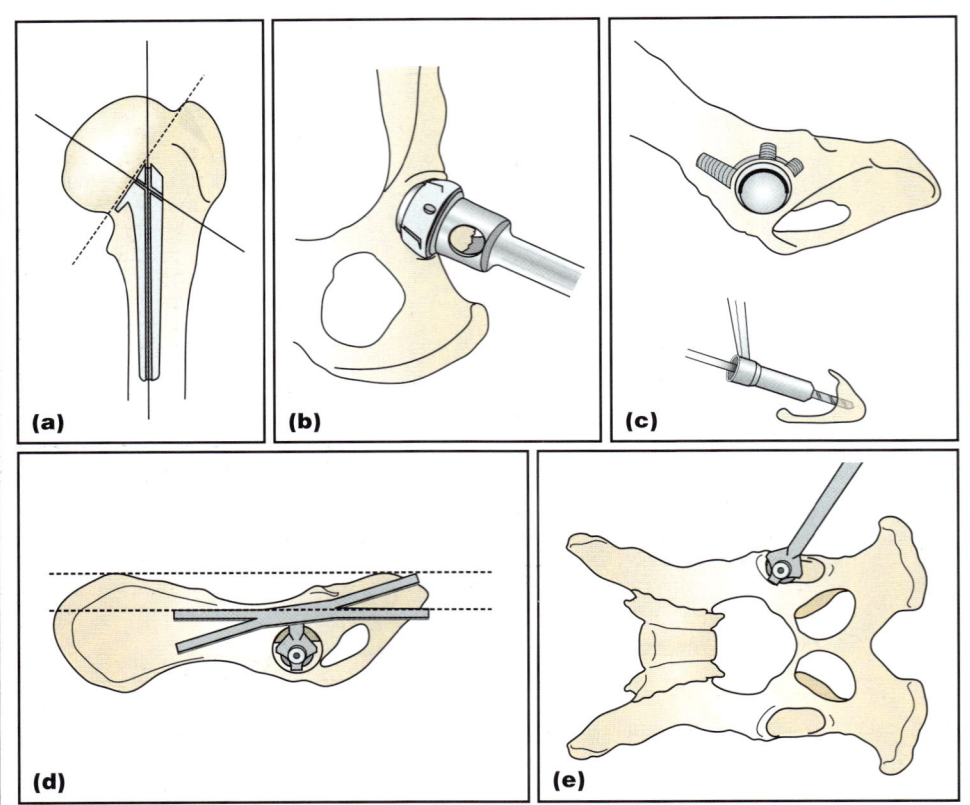

21.25 (a) The femoral cutting guide is placed such that the long axis runs parallel to the femur and the line of the cut aligns with the proximal border of the greater trochanter. (b) The appropriate reamer, chosen from templating and assessment at surgery, is used to remove cartilage and bone as far as the medial cortex of the acetabulum. The trial cup can be used to assess fit and there should be 90% coverage of the dorsal cup.
(c) Three to five drill holes are placed in the dorsal acetabular cancellous bone (use the same drill bit as that intended for preparation of the femur) to create 'undercut locks' for cement. These holes are joined with a Volkmann's curette to create a dorsal 'trench'.
(d) The alignment bar on the positioning aid should be parallel with a line joining the dorsal iliac spine with the tuber ischii. (e) The positioner should be angled 15–20 degrees caudally, to create a retroverted cup.

Chapter 21 The hip

OPERATIVE TECHNIQUE 21.8 continued
Cemented total hip arthroplasty

The femur is then externally rotated and positioned for preparation for endoprosthesis insertion (Figure 21.26a). The appropriately sized drill bit, reamer and finishing file are used sequentially to prepare the femoral canal for the cement and prosthesis (Figures 21.26b–d). Care is taken to ensure that the drill bit is centred on the long axis of the femur.

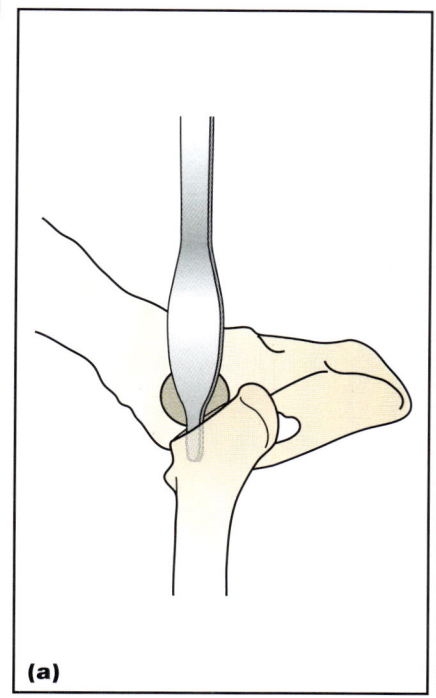

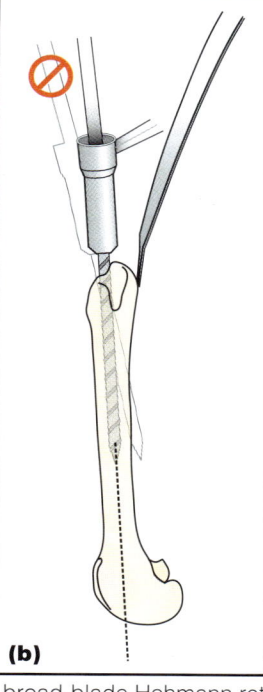

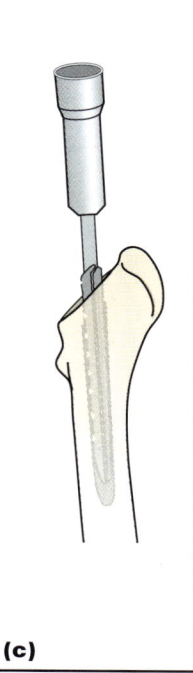

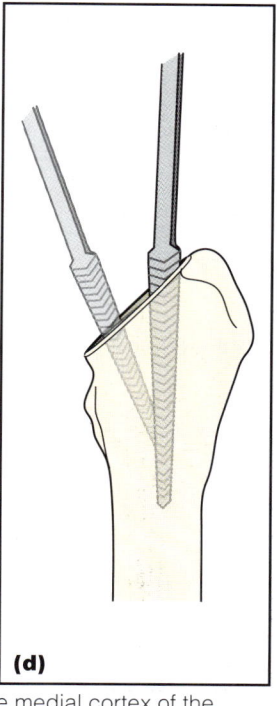

(a) **(b)** **(c)** **(d)**

21.26 (a) The femur is elevated with a broad-blade Hohmann retractor. If necessary, the medial cortex of the femur at the osteotomy site is removed with rongeurs to facilitate entry of the drill into the central axis of the femur. (b) Using the appropriate drill size, as determined from templating, a hole is drilled in the femur, using the tissue guard to protect muscles dorsal to the hip. The drill is carefully aimed along the axis of the femur. (c) The same size tapered reamer is used until it fully penetrates the femur to the level of the end of the cutting blades. (d) The 'finishing file' is used to remove cancellous bone in the neck area, especially along the medial edge of the greater trochanter and lateral to the calcar.

A trial femoral endoprosthesis is placed to ensure appropriate fit, positioning and osteotomy angle. The femoral canal is then copiously lavaged and suctioned. For size 8 femoral stems and upwards, a femoral canal restraining device is placed within the canal to allow optimal polymethylmethacrylate filling. The femoral canal is then filled with polymethylmethacrylate (containing cefazolin) and the appropriate femoral endoprosthesis (ideally with moulded centralizer fins in place) is placed within the femoral canal and held in position for 7–10 minutes to allow initial curing of the polymethylmethacrylate (Figure 21.27).

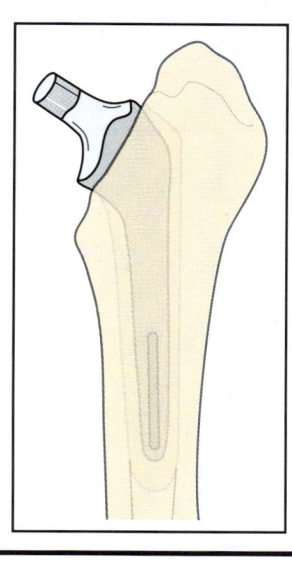

21.27 The trial femoral stem is inserted. There should be significant 'play' to allow easy insertion and some instability once inserted. The angle of the osteotomy cut is checked and adjusted if necessary. Cement is injected under pressure using a syringe extension tube and cement gun. The stem (with the moulded PMMA centralizer fins) is placed into the femur and the team waits until the cement has cured.

→

341

Chapter 21 The hip

> **OPERATIVE TECHNIQUE 21.8** *continued*
> **Cemented total hip arthroplasty**

A trial femoral head of the appropriate length is then placed on the femoral endoprosthesis and a trial reduction of the joint is performed (Figure 21.28). After assessment of hip range of motion and stability, the joint is luxated, the appropriate femoral head prosthesis is placed on the femoral endoprosthesis and the joint is again reduced.

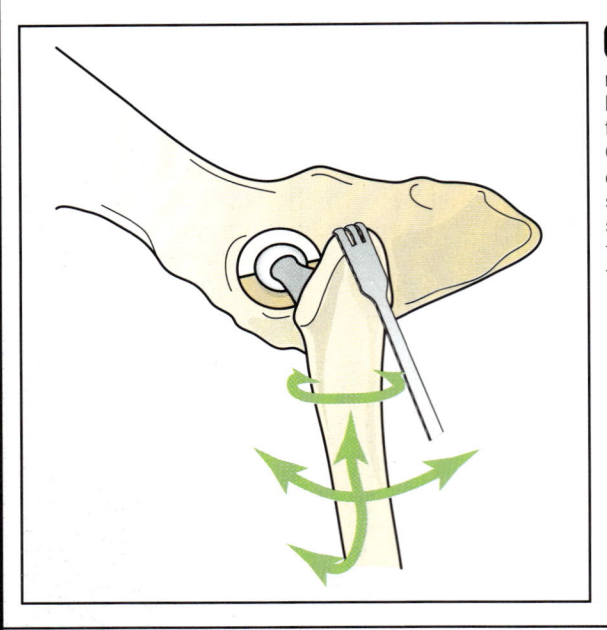

21.28 Trial femoral heads are used to assess hip stability and range of motion. Reduction is achieved by use of bone forceps on the greater trochanter and applying distal traction. Once the appropriate femoral head is chosen, the head is placed on the stem and covered with a clean gauze swab. The head impactor is placed on the femoral head and tapped three times with the plastic mallet.

Closure
Careful apposition with or without imbrication of the joint capsule is performed using monofilament absorbable 3.5 metric (0) or 3 metric (2/0) suture. The partial tenotomy of the deep gluteal tendon is repaired with one to two mattress sutures of 3.5 metric (0) or 3 metric (2/0) monofilament absorbable suture. The fascia, subcutaneous tissues and skin are closed routinely.

Postoperative care
For the first week after surgery, activity is restricted to lead walking with support of the hindlimbs. Activity restriction should continue for the first month, with a gradual return to function 10–12 weeks after surgery.

Complications
Complications include luxation, osteomyelitis, aseptic component loosening, femoral fractures, implant failure and sciatic neuropraxia.

Chapter 21 The hip

OPERATIVE TECHNIQUE 21.9
Non-cemented total hip arthroplasty

WARNING
Clinicians should not attempt these surgeries without first receiving practical training in their execution.

The details of the procedure described apply to the use of the Biomedtrix BFX non-cemented total hip implant. For other implants, follow the manufacturer's recommendations.

Templating
VD hip-extended and lateral (affected limb down) radiographs are taken to assess pathology and implant size. 10–15% magnification is assumed. The templates are used to estimate the implants that will best fit. Templating for the acetabulum is similar to that for the cemented system (Figure 21.29a). The intersection of the central axis of the implant with the caudal femoral neck is noted to inform the surgeon regarding the central axis of the femur and the starting point for femoral canal opening (Figures 21.29b,c). In addition, the requirement for removal of bone from the caudal femoral neck can be estimated by noting the intersection between the caudal aspect of the implant and the caudal border of the femoral neck.

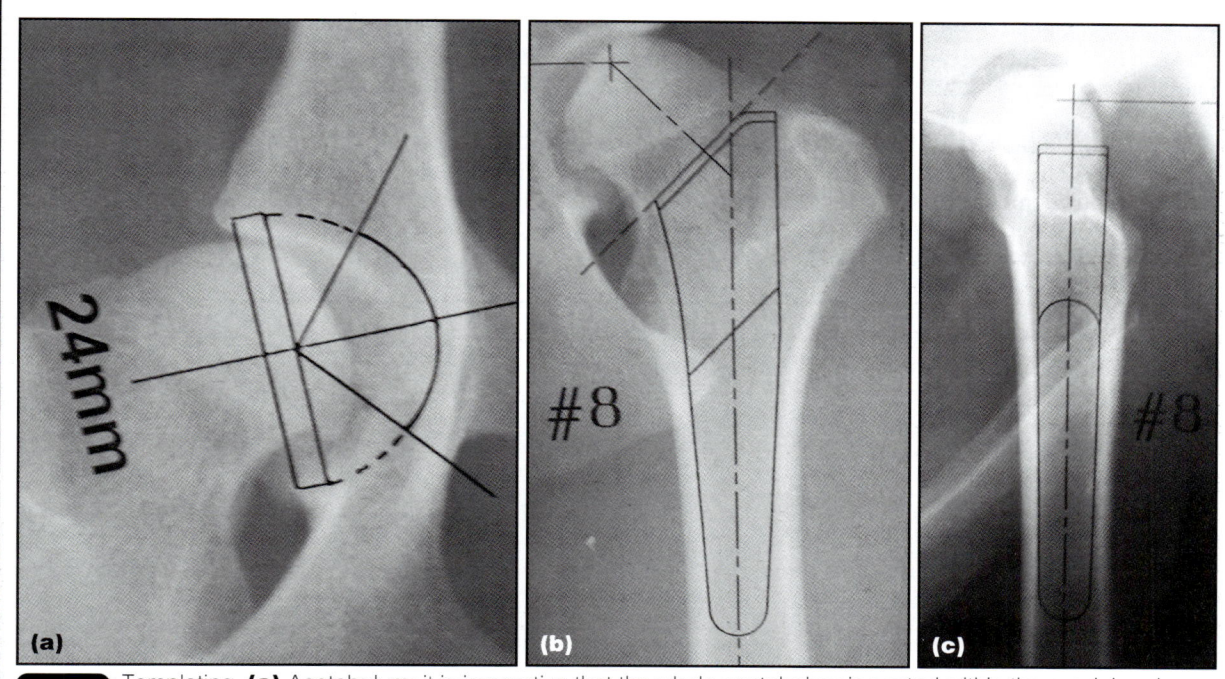

21.29 Templating. **(a)** Acetabulum: it is imperative that the whole acetabulum is seated within the cranial and caudal pillars. **(b)** Femur: craniocaudal view. The largest femoral component possible is templated. **(c)** Femur: mediolateral view.

Positioning
Lateral recumbency with the affected limb uppermost. Use the Biomedtrix positioning board to align the pelvis in relation to the floor. It is essential for accurate cup placement that the pelvis is aligned with the transaxial plane at 90 degrees to the floor.

Assistant
Essential; a four-person surgical team is ideal, including one person working the instrument trolley. Less assistance leads to less efficiency and longer surgical time.

Chapter 21 The hip

OPERATIVE TECHNIQUE 21.9 continued
Non-cemented total hip arthroplasty

Tray extras
Biomedtrix BFX total hip arthroplasty instrumentation system; sagittal saw; high-torque drill; Meyerding retractors; curettes; rongeurs; AO reduction forceps; large blunt-tip Hohmann retractor.

Surgical technique
After a craniolateral approach to the hip joint with partial tenotomy of the deep gluteal tendon, the joint capsule is incised and the femoral head and neck are exposed. The hip joint is luxated and the femur is externally rotated so that the cranial surface of the femoral head and neck are pointing laterally. The femoral osteotomy is then performed at the desired level along the surface of the cut template using an oscillating saw. The femoral cut is relatively low but trochanteric damage should be avoided. The femoral head and portion of the femoral neck are removed.

The acetabulum is exposed and soft tissue debris is removed. The acetabulum is then reamed in two stages: starter and finsher. The reaming is started with an under-sized 'starter' ('cheese-grater' style) reamer at an angle of approximately 15 degrees to the vertical to avoid dorsal migration of the reamer (Figure 21.30a). The reamer is then used in the correct anatomical position to create the correct depth. Depth is judged by looking for when the cranial and caudal borders of the reamer are recessed in the acetabulum (Figure 21.30b). The solid finishing reamer is designed to create the correct width for the cup by expanding the bone bed width; it will not add depth. The surgeon should ream at 45 degrees to the vertical and with approximately 20 degrees of retroversion. The reaming guide is placed on the positioning board columns to guide the surgeon during reaming (Figure 21.30c). The surgeon should stand still for reaming with feet apart, holding the reamer in the same axis to create the reamed tunnel accurately for the press-fit cup.

A trial cup is placed to assess the boundaries; there must be no interference from ventral osteophyte or capsule. The cup is placed and inserted along the reamed axis. The alignment of the impactor mimics the reamer. Small adjustments to cup alignment must be made early before full impaction. Eccentric taps with the impactor on the cup rim can adjust cup alignment. Impaction is performed until the pitch of the sound from the mallet increases to signal full impaction.

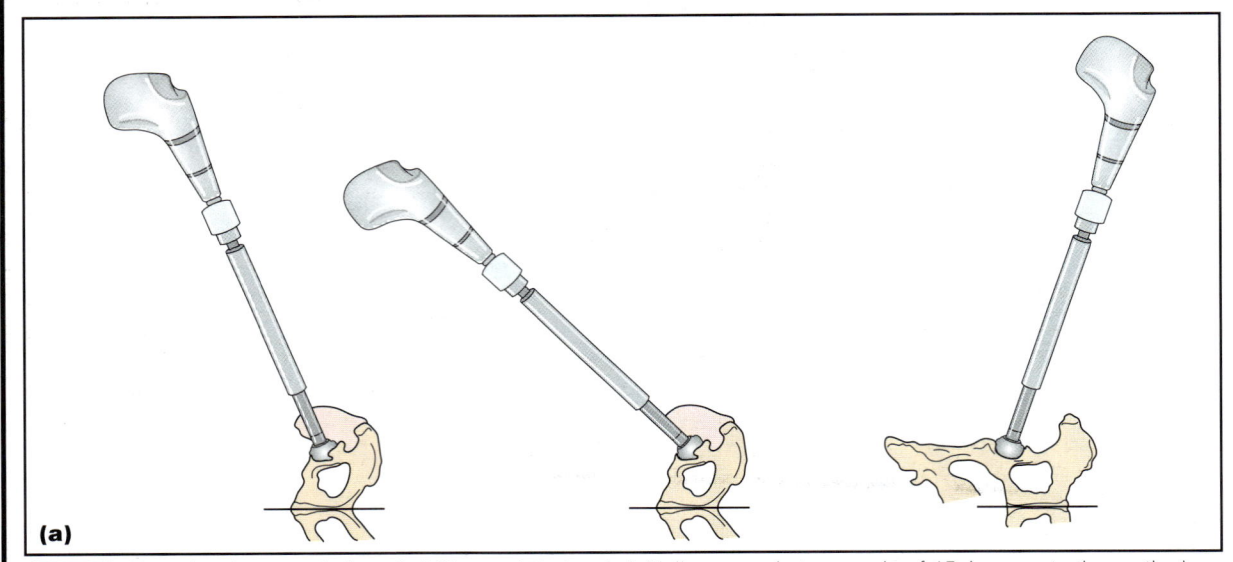

21.30 Reaming the acetabulum. **(a)** The acetabulum is initially reamed at an angle of 15 degrees to the vertical, then it is moved to the correct anatomical position with 10–15 degrees of retroversion. (continues)

Chapter 21 The hip

OPERATIVE TECHNIQUE 21.9 *continued*
Non-cemented total hip arthroplasty

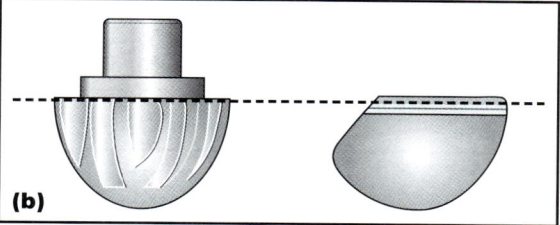

21.30 (continued) Reaming the acetabulum. **(b)** Reaming is sufficient when the reamer is fully submerged. **(c)** The surgeon reams with the reamer held in the correct anatomical alignment. The reaming guide is placed on the positioning columns to aid in correct alignment of reaming.

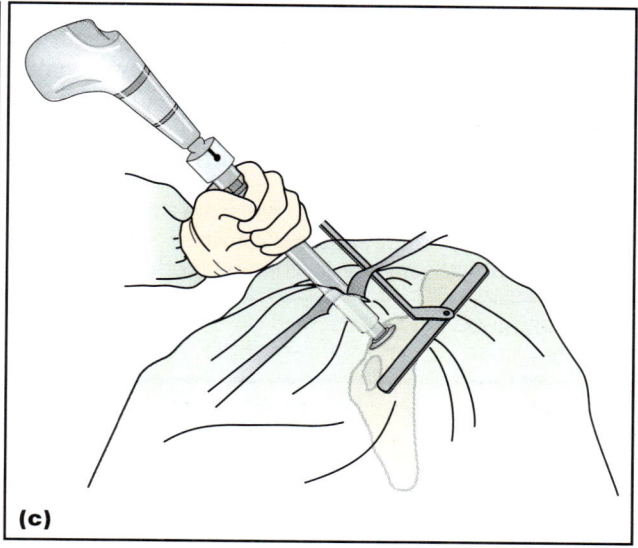

The femoral canal is opened using a 2.5 mm drill starting at the intertrochanteric fossa and working up to a 5 mm drill bit. A small spinal burr is used to remove the bone cranial to the fossa to facilitate the insertion of the reamer. This ensures that the femoral prosthesis is centred within the canal and minimizes the risk of varus insertion. The cancellous bone is preserved cranially and medially. Sequentially larger broaches are then used in conjunction with a mallet to achieve press-fit stabilization. The broach is removed along the axis of the femur and side-to-side motion is avoided. Once the appropriately sized broach has been inserted to the required depth, the femoral prosthesis is positioned and tapped into place to leave 1–2 mm of ingrowth surface protruding (Figure 21.31).

A trial femoral head of the appropriate length is then placed on the femoral endoprosthesis and a trial reduction of the joint is performed. If bone or osteophyte on the acetabular rim or greater trochanter interferes with hip motion, it should be removed with rongeurs. Cup position is also assessed at this stage because it cannot be accurately assessed on postoperative radiographs. With the limb held in a neutral weightbearing position, the flat surface on the back of the femoral component should be parallel with the plane of the cup. If necessary, cup position is corrected at this time. After assessment of hip range of motion and stability, the joint is luxated, the appropriate femoral head prosthesis is placed on the femoral endoprosthesis and the joint is again reduced.

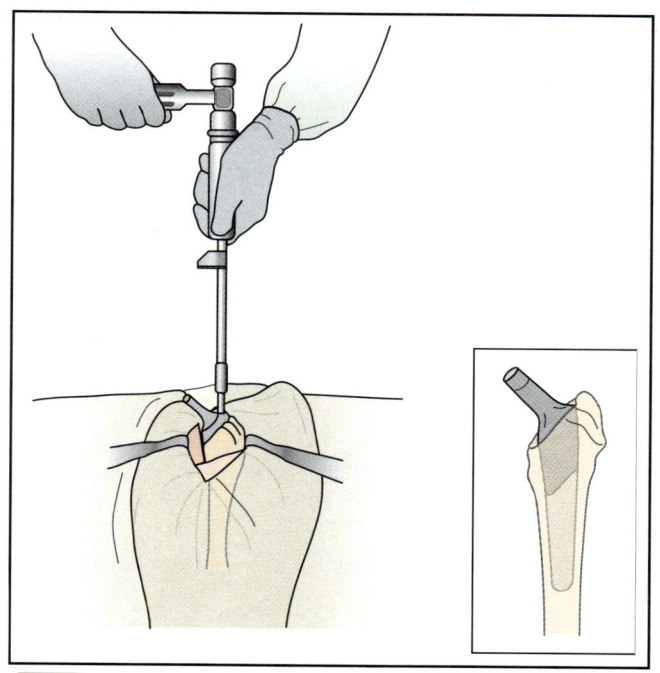

21.31 Once the largest broach has been inserted to the required depth, the femoral prosthesis is tapped in to leave the beaded section flush with the osteotomy.

Chapter 21 The hip

OPERATIVE TECHNIQUE 21.9 *continued*
Non-cemented total hip arthroplasty

Closure
The skin is closed with simple interrupted sutures. Careful apposition with or without imbrication of the joint capsule is performed using monofilament absorbable 3.5 metric (0) or 3 metric (2/0) suture. The partial tenotomy of the deep gluteal tendon is repaired with one to two mattress sutures of 3.5 metric (0) or 3 metric (2/0) monofilament absorbable suture. The fascia, subcutaneous tissues and skin are closed routinely.

Postoperative care
Radiographs must be taken for assessment of implant placement.
For the first week after surgery, activity is restricted to leash walking with support of the hindlimbs. Activity restriction should continue for the first month, with a gradual return to function 10–12 weeks after surgery.

Complications
Luxation.

Chapter 21 The hip

OPERATIVE TECHNIQUE 21.10
Capsulorrhaphy for craniodorsal hip luxation

Positioning
Lateral recumbency. The dog is tied to the operating table to facilitate traction on the luxated hip.

Assistant
Preferred but not essential.

Tray extras
Senn retractors; right-angled Gelpi retractors; large and small Weitlander retractors (or Myerding retractors if assistance available); periosteal elevator; Hohmann retractors; drill; appropriately sized (20–40 kg breaking strain) monofilament nylon for capsular prosthesis; either suture anchors with appropriate inserting equipment or appropriately sized drill bit, tap, screw and spiked washer.

Surgical technique
See Operative Technique 21.2 for approach. The acetabulum is cleared of debris and the hip is reduced. Holes are drilled in the acetabulum in the appropriate places. For a left hip these are at 10 o'clock and 1 o'clock; for a right hip these are at 11 o'clock and 2 o'clock. The drill holes should be placed in a direction to avoid penetration of the acetabular articular surface. A hole is drilled through the femoral neck to act as the femoral anchor point for the sutures. Two horizontal mattress sutures are placed linking each acetabular anchor point to the femoral neck tunnel. The limb is held in a neutral 'weightbearing' position and the sutures are tied such that the hip has a functional range of motion (Figure 21.32). Overtightening the sutures can limit adduction of the hip and may lead to early suture failure. The sutures are tied such that the knots do not interfere with joint motion. Following placement of the sutures, it should not be possible to luxate the femoral head.

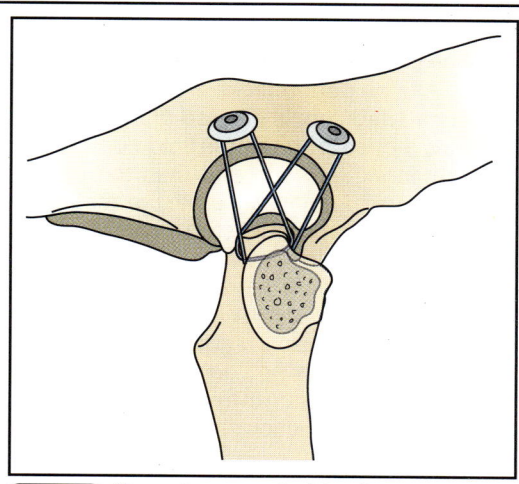

21.32 The sutures are tied to allow a functional range of motion.

Closure
The skin is closed with simple interrupted sutures.

Postoperative care
Strict rest is needed for 6 weeks to allow for capsular repair.

Complications
Failure of the prosthetic capsule can occur and revision surgery or salvage may then be necessary.

Chapter 21   The hip

OPERATIVE TECHNIQUE 21.11
Transarticular pinning for hip luxation

Positioning
Lateral recumbency. The patient is tied to the table to facilitate traction on the femoral head.

Assistant
Preferred but not essential.

Tray extras
See Operative Technique 21.2. Drill; aiming device; appropriately sized pin.

Surgical technique
See Operative Technique 21.2 for approach. The pin is drilled through the femoral neck to exit the femoral head at the insertion of the teres ligament. The pin should be inserted on the lateral aspect of the femur, just below the third trochanter. For larger pins, it is necessary to pre-drill the femoral tunnel with a drill bit slightly smaller than the intended pin. An aiming device can be useful to place the femoral tunnel accurately. Alternatively, pre-drilling can be performed in a retrograde manner prior to pin placement in a normograde fashion.

The acetabulum is cleared of debris and the hip is reduced. The limb is held in a neutral 'weightbearing' position and then the pin is driven across the joint space into the acetabulum. The surgeon should stop driving the pin as soon as it is felt to penetrate the transcortex of the acetabulum. If there is any doubt regarding the length of the pin, an unscrubbed assistant can perform a rectal examination to check that the pin is not too long. The range of flexion and extension of the hip are checked; adduction and abduction should be limited by the pin.

The free end of the pin is bent to stop pin migration and the free end is cut (Figure 21.33). The free end of the pin is rotated such that it lies parallel to the long axis of the femur and will not irritate the soft tissues.

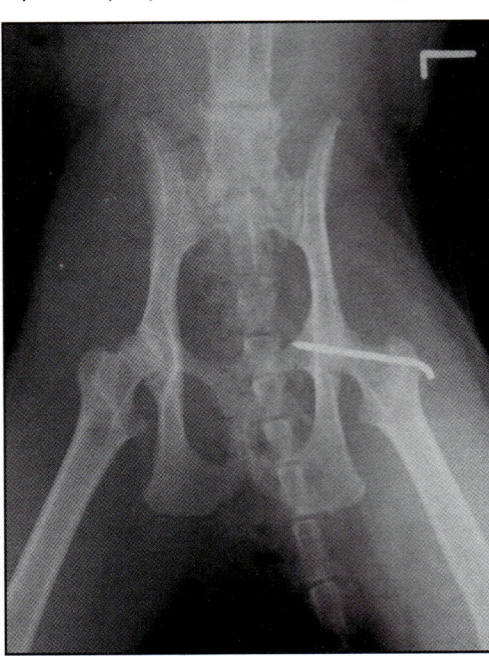

21.33 Transarticular pinning in a cat. The free end of the pin is bent and cut to prevent pin migration.

Closure
The skin is closed with simple interrupted sutures.

Postoperative care
Strict rest for 4 weeks. The pin is removed 4 weeks postoperatively.

Complications
Pin breakage; femoral head and neck fracture; pin migration (should be avoided by bending the free end of the pin); reluxation (revision surgery or salvage may then be necessary).

Chapter 21 The hip

OPERATIVE TECHNIQUE 21.12
Hip toggle for luxation

Positioning
Lateral recumbency. The patient is tied to the table to facilitate traction on the femoral head.

Assistant
Preferred but not essential.

Tray extras
See Operative Technique 21.3. Drill; drill guide; appropriately sized drill bit to drill the acetabulum to allow passage of the toggle; appropriately sized drill bit to drill the femoral head and neck tunnel to allow passage of the double suture; appropriately sized drill bit to drill the greater trochanter to allow passage of the single suture.

Surgical technique
Choose from Operative Technique 21.1 or 21.3 for approach.

The acetabulum is cleared of debris. A hole is drilled in the acetabular fossa to allow passage of the toggle. A tunnel is drilled in the femoral head and neck in a retrograde manner starting at the fovea capitis and exiting on the lateral aspect of the femur. The toggle with suture attached is placed in the acetabulum and the suture is locked behind the acetabulum. The double suture is passed along the femoral tunnel to exit laterally. The hip is reduced and the suture is pulled tight. A transverse bone tunnel is drilled in the greater trochanter to accept one of the free ends of the suture and the suture is tied on the lateral aspect of the femur with the limb held in a neutral 'weightbearing' position (Figure 21.34).

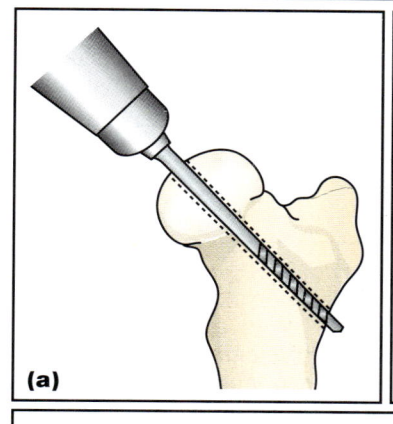

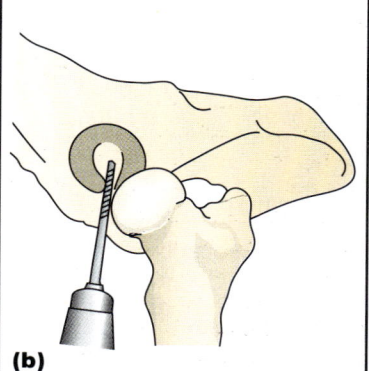

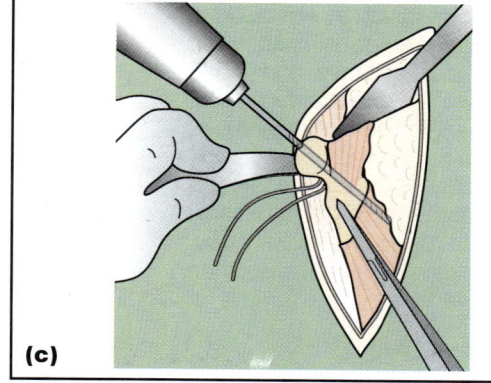

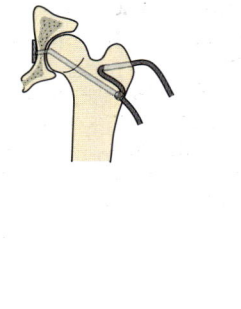

21.34 Hip toggle. **(a)** The femur is drilled from the insertion point of the teres ligament at the articular surface, along the femoral neck to exit laterally. **(b)** Whilst retracting the femoral head, the acetabulum is drilled at the origin of the teres ligament. **(c)** The suture is tied, with the limb held in a neutral weightbearing position.

Closure
See Operative Technique 21.3.

Postoperative care
Strict rest for 6–8 weeks.

Complications

- Suture failure and reluxation: revision surgery or salvage will then be required
- Infective arthritis: placement of a permanent suture inside a joint requires high levels of asepsis. Multifilament suture materials are more likely to be associated with this complication.

22

The stifle

W. Malcolm McKee and James L. Cook

Introduction

This chapter deals with the diagnosis and management of a number of developmental and acquired conditions of the canine and feline stifle. Surgical approaches to the stifle are described in Operative Techniques 22.1, 22.2 and 22.3. Fractures involving the stifle are covered in detail in the *BSAVA Manual of Small Animal Fracture Repair and Management*.

Arthroscopy

Arthroscopic procedures are the mainstay of knee surgery in human orthopaedics and are rapidly becoming a major component of veterinary joint surgery. The advantages of arthroscopic surgery over open arthrotomies are significant and well documented. In general, arthroscopic surgery provides increased inspection and access to the joint, while also resulting in less patient morbidity, shorter anaesthetic and surgery times, lower complication rates, shorter hospital stays and more rapid and functional recoveries. The disadvantages are few, and primarily involve the expertise and equipment required to perform arthroscopic surgery at an appropriate level. That said, arthroscopy of the canine stifle is relatively challenging when compared with arthroscopy of the shoulder or elbow joint. Inexperienced arthroscopists are advised to gain experience in other joints prior to attempting stifle arthroscopy.

Indications

Arthroscopic procedures routinely performed in the stifle of dogs currently include:

- Exploratory/diagnostic arthroscopy
- Osteochondrosis – flap removal, debridement, curettage/micropicking
- Cranial cruciate ligament – debridement/ablation of damaged ligament
- Meniscus – release, partial or total meniscectomy
- Debridement/wash-out for septic arthritis or osteoarthritis
- Trochleoplasty for selected patellar luxation cases
- Thermal capsulorrhaphy in selected cases.

Instrumentation

A 2.7 mm 30 degree fore-oblique arthroscope works well in nearly all canine stifles. Video arthroscopy is required. A motorized shaver is highly recommended for use in the stifle joint, in order to debride proliferative synovium and fat pad for creation of a viewing window. A variety of arthroscopic probes, graspers, basket forceps and knives are needed in order to be able to perform the full range of procedures listed for stifle arthroscopy. A radiofrequency generator and probes may be helpful in selected cases, but should be used with extreme caution to avoid thermal damage to intra-articular tissues.

Basic technique and portals

The affected limb is prepared for aseptic surgery using a hanging limb technique. The dog is placed in dorsal recumbency with the pelvic limbs extending past the edge of the operating table. In this manner, the surgeon can position the limb such that the paw is in contact with his or her torso, allowing flexion and extension of the stifle to be achieved while the hands are left free to manipulate the arthroscope and instruments (Figure 22.1). Arthroscopy of the stifle is typically performed through craniolateral and craniomedial portals (Operative Technique 22.4). The portals the authors suggest for the stifle are a modification of what has been reported. The portals are placed approximately 5–8 mm medial and lateral to the patellar tendon at a point slightly proximal to the midpoint of the patella-to-tibial tuberosity distance (Figure 22.2).

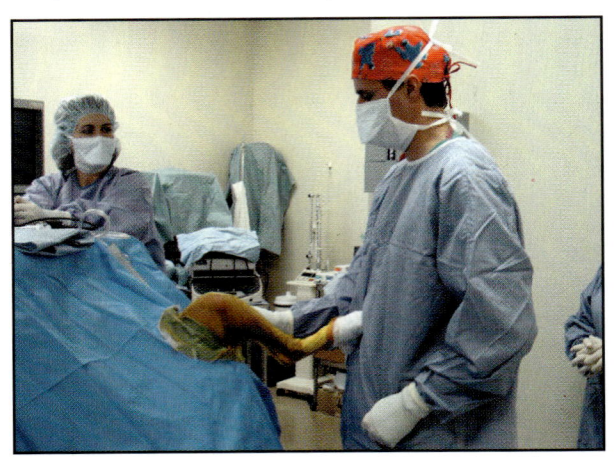

22.1 Recommended patient positioning for stifle arthroscopy. The dog is placed in dorsal recumbency with the pelvic limbs extending past the edge of the operating table such that the paw is in contact with the surgeon's torso, allowing flexion and extension of the stifle to be achieved while the hands are left free to manipulate the arthroscope and instruments.

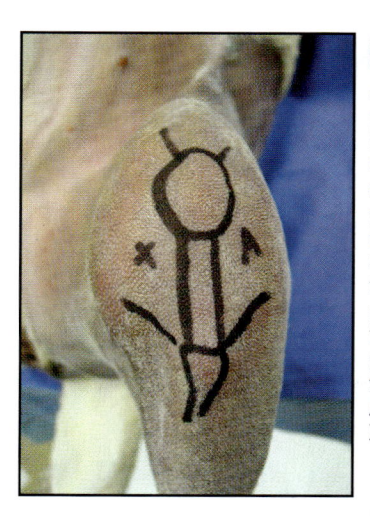

22.2 Arthroscopic portal placement as recommended by the author [JLC] for stifle arthroscopy. The portals are placed approximately 5–8 mm medial and lateral to the patellar tendon at a point slightly proximal to the midpoint of the patella-to-tibial tuberosity distance. A, arthroscope portal; X, instrument portal.

This allows maximum initial inspection, while minimizing the amount of fat pad that must be removed to access the relevant structures. Some arthroscopists employ the use of an egress cannula placed in the proximal aspect of the joint. However, the authors do not find this necessary or additive.

> **WARNING**
> **Debridement of the fat pad should be avoided, if possible, in cases in which the cranial cruciate ligament is intact (i.e. osteochondrosis, exploratory procedure), as a major component of cruciate ligament blood supply is associated with this structure.**

In the authors' experience, the central and caudal horns of the menisci can be adequately inspected only in cases with cranial cruciate ligament deficiency. Fortunately, nearly all meniscal lesions requiring treatment occur in association with cranial cruciate ligament pathology, making access possible when needed. In order to inspect and access the menisci arthroscopically, it is helpful to have an assistant place the stifle in a 'cranial draw' position. Alternatively, a small Hohmann retractor can be inserted into the joint through a separate portal and placed on the caudal aspect of the tibia to provide cranial translation and distraction of the tibia. Varus or valgus stress on the joint may also be helpful.

Osteochondrosis

Osteochondrosis of the stifle is the fourth most common location of occurrence (after shoulder, elbow and hock) of osteochondrosis in dogs (Montgomery *et al.*, 1994). Stifle osteochondrosis occurs most commonly on the medial aspect of the lateral condyle in growing large-breed dogs. Osteochondrosis lesions may also occur, separately or concurrently, on the lateral aspect of the medial condyle. The resultant incongruity and malarticulation result in dysfunction and inflammation that lead to pain and lameness. Osteoarthritis is the ultimate sequel. Recognition of associated clinical signs is important for early diagnosis and optimal treatment.

Aetiopathogenesis

Osteochondrosis is a developmental disorder of articular epiphyseal and physeal cartilage, characterized as a disturbance of normal endochondral ossification. More than a dozen disorders can be included within this disease complex. In small animal surgery, however, osteochondrosis is typically used to refer only to those disorders of endochondral ossification involving the articular surfaces of the shoulder, elbow, hock and stifle.

In developing articular cartilage, failure of normal endochondral ossification results in thickening of the cartilage. Thickened cartilage is less able to tolerate biomechanical load and less capable of receiving adequate nutrition via synovial fluid diffusion. Cartilage in the deeper zones of the tissue may become necrotic and fissure, causing formation of a detached articular cartilage flap: osteochondritis dissecans (OCD).

The aetiopathogenesis of osteochondrosis is not fully known and is thought to be multifactorial. Factors such as over-nutrition, genetic make-up and hormonal influences, which can promote rapid growth and weight gain, are thought to play pivotal roles (Guthrie and Pidduck, 1990; Slater *et al.*, 1991; Harari, 1998). Ischaemia and biomechanical forces are also likely to be involved in the disease process (Douglas and Rang, 1981; Carlson *et al.*, 1991). Primary cell and matrix abnormalities may also influence occurrence and progression of osteochondrosis (Tomlinson *et al.*, 2001; Kuroki *et al.*, 2002). Prevention and treatment should be aimed at all involved factors in order to optimize success.

Signalment and history

Stifle osteochondrosis most commonly occurs in large and giant breeds of dog, including Great Danes, Labrador Retrievers, Golden Retrievers, Newfoundlands and German Shepherd Dogs. Mastiffs, Samoyeds, Boxers and many other breeds can also be affected. A gender predisposition for males has been reported. Age at presentation typically ranges from 5–12 months of age. However, due to the developmental nature of the disorder and potential lack of recognition of clinical signs by the owner, age of onset may be much earlier.

Clinical findings

The most common clinical sign attributable to stifle osteochondrosis is insidious pelvic limb lameness, involving one or both limbs. The degree of lameness can range from very mild to non-weightbearing, and is often exacerbated by exercise or minor trauma (jump or fall). Joint effusion, resistance to flexion and extension, pain, crepitus and muscle atrophy may also be present. Differential diagnoses based on signalment, history, and clinical findings include patellar luxation, panosteitis, trauma (fracture, ligament, tendon, muscle damage) and infective arthropathy.

Radiography

Plain-film radiography typically provides the definitive diagnosis of stifle osteochondrosis (Figure 22.3). Craniocaudal and mediolateral views of the stifle should be obtained after sedation with analgesia. The radiographic findings associated with stifle osteochondrosis include:

Chapter 22 The stifle

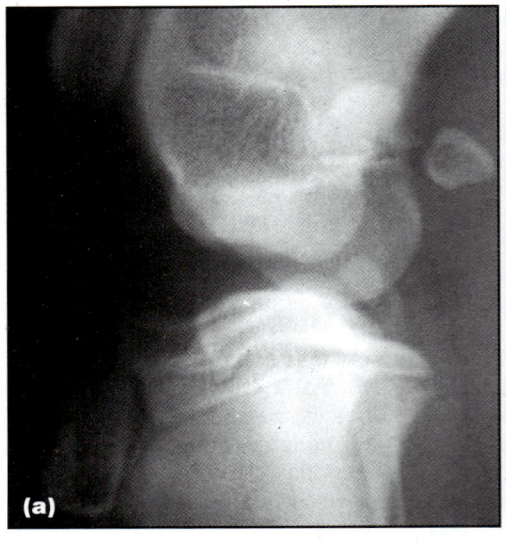

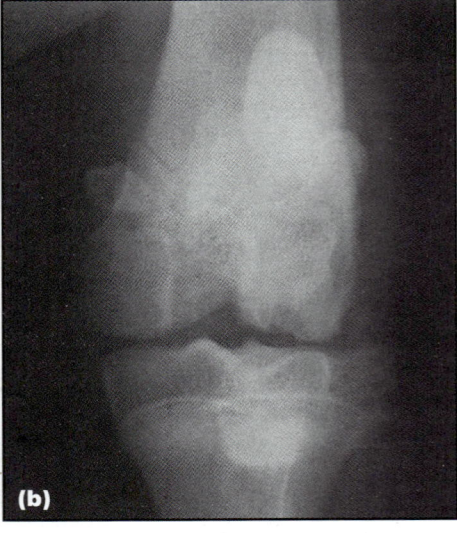

22.3 Mediolateral (a) and craniocaudal (b) radiographs, showing osteochondrosis of the lateral femoral condyle in a 6-month-old Bullmastiff.

- Radiolucent defects of the subchondral bone of the condyle(s)
- Sclerosis associated with the defect and affected condyle
- Joint effusion
- Calcified free bodies ('joint mice')
- Evidence of osteoarthritis (osteophytosis, sclerosis) may be present in more chronic cases.

> **PRACTICAL TIPS**
> - Radiographs should be taken of both stifles, even in dogs with unilateral clinical signs, as osteochondrosis is often bilateral and, therefore, health or disease of both stifles should be documented.
> - The normal radiographic appearance of the extensor fossa of the femur on the mediolateral radiograph can be mistaken for an osteochondrosis lesion.

Additional imaging techniques, including contrast arthrography, MRI, CT and arthroscopy, are rarely necessary, but may be useful in selected cases.

Non-surgical management
Non-surgical management has been advocated by some clinicians. The authors, however, recommend that it be reserved for only those cases in which the stifle osteochondrosis lesion was an incidental finding with no associated clinical signs, and cases in which anaesthesia or surgery are contraindicated for other reasons. Non-surgical management consists of weight and nutritional management, rest and recheck examinations until clinical and radiographic resolution are documented.

Surgical management
Surgical treatment is advocated for the majority of cases and should be performed as early as possible after diagnosis. Surgical therapy consists of:

- Removal of pathological cartilage (flaps, loose bodies, abnormal cartilage)
- Curettage, forage or micropicking of subchondral bone to stimulate bleeding in order to optimize fibrocartilage formation within the defect
- Joint lavage.

Inspection of, and access to, the osteochondrosis lesion can be accomplished via a lateral or medial parapatellar approach, or arthroscopically (Figure 22.4). Arthroscopic treatment of osteochondrosis lesions of the stifle may have advantages in terms of inspection, precision of treatment and postoperative morbidity.

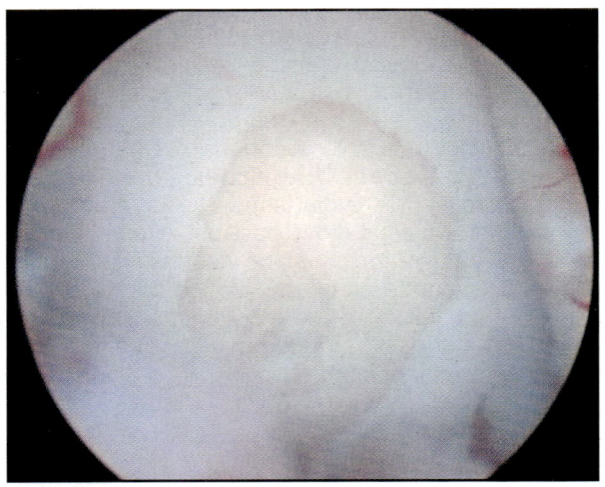

22.4 Arthroscopic view of an osteochondrosis lesion on the lateral femoral condyle of the stifle as seen from the craniomedial camera portal.

Recommended postoperative care includes:

- Analgesic therapy
- Soft padded bandaging (24–48 hours)
- NSAIDs and nutraceuticals
- Physical rehabilitation to promote fibrocartilage healing, muscle strength, range of motion and limb function.

Prognosis

The prognosis for return to full function in dogs with stifle osteochondrosis is dependent on type of therapy, duration of the problem, size and location of the lesion, and severity of osteoarthritis present. However, the prognosis is generally considered to be guarded for return to full function due to progression of osteoarthritis secondary to the articular cartilage pathology in osteochondrosis. Early diagnosis and treatment, along with physical rehabilitation, are likely to optimize the prognosis.

Patellar luxation

Patellar luxation is a common stifle condition in dogs that can result in pain, lameness and osteoarthritis. The condition has traditionally been recognized in toy and miniature breeds but appears to be increasing in prevalence in large-breed dogs, especially Labrador Retrievers. Patellar luxation is most commonly a developmental disorder associated with multiple anatomical abnormalities of the pelvic limb. Medial luxation is more frequently recognized than lateral luxation.

Anatomy and biomechanics

The patella is a sesamoid bone in the tendon of insertion of the quadriceps femoris muscle. It is ovate in shape and curved so as to articulate with the femoral trochlea. Parapatellar fibrocartilages on each side of the patella articulate with ridges of the trochlea. Lateral and medial femoropatellar ligaments exist as delicate bands of loose connective tissue connecting the patella to the fabella laterally and the periosteum of the femoral epicondyle medially.

The femoropatellar articulation greatly increases the mechanical efficiency of the quadriceps muscle group and facilitates stifle extension. The extensor mechanism is composed of the quadriceps femoris muscle, patella, trochlea, patellar tendon and tibial tuberosity (Figure 22.5). These structures should be in correct anatomical alignment to prevent patellar luxation or subluxation. The angle between the rectus femoris muscle, the patella and the patellar tendon is referred to as the quadriceps angle (Q-angle). It may be measured by magnetic resonance methods. There is a significant difference in the Q-angle in dogs with grade II and grade III congenital patellar luxation compared with that in dogs without patellar instability (Kaiser *et al.*, 2001a). With abnormal alignment of the extensor mechanism there is a reduced extensor moment of the stifle.

Aetiopathogenesis

Traumatic luxation of the patella is uncommon. The majority of patellar luxations are a result of developmental malalignment of the quadriceps mechanism. Patellar luxation should be considered as one aspect of a generalized deformity of the entire limb. In severe cases there can be marked angular and rotational deformity of the femoral and tibial bones. The over-representation of certain breeds supports the theory that patellar luxation is a genetic condition.

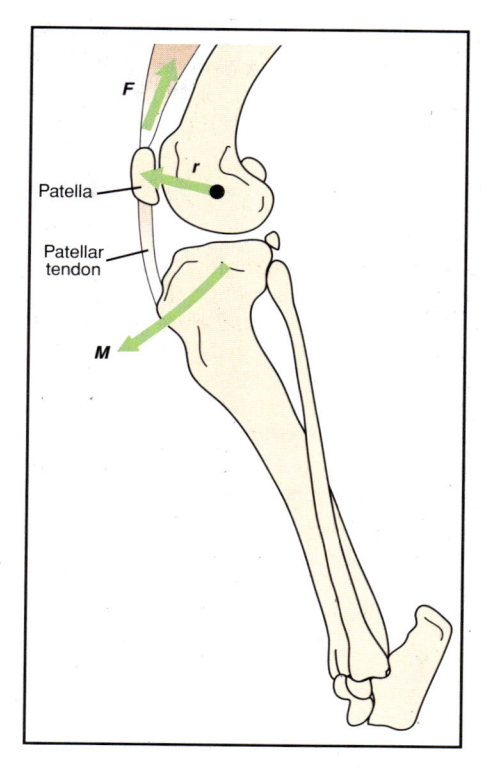

22.5 Anatomy and biomechanics of the quadriceps femoris extensor mechanism. Moment (***M***) = Force (***F***) x distance (***r***).

The pathogenesis of developmental patellar luxation remains speculative and controversial (Robins, 1990). Abnormal femoral head and neck angles of inclination and anteversion have been hypothesized as being key primary features affecting quadriceps alignment; however, they have not been proven (Kaiser *et al.*, 2001b). A variable degree of asymmetrical growth of the distal femoral and proximal tibial physes is recognized in many cases. When this occurs in very young dogs it may become a self-perpetuating problem with further retardation in growth on the compression aspect of the physes and acceleration of growth on the tension aspect of the physes. With medial patellar luxation this may result in marked lateral bowing of the distal femur and medial bowing of the proximal tibia. The limb has a resultant S-shaped conformation with tilting of the joint.

Failure of the luxated patella to articulate with the femoral trochlea results in loss of physiological pressure and accelerated growth in this area. The femoral condyle on the side of the patellar luxation may be hypoplastic. Repetitive luxation of the patella damages the articular surfaces of the patella and femoral condyle. This may result in further flattening of the condyle, so facilitating further luxation. Proximal location of the patella (patella alta) has been hypothesized as a possible predisposing factor to lateral patellar luxation in humans and may play a role in dogs, since many luxations tend to occur when the stifle is extended.

Although the majority of cases present with complete femoropatellar luxation, subluxation is also possible. Dogs with patellar subluxation tend to be presented when adults due to chronic abnormal tracking of the patella causing ulceration of patellar and trochlear ridge articular cartilage. Chronic patellar luxation may be associated with concomitant cranial cruciate

Chapter 22 The stifle

ligament rupture. It has been hypothesized but not proven that abnormal stifle joint biomechanics with excessive internal rotation is the cause of the cranial cruciate ligament degeneration and rupture.

Medial patellar luxation

Signalment and history
Medial patellar luxation is most commonly recognized in toy and miniature breeds, e.g. Miniature Poodle, Yorkshire Terrier. Also commonly presented are English and Staffordshire Bull Terriers and English Bulldogs. Of the larger breeds, the Labrador Retriever and Mastiff appear to be over-represented. Many dogs are presented when 6–12 months of age; however, in some mild cases lameness may only become a feature later in life or following cranial cruciate ligament rupture. Unilateral medial patellar luxation often presents as an intermittent lameness. Sudden luxation may result in acute lameness with non-weightbearing. The patella may spontaneously relocate and the lameness immediately resolve.

Clinical findings
The clinical signs of medial patellar luxation vary according to the degree of deformity, duration of the condition and whether one or both stifles are affected. Genu varum or a 'bow-legged' conformation is a feature in some dogs. The position of the tibial tuberosity should be assessed during weightbearing with the patella reduced. Tracking of the patella and the angle of the femorotibial joint when the patella luxates should be determined. Integrity of the cranial cruciate ligaments, evidence of femoropatellar crepitus or pain, and any reduced range of stifle extension should be noted.

Grading patellar luxations is useful for monitoring progression of the condition and response to surgery. The following clinical grades have been proposed:

- Grade I: The patella can be manually luxated when the stifle is extended; however, when released it returns to the trochlea. Internal rotation of the tibia and displacement of the tibial tuberosity are minimal.
- Grade II: The patella is frequently located medially with flexion of the stifle joint; however, it is easily reduced when the stifle is extended and the tibia externally rotated. The tibial tuberosity is displaced medially. Mild angular deformity of the femur and tibia may be present
- Grade III: The patella is permanently luxated. It may be reduced, but luxation recurs immediately. Angular and rotational deformities of the femur and tibia are common. The trochlea is usually shallow or flat
- Grade IV: The patella is permanently luxated and it is not possible manually to reposition it in the trochlea. Muscle contracture reduces the range of stifle extension. Angular and rotational deformity of the femur and tibia are generally marked and the tibial tuberosity is displaced 60–90 degrees medially. Concurrent external rotation of the distal tibia may result in reasonable alignment of the hock and hind paw. The trochlea is flat or convex.

Radiography
Mediolateral and caudocranial radiographs enable assessment of femoral and tibial deformity. Apparent angular and rotational deformities should be interpreted with caution since positioning may have a profound influence (Figure 22.6). Tangential ('skyline') views of the flexed stifle enable assessment of the femoral trochlea and femoropatellar congruence. Periarticular new bone (indicative of secondary osteoarthritis), and cranial displacement of the infrapatellar fat pad and caudal displacement of the joint capsule (consistent with a joint effusion) are common features.

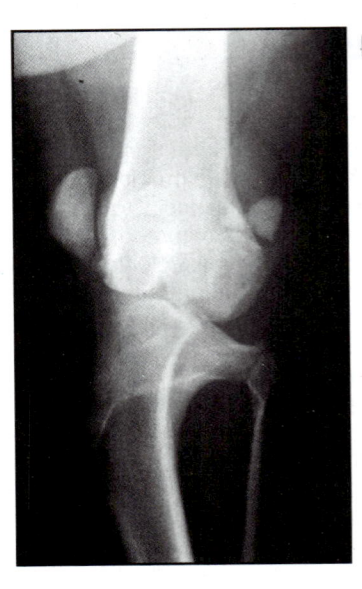

22.6 Caudocranial radiograph, showing medial luxation of the patella in a 4-year-old Labrador Retriever.

Surgical management
Surgical management of medial patellar luxation in asymptomatic small-breed dogs is controversial and is generally not necessary. However, surgery is indicated in medium and large breeds and in all dogs with persistent lameness. It is essential that intervention is not delayed in immature cases, especially with Grade III and IV luxations where realignment of the quadriceps mechanism during growth may retard the progression of angular and rotational deformity.

> **The aim of surgery is to restore normal stifle biomechanics and eliminate repeated trauma to articular cartilage by realigning the quadriceps mechanism and stabilizing the femoropatellar joint.**

The surgical techniques that are most commonly employed include:

- Deepening the femoral trochlea
- Tibial tuberosity transposition
- Medial soft tissue release
- Lateral soft tissue tightening.

Other procedures, such as transplantation of the origin of the rectus femoris muscle, corrective osteotomy and patellectomy, are rarely necessary. The authors perform a tibial tuberosity transposition in all cases. It is generally necessary to release the medial soft tissues and tighten the lateral soft tissues. If there is any doubt regarding the depth of the femoral trochlea, it should be deepened.

> **PRACTICAL TIP**
> Surgery should be performed in a logical stepwise fashion, addressing each abnormality present and evaluating tracking and stability of the patella after each procedure.

> **WARNING**
> Over-reliance on derotational sutures and soft tissue tightening procedures in the absence of tibial tuberosity transposition should be avoided, as patellar stability is invariably temporary.

Deepening the femoral trochlea (trochleoplasty): Many techniques have been described for deepening the femoral trochlea. Rectangular recession trochleoplasty and wedge recession trochleoplasty are the only methods available that can recess the trochlea while preserving articular cartilage in adult animals. The authors favour the former technique.

> **WARNING**
> Trochleoplasty techniques that remove hyaline articular cartilage should be avoided, since postoperative morbidity is higher than in techniques that maintain hyaline cartilage.

Rectangular recession trochleoplasty (Operative Technique 22.5): Rectangular recession trochleoplasty (or trochlear block recession) utilizes a rectangular osteochondral autograft that is harvested from the trochlea and replaced into the deepened recipient bed (Talcott et al., 2000). The technique preserves maximum hyaline articular cartilage. However, harvesting the rectangular autograft is more technically demanding than harvesting a wedge.

Wedge recession trochleoplasty (Operative Technique 22.6): One potential disadvantage of this technique is the articular surface shape of the osteochondral wedge, which tapers to a point proximally and distally. This may prevent adequate recession of the proximal trochlea. As the stifle is extended and the patella moves proximally, the patella may articulate with the non-recessed proximal femoral trochlea instead of the recessed wedge, resulting in decreased patellar depth.

Using a cadaver model Johnson *et al.* (2001) compared rectangular recession trochleoplasty and wedge recession trochleoplasty. Computed tomography (CT) and biomechanical evaluations were performed pre- and postoperatively. The change in trochlear depth was not significantly different between groups. In the extended stifle position (patella proximally), patellar depth and patellar articular contact with the recessed trochlea were significantly greater after rectangular recession trochleoplasty than after wedge recession trochleoplasty. In addition, a smaller percentage of the patellae luxated with internal rotation of the tibia after rectangular recession trochleoplasty than after wedge recession trochleoplasty.

Trochlear chondroplasty: Preservation of articular cartilage may be achieved in dogs under 6 months of age by creating a flap of cartilage (which is left attached distally), removing subchondral bone and then replacing the layer of articular cartilage.

Tibial tuberosity transposition (Operative Technique 22.7): The tibial tuberosity should be transposed in all surgical cases to improve quadriceps alignment. Failure to do so will result in a high incidence of reluxation following surgery.

> **WARNING**
> The potential for complications with this technique should not be underestimated, especially in large dogs.

Medial soft tissue release: A varying degree of release of medial soft tissues is often necessary to enable normal patellar tracking, especially at the proximal aspect of the trochlea where there may remain a tendency for the patella to displace medially. Sequential sectioning of the femoral fascia, medial femoropatellar ligament, joint capsule, insertion of the cranial sartorius muscle and vastus medialis muscle may be necessary.

Lateral soft tissue tightening: The lateral joint capsule and fascia lata should be tightened following stabilization of the patella. Care should be taken to avoid excessive tightening, since this may result in lateral patellar luxation. Pre-placement of sutures should be considered. Occasionally it is necessary to place a non-absorbable suture or strip of fascia lata from the lateral fabella to the patella to augment other stabilizing procedures, especially in dogs with increased internal rotational laxity.

Transplantation of the origin of the rectus femoris muscle: Slocum and Slocum (1998) advocated transplantation of the origin of the rectus femoris muscle in dogs with marked genu varum. The rectus femoris muscle originates on the shaft of the ilium, just cranial to the hip, and inserts on the medial aspect of the patellar fascia. The origin is freed with a section of bone and transplanted to a position close to the insertion of the deep gluteal muscle, to redirect the forces within the quadriceps. There are no reports on the results of this procedure.

Corrective osteotomy: In cases with severe deformity of the distal femur and, or, proximal tibia, the above techniques may fail to provide femoropatellar stability. It may be necessary to consider corrective osteotomies of one, or generally both, bones. Preoperative radiographic planning is critical. Such procedures are rarely indicated.

Patellectomy: Patellectomy is rarely indicated, despite the frequent finding of ulceration of patellar articular cartilage. It is only performed when there is intractable femoropatellar pain. The function of the stifle following patellectomy appears to be satisfactory.

Chapter 22 The stifle

Grade IV luxations in puppies: Deepening of the femoral trochlea may be performed via a chondroplasty technique. A radical medial fascial release is generally necessary to enable reduction of the luxation. Two mattress sutures are placed from the lateral femoral condyle: one around the patella and the other through the tibial tuberosity. The tibia is externally rotated as the sutures are tightened. Suture breakage or pull-through is inevitable within a few weeks; however, the results of surgery are often satisfactory. The objective of early treatment is to avoid the severe structural changes that would occur during growth and make conventional therapy unrewarding.

Concomitant cranial cruciate ligament rupture: Correction of femoropatellar instability by the above methods is generally more important than management of the cranial cruciate ligament rupture. Affected joints often have significant osteoarthritis and the associated periarticular fibrosis reduces femorotibial instability. When significant cranial draw is present a lateral fabellotibial suture may provide temporary stability. The Kirschner wires stabilizing the tibial tuberosity transposition may be used as the distal anchor. Meniscal inspection is mandatory. Tibial plateau levelling techniques may be used to manage medial patellar luxation and concomitant cranial cruciate ligament rupture. With the TPLO procedure the craniodistal fragment, including the tibial tuberosity, is externally rotated in order to realign the quadriceps mechanism. With tibial wedge osteotomy surgery it is necessary independently to transpose the tibial tuberosity laterally.

Prognosis
The prognosis following patellar luxation surgery is generally good, though the development and progression of osteoarthritis remain inevitable. It is worth considering that in one study of 34 dogs (52 stifles), 48% of the patellae reluxated; 68% of these recurrences were Grade I. Only 12% had any permanent lameness and these were mainly associated with concomitant cranial cruciate ligament injury (Willauer and Vasseur, 1987). Recurrence of patellar luxation is generally due to failure to transpose the tibial tuberosity. The prognosis may become more guarded with increasing deformity. Denny and Minter (1973) observed poor outcomes in cases with marked anatomical deformities. Contraction of the soft tissues caudal to the stifle may result in inability to extend the joint fully and persistent lameness.

Lateral patellar luxation
Lateral patellar luxation is primarily recognized in large and giant breeds in association with genu valgum ('knock knees'). Changes that may be present include a shallow acetabulum, increased anteversion of the femoral neck, increased angle of inclination (coxa valga), medial bowing of the distal femur, shallow trochlea, lateral displacement of the tibial tuberosity, lateral bowing of the tibia and external rotation of the paw (Figure 22.7).

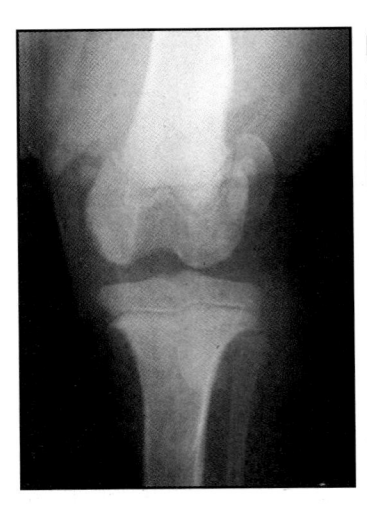

22.7 Caudocranial radiograph, showing lateral luxation of the patella in a 5-month-old Flat-coated Retriever.

Treatment
Lateral patellar luxation, when associated with severe limb deformities, is a complex disorder with a guarded prognosis. In the immature dog, with significant remaining growth potential, hemicircumferential elevation of the periosteum of the lateral aspect of the distal femur and transphyseal bridging may be employed. In mature dogs, the principles of surgical management are similar to those described for medial patellar luxation.

Patellar luxation in the cat
Congenital medial patellar luxation is uncommon in the cat and lateral luxation is even less common (Houlton and Meynink, 1989). It has been reported in numerous breeds, including Devon Rex, Siamese and Domestic Shorthair, and is often found in association with hip dysplasia. It is frequently an incidental finding, since the majority of cats with patellar luxation are not lame. Smith *et al.* (1999) studied 78 cats of which 11 had clinical signs of disease in the pelvic limbs. Medial patellar luxation (Figure 22.8) was found in 45 cats (78% grade I) and medial patellar subluxation in 33 cats. Hip dysplasia was diagnosed radiographically in 25 cases. Concurrent medial patellar luxation and hip dysplasia were detected in 24% of cats. There was a weak association between the two conditions: cats were three times more likely to have both than to have either condition alone.

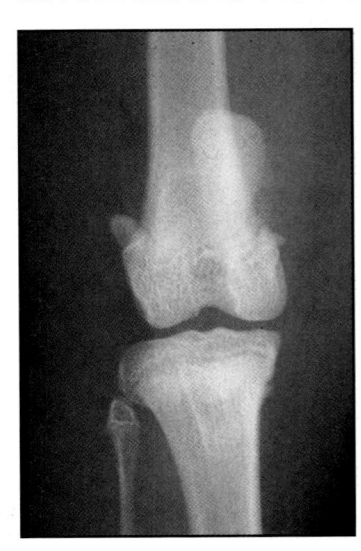

22.8 Caudocranial radiograph, showing medial luxation of the patella in a 14-month-old Maine Coon cat.

Chapter 22 The stifle

Treatment
Skeletal deformity is generally less severe than in dogs. When patellar luxation results in lameness, surgical correction is indicated (Houlton and Meynink, 1989). Tibial tuberosity transposition, with or without a recession trochleoplasty technique, is often necessary. The prognosis is generally good with a marked improvement in the degree of lameness.

Cranial cruciate ligament disease and meniscal injury

Cranial cruciate ligament disease, with or without concomitant meniscal injury, is the most common cause of lameness in the dog. Isolated rupture of the cranial cruciate ligament is uncommon in cats. The term 'disease' is used to cover a spectrum of pathology that may range from stretching to partial or complete rupture. Stifle joint osteoarthritis is invariably a feature with this condition. There is still considerable controversy with regard to the aetiology, pathogenesis and most appropriate method of management of cranial cruciate ligament disease in the dog.

Anatomy and function
The cranial cruciate ligament originates on the caudomedial aspect of the lateral femoral condyle and inserts on the cranial intercondylar region of the tibial plateau (Figure 22.9). It crosses the intercondylar notch caudally to cranially and laterally to medially. The cranial cruciate ligament is covered by a layer of synovial membrane and is thus intra-articular but extrasynovial. It is composed of numerous bundles of collagen fibres separated by columns of connective tissue cells. Collagen bundles are arranged into fascicles separated by thin membranous sheets containing blood vessels and nerves. Vascularization is from the overlying synovial vessels that emanate from the infrapatellar fat pad and caudal soft tissues. The central core of the midsection of the cranial cruciate ligament is relatively poorly vascularized (Vasseur et al., 1985). Mechanoreceptors in the ligament detect increased strain and initiate neural reflex arcs that result in contraction of the caudal thigh muscles and simultaneous relaxation of the quadriceps muscles. This is a protective mechanism that contributes to joint stability.

The cranial cruciate ligament functions as an important stabilizer to cranial displacement of the tibia and also prevents hyperextension of the stifle joint. In conjunction with the caudal cruciate ligament and collateral ligaments it has a secondary role of preventing excessive internal rotation of the tibia (Arnoczky and Marshall, 1977). It prevents excessive varus or valgus movement when the stifle is flexed.

The cranial cruciate ligament can be regarded as being composed of two functional components: the craniomedial band (narrow); and the caudolateral band (broad). This is an oversimplification of the complex structure and functional relationships but is relevant in the diagnosis of partial rupture of the ligament. The craniomedial band remains taut in all positions of the joint in contrast to the caudolateral band, which is only taut when the joint is extended.

Cranial tibial thrust
Knowledge of the forces that act within the stifle joint is important in order to understand the aetiopathogenesis and management concepts of cranial cruciate ligament disease. The stifle is subjected to external ground reaction forces that are applied to the limb during weightbearing and internal forces generated by muscle contraction (Figure 22.10). The quadriceps and gastrocnemius muscles exert a cranial force on the tibia, while the hamstring and biceps femoris muscles exert a caudal force. External and internal forces not only compress the femoral and tibial articular surfaces together, they also generate a cranially orientated shear force in the tibia, termed 'cranial tibial thrust' (Slocum and Devine, 1983). This is because the tibial plateau is not perpendicular to a line joining the centre of motion of the stifle and hock joints but is oriented caudodistally. The tibial plateau angle in the Greyhound is approximately 22 degrees and the standing

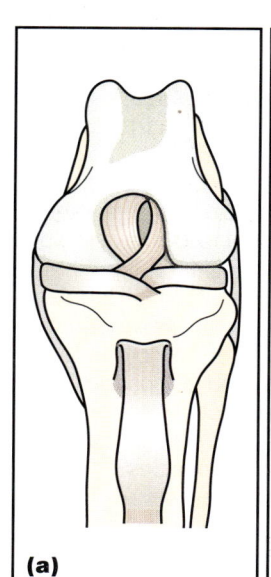

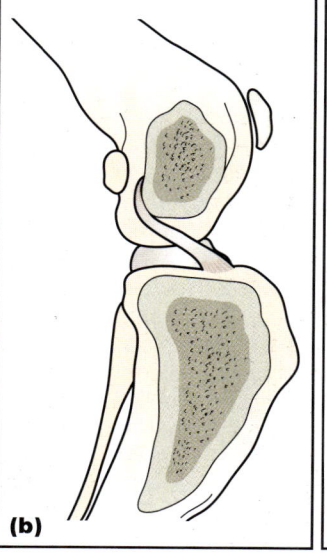

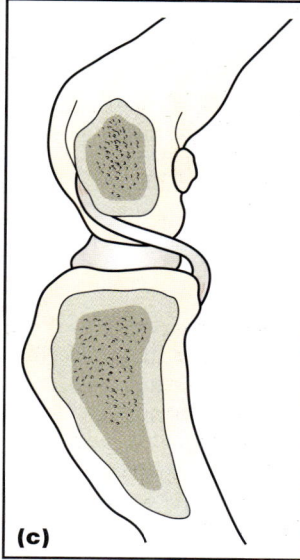

22.9 Anatomy of the cruciate ligaments. **(a)** The cranial cruciate dominates the cranial view. **(b)** The cranial cruciate arises on the medial aspect of the lateral condyle and inserts in the intercondylar region. **(c)** The caudal cruciate arises from the lateral aspect of the medial condyle and inserts on the caudal aspect of the tibia.

Chapter 22 The stifle

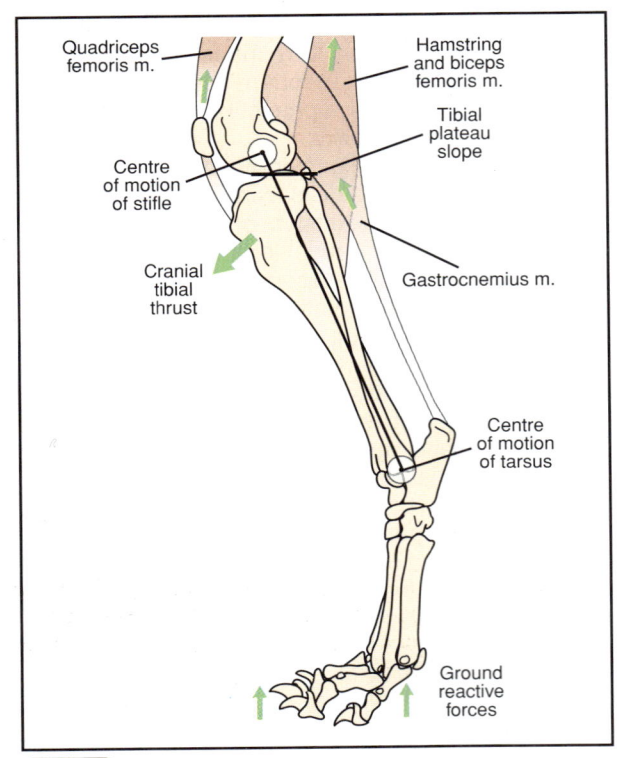

22.10 Stifle joint forces and cranial tibial thrust.

plateau angle (i.e. the angle relative to the ground) is approximately 1.5 degrees (Wilke *et al.*, 2002). Cranial tibial thrust is opposed passively by the cranial cruciate ligament and actively by the hamstring and biceps femoris muscles. Rupture of the cranial cruciate ligament results in cranial translation of the tibia when the joint is loaded (Korvick *et al.*, 1994). This is the basis of the tibial compression test (see below). The greater the tibial plateau angle, the greater the cranial tibial thrust (Warzee *et al.*, 2001).

Aetiopathogenesis

Acute traumatic rupture of a normal cranial cruciate ligament is very uncommon. In the dog the vast majority of partial and complete cranial cruciate ruptures do not involve significant trauma. Histopathological examination of these ligaments reveals degenerative changes and examination of the joint generally reveals evidence of osteoarthritis that has been present longer than the duration of the lameness. Often the contralateral cranial cruciate ligament and stifle joint have pathological changes. A conservative estimate of the incidence of clinically significant bilateral cranial cruciate disease is 30% (Doverspike *et al.*, 1993).

> **Cranial cruciate ligament disease in the dog is generally a degenerative condition rather than a traumatic condition. This has important implications regarding the management and prognosis.**

The strength of the cranial cruciate ligament decreases with ageing, in association with degeneration of collagen fibres and cellular elements; these changes are more dramatic and occur at a younger age in large dogs. This agrees with the observation that large dogs tend to rupture the ligament earlier in life than small dogs (Bennett *et al.*, 1988). Partial rupture of the cranial cruciate ligament is not uncommon. These joints may be more inflamed than joints with complete ligament rupture (Griffin and Vasseur, 1992).

The cause of cranial cruciate ligament degeneration and rupture is poorly understood. Abnormal conformation and gait, increased tibial plateau angle (Read and Robins, 1982; Morris and Lipowitz, 2001; Macias *et al.*, 2002), obesity (Vasseur *et al.*, 1985; Lampman *et al.*, 2003) and lack of fitness (Bennett *et al.*, 1988) may adversely affect cranial tibial thrust and play an important role. Some dogs have a varus ('bow-legged') deformity with internal rotation of the tibia that may increase stress on the cranial cruciate ligament and contribute to degeneration and rupture. The mean tibial plateau angle of dogs with cranial cruciate ligament rupture was reported to be significantly greater than the mean tibial plateau angle of dogs with intact cranial cruciate ligaments (Morris and Lipowitz, 2001). These findings were, however, not supported in other studies (Wilke *et al.*, 2002; Reif and Probst, 2003). Obesity and poor physical condition may hamper the protective action of the hamstring and biceps femoris muscles and thus indirectly increase stress on the cranial cruciate ligament.

A number of other factors may contribute to cranial cruciate ligament degeneration, including breed variation in the mechanical and physical properties of the cranial cruciate ligament, patellar luxation, intercondylar notch deformity (Aiken *et al.*, 1995), immune-mediated disease (Niebauer, 1982; Galloway and Lester, 1995) and vascular disease (Vasseur *et al.*, 1985). It is probable that a number of these factors are interrelated. Interestingly, a study *in vitro* showed that only half the load per unit body mass was required to cause rupture of the ligament in the Rottweiler compared with that in the Greyhound (Wingfield *et al.*, 2000).

Meniscal anatomy and pathology

The medial and lateral menisci are semilunar fibrocartilaginous structures interposed between the articular surfaces of the femur and tibia. They are wedge-shaped in cross-section with the thicker peripheral border attached to the joint capsule (Figure 22.11). Short ligaments attach the cranial and caudal aspects of the medial and lateral menisci to the tibia. An additional ligament attaches the caudal aspect of the lateral meniscus to the axial aspect of the medial femoral condyle. The medial meniscus has a peripheral attachment to the adjacent collateral ligament in contrast to the lateral meniscus. An intermeniscal ligament loosely attaches the cranial aspects of the menisci. The menisci play an important role in femorotibial stability, load distribution and lubrication. Their sensory function may contribute to joint proprioception and help protect ligaments from excessive loading via neural reflex arcs involving regional muscles. Meniscal horns are richly supplied with blood vessels and nerves. Only the peripheral 15% of the meniscal body is vascularized from the joint capsule. The central zone is avascular and thus healing following injury is poor.

Chapter 22 The stifle

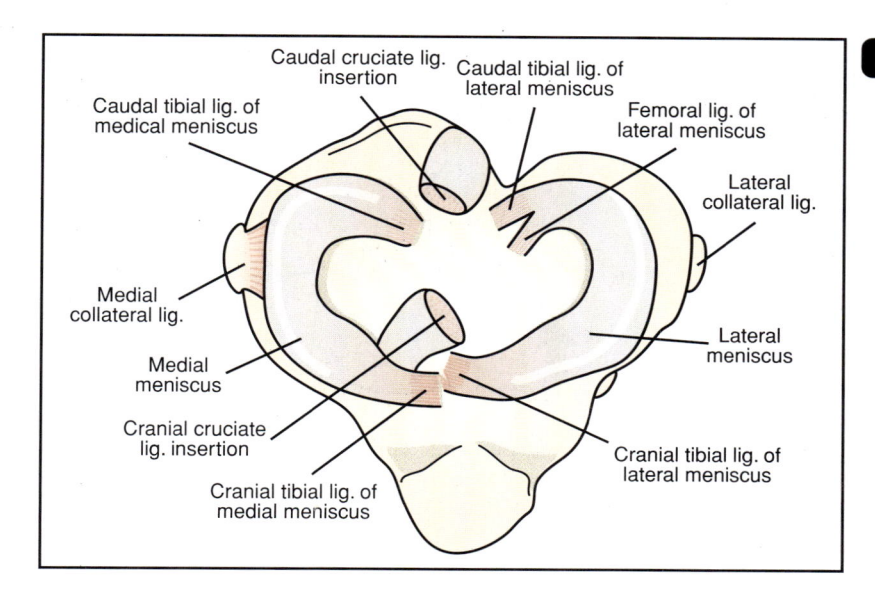

22.11 Anatomy of the medial and lateral menisci.

In referral practice approximately 50% of dogs with cranial cruciate ligament rupture have concomitant meniscal injuries. Dogs with partial ligament rupture and small dogs have a lower incidence (Bennett et al., 1988). The medial meniscus is particularly prone to injury and the lateral meniscus is rarely involved. The medial meniscus is firmly attached to the medial collateral ligament and it does not have an attachment to the femur. As a result it moves cranially with the tibia during weightbearing and becomes crushed between the medial femoral condyle and tibial plateau. The most common injury is a longitudinal tear at the periphery of the caudal horn. The axial aspect often displaces cranially and centrally, remaining attached at either end, forming the so-called 'bucket handle tear'.

Signalment
Any breed of dog or cat may be presented with cranial cruciate ligament disease, but large- and giant-breed dogs (Golden Retriever, Rottweiler, Boxer, Mastiff, St Bernard, Great Dane, Chow Chow) appear to be over-represented. The condition has primarily been recognized in older animals, although the incidence in young dogs seems to be increasing (Bennett et al., 1988). It is not uncommon for large- and giant-breed dogs to be presented with bilateral cranial cruciate ligament disease when under 2 years of age. Numerous studies have reported a higher incidence in spayed females.

History
Acute-onset severe pelvic limb lameness, perhaps associated with minor trauma, may be reported in dogs with sudden rupture of a degenerate cranial cruciate ligament. Meniscal injury is the other key possibility in these cases. In many dogs, however, the onset of lameness is insidious. Stiffness after rest is a common feature, especially following a period of exercise. The majority of dogs with cranial cruciate ligament disease will not sit in a symmetrical position with full flexion of the stifle. Owners may report reduced weightbearing on one or both pelvic limbs when standing ('toe touching') or an audible click. Bilateral rupture may result in difficulty rising from a lying position, difficulty in jumping and climbing, or poor exercise tolerance; the dog may have an arched back and may mistakenly be thought to have a spinal disorder.

Clinical examination

Acute traumatic cranial cruciate ligament rupture generally causes severe lameness or non-weightbearing. In contrast to degenerative cranial cruciate ligament disease, muscle atrophy and joint thickening are not features at the time of injury.

Gait should be analysed for evidence of bilateral lameness and the degree of lameness recorded. The latter may be extremely variable. Conformation and posture should be carefully evaluated. Examination of the entire limb and lumbosacral spine is important to detect other possible causes of lameness. Femoropatellar stability should be assessed. Quadriceps muscle atrophy is invariably a feature with degenerative cranial cruciate ligament disease. Thickening of the medial aspect of the proximal tibia is common in chronic cases. A joint effusion is often present and may be detected on either side of the patellar tendon where the edges are less distinct. Flexion and extension of the stifle may cause pain and crepitus may be palpable. A reduction in range of joint flexion and extension may be evident, especially in chronic cases with advanced osteoarthritis and occasionally in dogs with displaced meniscal injuries. An audible or palpable 'click' may be detected and may be associated with a meniscal injury; however, this is not always the cause and the absence of a click does not exclude the possibility of meniscal damage.

Many, but not all, dogs with cranial cruciate ligament disease have femorotibial instability, demonstrable by either the cranial draw or the tibial compression test. These tests may be performed with the dog either standing or lying in lateral recumbency with the affected limb uppermost. Sedation or anaesthesia may be necessary if pain, anxiety or aggressiveness make a thorough examination impossible.

Chapter 22   The stifle

Cranial draw test
The index finger is placed on the patella, and the thumb of the same hand is placed on the lateral fabella. With the other hand the index finger is placed on the tibial crest and the thumb is placed on the head of the fibula. A cranial force is applied to the tibia with the joint in full extension and in 30–60 degrees of flexion to aid detection of partial ruptures (Figure 22.12). With complete rupture of the cranial cruciate ligament, abnormal cranial draw motion is evident when the joint is extended and flexed. When the craniomedial band of the ligament is ruptured in isolation, cranial draw is only detected when the joint is flexed, since the intact caudolateral band is taut when the joint is extended. Isolated rupture of the caudolateral band is not associated with cranial draw since the intact craniomedial band prevents abnormal motion regardless of the position of the joint.

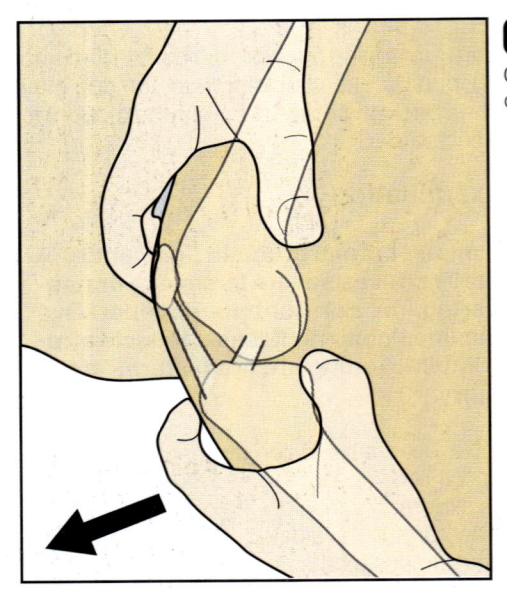

22.12 Cranial draw test.

22.13 Tibial compression test.

Pain may be a feature when performing the cranial draw test. This should alert the clinician to the possibility of cranial cruciate ligament disease in the absence of femorotibial instability. Comparison should be made with the contralateral stifle, remembering the possibility of bilateral symmetrical disease. Periarticular fibrosis and meniscal injury, with the caudal horn of the medial meniscus wedged between the femoral condyle and tibial plateau, may prevent cranial draw in a cranial cruciate ligament deficient stifle. A short cranial draw motion with a sharp end point may be detected in young animals and is normal.

Tibial compression test
The hock joint is slowly flexed with one hand as the stifle joint is maintained in a slight degree of flexion, while the other hand palpates the tibial tuberosity for cranial subluxation (Figure 22.13). This test mimics the loading conditions that generate cranial tibial thrust. The tibial compression test may cause less discomfort than the cranial draw test but it may be less sensitive at detecting partial cranial cruciate ligament ruptures.

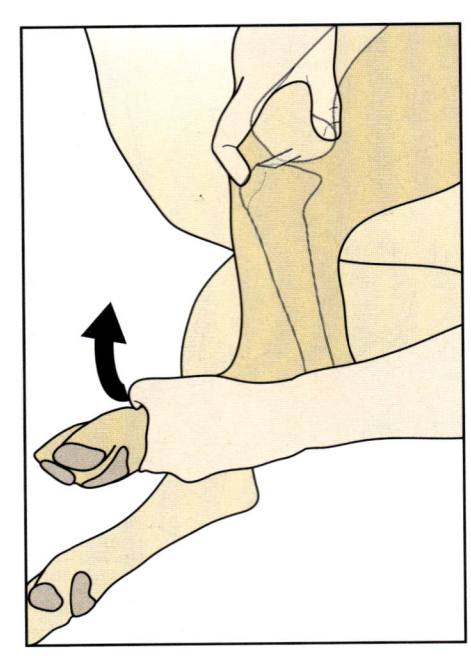

> Not all dogs with pelvic limb lameness due to cranial cruciate ligament disease have femorotibial instability that can be detected by the cranial draw or tibial compression test.

Radiography
Radiographs of the stifle in dogs and cats with cranial cruciate ligament disease have conventionally been obtained in order to detect evidence of osteoarthritis and to exclude other possible causes of lameness such as bone or joint neoplasia. Due to recent understanding of the importance of the tibial plateau angle and conformational abnormalities, it is recommended that specific orthogonal views of both pelvic limbs be obtained to enable these features to be assessed.

> **PRACTICAL TIP**
> Mediolateral and caudocranial radiographs that enable assessment of the tibial plateau angle and angular and rotational limb deformities should be obtained in all dogs prior to possible surgery for cranial cruciate ligament disease.

Positioning

Mediolateral view: Superimposition of the femoral condyles is critical for accurate measurement of the tibial plateau angle. The patient is positioned in lateral recumbency with the affected limb on the table and the contralateral pelvic limb secured cranially. If the latter is positioned too far cranially, it will result in external rotation of the affected limb; if it is positioned caudally, it will result in internal rotation of the affected limb. In both these scenarios the femoral condyles will not be superimposed. It is helpful to elevate the proximal limb and lumbosacral spine to the same height as the tabletop X-ray film cassette. The X-ray beam is centred on the stifle and collimated to include the tibia and talocrural joint (Figure 22.14).

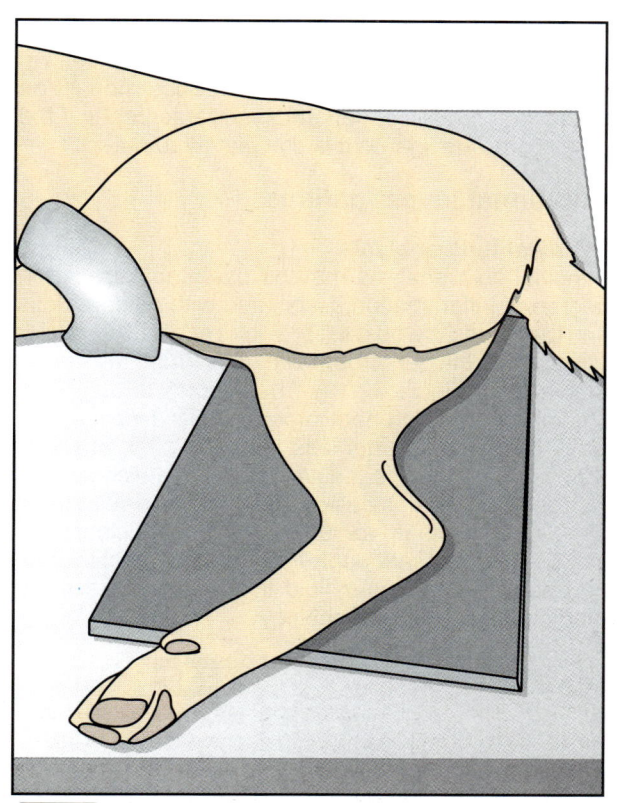

Chapter 22 The stifle

22.14 Radiographic positioning for mediolateral view of the stifle, tibia and tarsus.

Caudocranial view: Symmetrical positioning of the femoral condyles, fabellae and patella is critical for assessment of angular and rotational limb deformities. The patient is positioned in lateral recumbency, as for the mediolateral view, and the affected limb is extended caudally. Supporting the groin on sandbags and securing the contralateral limb cranially is helpful. The X-ray beam is centred on the stifle and collimated to include the femur, tibia and talocrural joint (Figure 22.15).

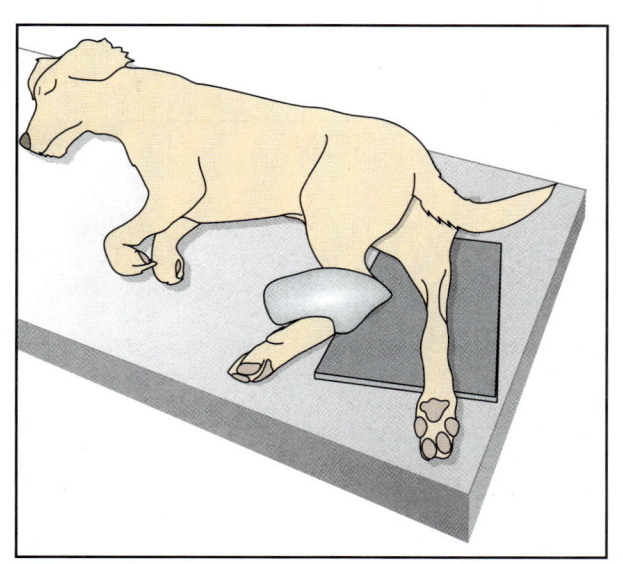

22.15 Radiographic positioning for caudocranial view of the femur, stifle, tibia and tarsus.

Interpretation

Periarticular osteophytes and enthesophytes: Periarticular new bone formation may be seen around the margins of the femoral trochlea, the poles of the patella, the tibial plateau and around the fabellae (Figure 22.16). It is a feature of osteoarthritis. There is, however, poor correlation between radiographic evidence of osteoarthritis (i.e. periarticular new bone) and limb function (Gordon *et al.*, 2003).

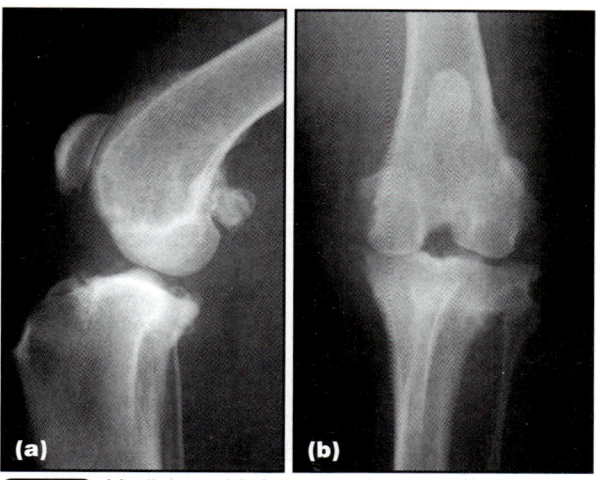

22.16 Mediolateral **(a)** and caudocranial **(b)** radiographs, showing periarticular osteophyte and enthesophyte formation. Note the reduction in size of the infrapatellar fat pad consistent with a joint effusion.

> **PRACTICAL TIP**
> Dogs with radiographic evidence of osteoarthritis in the contralateral stifle joint have an increased likelihood of cranial cruciate ligament rupture, compared with dogs with radiographically normal contralateral joints (Doverspike *et al.*, 1993).

Joint effusion: A joint effusion may be recognized by reduction in size of the infrapatellar fat pad (see Figure 22.8), displacement of the caudal joint capsule and/or loss of the fascial planes caudal to the joint. It should be considered that thickening of the joint capsule and soft tissue masses may cause similar radiographic changes.

Tibial plateau angle: The patient is positioned in lateral recumbency with the affected limb on the table and the contralateral pelvic limb secured cranially. It is helpful to elevate the proximal limb and lumbosacral spine to the same height as the tabletop X-ray cassette. The X-ray beam is centred on the stifle and collimated to include the tibia and talocrural joint.

The tibial plateau angle is measured by comparing the functional axis of the tibia and the axis of the medial tibial condyle (Figure 22.17). Tibial plateau angle reference limits for various breeds of dogs are approximately 20–25 degrees (Morris and Lipowitz, 2001; Wilke *et al.*, 2002; Fettig *et al.*, 2003; Reif and Probst, 2003).

Chapter 22 The stifle

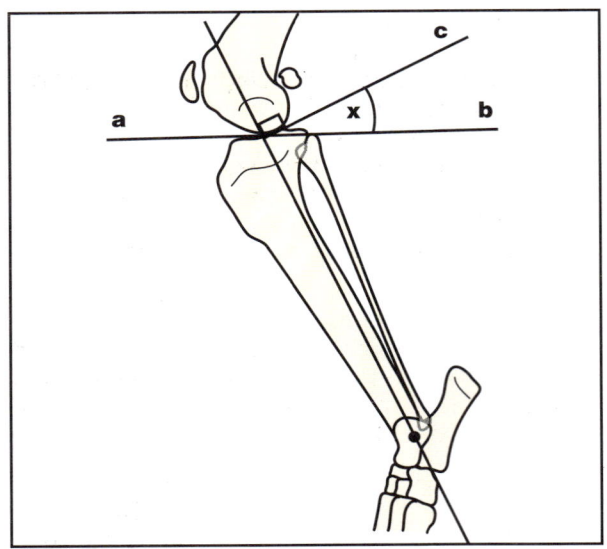

22.17 Tibial plateau angle. On a radiograph, a line representing the functional axis of the tibia (a) is drawn through the midpoint of the tibial intercondylar eminences and the centre of the talus. A second line representing the axis of the medial tibial condyle (b) is drawn through the cranial and caudal margins of the tibial plateau. The tibial plateau angle (x) is measured from a line (c) drawn perpendicular to the functional axis of the tibia and intersecting the line defining the tibial plateau.

Limb deformity: Angular limb deformity may be assessed and quantified on the caudocranial radiograph by drawing lines through the mid femur and mid crus. Rotational deformity may be assessed but not quantified on the caudocranial radiograph by evaluating the position of the calcaneus relative to the distal tibia (Figure 22.18). In a normal dog the medial aspect of the calcaneus should bisect the articular surface of the tibia.

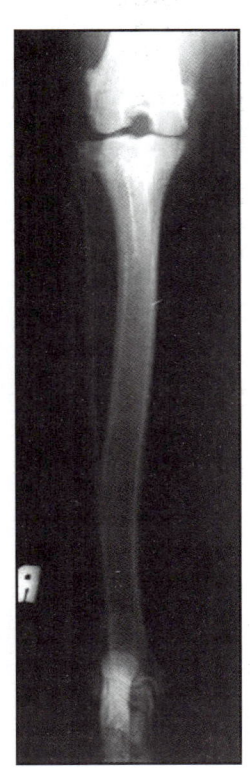

22.18 Caudocranial radiograph, showing assessment of angular and rotational deformity. Note the medial aspect of the calcaneus bisects the articular surface of the tibia.

Other abnormalities: Subchondral bone sclerosis and areas of soft tissue mineralization may be seen in advanced osteoarthritis. The tibia may occasionally be displaced cranially in non-stressed radiographs if the cranial cruciate ligament is completely ruptured.

Additional investigations

Synovial fluid analysis

Synovial fluid analysis may be useful to assess the degree of inflammation associated with osteoarthritis and to exclude the possibility of joint sepsis. It is easier to aspirate the femoropatellar joint than the femorotibial joint (Figure 22.19). The majority of dogs with cranial cruciate ligament rupture have synovial fluid white blood cell counts less than $5 \times 10^9/l$, of which >90% are mononuclear. These features are consistent with osteoarthritis. Occasionally white blood cell counts of $12 \times 10^9/l$, with up to 30% polymorphonuclear cells can be detected. Although fragments of menisci may be detected in synovial fluid this is not an accurate predictor of meniscal pathology.

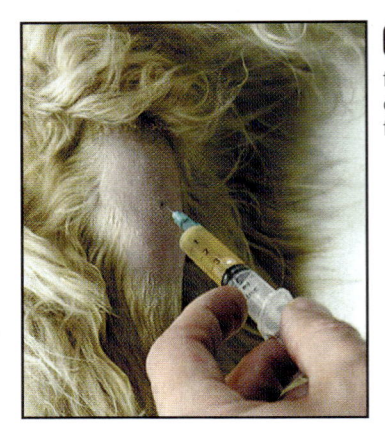

22.19 Aspiration of synovial fluid from the lateral compartment of the femoropatellar joint.

Arthroscopy

Arthroscopic examination of the stifle joint may be employed to evaluate the cranial cruciate ligament and menisci (Figure 22.20). Removal of the infrapatellar fad pad with a shaver is generally necessary. Arthroscopic meniscectomy is challenging. It is likely that this diagnostic and therapeutic tool will be increasingly employed.

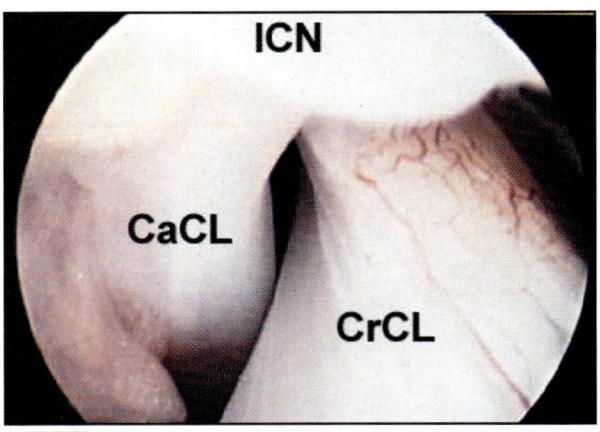

22.20 Arthroscopic view of the cruciate ligaments. CaCL, caudal cruciate ligament; CrCL, cranial cruciate ligament; ICN, intercondylar notch.

Magnetic resonance imaging

MRI may be used to assess meniscal injuries (Banfield and Morrison, 2000), though its sensitivity and specificity have not been well documented. Small lesions may not be detected.

Treatment

The treatment of cranial cruciate ligament disease in the dog remains a subject of considerable controversy and the recommendations in this chapter reflect the authors' current clinical opinion and philosophy. Non-surgical management is appropriate in selected cases and many surgical techniques have been described. The key features that influence decision-making are:

- Lameness
- Tibial plateau angle
- Degree of periarticular fibrosis (femorotibial stability)
- Meniscal pathology
- Bodyweight and age
- Unilateral or bilateral lameness
- Underlying primary arthropathy (e.g. immune-mediated disease)
- Response to non-surgical management.

Additional factors, such as available equipment and expertise, intended function of the dog, patient and owner compliance, and finance, should also be considered. Approaches to the management of cranial cruciate ligament disease in dogs of varying weight are presented in Figures 22.21 to 22.23.

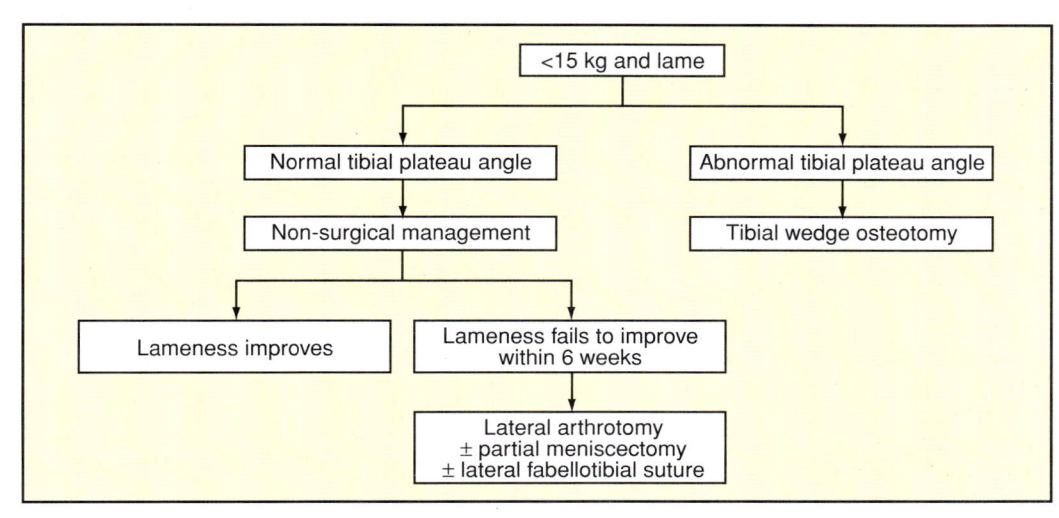

22.21 Approach to the management of cranial cruciate ligament disease causing lameness in a dog weighing <15 kg.

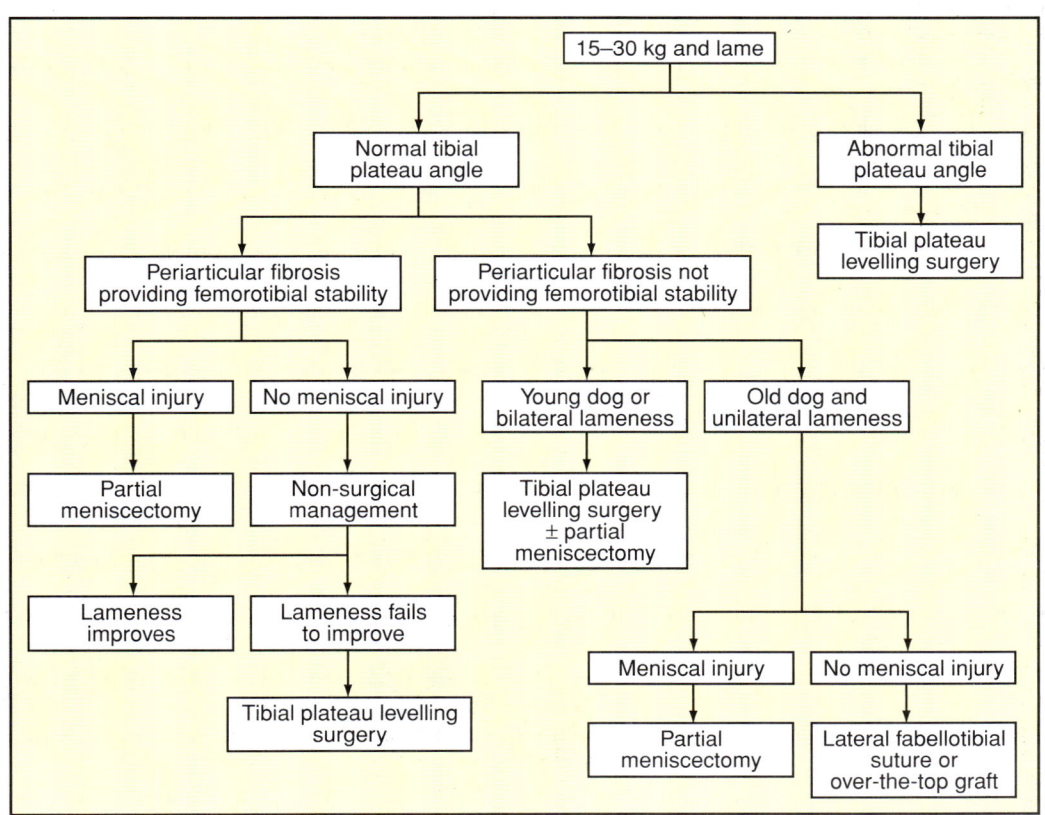

22.22 Approach to the management of cranial cruciate ligament disease causing lameness in a dog weighing 15–30 kg.

363

Chapter 22 The stifle

22.23 Approach to the management of cranial cruciate ligament disease causing lameness in a dog weighing >30 kg.

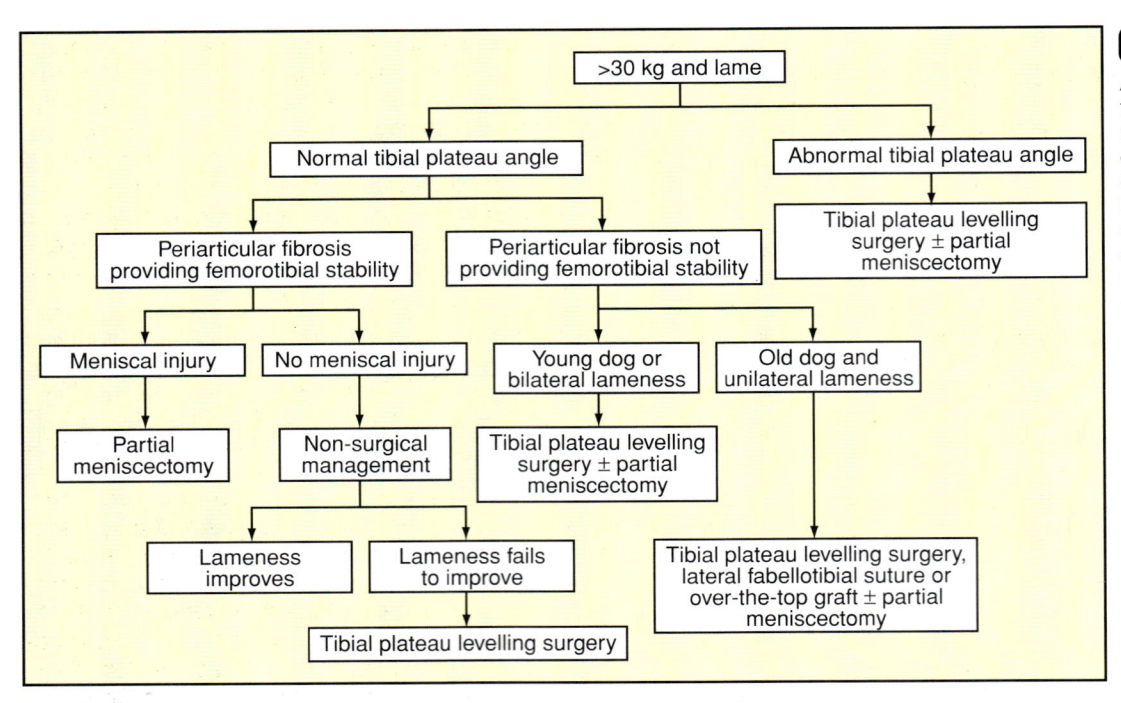

```
>30 kg and lame
├── Normal tibial plateau angle
│   ├── Periarticular fibrosis providing femorotibial stability
│   │   ├── Meniscal injury → Partial meniscectomy
│   │   └── No meniscal injury → Non-surgical management
│   │       ├── Lameness improves
│   │       └── Lameness fails to improve → Tibial plateau levelling surgery
│   └── Periarticular fibrosis not providing femorotibial stability
│       ├── Young dog or bilateral lameness → Tibial plateau levelling surgery ± partial meniscectomy
│       └── Old dog and unilateral lameness → Tibial plateau levelling surgery, lateral fabellotibial suture or over-the-top graft ± partial meniscectomy
└── Abnormal tibial plateau angle → Tibial plateau levelling surgery ± partial meniscectomy
```

Non-surgical management

Non-surgical management is appropriate in the following situations:

- Cranial cruciate ligament disease and osteoarthritis are not causing lameness
- Lameness is mild and intermittent
- Small dogs (<15 kg), provided the lameness improves within 6 weeks
- There is a contraindication to surgery (e.g. patient receiving high-dose glucocorticoid therapy for immune-mediated polyarthritis)
- Financial restrictions.

The key aspects of non-surgical management are:

- Weight control
- Exercise regulation
- Physiotherapy (including hydrotherapy) (see Chapter 16)
- Analgesia (if necessary) (see Chapter 16).

Dogs that are overweight should be placed on a diet and their weight monitored. Exercise should be regular and controlled on a lead. Jumping and climbing should be avoided. Hydrotherapy and range-of-motion exercises are excellent forms of physiotherapy. There may be a threshold of duration and type of activity beyond which lameness increases. Non-steroidal anti-inflammatory drugs should be administered if considered necessary. Once a drug has been shown to be beneficial it should be reduced to the lowest possible dose and given as infrequently as possible. Femorotibial instability gradually reduces as periarticular fibrosis develops (generally 6–12 months). The development and progression of osteoarthritis are inevitable (Vasseur, 1984).

Prognosis: Despite the inevitable progression of osteoarthritis, the prognosis for non-surgical management in small dogs (<15 kg) is generally good to excellent (Pond and Campbell, 1972; Vasseur, 1984). Possible reasons for persistent lameness include meniscal injury, partial cranial cruciate ligament rupture (may be more painful than complete rupture), abnormal tibial plateau angle (Macias *et al.*, 2002) and concomitant joint sepsis. Radiography and synovial fluid analysis should be performed in cases with chronic lameness. Surgical inspection of the menisci and femorotibial stabilization may be necessary.

The prognosis for non-surgical management in large dogs (>15 kg) is generally poor. In one study, lameness persisted or progressed in 46 of 57 dogs (Vasseur, 1984).

Surgical management

The aims of surgery have been to:

- Remove injured tissue (cranial cruciate ligament, meniscal)
- Stabilize the femorotibial joint
- Reduce cranial tibial thrust
- Prevent future meniscal injury
- Prevent or retard osteoarthritis.

With all surgical techniques the cranial cruciate ligament and menisci should be inspected by medial or lateral arthrotomy, or, alternatively, arthroscopically.

Treatment of the partially ruptured cranial cruciate ligament is under debate (Scavelli *et al.*, 1990). The remaining ligament is often weak and easily torn. Progressive rupture is likely, especially with surgical techniques that attempt to provide femorotibial stability. As a result it is probably best to excise any remaining ligament unless the tear is small and surgery is performed to reduce cranial tibial thrust.

Chapter 22 The stifle

> **PRACTICAL TIP**
> Pre-emptive analgesia with intra-articular bupivacaine should be considered in all surgical cases. Synovial fluid can be evaluated at the same time.

Meniscal injury: It is mandatory that the menisci be examined in all surgical procedures, since failure to remove injured tissue is likely to result in persistent lameness. The surgical approach may be via a medial or lateral arthrotomy, depending on what other procedure, if any, is being performed. Arthroscopic examination is an alternative. The use of a stifle distractor greatly assists examination of the caudal aspect of the medial meniscus. Occasionally a Hohmann retractor is also helpful to lever the tibia cranially. Damaged portions of meniscus should be removed (partial meniscectomy) (see Operative Technique 22.8).

Femorotibial joint stabilization

> Numerous intra- and extra-articular procedures that attempt to mimic the restraint normally provided by the intact cranial cruciate ligament have been reported. No technique, however, satisfactorily stabilizes the femorotibial joint or prevents progressive osteoarthritis. The procedures do not attempt to address cranial tibial thrust.

Intra-articular techniques: The challenge is to replace the cranial cruciate ligament, as closely as possible to its normal anatomical position, with a graft or prosthesis whose final biomechanical properties are the same as the normal ligament. Autogenous grafts are preferable and a composite graft using the lateral third of the patellar tendon and fascia lata has been most commonly advocated (see Operative Technique 22.9). Intra-articular grafts undergo avascular necrosis, and neovascularization may take 12–14 weeks. During this period intra-articular grafts are weak and have a tendency to break or tear from their anchor points. Attempts may be made to protect the graft during this period, for example, by combining the technique with an extra-articular procedure. Although femorotibial instability is often abolished immediately postoperatively, palpation a few weeks later invariably reveals recurrent instability. It is possible that long-term femorotibial stability is primarily due to periarticular fibrosis rather than the intra-articular graft.

Extra-articular techniques: Anchoring a loop of material around the lateral fabella and through a tunnel in the tibial crest is commonly performed as a sole procedure or to augment intra-articular grafts; it is referred to as a lateral fabellotibial suture. Materials used are generally non-absorbable, such as monofilament nylon, polypropylene and monofilament wire. The biomechanical properties of large diameter monofilament nylon leader line have been studied (Caporn and Roe, 1996). A self-locking knot aids tightening and tying of the material (McKee and Miller, 1999) (see Operative Technique 22.10). Alternatively, a crimp clamp may be employed (Peycke et al., 2002).

Femorotibial stability immediately following lateral fabellotibial suture placement is generally good. Within a few weeks, however, a cranial draw invariably returns, presumably due to the suture breaking, displacing from its anchor points, or cutting through regional soft tissues. Follow-up radiographs when wire has been used reveal that the material is generally broken or fabellar anchorage is lost within 6 weeks of surgery. As with intra-articular procedures, long-term femorotibial stability may be the result of periarticular fibrosis rather than the extra-articular suture.

Cranial tibial thrust reduction: In 1983 Slocum hypothesized that 'levelling' the tibial plateau would provide functional femorotibial stability during weightbearing by reducing cranial tibial thrust (Slocum and Devine, 1983). He proposed two surgical procedures to reduce the tibial plateau slope angle and, thus, cranial tibial thrust. The initial technique involved a proximal cranial tibial wedge osteotomy (Slocum and Devine, 1984) (see Operative Technique 22.11). Subsequently, the tibial plateau levelling osteotomy procedure (TPLO) was developed and patented (Slocum and Devine, 1993) (see Operative Technique 22.12). The TPLO is performed by making a crescent-shaped osteotomy caudal to the insertion of the patellar tendon. With both techniques the tibial plateau angle is reduced to approximately 6 degrees, i.e. not completely levelled (Warzee et al., 2001). Over-rotation of the tibial plateau (<6 degrees) may result in caudal tibial thrust and caudal cruciate ligament injury (Reif et al., 2002). The relative effectiveness of the TPLO and tibial wedge osteotomy has not been reported.

Prevention of future meniscal injury: With extra-articular and intra-articular techniques the incidence of postsurgical ('late') meniscal injuries is 15–20% (Metalman et al., 1995). Slocum and Devine Slocum (1998) advocated performing a medial meniscal release in dogs with normal menisci to prevent them becoming injured postsurgically. They proposed that releasing the caudal horn of the medial meniscus may allow it to remain in the caudal compartment of the joint during cranial translation of the tibia. The medial meniscus can be released either by cutting the caudal tibial ligament or by sectioning the meniscal body just caudal to the medial collateral ligament (see Operative Technique 22.8). The former technique may be preferable, but studies documenting the long-term effects of these procedures are lacking.

Retardation of osteoarthritis: Regardless of the technique chosen, intra-articular and extra-articular techniques fail to stop the progression of osteoarthritis (Innes et al., 2000). A poor understanding of the aetiopathogenesis of degenerative cranial cruciate ligament disease and failure to reduce cranial tibial thrust and provide functional joint stability are possible reasons. Recent studies suggest that the incidence and severity of radiographic progression of osteoarthritis following TPLO are comparable to those of other surgical techniques (Lazar et al., 2001; Rayward et al., 2004).

Postoperative rehabilitation: This is extremely important following cranial cruciate ligament surgery. A recent study demonstrated the value of early postoperative physiotherapy on limb function following cranial cruciate ligament surgery (lateral fabellotibial suture technique) (Marsolais *et al.*, 2002). Twenty-five dogs were included in a postoperative rehabilitation group and 26 dogs were included in an exercise-restricted group. Rehabilitation consisted of hydrotherapy, stretching and passive range-of-motion exercises and lead walking. Vertical forces were measured using force plate gait analysis preoperatively and 6 months after surgery. Prior to surgery vertical forces were statistically similar between groups. Six months after surgery vertical forces in dogs in the physiotherapy group were significantly greater than in dogs in the exercise restriction group. Peak vertical force was 18.5% greater and vertical impulse was 13.9% greater in the former group.

Kinematic studies in dogs following cranial cruciate ligament surgery have demonstrated that hydrotherapy results in a significantly greater range of motion of the stifle joint compared with slow or fast walking, primarily because of greater flexion of the joint (Marsolais *et al.*, 2003). The authors concluded that if range of motion is a factor in the rate or extent of return to function then hydrotherapy would probably result in a better overall outcome than walking alone.

Complications: Although cranial cruciate ligament surgery is commonly performed in primary care practice, the possibility of complications with intra-articular, extra-articular and tibial plateau levelling procedures is often under-rated. Careful attention to detail is essential in order to limit these potential problems.

Intra-articular techniques: Peroneal nerve, popliteal artery and caudal cruciate ligament injury are possible with inappropriate placement of the intra-articular graft passer. Ensuring the graft passer remains in close contact with the caudal and medial aspects of the lateral femoral condyle reduces the risk of injury.

Extra-articular techniques: Aseptic technique is necessary with extra-articular suture procedures to minimize the possibility of sepsis. In a prospective study (Dulisch, 1981), suture-related complications developed in 12 of 66 stifles, 6 of which had draining sinuses. The complication rate correlated with the surgeon's experience. It has been suggested that the use of braided suture materials is associated with an increased incidence of infection. Peroneal nerve injury is an additional complication with extra-articular techniques; it may result from inappropriate placement of the suture around the lateral fabella.

Tibial plateau levelling techniques: Complication rates of 20.6% (Priddy *et al.*, 2003) and 28% (Pacchiana *et al.*, 2003) have been reported following TPLO surgery. Most problems resolve with non-surgical management and do not appear to affect long-term outcome. Sepsis, tibial tuberosity fracture, fibular fracture, patellar tendon injury and intra-articular screw placement are the most common complications.

Prognosis: Clinical results of intra-articular and extra-articular surgery have been reported as good to excellent in 80–90% of cases, despite the consistent inability to provide long-term joint stability, to stop the progression of osteoarthritis and to prevent future meniscal injury. However, a more critical appraisal would suggest that only approximately 50% of dogs are actually sound (Moore and Read, 1995). In a prospective clinical trial comparing TPLO and extra-articular imbrication, the former technique consistently yielded subjectively better outcomes for all parameters evaluated (Schwarz, 1999). Other work has not supported this claim (Conzemius *et al.*, 2002). Radiographic assessment of osteoarthritis should not be used as a predictor of clinical outcome since there is a poor correlation between radiographic findings and clinical function (Gordon *et al.*, 2003).

Flare-up in lameness

Dogs with cranial cruciate ligament disease and osteoarthritis, whether managed surgically or non-surgically, may have bouts of increased lameness. Possible causes include:

- Further rupture of a partially torn ligament
- Meniscal injury
- Sepsis
- Other ligament strain
- 'Flare-up' in osteoarthritis (e.g. following strenuous exercise).

If lameness persists in dogs with no previous meniscal injury and sepsis has been excluded, a meniscal injury is probable. An exploratory arthrotomy is often justified, especially if arthroscopy, ultrasonography or MRI is not readily available.

Traumatic cranial cruciate ligament rupture

Hyperextension of the stifle (e.g. due to trapping the pelvic limb in a fence) and excessive internal rotation are the major forces that may overload the cranial cruciate ligament and result in traumatic rupture. In immature animals such forces are more likely to result in an avulsion fracture at the insertion of the ligament.

Lameness is usually severe initially with minimal weightbearing. Treatment depends on a number of factors, such as bodyweight. Non-surgical management or lateral fabellotibial stabilization may be appropriate in small dogs. Since cranial cruciate ligament rupture is traumatic rather than degenerative, an intra-articular graft augmented with a lateral fabellotibial suture may be considered in larger dogs. Avulsion fractures may be repaired with a lag screw or wire suture if the fragment is large enough. The role of tibial plateau levelling procedures in traumatic cranial cruciate ligament rupture has not been evaluated.

Cranial cruciate ligament disease in the cat

Rupture of the cranial cruciate ligament in the cat is generally associated with trauma; however, unilateral and bilateral rupture may occur in the absence of any significant trauma, implying that there may be pre-existing degenerative pathology in some cases. The prognosis with non-surgical management tends to be good, provided concomitant meniscal injury is not a feature (Scavelli and Schrader, 1987). Extra-articular stabilization may give a more rapid recovery, especially in cats with bilateral rupture.

Caudal cruciate ligament rupture

Anatomy and function
The caudal cruciate ligament arises within the intercondylar fossa from the lateral aspect of the medial femoral condyle and extends caudodistally to the lateral edge of the popliteal notch of the tibia (see Figure 22.1). It is covered by a layer of synovial membrane and is thus intra-articular but extrasynovial. There are two functional components; the relatively larger cranial portion that is taut in flexion and lax in extension and the caudal portion that is taut in extension and lax in flexion. The caudal cruciate ligament prevents caudal translation of the tibia relative to the femur and helps limit internal rotation of the tibia during joint flexion by twisting together with the cranial cruciate ligament. It is a secondary restraint to hyperextension and helps limit varus and valgus movement when the stifle is flexed.

Clinical features
Rupture of the caudal cruciate ligament is uncommon and usually occurs with concomitant traumatic rupture of the cranial cruciate ligament. Isolated caudal cruciate ligament rupture is a rare injury generally diagnosed in young, large dogs that have sustained severe trauma. Avulsion from the femoral attachment site is a frequent finding. Reduced prominence of the tibial tuberosity and a caudal draw are the key clinical features.

Treatment
Non-surgical management should be attempted initially, since caudal cruciate ligament rupture causes minimal secondary damage within the stifle joint and dogs studied experimentally all recovered a normal gait (Harari et al., 1987). Exploration of the joint and extra-articular stabilization may be considered after 6 weeks if lameness fails to improve. Acute avulsion injuries are managed surgically with fixation of the avulsed fragment with a lag screw or wire suture. The prognosis is generally good.

Proximal tibial deformity

Deformity of the proximal tibia with an increased tibial plateau angle can be associated with cranial cruciate ligament rupture and osteoarthritis of the stifle in the dog. It is an uncommon condition, primarily recognized in small breeds, although it has been reported in large dogs (Read and Robins, 1982).

Aetiopathogenesis
Read and Robins (1982) suggested that retardation of growth of the caudal aspect of the proximal tibial physis was responsible for the proximal tibia deformity. The fact that many cases are bilateral suggests a developmental aetiology. Trauma to the proximal tibial physis is also possible. Interestingly, Terriers appear to be over-represented in proximal tibial deformity and proximal tibial physeal fractures (Pratt, 2001; Macias et al., 2002; Clements et al., 2003). An increased tibial plateau angle is a significant feature of proximal tibial deformity. The resultant increased cranial tibial thrust is thought to cause secondary osteoarthritis of the stifle and cranial cruciate ligament rupture. Concomitant meniscal injury is uncommon.

Signalment and history
In the United Kingdom terrier breeds appear to be over-represented (Macias et al., 2002), whereas all the dogs reported from Brazil were Poodles or Poodle crosses (Selmi and Padilha Filho, 2001). Read and Robins (1982) described the condition in five large dogs. The age at onset of lameness appears to be related to size. Small dogs are often 3–6 years of age (Selmi and Padilha Filho, 2001; Macias et al., 2002) in contrast to larger dogs that are often less than 18 months old (Read and Robins, 1982). The incidence in males and females is similar.

A gradual onset, progressive pelvic limb lameness may be reported or alternatively lameness may be sudden in onset associated with cranial cruciate ligament rupture. There is often a poor response to restricted exercise and NSAID therapy. Inability to jump and climb may be a feature in dogs with bilateral lameness.

Clinical findings
The severity of pelvic limb lameness is variable. Intermittent 'skipping' may be evident. Quadriceps muscle atrophy is a common feature. Cranial prominence of the tibial tuberosity is palpable. A cranial draw is demonstrable in dogs with cranial cruciate ligament rupture. This manipulation is often painful, especially in dogs with partial cranial cruciate ligament rupture. Occasionally the proximal tibial deformity results in persistent cranial subluxation of the tibia. It is necessary to reduce the subluxation prior to performing the cranial draw test in these cases. The contralateral stifle joint should be examined for evidence of deformity, thickening, instability and pain.

Radiography
Orthogonal views that enable measurement of the tibial plateau angles (see Figure 22.17) should be obtained of both stifles. Examination reveals the tibial tuberosity to be prominent cranially and the tibial crest to be barely distinguishable from the cranial diaphysis of the tibia (Figure 22.24). Caudal bowing of the proximal fibula may be detected. The tibial plateau angle is generally >30 degrees (Macias et al., 2002). Cranial subluxation of the tibia may be evident.

Chapter 22 The stifle

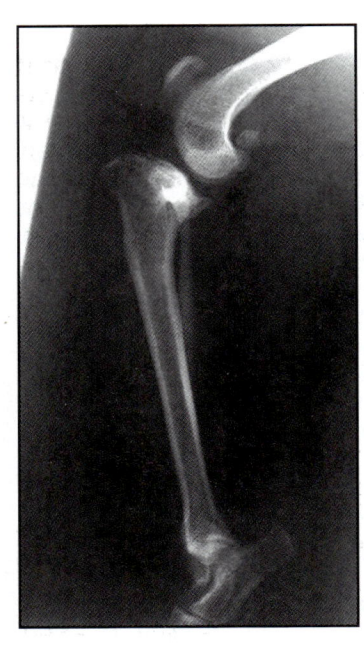

22.24 Mediolateral non-stressed radiograph, showing proximal tibial deformity in a 2.5-year-old West Highland White Terrier with cranial cruciate ligament disease and stifle osteoarthritis. There is subluxation of the femorotibial joint.

Surgical management
Surgery is warranted in dogs that are lame, since the response to non-surgical management is poor (Read and Robins, 1982; Macias *et al.*, 2002). A corrective cranial tibial wedge osteotomy is indicated (see Operative Technique 22.11). Reducing the angle of the tibial plateau to between 10 and 20 degrees appears to be appropriate (Macias *et al.*, 2002). Single bone plate fixation augmented with a Kirschner wire or figure-of-eight orthopaedic wire enables predictable osteosynthesis. Selmi and Padilha Filho (2001) recommended additional lateral fabellotibial suture stabilization, but this is probably not necessary (Macias *et al.*, 2002). Although the incidence of meniscal injury is low, inspection is recommended. Examination of the menisci is technically difficult due to the small size of many of these dogs and the abnormal tibial plateau angle.

Prognosis
The prognosis following corrective tibial osteotomy surgery appears to be good, despite the concomitant osteoarthritis.

Collateral ligament rupture

Collateral ligament injuries in the stifle joint most often occur in conjunction with major trauma to the animal. Therefore, complete patient assessment and comprehensive treatment are vital in these cases. When collateral ligament injury occurs in the stifle, other structures of the joint are usually injured and luxation of the joint may occur (see Stifle luxation).

Anatomy and function
The collateral ligaments act as major stabilizers of the stifle joint counteracting varus/valgus, rotational and translational instabilities. The medial collateral ligament originates on the medial femoral epicondyle and courses distally to insert on the proximal aspect of the medial tibia. Attachments between the medial collateral ligament and the medial joint capsule and medial meniscus are present. The cranial fibres of the medial collateral ligament remain taut throughout the range of motion of the stifle, while the caudal fibres become lax in flexion. The lateral collateral ligament originates on the lateral femoral epicondyle and inserts on the lateral aspect of the fibular head. There are no distinct, fibrous attachments between the lateral collateral ligament and lateral meniscus or joint capsule. The entire lateral collateral ligament becomes relatively lax when the stifle is in flexion and is taut in extension.

Aetiopathogenesis
Isolated injuries of the collateral ligaments of the stifle are rare, but can occur from athletic trauma, slips or falls or iatrogenic surgical damage. Most often, collateral ligament injuries result from violent trauma and are seen in conjunction with deranged joints. Ligamentous injuries are designated sprains and are categorized as follows:

- First degree – mild stretching of ligament fibres causing minimal instability
- Second degree – moderate stretching with some tearing of ligament fibres causing moderate instability (ligament remains grossly intact)
- Third degree – complete rupture or avulsion of the ligament with gross instability.

Signalment and history
Any age, gender and breed of dog or cat can experience collateral ligament injuries. However, athletic dogs (i.e. racing Greyhounds) and dogs most subject to trauma (i.e. young males) are more likely to be affected.

Clinical findings
The clinical findings associated with collateral ligament injuries of the stifle will vary depending on involvement, severity and duration of the injury. The symptoms may range from mild, intermittent lameness with first-degree sprains to non-weightbearing lameness with marked swelling and limb angulation for third-degree, multi-ligament problems. Marked periarticular fibrosis may be present in cases of chronic injury with instability.

After sedation with analgesia, palpation should be performed to assess involvement and extent of injury. Varus and valgus stress tests of the stifle should be performed with the limb held in extension to assess the integrity of the lateral collateral ligament and medial collateral ligament, respectively.

> When collateral ligament injuries of the stifle are diagnosed, comprehensive palpation of the joint is vital to assess all other aspects of stifle joint function, as injuries to the cruciate ligaments, menisci, articular cartilage, patellar tendon, long digital extensor tendon and other associated structures often occur in conjunction with collateral ligament injuries.

Radiography

Plain film orthogonal radiographic views of the stifle should be obtained after sedation with analgesia, or general anaesthesia, to help define the extent of trauma, including avulsion fractures and concurrent injuries. Stressed radiographic views may be helpful to document instability (Figure 22.25).

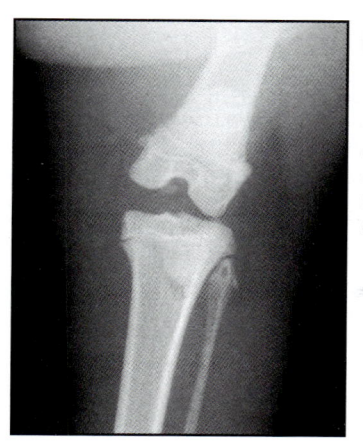

22.25 Caudocranial valgus stressed-view radiograph of a 2-year-old Domestic Shorthair cat with isolated rupture of the medial collateral ligament.

Management

First-degree sprains may be amenable to non-surgical therapy, consisting of strict rest and/or support bandages, with rehabilitation and re-evaluation. However, the majority of collateral ligament injuries diagnosed result in joint instability and will require surgical intervention. Because surgical inspection provides the definitive assessment of all potentially involved structures, exploration of the stifle joint is generally recommended, requiring a lateral or medial parapatellar approach, or exploratory arthroscopy. In the rare cases when isolated collateral ligament injury can be assured, a lateral or medial approach directly over the affected ligament can be used, and arthrotomy avoided.

The goal of surgical treatment for collateral ligament injury is to re-establish the functional length of the ligament and attain adequate joint stability and function through healing with fibrous tissue formation. This goal can be accomplished by various means:

- Ligament imbrication
- Primary suture repair
- Tissue anchors
- Synthetic ligament replacement using screw/tissue anchor and suture
- Reattachment of avulsed fragments.

Choice of technique will depend on the extent, severity and duration of the injuries, patient signalment, intended purpose of the patient and surgeon capabilities and preference.

External coaptation, in the form of a splint or cast, or external skeletal fixation is recommended for 2–12 weeks after surgery, depending on the extent and severity of the trauma, type of treatment, the temperament of the patient and the compliance of the owner. After surgical repair, analgesic therapy and NSAIDs are instituted. A physical rehabilitation programme should be started, to promote functional periarticular fibrosis, muscle strength, range of motion and limb function.

Prognosis

The prognosis for patients with collateral ligament injuries of the stifle will vary markedly, depending on the nature of the damage. With appropriate surgical treatment and physical rehabilitation, the prognosis for functional limb use is generally good. Mild loss of range of motion, intermittent lameness and osteoarthritis should be expected in cases requiring surgery. Owners should be warned that athletic and working dogs are not likely to return to pre-injury levels of performance.

Stifle luxation

Stifle luxation, also referred to as derangement of the stifle, is a relatively uncommon, severe injury in dogs and cats. Typically, three or more of the major transarticular ligaments, the joint capsule and one or both menisci are damaged. It is imperative that complete patient assessment be performed in light of the violent nature of the trauma required to luxate the joint.

Aetiology

The most common combination of injuries associated with stifle luxation is cranial cruciate ligament rupture, caudal cruciate ligament rupture, medial collateral ligament sprain or rupture and joint capsule tears. The anatomy and soft tissue support of the stifle joint make fractures much more likely than luxation. When luxation does occur, it is most often the result of a direct, violent, blunt blow (vehicular trauma) to the joint while the limb is bearing weight. Because the lateral side of the joint is more exposed to this type of trauma, the force is often incurred on the lateral side, explaining the involvement of the medial collateral ligament in the majority of cases.

> The neurological and vascular function of the limb must be assessed carefully in cases of stifle luxation. Due to the extremely violent nature of the trauma required to luxate the stifle joint, periarticular injury can extend to vessels and nerves.

Signalment and history

Any age, gender and breed of dog or cat can experience stifle luxation. However, dogs experiencing vehicular trauma are more likely to be affected; therefore, it is seen most frequently in young, male, large-breed dogs.

Clinical findings

Diagnosis is based on visual inspection and palpation. Typically, stifle swelling, bruising, malalignment and angulation (genu valgum) are evident on initial examination. After sedation with analgesia, palpation for varus, valgus, cranial and caudal draw and rotational instability can be performed to confirm the diagnosis and make an initial assessment of the extent of damage.

Chapter 22 The stifle

> A minimum database for trauma patients, including complete physical and neurological examinations, electrocardiogram, thoracic, abdominal, and pelvic radiographs, complete blood count, serum biochemical analysis and urinalysis is strongly recommended.

Radiography
Plain film orthogonal radiographic views of the stifle should be obtained after sedation with analgesia, or under general anaesthesia. Radiographs help further to define the extent of trauma, including avulsion fractures, concurrent injuries and displacement. Stressed radiographic views may be helpful to document instability if necessary (Figure 22.26).

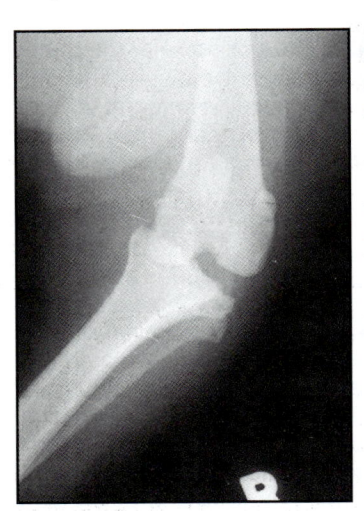

22.26 Caudocranial varus stressed-view radiograph of a 3.5-year-old Border Collie, showing femorotibial luxation associated with rupture of the medial and lateral collateral and cranial cruciate ligaments.

Surgical management
Surgical exploration provides the definitive assessment of involvement and severity of the damage. The surgical approach must provide access to both the medial and lateral compartments of the joint. Therefore, a lateral or medial parapatellar approach with extension of the skin incision and dissection of the subcutaneous tissues is most often performed to provide appropriate exposure.

> **PRACTICAL TIP**
> The joint must be explored thoroughly and all intra- and periarticular structures inspected. Trauma to the meniscal attachments, long digital extensor tendon of origin, trochlear ridges, patella and patellar tendon can be missed if assessment is not complete.

Each structure that is damaged needs to be addressed in some manner, whether by debridement, resection, primary repair, replacement, functional augmentation or external coaptation. Figure 22.27 shows treatment options for each of the major structures potentially involved in stifle luxation.

External skeletal fixation, or external coaptation in the form of a splint or cast, is recommended for 2–12 weeks after surgery, depending on the extent and severity of the trauma, type of treatment, the temperament of the patient and the compliance of the owner. Hinged transarticular skeletal fixation systems are commercially available and can be very advantageous in stifle luxation cases for providing stability and protection while allowing for increased joint range of motion and limb use (Figure 22.28).

Structure	Primary method(s) of repair	Secondary method(s) of repair
Collateral ligaments	Primary suture repair Screw and washer reattachment Screw and spiked plate reattachment Divergent Kirschner wire reattachment	External skeletal fixation External coaptation Transarticular pin(s)
Cranial cruciate ligament	Screw or Kirschner wire reattachment of avulsion Tibial plateau levelling osteotomy Fabellotibial suture(s)	External skeletal fixation External coaptation Transarticular pin(s) Fascial imbrication
Caudal cruciate ligament	Screw or Kirschner wire reattachment of avulsion	External skeletal fixation External coaptation Transarticular pin(s) Fascial imbrication
Menisci	Primary repair in very select cases Partial meniscectomy	Total meniscectomy
Patellar tendon	Primary suture repair Lag screw reattachment Pin and tension band reattachment	Fascial, synthetic or biomaterial graft External skeletal fixation External coaptation Transarticular pin(s)
Articular cartilage	Fragment reattachment by screws or Kirschner wires	Debridement and curettage
Long digital extensor tendon	Screw or Kirschner wire reattachment of avulsion Primary repair	Tenodesis to proximal tibia Fascial, synthetic or biomaterial graft
Joint capsule	Primary repair Fascial, synthetic or biomaterial graft	External skeletal fixation External coaptation

22.27 Treatment options for the major structures potentially involved in stifle luxation.

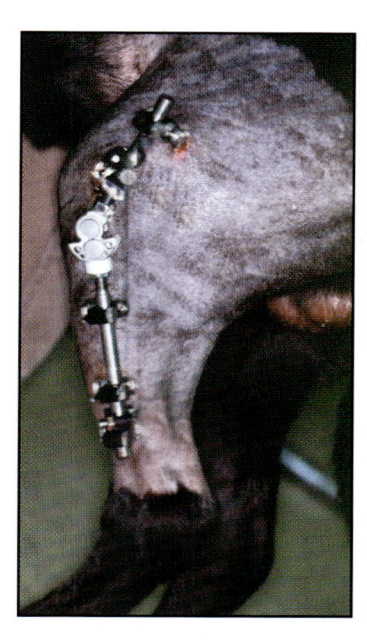

Chapter 22 The stifle

22.28 Hinged transarticular external skeletal fixator (IMEX, Longview, Texas) placed on the lateral aspect of the femur and tibia to aid in treatment of stifle luxation, instability or patella–patellar ligament complex pathology.

22.29 Mediolateral radiograph of a 5-year-old mixed breed dog with rupture of the patellar tendon. There is proximal displacement of the patella.

After surgical repair, analgesic therapy and NSAIDs are provided. A physical rehabilitation programme should be instituted to promote functional periarticular fibrosis, muscle strength, range of motion and limb function.

Stifle arthrodesis and amputation are salvage procedures. They may be indicated if functional repair cannot be accomplished, or concurrent or subsequent orthopaedic, neurological or vascular pathology dictate futility of repair.

Prognosis

With appropriate surgical treatment and physical rehabilitation, the prognosis for functional limb use is good. Mild loss of range of motion, intermittent lameness and secondary osteoarthritis should be expected. Athletic and working dogs are unlikely to return to pre-injury levels of performance.

Patellar tendon rupture

Injuries to the patellar tendon can result from laceration, blunt trauma or supraphysiological load transmitted through the quadriceps–patellar complex as a result of a fall or athletic injury. The resultant lesion can occur anywhere along the length of the tissue from the musculotendinous junction to the insertion on the tibial tuberosity. Fracture of the patella and/or tibial tuberosity avulsion may occur concurrently.

There is no reported age, gender or breed predilection. Clinical signs associated with these injuries include lameness, localized swelling and patellar displacement. The degree of lameness is variable, and the patella can be proximally (patella alta) or distally (patella baja) displaced depending on the location of the lesion. Patellar displacement can be determined by palpation and radiography with comparison to the contralateral stifle (Figure 22.29). Ultrasonographic evaluation of the tendon with comparison to the contralateral side may also aid in diagnosis.

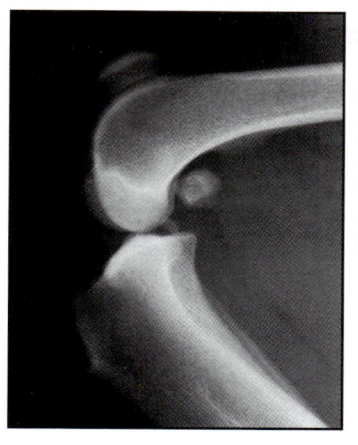

Non-surgical management

Treatment will depend on the degree and location of the pathology. First-degree strains and sprains often respond well to strict rest and anti-inflammatory medications. Strict cage rest should be enforced for a minimum of 3 weeks, followed by a very progressive return to function with appropriate physical rehabilitation and careful monitoring of healing.

Surgical management

Failure of non-surgical therapy to resolve the problem completely indicates that surgical therapy may be required for a successful outcome. More severe injuries typically require surgery. Primary suture repair of tears and lacerations at the musculotendinous junction or midsubstance of the tendon is recommended to restore the functional length of the quadriceps–patellar mechanism. Insertional avulsions of the tendon can be repaired using suture and bone tunnels, suture/tissue anchors, screw and tissue washer or bone staples. Augmentation of tendon repairs with fascia, biomaterials or synthetic implants may be advantageous, especially when defects are present or healing may be compromised.

Protection of the repair must be addressed, because of the tremendous amount of tension placed on the tendon during the healing period. The tendon can be protected by using internal and/or external methods. Internal methods include tension-distributing techniques, such as musculotendinous–tibial tuberosity or patellar–tibial tuberosity orthopaedic wire (this wire will inevitably break at some point after surgery and may need to be removed). External techniques include casts, splints and transarticular external skeletal fixators (fixed or hinged). The repair should be protected for a minimum of 4 weeks and some cases will require protection for 12 weeks or more.

Postoperative care includes strict exercise restriction and maintenance of the protective devices, careful monitoring of progress and physical rehabilitation after removal of protection.

Prognosis

The prognosis for isolated patellar tendon injuries is good if quadriceps–patellar (extensor) mechanism function is restored. However, it is important to remember that original tissue strength is never restored and the tendon will always be predisposed to re-injury.

Chapter 22 The stifle

Long digital extensor tendon avulsion

The long digital extensor tendon originates in the extensor fossa of the lateral femoral condyle and nearly the entire tendon is intra-articular. The long digital extensor muscle traverses the length of the tibia and hock to insert on digits II–V and functions to flex the hock and extend the digits.

Long digital extensor tendon avulsion has been reported to occur most commonly in immature, large-breed dogs, most likely as the result of low-grade trauma (e.g. jumping, falling). Avulsion with or without a bone attachment is the typical lesion. The initiating trauma is often not observed and, therefore, the diagnosis is not often made until a chronic weightbearing lameness is noticed by the owner. Iatrogenic laceration or detachment of the tendon can also occur during stifle surgery.

Diagnosis is based on palpation of stifle effusion and the ability simultaneously to flex the stifle completely, extend the hock completely, and flex the digits completely without tension. Radiographic findings may include evidence of bone avulsion, joint effusion and bone proliferation involving the lateral femoral condyle. Exploratory arthrotomy or arthroscopy may be required for definitive diagnosis.

Surgical management

The treatment of choice for long digital extensor tendon avulsion is surgical reattachment of the tendon at its natural origin. This can be accomplished via:

- Screw or divergent Kirschner wire fixation of an avulsed bone fragment
- Screw and tissue washer fixation of the avulsed tendon.

If appropriate reattachment at the origin cannot be accomplished, tenodesis on the proximal tibia should be performed via bone tunnel or suture, tissue anchor, screw and tissue washer or staple fixation.

Postoperatively, the repair should be protected by strict exercise restriction and prevention of stifle flexion using a soft padded bandage, splint or cast for 2–3 weeks. Physical rehabilitation should be employed over the next 4–6 weeks to optimize healing and function. The prognosis is good if reattachment can be accomplished soon after trauma. Complications include osteoarthritis, failure of repair and recurrence.

Popliteal tendon avulsion

The popliteal tendon originates on the lateral femoral condyle medial to the lateral collateral ligament, and contains a sesamoid bone. The tendon continues caudally to unite with the muscle belly on the caudal aspect of the stifle. The popliteus muscle acts to flex the stifle joint and rotate the tibia internally. Avulsion of the tendon of origin as an isolated injury is thought to occur due to athletic injuries, falls or jumps, but the causal event is typically not observed. Clinical signs include a weightbearing lameness with localized swelling and pain. Radiographs reveal distal displacement of the popliteal sesamoid.

Surgical management

The treatment of choice is surgical reattachment of the avulsed tendon at its natural origin. Reattachment can be accomplished via:

- Direct suture–soft tissue repair
- Suture–bone tunnel repair
- Suture–tissue anchor fixation
- Screw and tissue washer fixation.

With the suturing techniques, passing the suture around the displaced popliteal sesamoid is recommended.

Postoperatively, strict exercise restriction and restriction of stifle range of motion using a soft padded bandage, splint or cast should be maintained for 2–3 weeks. Physical rehabilitation should be employed over the subsequent 4–6 weeks.

The prognosis for successful reattachment of isolated popliteal tendon avulsions is very good. Complications include failure of repair and recurrence.

Gastrocnemius muscle avulsion

The muscle bellies (medial and lateral) of the gastrocnemius originate on the medial and lateral supracondylar tuberosities and combine distally to comprise the major components of the common calcanean tendon. The gastrocnemius acts to flex the stifle and extend the hock. Each gastrocnemius muscle head contains a sesamoid bone (fabella) within its origin, which has ligamentous attachments to and articulates with the respective femoral condyle. Avulsion of the origin of the gastrocnemius muscle inevitably includes avulsion of the associated fabella. This injury probably occurs most often as the result of unobserved low-grade trauma. Clinical presentation is usually that of a weightbearing lameness with varying degrees of hyperflexion of the hock (plantigrade stance). Localized swelling and pain may be present. Radiographs reveal distal displacement of one or both fabellae with associated soft tissue swelling.

Surgical management

The treatment of choice for gastrocnemius muscle avulsion is surgical reattachment of the muscle at its natural origin. This can be accomplished via:

- Direct suture–soft tissue repair
- Suture–bone tunnel repair
- Suture–tissue anchor(s) fixation
- Screw and tissue washer fixation.

With the suturing techniques, passing the suture around the displaced fabella is recommended.

Postoperatively, strict exercise restriction and prevention of stifle flexion using a soft padded bandage, splint or cast should be maintained for 2–3 weeks. Physical rehabilitation should be employed over the subsequent 4–6 weeks to optimize healing and function.

The prognosis is good with successful reattachment and appropriate postoperative management. Complications include failure of repair and recurrence.

Arthrodesis of the stifle

Stifle arthrodesis is indicated for end-stage conditions when no other means for preserving pain-free limb function are possible. When stifle arthrodesis is performed, ambulation is maintained by providing a fixed, functional joint angle with compensatory changes in hip and hock range of motion. Currently, this is the only salvage procedure routinely performed for the stifle. Careful attention should be given to removal of all articular cartilage and menisci, and condylectomy and patellectomy are recommended. The recommended angle of fixation is 130–140 degrees. Fixation can be achieved by use of plates, screws, pins and/or external skeletal fixation (Cofone et al., 1992; McLaughlin, 1993; Cook and Payne, 1997).

With appropriate surgical technique, maintenance of fixation and postoperative rehabilitation, one can expect a relatively good success rate for bony fusion. Abnormalities in the gait will be present, but pain-free limb use can typically be achieved. Complications include failure of fusion, infection, lameness and fracture. In addition, biomechanical alterations caused by compensation in the hip and tarsus can result in abnormal stresses on these joints, potentiating the risk for soft tissue and skeletal trauma, and osteoarthritis.

References and further reading

Aiken SW, Kass PH and Toombs JP (1995) Intercondylar notch width in dogs with and without cranial cruciate ligament injuries. *Veterinary and Comparative Orthopaedics and Traumatology* **8**, 128–132

Arnoczky SP and Marshall JL (1977) The cruciate ligaments of the canine stifle: an anatomical and functional analysis. *American Journal of Veterinary Research* **38**, 1807–1814

Banfield CM and Morrison WB (2000) Magnetic resonance arthrography of the canine stifle joint: technique and applications in eleven military dogs. *Veterinary Radiology and Ultrasound* **41**, 200–213

Bennett D, Tennant B, Lewis DG et al. (1988) A reappraisal of anterior cruciate ligament disease in the dog. *Journal of Small Animal Practice* **29**, 275–297

Caporn TM and Roe SC (1996) Biomechanical evaluation of the suitability of monofilament nylon and leader line for extra-articular stabilisation of the canine cranial cruciate-deficient stifle. *Veterinary and Comparative Orthopaedics and Traumatology* **9**, 126–133

Carlson CS, Meuten DJ and Richardson DC (1991) Ischemic necrosis of cartilage in spontaneous and experimental lesions of osteochondrosis. *Journal of Orthopaedic Research* **9**, 317–329

Clements DN, Gemmill T, Corr SA, Bennett D and Carmichael S (2003) Fracture of the proximal tibial epiphysis and tuberosity in 10 dogs. *Journal of Small Animal Practice* **44**, 355–358

Cofone MA, Smith GK, Lenehan TM, Newton CD (1992) Unilateral and bilateral stifle arthrodesis in 8 dogs. *Veterinary Surgery* **21**, 299

Conzemius MG, Gordon WJ, Besancon MF et al. (2002) The effect of surgical technique on limb function after surgery for cranial cruciate ligament disease in the Labrador Retriever. ACVS abstract. *Veterinary Surgery* **31**, 479

Cook JL and Payne JT (1997) Surgical treatment of osteoarthritis. *Veterinary Clinics of North America: Small Animal Practice* **27(4)**, 931–944

Coughlan A and Miller A (2006) *BSAVA Manual of Small Animal Fracture Repair and Management (revised reprint)*. BSAVA Publications, Gloucester

Denny HR and Minter HM (1973) Canine stifle surgery. *Journal of Small Animal Practice* **14**, 695–713

Douglas G and Rang M (1981) The role of trauma in the pathogenesis of osteochondrosis. *Clinical Orthopaedics* **158**, 28–32

Doverspike M, Vasseur PB, Harb MF and Walls CM (1993) Contralateral cranial cruciate ligament rupture: Incidence in 114 dogs. *Journal of the American Animal Hospital Association* **29**, 167–170

Dulisch ML (1981) Suture reaction following extra-articular stifle stabilization in the dog – part II: a prospective study of 66 stifles. *Journal of the American Animal Hospital Association* **17**, 572–574

Fettig AA, Rand WM, Sato AF et al. (2003) Observer variability of tibial plateau slope measurement in 40 dogs with cranial cruciate ligament-deficient stifle joints. *Veterinary Surgery* **32**, 471–478

Galloway RH and Lester SJ (1995) Histopathological evaluation of canine stifle joint synovial membrane collected at the time of repair of cranial cruciate ligament rupture. *Journal of the American Animal Hospital Association* **31**, 289–294

Gordon WJ, Conzemius MG, Riedesel E et al. (2003) The relationship between limb function and radiographic osteoarthrosis in dogs with stifle osteoarthrosis. *Veterinary Surgery* **32**, 451–454

Griffin DW and Vasseur PB (1992) Synovial fluid analysis in dogs with cranial cruciate ligament rupture. *Journal of the American Animal Hospital Association* **28**, 277–281

Guthrie S and Pidduck HG (1990) Heritability of elbow osteochondrosis within a closed population of dogs. *Journal of Small Animal Practice* **31**, 93–96

Harari J (1998) Osteochondrosis of the femur. *Veterinary Clinics of North America: Small Animal Practice* **28**, 87–94

Harari J, Johnson AL, Stein LE, Kneller SK and Pijanowski G (1987) Evaluation of experimental transection and partial excision of the caudal cruciate ligament in dogs. *Veterinary Surgery* **16**, 151–154

Houlton JEF and Meynink SE (1989) Medial patellar luxation in the cat. *Journal of Small Animal Practice* **30**, 349–352

Innes JF, Bacon D, Lynch C and Pollard A (2000) Long-term outcome of surgery for dogs with cranial cruciate ligament deficiency. *Veterinary Record* **147**, 325–328

Johnson AL, Probst CW, DeCamp CE et al. (2001) Comparison of trochlear block recession and trochlear wedge recession for canine patellar luxation using a cadaver model. *Veterinary Surgery* **30**, 140–150

Kaiser S, Cornely D, Golder W et al. (2001a) Magnetic resonance measurements of the deviation of the angle of force generated by contraction of the quadriceps muscle in dogs with congenital patellar luxation. *Veterinary Surgery* **30**, 552–558

Kaiser S, Cornely D, Golder W et al. (2001b) The correlation of canine patellar luxation and the anteversion angle as measured using magnetic resonance images. *Veterinary Radiology and Ultrasound* **42**, 113–118

Korvick DL, Pijanowski GJ and Schaeffer DJ (1994) Three-dimensional kinematics of the intact and cranial cruciate ligament-deficient stifle of dogs. *Journal of Biomechanics* **27**, 77–87

Kuroki K, Cook JL, Tomlinson JL and Kreeger JM (2002) In vitro characterization of chondrocytes isolated from naturally occurring osteochondrosis lesions of the humeral head of dogs. *American Journal of Veterinary Research* **63**, 186–193

Lampman TJ, Lund EM and Lipowitz AJ (2003) Cranial cruciate disease: current status of diagnosis, surgery and risk for disease. *Veterinary and Comparative Orthopaedics and Traumatology* **16**, 122–126

Lazar TP, Berry CR, deHann JJ and Peck JN (2001) Long-term comparison of stifle osteoarthritis in dogs with surgical repair of cranial cruciate ligament injury utilizing tibial plateau leveling osteotomy versus extracapsular stabilization. ACVS Abstracts. *Veterinary Surgery* **30**, 498

Macias C, McKee WM and May C (2002) Caudal proximal tibial deformity and cranial cruciate ligament rupture in small breed dogs. *Journal of Small Animal Practice* **43**, 433–438

Marsolais GS, Dvorak G and Conzemius MG (2002) Effects of postoperative rehabilitation on limb function after cranial cruciate ligament repair in dogs. *Journal of the American Veterinary Medical Association* **220**, 1325–1330

Marsolais GS, McLean S, Derrick T and Conzemius MG (2003) Kinematic analysis of the hind limb during swimming and walking in healthy dogs and dogs with surgically corrected cranial cruciate ligament rupture. *Journal of the American Veterinary Medical Association* **222**, 739–743

McKee WM and Miller A (1999) A self-locking knot for lateral fabellotibial suture stabilisation of the cranial cruciate ligament deficient stifle in the dog. *Veterinary and Comparative Orthopaedics and Traumatology* **12**, 78–80

McLaughlin R (1993) Intra-articular stifle fractures and arthrodesis. *Veterinary Clinics of North America: Small Animal Practice* **23(4)**, 877–895

Metalman LA, Schwarz M, Salman M and Alvis MR (1995) An evaluation of three different cranial cruciate ligament surgical stabilization procedures as they relate to postoperative meniscal injuries: a retrospective study of 665 stifles. *Veterinary and Comparative Orthopaedics and Traumatology* **8**, 118–123

Montgomery RD, Milton JL, Hathcock JT and Fitch RB (1994) Osteochondritis dissecans of the canine tarsal joint. *Compendium on Continuing Education for the Practicing Veterinarian* **16**, 835–844

Moore KW and Read RA (1995) Cranial cruciate ligament rupture in the dog: a retrospective study comparing surgical techniques. *Australian Veterinary Journal* **72**, 281–285

Chapter 22 The stifle

Morris E and Lipowitz AJ (2001) Comparison of tibial plateau angles in dogs with and without cranial cruciate ligament injuries. *Journal of the American Veterinary Medical Association* **218**, 363–366

Niebauer GW (1982) Immunological changes in canine cruciate ligament rupture. *Research in Veterinary Science* **32**, 235–241

Pacchiana PD, Morris E, Gillings SL, Jessen CR and Lipowitz AJ (2003) Surgical and postoperative complications associated with tibial plateau leveling osteotomy in dogs with cranial cruciate ligament rupture: 397 cases (1998–2001). *Journal of the American Veterinary Medical Association* **222**, 184–193

Peycke LE, Kerwin SC, Hosgood G and Metcalf JB (2002) Mechanical comparison of six loop fixation methods with monofilament nylon leader line. *Veterinary and Comparative Orthopaedics and Traumatology* **15**, 210–214

Pond MJ and Campbell JR (1972) The canine stifle joint: I. Rupture of the cranial cruciate ligament – an assessment of conservative and surgical treatment. *Journal of Small Animal Practice* **13**, 1–10

Pratt JNJ (2001) Avulsion of the tibial tuberosity with separation of the proximal tibial physis in seven dogs. *Veterinary Record* **149**, 352–356

Priddy NH, Tomlinson JL, Dodam JR and Hornbostel JE (2003) Complications with and owner assessment of the outcome of tibial plateau levelling osteotomy for treatment of cranial cruciate ligament rupture in dogs: 193 cases (1997–2001). *Journal of the American Veterinary Medical Association* **222**, 1726–1732

Rayward RM, Thomson DG, Davies JV, Innes JF and Whitelock RG (2004) Progression of osteoarthritis following TPLO surgery: a prospective radiographic study of 40 dogs. *Journal of Small Animal Practice* **45**, 92–97

Read RA and Robins GM (1982) Deformity of the proximal tibia in dogs. *Veterinary Record* **111**, 295–298

Reif U, Hulse DA and Hauptman JG (2002) Effect of tibial plateau leveling on stability of the canine cranial cruciate deficient stifle joint: an in vitro study. *Veterinary Surgery* **31**, 147–154

Reif U and Probst CW (2003) Comparison of tibial plateau angles in normal and cranial cruciate deficient stifles of Labrador Retrievers. *Veterinary Surgery* **32**, 385–389

Robins GM (1990) The canine stifle joint. In: *Canine Orthopaedics, 2nd edn*, ed. WG Whittick, pp. 693–760. Lea & Febiger, Philadelphia

Scavelli TD and Schrader SC (1987) Nonsurgical management of rupture of the cranial cruciate ligament in 18 cats. *Journal of the American Animal Hospital Association* **23**, 337–340

Scavelli TD, Schrader SC, Matthiesen DT and Skorup DE (1990) Partial rupture of the cranial cruciate ligament of the stifle in dogs: 25 cases (1982–1988). *Journal of the American Veterinary Medical Association* **196**, 1135–1138

Schwarz PD (1999) Tibial plateau leveling osteotomy (TPLO): a prospective clinical comparative study. Proceedings of the 9th American College of Veterinary Surgeons Symposium, San Francisco, p. 379

Selmi AL and Padilha Filho JG (2001) Rupture of the cranial cruciate ligament associated with deformity of the proximal tibia in five dogs. *Journal of Small Animal Practice* **42**, 390–393

Slater MR, Scarlett JM, Kaderly RE and Bonnett BN (1991) Breed, gender, and age risk factors for canine osteochondritis dissecans. *Veterinary and Comparative Orthopaedics and Traumatology* **4**, 100–106

Slocum B and Devine T (1983) Cranial tibial thrust: a primary force in the canine stifle. *Journal of the American Veterinary Medical Association* **183**, 456–459

Slocum B and Devine T (1984) Cranial tibial wedge osteotomy: a technique for eliminating cranial tibial thrust in cranial cruciate ligament repair. *Journal of the American Veterinary Medical Association* **184**, 564–569

Slocum B and Devine T (1993) Tibial plateau leveling osteotomy for repair of cranial cruciate ligament rupture in the canine. *Veterinary Clinics of North America: Small Animal Practice* **23**, 777–795

Slocum B and Devine Slocum T (1998) Meniscal release. In: *Current Techniques in Small Animal Surgery, 4th edn*, eds. MJ Bojrab, GW Ellison and B Slocum, pp. 1197–1199. Williams & Wilkins, Philadelphia

Slocum B and Slocum TD (1998) Rectus femoris transplantation for medial patellar luxation. In: *Current Techniques in Small Animal Surgery, 4th edn*, eds. MJ Bojrab, GW Ellison and B Slocum, pp. 1234–1237. Williams & Wilkins, Philadelphia

Smith GK, Langenbach A, Green PA, Rhodes WH and Gregor TP (1999) Evaluation of the association between medial patellar luxation and hip dysplasia in cats. *Journal of the American Veterinary Medical Association* **215**, 40–45

Talcott KW, Goring RL and deHaan JJ (2000) Rectangular recession trochleoplasty for treatment of patellar luxation in dogs and cats. *Veterinary and Comparative Orthopaedics and Traumatology* **13**, 39–43

Tomlinson JT, Cook JL, Kuroki K, Kreeger JM and Anderson MA (2001) Biochemical characterization of cartilage affected by osteochondritis dissecans in the humeral head of dogs. *American Journal of Veterinary Research* **62**, 876–881

Vasseur PB (1984) Clinical results following non-operative management of rupture of the cranial cruciate ligament in dogs. *Veterinary Surgery* **13**, 243–246

Vasseur PB, Pool RR, Arnoczky SP and Lau RE (1985) Correlative biomechanical and histologic study of the cranial cruciate ligament in dogs. *American Journal of Veterinary Research* **46**, 1842–1854

Warzee CE, Dejardin LM, Arnoczky SP and Perry RL (2001) Effect of tibial plateau leveling on cranial and caudal tibial thrusts in canine cranial cruciate-deficient stifles: an in vitro experimental study. *Veterinary Surgery* **30**, 278–286

Watt PR, Sommerlad SM and Robins GM (2001) Tibial wedge osteotomy for treatment of cranial cruciate rupture. ACVS abstract. *Veterinary Surgery* **29**, 478

Wheeler JL, Cross AR and Gingrich W (2003) In vitro effects of osteotomy angle and osteotomy reduction on tibial angulation and rotation during the tibial plateau-leveling osteotomy procedure. *Veterinary and Comparative Orthopaedics and Traumatology* **32**, 371–377

Wilke VL, Conzemius MG, Besancon MF, Evans RB and Ritter M (2002) Comparison of tibial plateau angle between clinically normal Greyhounds and Labrador Retrievers with and without rupture of the cranial cruciate ligament. *Journal of the American Veterinary Medical Association* **221**, 1426–1429

Willauer CC and Vasseur PB (1987) Clinical results of surgical correction of medial luxation of the patella in dogs. *Veterinary Surgery* **16**, 31–36

Wingfield C, Amis AA, Stead AC and Law HT (2000) Comparison of the biomechanical properties of rottweiler and racing greyhound cranial cruciate ligaments. *Journal of Small Animal Practice* **41**, 303–307

Chapter 22 The stifle

OPERATIVE TECHNIQUE 22.1
Lateral parapatellar approach

Positioning
Dorsolateral recumbency with the affected limb positioned caudally.

Assistant
No.

Tray extras
Gelpi retractors.

Surgical technique
The skin is incised on the craniolateral aspect of the stifle and distal femur. Fascia lata and lateral fascia of the stifle are exposed. Another incision is made along the cranial border of the biceps femoris muscle. This is continued distally a few millimetres lateral and parallel to the patella and patellar tendon (Figure 22.30a). The biceps femoris muscle and attached fascia lata are retracted caudally. Distally it is necessary to separate these structures from the femur. The blood vessels in this area may need to be ligated. A curvilinear incision is made in the joint capsule from the lateral fabella to the tibial tuberosity (Figure 22.30b). With the stifle joint extended the patella is luxated medially. Flexion of the joint exposes the intra-articular structures. Retraction of the infrapatellar fat pad with Gelpi retractors placed between the fat pad and the tendon of the long digital extensor muscle aids inspection of the intra-articular structures (Figure 22.30c).

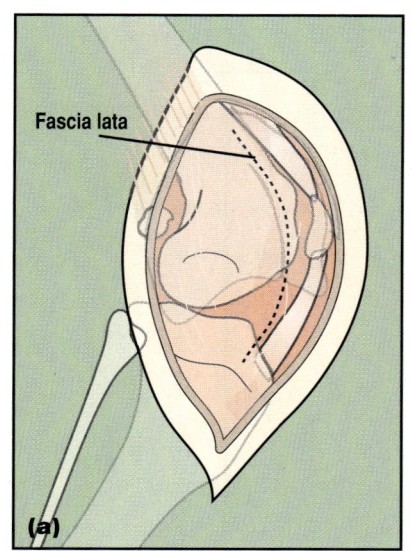

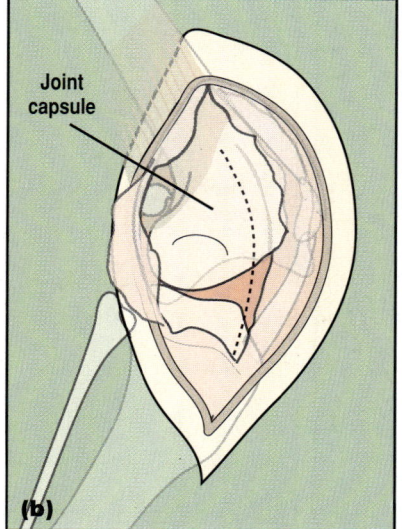

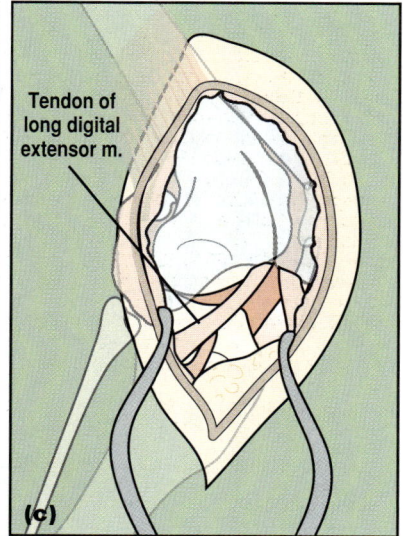

22.30 Lateral parapatellar approach. **(a)** Incision along the cranial border of the biceps femoris. **(b)** The biceps femoris muscle and fascia lata are retracted. **(c)** Retraction of the infrapatellar fat pad exposes the intra-articular structures.

Closure
The joint capsule and fascia lata are closed in separate layers with absorbable continuous sutures. Remaining wound closure is routine.

Postoperative care
See appropriate operative technique.

Complications
Medial patellar luxation if wound breakdown occurs.

Chapter 22   The stifle

OPERATIVE TECHNIQUE 22.2
Medial parapatellar approach

Positioning
Dorsolateral recumbency with the affected limb towards the surgical table.

Assistant
No.

Tray extras
Gelpi retractors.

Surgical technique
The skin is incised on the craniomedial aspect of the stifle and distal femur and the deep fascia is identified. Another incision is made in the medial fascia and medial joint capsule caudal to the patella. It is extended proximally into the cranial sartorius and vastus medialis muscles and distally to the tibial tuberosity (Figure 22.31a). With the stifle joint extended the patella is luxated laterally. Flexion of the joint exposes the intra-articular structures (Figure 22.31b). Retraction of the infrapatellar fat pad with Gelpi retractors aids inspection of the intra-articular structures.

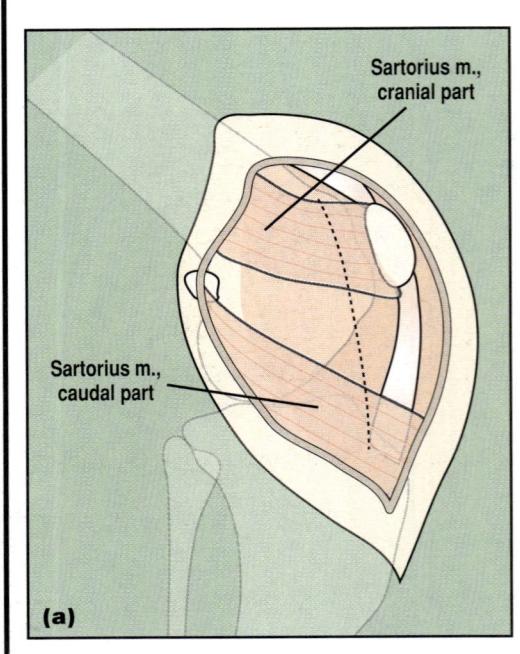

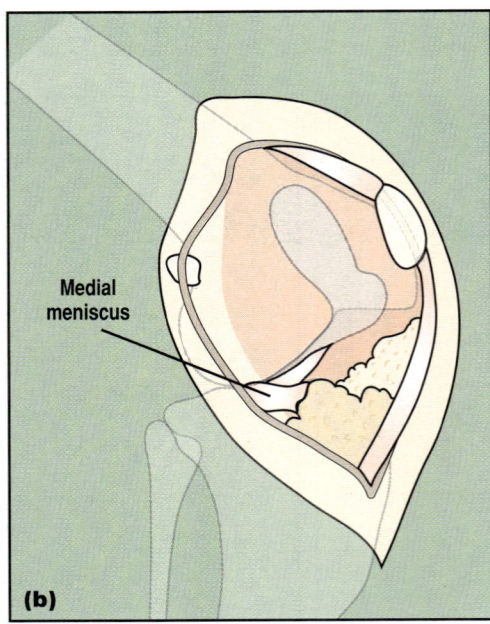

22.31 Medial parapatellar approach. **(a)** Incision into the sartorius muscle. **(b)** Luxation of the patella and stifle flexion exposes the intra-articular structures.

Closure
The joint capsule and medial fascia are closed in one layer with an absorbable continuous suture. Proximally the vastus medialis and cranial sartorius muscles are repaired in a similar manner. Remaining wound closure is routine.

Postoperative care
See appropriate operative technique.

Complications
Lateral patellar luxation if wound breakdown occurs.

Chapter 22 The stifle

OPERATIVE TECHNIQUE 22.3
Limited medial approach

Positioning
Dorsolateral recumbency with the affected limb towards the surgical table.

Assistant
No.

Tray extras
Gelpi retractors; stifle distractor.

Surgical technique
The skin is incised on the craniomedial aspect of the stifle from the patella to the tibial plateau. Another incision is made in the medial fascia and medial joint capsule caudal to the patellar tendon. This incision extends from the distal pole of the patella to the tibial tuberosity. Retraction of the infrapatellar fat pad with Gelpi retractors aids inspection of the intra-articular structures (Figure 22.32). Placement of a stifle distractor from the intercondylar notch to the tibial plateau is extremely helpful in improving the view of the joint.

> **PRACTICAL TIP**
> A head-mounted focal light source greatly assists meniscal inspection. Suction to evacuate haemorrhage and irrigation fluid is useful.

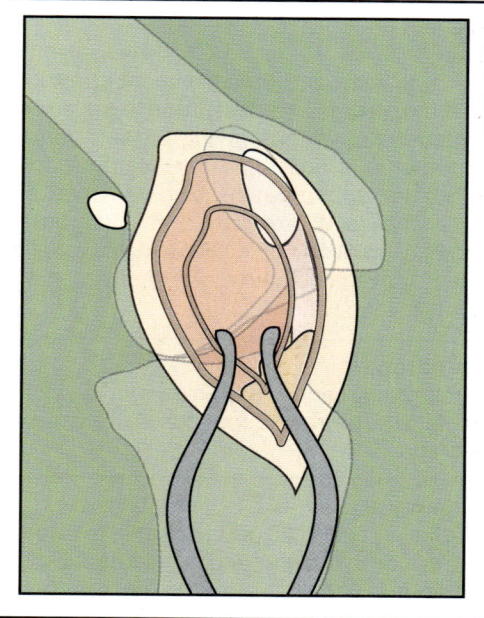

22.32 Limited medial approach.

Closure
The joint capsule and medial fascia are closed in one layer with an absorbable continuous suture. Remaining wound closure is routine.

Postoperative care
See appropriate operative technique.

Complications
Very uncommon.

Chapter 22 The stifle

> ## OPERATIVE TECHNIQUE 22.4
> ### Arthroscopy of the stifle
>
> **Positioning**
> The imaging tower is positioned to the side of the patient with the screen angled caudally. The surgeon stands or sits caudal to the patient.
>   The limb is prepared as for an open arthrotomy. Best results will be obtained through a hanging limb preparation. The dog is positioned in dorsal recumbency but leaning and supported away from the index side such that the index stifle joint is uppermost.
>
> **Assistant**
> Desirable for diagnostic arthroscopy, essential for operative arthroscopy
>
> **Tray extras**
> Arthroscopy tower with light source, camera unit, monitor; 2.7 mm 30-degree arthroscope with sleeve and blunt obturator (2.4 mm in small breeds, 4 mm in giant-breed dogs); two 25–37 mm (1–1.5 inch) 20 gauge needles; two 10 ml hypodermic syringes; giving set; sufficient quantity of Hartmann's solution (usually 5 l); an assortment of hand instruments is necessary for examination, biopsy or treating pathological lesions. Recommended instruments include appropriately sized cannulas, switching stick, a small probe, small joint graspers, a small joint curette, a small joint hand burr, and small joint biopsy forceps. Very desirable is a motorized shaver and/or radiofrequency ablation unit. Often synovial proliferation in the region of the fat pad is such that the viewing field in the joint space is obscured. A motorized shaver or ablation unit is helpful in removing synovial villi and fat to create a viewing window.
>
> **Clipping and draping**
> A hanging limb preparation is preferred with the clip extending from just distal to the hip to just proximal to the tarsus. Four field drapes and a foot drape are used and covered by a sterile impervious transparent adhesive disposable drape.
>
> **Surgical technique**
> To begin, a 25 mm (1 inch) 20 gauge needle is inserted into the femorotibial joint and the joint is distended with fluid. Portals are craniolateral and craniomedial and are located either side of the patellar tendon. A push-through technique is used to establish an egress portal with a drainage cannula. A No. 11 blade is inserted into the medial (or lateral) femorotibial joint to create the first portal, a switching stick is inserted into this portal and this is passed proximally through the femoropatellar joint such that it passes through the joint capsule proximally and out through the tissue under the skin. The skin is cut to allow the stick to protrude and the cannula is placed over the stick and inserted. The stick is removed to leave the cannula in position. Some surgeons prefer a medial cannula, some a lateral.
>   The arthroscope sheath and obturator are inserted through the portal into the joint. The arthroscope and light post are positioned to view the area of interest. It is best to start the arthroscope in the femoropatellar joint and use the patella as a landmark. The stifle joint is held extended for this. As the arthroscope is moved distally, the stifle joint is flexed.
>   If visualization of the cartilage surface is difficult due to synovial proliferation, the joint should be distended further by temporarily occluding egress of fluid. If the view remains obstructed, an instrument portal is established (see below) and a motorized shaver blade (full radius cutting blade on oscillate at 1000–1200 rpm) or radiofrequency unit is inserted to perform a synovectomy. Haemorrhage is controlled by ingress fluid pressure for tamponade, electrocoagulation or ablation with a radiofrequency unit.
>   An instrument portal is established if the viewing window is obscured by synovial villi, a biopsy of intra-articular tissue is desired or if treatment of joint pathology is required. The instrument portal is established adjacent to the patellar tendon, opposite the arthroscope. Hand instruments, a shaver blade (motorized shaver) or radiofrequency probe can now easily be inserted, withdrawn and re-inserted into the joint space.
>   Complete exploration of the joint can be performed by moving the arthroscope and changing the direction of view with the 30-degree fore oblique scope. The stifle joint is typically explored in the following order:
>
> →

OPERATIVE TECHNIQUE 22.4 continued
Arthroscopy of the stifle

1. Medial articular compartment (medial femoral and tibial condyles, cranial horn of medial meniscus)
2. Medial joint pouch (medial trochlear ridge and joint capsule)
3. Intercondylar notch (cruciate ligament, notch) – often requires debridement of fat pad and proliferative synovium
4. Lateral articular compartment (lateral femoral and tibial condyles, cranial horn of lateral meniscus)
5. Lateral joint pouch (lateral trochlear ridge, joint capsule, long digital extensor tendon of origin)
6. Proximal compartment (patella, trochlear groove).

> **PRACTICAL TIP**
> The instrument portal and arthroscope portal are interchangeable, depending on which compartment of the stifle joint needs to be examined.

Removal of stifle OCD lesions
The arthroscope and instrument portals are located appropriately. If the osteochondral tissue is still attached at one or more sites, a probe or small elevator is inserted to free the edge of the flap partially. The osteochondral flap is not freed completely but is left attached at one site. Grasping forceps are inserted and the free osteochondral flap removed. The cartilage flap may be removed as a single large fragment or, as is often the case, in two to three smaller pieces. A curette is used to debride the edges of the lesion. The subchondral bone surface of the lesion is treated with abrasion using a handheld curette, handheld burr or motorized shaver. The surface is lightly abraded until the underlying bone bleeds freely. Abrasion arthroplasty should be halted once multifocal pinpoint bleeding is observed. Further abrasion leads to a deepening of the defect, which may increase instability. Upon completion of surface abrasionplasty or microfracture, small bone or cartilage fragments are flushed from the joint by increasing the ingress flow.

Arthroscopic meniscectomy
Appropriate locking grasping forceps are essential for this procedure. The loose meniscal tissue is grasped and passed to an assistant. A Smillie knife, hooked blade or mini-radiofrequency probe is directed parallel to the forceps and the loose meniscus is cut free from the remaining tissue. Small amounts of damaged meniscal tissue may be removed with radiofrequency but care must be taken to avoid iatrogenic injury to other tissues.

Closure
Single skin sutures are placed in the portal sites.

Postoperative care
See appropriate operative technique. Generally 48 hours' rest is required following diagnostic arthroscopy. If operative procedures are used, the period of rest is extended as appropriate to each individual procedure.

Complications
Accumulation of subcutaneous fluid can occur during the procedure; this can cause some joint space collapse; it resolves within 48–72 hours.

Chapter 22 The stifle

OPERATIVE TECHNIQUE 22.5
Rectangular recession trochleoplasty

Preoperative planning
The location of the patella in relation to the femoral trochlea when it (sub)luxates should be determined by palpation. Tangential ('skyline') views of the flexed stifle enable assessment of the morphology of the femoral trochlea; however, the decision as to whether or not to deepen the trochlea is generally based on intra-operative findings.

Positioning
Dorsolateral recumbency with the affected limb uppermost.

Assistant
Useful when preparing the osteochondral block.

Tray extras
Hobby saw (fine-toothed); various sizes of sharp chisels or osteotomes; mallet.

Surgical approach
- Medial patellar luxation: lateral parapatellar approach (see Operative Technique 22.1)
- Lateral patellar luxation: medial parapatellar approach (see Operative Technique 22.2).

Surgical technique
Parallel incisions are made on the medial and lateral trochlear ridges with a scalpel blade to define the size of the block. The width of the cut should be wide enough to accept the patella, and the trochlear ridges should be maintained. Each cut is angled approximately 10 degrees axially toward the sagittal plane of the femur (Figure 22.33a). This ensures compression between the autograft and recipient bed. The cuts extend from the proximal trans-trochlear margin to the intercondylar fossa. The rectangular block is separated using a fine osteotome or oscillating saw. Care is necessary to avoid fracturing the osteochondral segment. Cancellous bone is removed from the base and the edges of the defect to enable recession of the block. Resected cancellous bone should be stored in a blood-soaked swab and used with the tibial tuberosity transposition. Following replacement of the osteochondral block (22.33b) the patella is reduced and tracking examined (Figure 22.34).

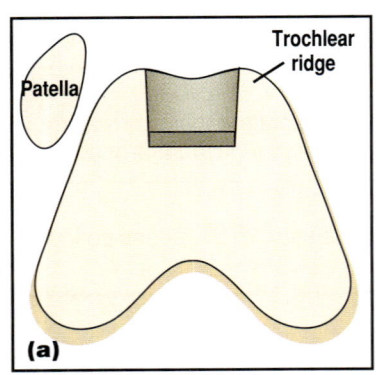

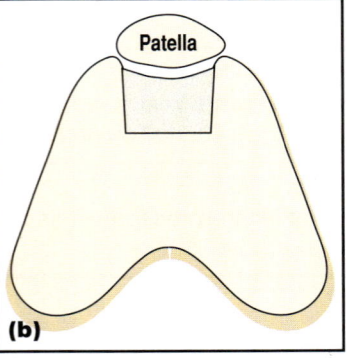

22.33 Rectangular recession trochleoplasty. **(a)** Parallel incisions in the trochlear ridges, angled at approximately 10 degrees axially. **(b)** Following resection of cancellous bone, the osteochondral block is replaced.

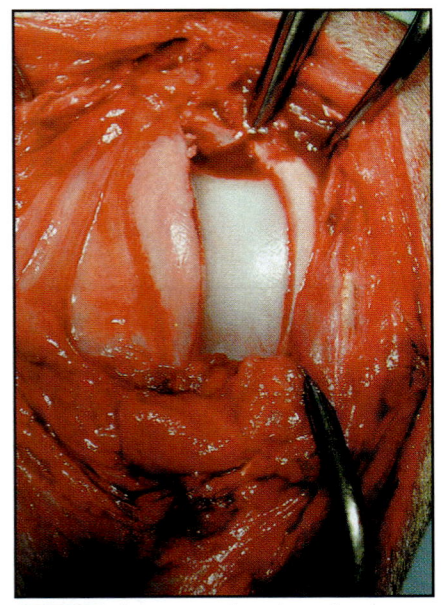

22.34 Intraoperative view of a block recession.

OPERATIVE TECHNIQUE 22.5 continued
Rectangular recession trochleoplasty

PRACTICAL TIP
A preferential amount of bone may be removed proximally or distally depending on where the patella is (sub)luxating, such that the the trochlea is recessed asymmetrically.

WARNING
Overzealous removal of bone from the recipient bed should be avoided since excessive recession of the trochlea will prevent femoropatellar contact.

Closure
- Medial patellar luxation: medial soft tissue release and lateral soft tissue tightening is generally necessary.
- Lateral patellar luxation: lateral soft tissue release and medial soft tissue tightening is generally necessary.

PRACTICAL TIP
Patella tracking and stability should be regularly evaluated during wound closure.

Postoperative care
Strict rest for 2 weeks, followed by a gradual increase in regular, controlled lead exercise for 2 months. Twice-weekly hydrotherapy may be started 2–4 weeks postoperatively.

Complications
Complications include fracture of the osteochondral block; postoperative fracture of the medial or lateral trochlear ridge; and poor femoropatellar tracking (excessive block recession, inadequate block recession, recessed block too narrow).

Chapter 22 The stifle

OPERATIVE TECHNIQUE 22.6
Wedge recession trochleoplasty

Preoperative planning
The location of the patella in relation to the femoral trochlea when it (sub)luxates should be determined by palpation. Tangential ('skyline') views of the flexed stifle enable assessment of the morphology of the femoral trochlea. However, the decision as to whether or not to deepen the trochlea is generally based on intra-operative findings.

Positioning
Dorsolateral recumbency with the affected limb uppermost.

Assistant
No.

Tray extras
Hobby saw (fine toothed); rongeurs or bone cutters.

Surgical approach
- Medial patellar luxation: lateral parapatellar approach (see Operative Technique 22.1)
- Lateral patellar luxation: medial parapatellar approach (see Operative Technique 22.2).

Surgical technique
Marks are made on the medial and lateral trochlear ridges with a scalpel blade to define the maximum width of the wedge. A fine-toothed saw is used to create a wedge-shaped segment, which is carefully stored, as a second cut is made parallel to the first on the side opposite the direction of the patellar luxation (Figure 22.35a). The osteotomy must be made so that the two oblique planes of the cuts intersect proximally at the proximal edge of the trochlear articular cartilage and distally at the intercondylar notch. The wedge is replaced in the deepened defect (Figure 22.35b). Removal of the ridge of bone on the caudal aspect of the wedge is often beneficial in ensuring a secure fit. Resected cancellous bone should be stored in a blood-soaked swab and used with the tibial tuberosity transposition. Occasionally, rotating the wedge 180 degrees can be beneficial. Following replacement of the wedge the patella is reduced and tracking examined (Figure 22.36).

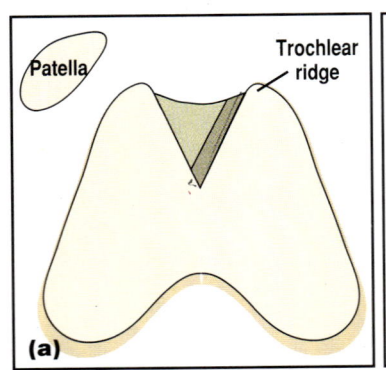

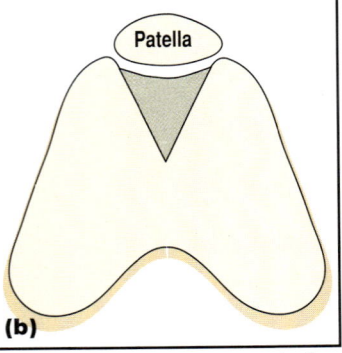

22.35 Wedge recession trochleoplasty. **(a)** Following removal of a wedge-shaped section, a parallel cut is made in the side opposite the direction of patellar luxation. **(b)** After removal of the second section, the original wedge is replaced. The caudal ridge has been removed to secure a tight fit.

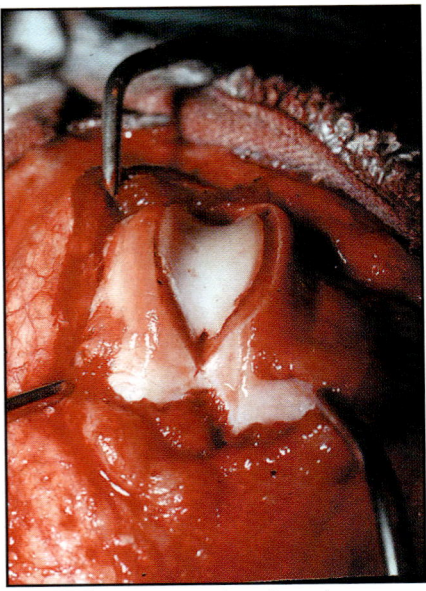

22.36 Intraoperative view of a wedge recession.

OPERATIVE TECHNIQUE 22.6
Wedge recession trochleoplasty

PRACTICAL TIP
In cases where the patella is (sub)luxating at the proximal aspect of the trochlea it may be necessary to increase the width and depth of the trochlea in this region by removing articular cartilage and subchondral bone, i.e. perform a limited excisional trochleoplasty.

WARNING
Overzealous removal of bone from the wedge defect should be avoided since excessive recession of the trochlea will prevent femoropatellar contact.

Closure
- Medial patellar luxation: medial soft tissue release and lateral soft tissue tightening is generally necessary
- Lateral patellar luxation: lateral soft tissue release and medial soft tissue tightening is generally necessary.

PRACTICAL TIP
Patella tracking and stability should be regularly evaluated during wound closure.

Postoperative care
Strict rest for 2 weeks, followed by gradual increase in regular, controlled lead exercise for 2 months. Twice-weekly hydrotherapy may be started 2–4 weeks postoperatively.

Complications
Complicatons include recession of the medial or lateral trochlear ridges, due to the wedge being too wide, and poor femoropatellar tracking (excessive wedge recession, inadequate wedge recession, recessed wedge too narrow).

Chapter 22 The stifle

OPERATIVE TECHNIQUE 22.7
Tibial tuberosity transposition (medial patellar luxation)

Preoperative planning
If possible the position of the tibial tuberosity should be assessed relative to the quadriceps muscle group and femoral trochlea during weightbearing, with the patella reduced.

Positioning
Dorsolateral recumbency with the affected limb uppermost.

Assistant
No.

Tray extras
Periosteal elevator; Allis tissue forceps; hacksaw or bone cutters; rongeurs; drill; Kirschner wires; orthopaedic wire; pin cutters.

Surgical approach
See Operative Technique 22.1.

Surgical technique
The cranial tibial muscle is reflected from the craniolateral aspect of the proximal tibia and the tuberosity is separated, preferably using a hacksaw (Figure 22.37). Care is taken to preserve a periosteal attachment distally, although in severe cases it is often necessary to detach the tuberosity completely. Cortical bone on the caudolateral aspect of the osteotomy site may be removed to expose cancellous bone and provide a level bed for the transposed tuberosity. The tibial tuberosity is rotated laterally and stabilized with one or two Kirschner wires. In active dogs, those with bilateral lameness and all medium and large dogs, a tension-band wire is strongly recommended (Figure 22.38). Femoropatellar stability is assessed by flexing and extending the stifle while internally and externally rotating the distal limb. In cases of suspected patella alta (where the patella is located proximally and luxating when the stifle is extended) the tuberosity may be transposed distally in addition to laterally. If a recession trochleoplasty technique has been performed the excised cancellous bone is transferred and packed around the tibial tuberosity.

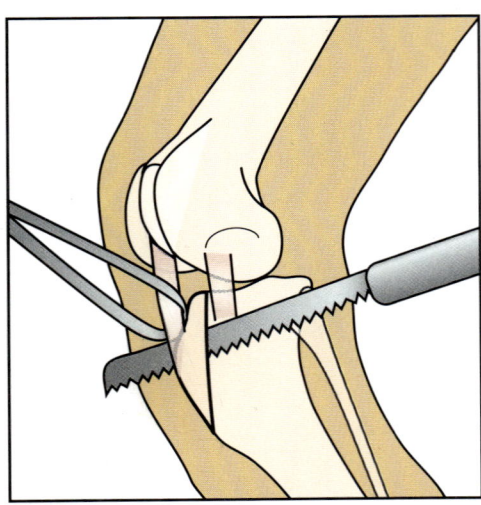

22.37 A hacksaw is used to separate the tibial tuberosity.

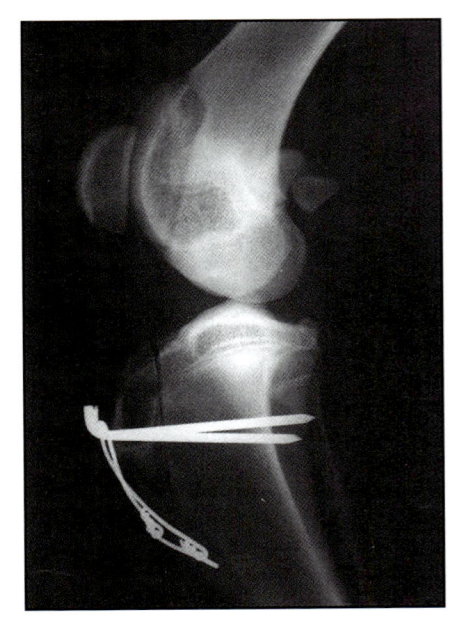

22.38 Tibial tuberosity transposition stabilized with two Kirschner wires and a tension-band wire in a 2.5-year-old Labrador Retriever. There is evidence of a rectangular recession trochleoplasty.

384

Chapter 22 The stifle

OPERATIVE TECHNIQUE 22.7 continued
Tibial tuberosity transposition (medial patellar luxation)

PRACTICAL TIP
Pre-drilling the tibial tuberosity prior to performing the osteotomy simplifies fixation.

WARNINGS
- Failure to protect the patellar tendon, with, for example, Allis tissue forceps, may result in iatrogenic laceration of the tendon by the top edge of the hacksaw.
- When using a tension band wire, care is needed to avoid trapping the patellar tendon between the tension band wire and the Kirschner wire(s).

Closure
See Operative Technique 22.5.

Postoperative care
Strict rest for 2 weeks. Gradual increase in regular, controlled lead exercise for 6 weeks. Twice-weekly hydrotherapy starting 2–4 weeks postoperatively.

Complications
Recurrence of medial patellar luxation due to inadequate transposition; lateral patellar luxation due to excessive transposition; implant failure or loosening; patellar tendon injury; tibial tuberosity avulsion, fracture or non-union.

Chapter 22   The stifle

OPERATIVE TECHNIQUE 22.8
Meniscal inspection, partial meniscectomy and medial meniscal release

Preoperative planning
The possible need for an intra-articular or extra-articular stabilization or a tibial plateau levelling technique should be considered, as this will influence the surgical approach.

Positioning
Dorsolateral recumbency with the affected limb on the surgical table if only meniscal surgery or possible concomitant tibial plateau levelling procedure to be performed. Dorsolateral recumbency with the affected limb positioned caudally if concomitant intra-articular or extra-articular stabilization technique to be performed.

Assistant
No.

Tray extras
Small and large stifle distractors; Hohmann and Gelpi retractors; Beaver knife and blades; Dandy nerve hook.

Surgical approach
Limited medial approach (see Operative Technique 22.3) if meniscal surgery and/or tibial plateau levelling procedure being performed. Lateral parapatellar approach (see Operative Technique 22.1) if concomitant intra-articular or extra-articular stabilization technique needed.

Surgical technique

Meniscal inspection
Placing a stifle distractor in the joint aids inspection of the menisci, especially the caudal horn of the medial meniscus. Alternatively a Hohmann retractor may be used. The axial border of the caudal horn of the medial meniscus may be gently tugged with a small pair of mosquito forceps to ensure there is not a non-displaced peripheral tear.

> **PRACTICAL TIPS**
> - A head-mounted focal light source greatly assists meniscal inspection, especially when a limited medial arthrotomy has been performed. Suction to evacuate haemorrhage and irrigation fluid is useful.
> - A Dandy nerve hook is helpful when examining the menisci. It helps to exteriorize bucket handle tears and in meniscal release.

Partial meniscectomy
The menisci should be examined carefully using a Dandy nerve hook or similar instrument to check for peripheral detachments and non-displaced tears. The caudal horn of the medial meniscus is most commonly injured. Removal of the caudal horn necessitates two incisions with a Beaver or No. 15 scalpel blade. First, the caudal tibial ligament of the medial meniscus is sectioned, taking care to avoid the caudal cruciate ligament. Secondly, a radial cut is made at the cranial extent of the injured section of meniscus (Figure 22.39). Small forceps are used to remove the damaged portion of the meniscus from the joint. Axial tears are managed by resection of the regional peripheral meniscus.

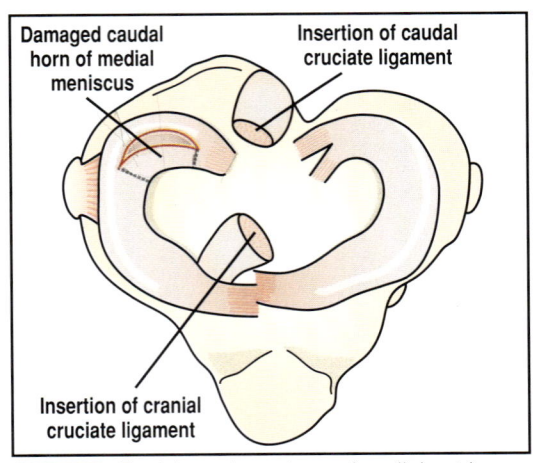

22.39 Partial meniscectomy. A radial cut is made at the cranial extent of the injured section of meniscus.

→

Chapter 22 The stifle

OPERATIVE TECHNIQUE 22.8 *continued*
Meniscal inspection, partial meniscectomy and medial meniscal release

Medial meniscal release

Technique A
Meniscal ligament release is performed via a limited medial arthrotomy. The caudal tibial ligament of the medial meniscus is sectioned with a Beaver blade, taking care to avoid injury to the caudal cruciate ligament. A Dandy nerve hook may be used to tension the ligament prior to cutting.

Technique B
Meniscal body release may be performed through the inspection arthrotomy or via a separate arthrotomy caudal to the medial collateral ligament. A Beaver blade is used to create a radial incision through the body of the meniscus. With the caudomedial approach the blade is directed craniolaterally.

Closure
Wound closure is routine.

Postoperative care
When stabilization or tibial plateau levelling procedures have not been performed, rehabilitation can be quite rapid. There should be a gradual increase in regular, controlled lead exercise for 6 weeks. Twice-weekly hydrotherapy may start 2 weeks postoperatively.

Complications
Complications following partial meniscectomy are uncommon. The long-term effects of meniscal release have not been studied.

Chapter 22 The stifle

OPERATIVE TECHNIQUE 22.9
Over-the-top graft

Preoperative planning
Measure tibial plateau angle (see Figure 22.17) to ensure it is not >25 degrees.

Positioning
Dorsolateral recumbency with affected limb positioned caudally.

Assistant
No.

Tray extras
Hohmann retractors; graft passers.

Surgical technique
For approach, see Operative Technique 22.1.

A cranial skin incision is made from the mid-femur to just distal to the tibial tuberosity. A 1.0–1.5 cm width of fascia lata and lateral third of the patellar tendon is dissected free of the quadriceps muscle, patella and joint capsule. The graft is left attached to the tibial tuberosity (Figure 22.40a). The joint is opened via a lateral curvilinear arthrotomy extending from the lateral fabella to the tibial tuberosity. Remnants of the cranial cruciate ligament are resected and osteophytes in the intercondylar region are removed.

The graft is placed under the infrapatellar fat pad and into the joint with curved mosquito forceps. A graft passer is placed through the caudal joint capsule lateral to the caudal cruciate ligament. The end of the graft is placed into the tip of the graft passer and pulled through the joint (Figure 22.40b). It is gently tensioned until cranial draw is eliminated. The graft is sutured to the regional periosteum and fascia (Figure 22.40c).

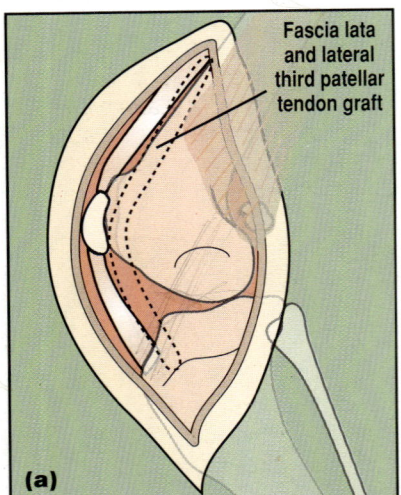

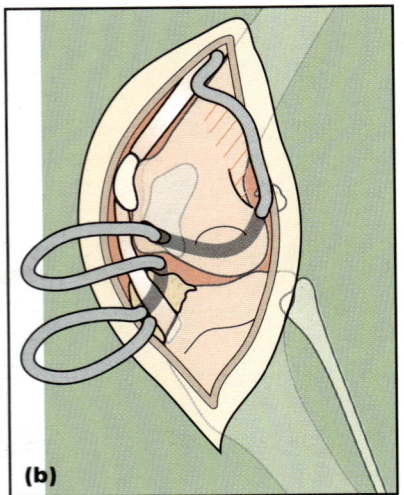

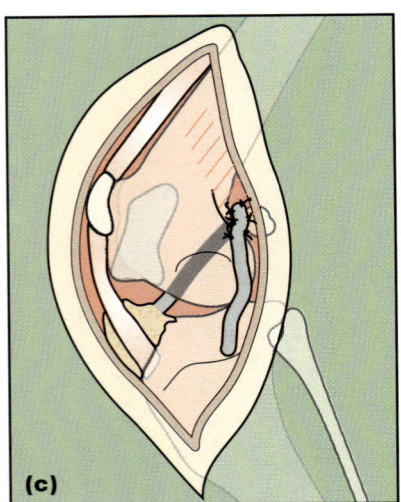

22.40 Over-the-top graft. **(a)** Graft is prepared. **(b)** The graft is pulled through the joint using a graft passer. **(c)** The graft is sutured to periosteum and fascia.

Closure
The joint capsule is sutured from proximally to distally whilst incorporating the remaining graft. Fascia lata, superficial fascia and skin are closed routinely in layers.

Postoperative care
Strict rest for 2 weeks. Gradual increase in regular, controlled lead exercise for 6 months. Twice-weekly hydrotherapy starting 2–4 weeks postoperatively.

Complications
Late meniscal injury; sepsis; iatrogenic injury to the caudal cruciate ligament, peroneal nerve or popliteal artery.

Chapter 22 The stifle

OPERATIVE TECHNIQUE 22.10
Lateral fabellotibial suture with self-locking knot

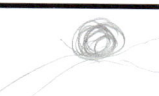

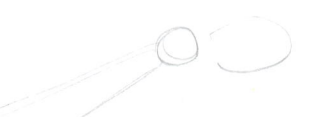

Preoperative planning
Measure tibial plateau angle (see Figure 22.17) to ensure it is not >25 degrees.

Positioning
Dorsolateral recumbency with affected limb positioned caudally.

Assistant
No.

Tray extras
Hohmann retractors; small graft passer; heavy-gauge semicircular needles; monofilament nylon leader line (22.7 kg (50 lb), 36 kg (80 lb), 45.4 kg (100 lb)); drill and drill bits; 16 gauge hypodermic needle.

Surgical technique
For approach see Operative Technique 22.1.

The tip of a Hohmann retractor is placed caudal to the lateral fabella to retract the biceps muscle. A small graft passer or heavy-gauge needle is passed around the lateral fabella, if possible, from cranioproximal to caudodistal. The two ends of a 40 cm length of monofilament nylon are passed 1 cm through the hole in the end of the instrument and pulled around the fabella until a small loop of material remains. The ends of the material are passed from lateral to medial through a hypodermic needle that is positioned caudal to the patellar tendon. A hole is drilled in the cranioproximal aspect of the tibial tuberosity from medial to lateral and the two ends of the suture material are passed through this hole to exit laterally (Figure 22.41a).

The stifle is positioned at a weightbearing angle. The loop of material in the region of the lateral fabella is reflected craniodistally and the ends of the material which have been passed through the tibial tuberosity are passed through the loop from lateral to medial (Figure 22.41b). Caudoproximal traction on the two ends reduces the size of the loop. The direction of the traction is then reversed towards the tibial tuberosity (craniodistally). The caudoproximal and craniodistal manoeuvres are repeated if necessary to ensure that the knot is tied in the region of the lateral fabella. The first throw of a square knot is placed lateral to the two strands of material passing through the loop (Figure 22.41c). If necessary, tension on the fabellotibial suture is increased by applying craniodistal traction and simultaneously tightening the first throw. When the suture is tightened sufficiently, as assessed by cranial draw estimation, four additional square throws are applied to the knot.

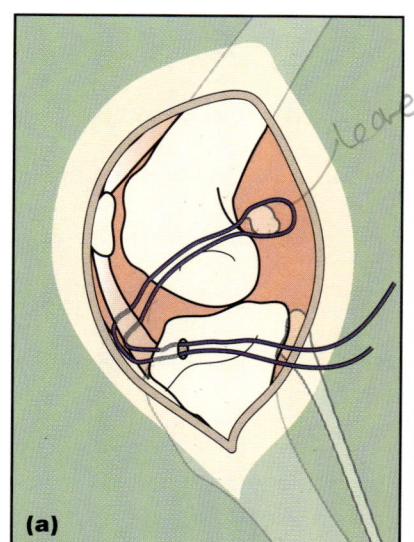

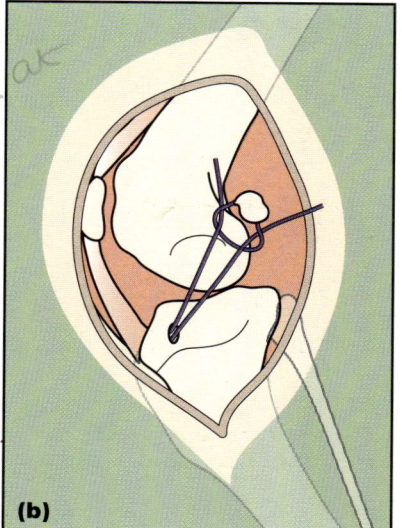

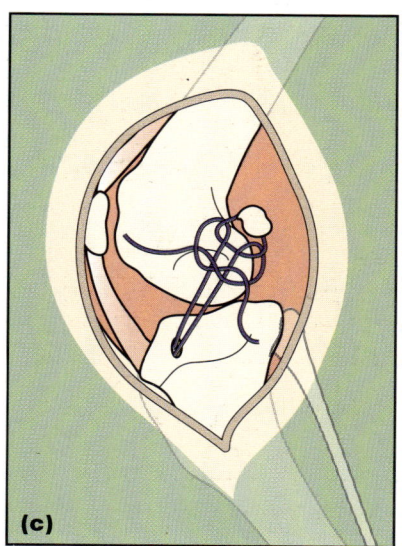

22.41 Lateral fabellotibial suture with self-locking knot.

Chapter 22 The stifle

OPERATIVE TECHNIQUE 22.10
Lateral fabellotibial suture with self-locking knot

Closure
The fascia lata incision is closed with an absorbable suture material in a continuous pattern from distally to proximally, locking the suture upon itself every 2–3 cm. Closure of the superficial fascia, subcutaneous tissues and skin is routine.

Postoperative care
Strict rest for 2 weeks. Gradual increase in regular, controlled lead exercise for 6 months. Twice-weekly hydrotherapy starting 2–4 weeks postoperatively.

Complications
Late meniscal injury; sepsis (soft tissue, joint); peroneal nerve injury; restriction in range of motion; fabella displacement.

OPERATIVE TECHNIQUE 22.11
Tibial wedge osteotomy

Preoperative planning
Measure tibial plateau angle (see Figure 22.9); calculate the angle of the wedge that needs to be removed; assess any angular or rotational limb deformity.

Positioning
Dorsolateral recumbency with the affected limb on the surgical table.

Assistant
Useful.

Tray extras
Periosteal elevator; drill; oscillating saw and blades; goniometer; dynamic compression plates; plate benders; screws and corresponding instrumentation for insertion; rongeurs.

Surgical approach
Medial approach with elevation and caudal retraction of the cranial part of the sartorius muscle. The insertion of the popliteus muscle is elevated from the caudal aspect of the proximal tibia at the level of the osteotomy. Similarly the muscles on the lateral aspect of the proximal tibia are elevated at the level of the osteotomy. This approach is combined with a medial arthrotomy approach to allow joint inspection, redundant cranial cruciate ligament debridement and appropriate action on any meniscal injury.

Surgical technique
A 21-gauge hypodermic needle is placed in the medial femorotibial joint to identify the proximal aspect of the tibial plateau. A six-hole dynamic compression plate is contoured to the caudomedial aspect of the proximal tibia, ensuring that the plate is positioned as proximally as possible. Adjustments may be made with plate contouring in an attempt to correct any angular or rotational deformity. The third screw hole is drilled, measured and tapped. A closing wedge osteotomy is performed distal to the prepared screw hole and the insertion of the medial collateral ligament and patellar tendon using an oscillating saw (Figure 22.42a). The osteotomy gap is accurately closed and the fourth screw placed in compression. In medium and large-breed dogs a second dynamic compression plate is contoured and applied to the craniomedial aspect of the proximal tibia (Figures 22.42b and 22.43). The remaining screws are placed in the plate. In small breed dogs a Kirschner wire or figure-of-eight orthopaedic wire may be used to augment single plate fixation (Figure 22.44) (Macias *et al.*, 2002). The excised bone is fragmented with rongeurs and placed at the lateral aspect of the osteotomy.

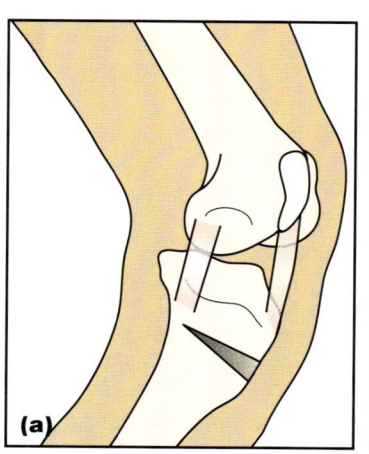

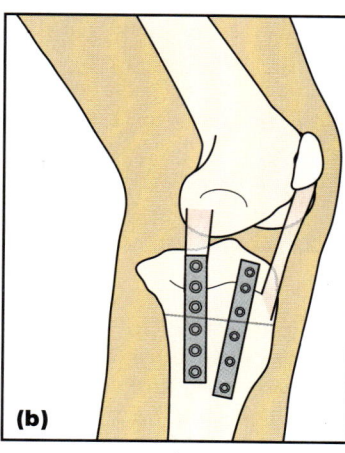

22.42 Tibial wedge osteotomy. **(a)** Closing wedge osteotomy. **(b)** Fixation with plates and screws.

OPERATIVE TECHNIQUE 22.11 continued
Tibial wedge osteotomy

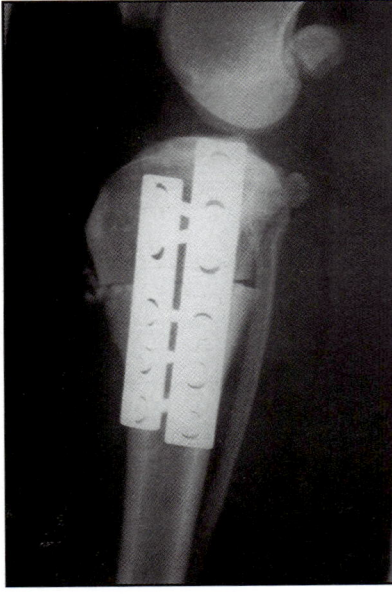

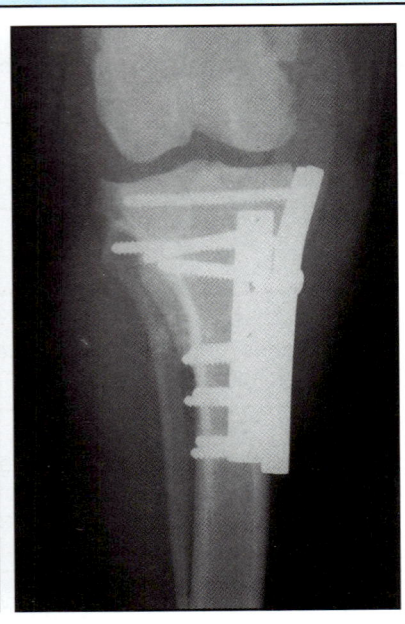

22.43 Tibial wedge osteotomy stabilized with two bone plates in a 2.5-year-old Rottweiler with cranial cruciate ligament disease. The postoperative tibial plateau angle measured 7 degrees. Note the caudal bowing of the proximal fibula.

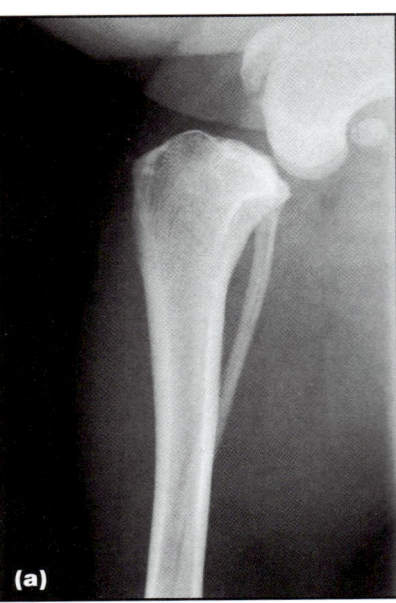

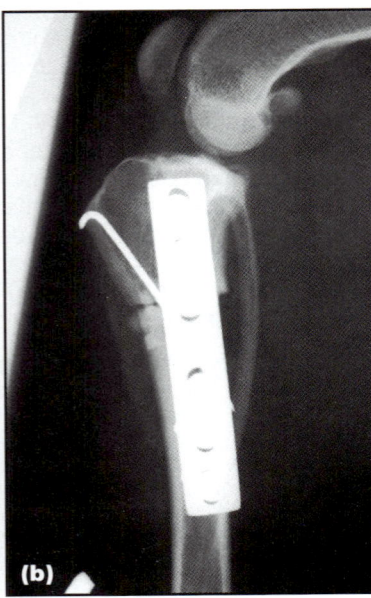

22.44 **(a)** Proximal tibial deformity and concomitant cranial cruciate ligament disease in a 4.5-year-old Cairn Terrier. Note the subluxation of the femorotibial joint on the non-stressed preoperative radiograph. **(b)** Tibial wedge osteotomy stabilized with a bone plate and a Kirschner wire. Tibial plateau angles before and after surgery were 34 and 12 degrees, respectively.

PRACTICAL TIPS
- The two osteotomies should converge just cranial to the caudal cortex of the tibia and the ostectomy is completed with a single saw cut through the caudal cortex. This will reduce the possibility of the intact fibula being relatively long and creating a varus deformity.
- The fibular head is used as a landmark when placing the proximal screws to avoid penetrating the femorotibial joint. Its precise location relative to the femorotibial joint space should be confirmed on a caudocranial radiograph.

OPERATIVE TECHNIQUE 22.11 *continued*
Tibial wedge osteotomy

Closure
The insertions of the popliteus and sartorius muscles are repaired and the deep fascia sutured over the implants. Remaining wound closure is routine.

Postoperative care
Strict rest for 2 weeks. Gradual increase in regular, controlled lead exercise for 12 weeks. Twice-weekly hydrotherapy starting 2–4 weeks postoperatively.

Complications
Intra-articular screw placement; distal limb oedema, sepsis (soft tissue, bone, joint); late meniscal injury; caudal cruciate ligament injury; delayed union; implant failure; fibular fracture; tibial fracture; angular and rotational limb deformity (Watt *et al.*, 2001).

Chapter 22 The stifle

> # OPERATIVE TECHNIQUE 22.12
> Tibial plateau levelling osteotomy (TPLO)

Preoperative planning
Measure tibial plateau angle (see Figure 22.17); calculate the distance the tibial plateau needs to be moved from tables; assess any angular or rotational limb deformity.

Positioning
Dorsolateral recumbency with the affected limb on the surgical table or dorsal recumbency with affected limb positioned caudally.

Assistant
Useful.

Tray extras
Periosteal elevator; tibial gig; Ellis pins; Kirschner wires; pointed reduction forceps; drill; oscillating saw; bi-radial TPLO saw blades (18 mm, 24 mm, 30 mm); ruler; left and right TPLO plates (2.7 mm and 3.5 mm); plate benders; screws and corresponding instrumentation for insertion.

Surgical approach
Medial approach with elevation and caudal retraction of the cranial part of the sartorius muscle. The insertion of the popliteus muscle is elevated from the caudal aspect of the proximal tibia at the level of the osteotomy. Similarly the muscles on the lateral aspect of the proximal tibia are elevated through a small incision at the distal aspect of the tibial tuberosity. This approach is combined with a medial arthrotomy approach to allow joint inspection, redundant cranial cruciate ligament debridement and appropriate action on any meniscal injury.

Surgical technique
A 21-gauge hypodermic needle is placed in the medial femorotibial joint to identify the proximal aspect of the tibial plateau. The gig is attached to the tibia, ensuring the fixation pins are parallel to the tibial plateau and perpendicular to the sagittal plane of the tibia in the craniocaudal direction. A TPLO saw (Slocum Enterprises) is used to perform the osteotomy from medial to lateral. The saw blade is positioned parallel to the proximal gig pin, with the proximal edge of the blade caudal to the patellar tendon. A pin is placed in the proximal tibial segment to enable rotation of the tibial plateau to an angle of approximately 6 degrees. The rotated fragments are temporarily stabilized with a pin and pointed reduction forceps. An attempt may be made to correct angular or rotational deformity by adjusting the jig. A six-hole TPLO plate (Slocum Enterprises) is contoured and applied to the proximal tibia (Figure 22.45). The gig, rotation pin and osteotomy fixation pin are removed.

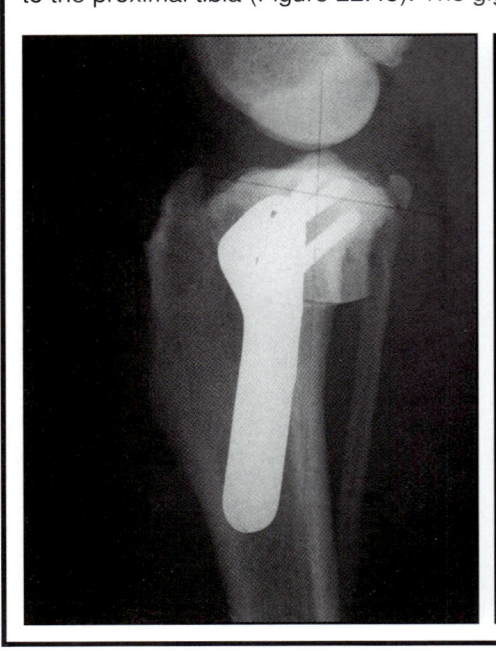

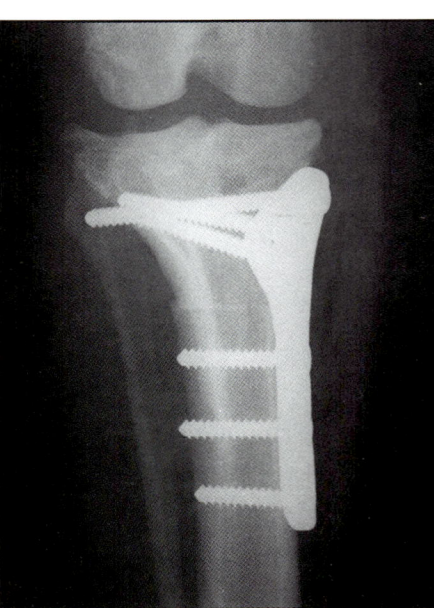

22.45 Tibial plateau levelling osteotomy stabilized with a Slocum TPLO plate in a 4-year-old Labrador Retriever with cranial cruciate ligament disease. The postoperative tibial plateau angle measured 8 degrees.

OPERATIVE TECHNIQUE 22.12 *continued*
Tibial plateau levelling osteotomy (TPLO)

WARNING
No attempt should be made to align the medial cortex of the tibial plateau segment with the medial cortex of the tibial metaphysis as this may result in angular and rotational limb deformity (Wheeler *et al.*, 2003).

PRACTICAL TIPS
- The osteotomy fixation pin is placed proximal to the insertion of the patellar tendon to avoid a stress riser and increased risk of tibial tuberosity fracture.
- The fibular head is used as a landmark when placing the proximal screws to avoid penetrating the femorotibial joint. Its precise location relative to the femorotibial joint space is confirmed on a caudocranial radiograph.

Closure
The insertions of the popliteus and sartorius muscles are repaired and the deep fascia sutured over the implants. Remaining wound closure is routine.

Postoperative care
Strict rest for 2 weeks. Gradual increase in regular, controlled lead exercise for 12 weeks. Twice-weekly hydrotherapy starting 2–4 weeks postoperatively.

Complications
Intra-articular screw placement; distal limb oedema, sepsis (soft tissue, bone, joint); late meniscal injury; caudal cruciate ligament injury; delayed union; implant failure; tibial tuberosity fracture; fibular fracture; patellar tendon strain; patellar fracture; angular and rotational limb deformity (Pacchiana *et al.*, 2003; Priddy *et al.*, 2003).

23

The tarsus

Andrew Miller and Don Hulse

Surgical anatomy

The tarsus (hock) is a compound joint consisting of seven named tarsal bones that form three irregular rows and four major joints: the talocrural joint, the proximal intertarsal joint, the distal intertarsal (centrodistal) joint and the tarsometatarsal joint (Figure 23.1). There are also numerous intertarsal joints between individual tarsal bones.

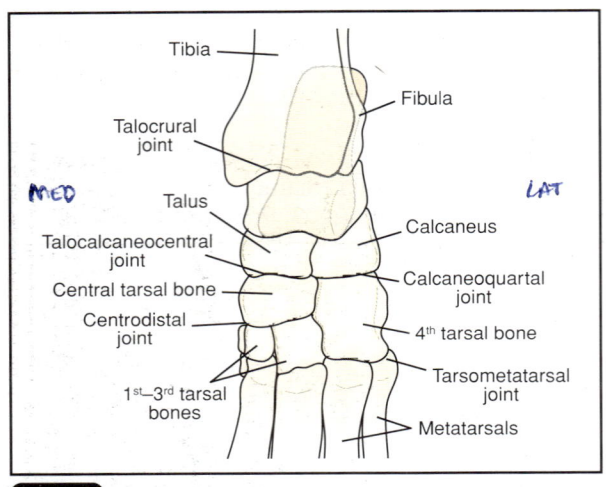

23.1 The bones and joints of the canine tarsus.

The talocrural joint

Most tarsal movement occurs at the talocrural joint, which is the articulation of the distal tibia and fibula with the talus (tibial tarsal bone). Movement is primarily flexion and extension. The normal tarsus will flex to an angle of around 15–25 degrees (such that the dorsum of the metatarsus almost contacts the cranial tibia) and extend to an angle of around 180–190 degrees.

Mediolateral stability is provided principally by the collateral ligaments (Figure 23.2), both of which have long and short components. Both ligaments originate on the respective malleoli. The short component of the medial ligament courses caudally and inserts on the medial aspect of the plantar end of the medial ridge of the talus, while the long component courses distally and has an attachment to the talus before finally inserting on the first tarsal bone. The short component of the lateral collateral ligament again courses caudally and inserts on the calcaneus. The long component passes over and attaches to the calcaneus and fourth tarsal bone and finally inserts on the head of the fifth metatarsal bone.

The Achilles (common calcaneal) tendon inserts on the tuber calcaneus. It comprises the tendon of insertion of the gastrocnemius and the combined tendon of the gracilis, biceps femoris and semitendinosus muscles. The superficial digital flexor tendon is associated with the Achilles tendon before passing distally over the tuber calcaneus, to which it has medial and lateral retinacular attachments.

23.2 The ligaments of the canine tarsus.

The proximal intertarsal joint

The proximal intertarsal joint comprises the calcaneoquartal and talocalcaneocentral articulations. The joint is supported on the plantar aspect by ligaments spanning the joint from the calcaneus to the fourth and central tarsal bones before passing distally to contribute to the plantar tarsal fibrocartilage. Mediolateral support is provided by the long components of the collateral ligaments. There are also dorsal intertarsal ligaments, but these are of little clinical significance.

The centrodistal/distal intertarsal joint

This is the articulation between the central tarsal bone and tarsal bones I to III. It is spanned laterally by tarsal bone IV, which helps to protect it from injury.

The tarsometatarsal joint

This joint consists of the articulations between the distal tarsal bones and the metatarsals. It is supported by distal extensions of the collateral and plantar ligaments and the plantar fibrocartilage.

Examination of the tarsus

Signs of tarsal lameness

Small animal patients with tarsal lameness may show some or all of the following signs:

- Postural abnormality (Figure 23.3), e.g. hyperextension in osteochondritis dissecans (OCD) or hyperflexion following Achilles tendon injury or intertarsal subluxation
- Periarticular swelling, usually visible upon inspection
- Altered range of motion, e.g. reduction in flexion of the talocrural joint in OCD
- Joint instability, e.g. hyperextension of the proximal intertarsal joint
- Pain upon palpation.

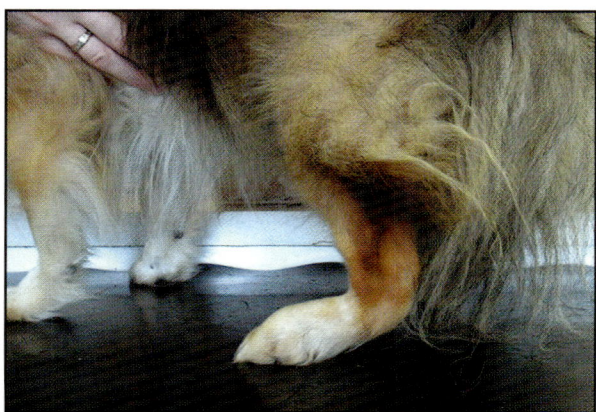

23.3 Hyperextension of the proximal intertarsal joint in a Shetland Sheepdog. Note the abnormal dropped posture of the hock, the mid-tarsal angulation and the absence of a visible calcaneus projecting caudally.

Physical examination of the tarsus

Physical examination of the tarsus is facilitated by a lack of bulky soft tissues surrounding the joint. Physical examination should include assessment of the following features.

- Palpation for talocrural joint swelling. This can be appreciated by palpation for the talar ridges during flexion (plantar limits of the talar ridges) and extension (dorsal limits). The plantar medial talar ridge, especially, is normally palpable and, if not, it is likely that there is abnormal swelling (Figure 23.4). More generalized tarsal swelling can usually be detected by palpation for anatomical landmarks and comparison with the contralateral limb, unless there is bilateral disease.
- Palpation of the Achilles tendon. This should normally be well defined and should be taut during weightbearing (Figure 23.5). Abnormal thickening and pain upon palpation may indicate Achilles tendinopathy. Lack of tension upon weightbearing or forced flexion against an extended stifle may indicate Achilles tendon rupture or avulsion.
- Examination for joint instability. This should include mediolateral angulation of the talocrural and tarsometatarsal joints and dorsoplantar angulation of the proximal intertarsal and tarsometatarsal joints especially.
- Examination for pain. Pain in tarsal lameness may be elicited by forced flexion (e.g. OCD), during examination for joint instability, or by direct palpation (e.g. tarsal bone fractures). Intertarsal rotation may elicit pain in cases of centrodistal lameness (Guilliard, 2005).

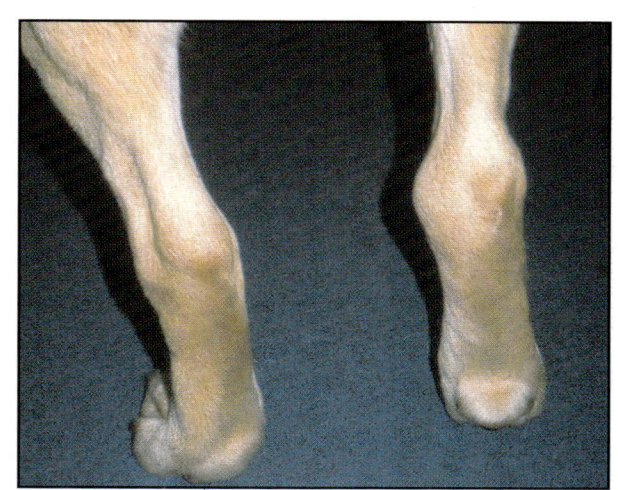

23.4 Swelling of the caudomedial aspect of the right talocrural joint in OCD of the medial ridge of the talus.

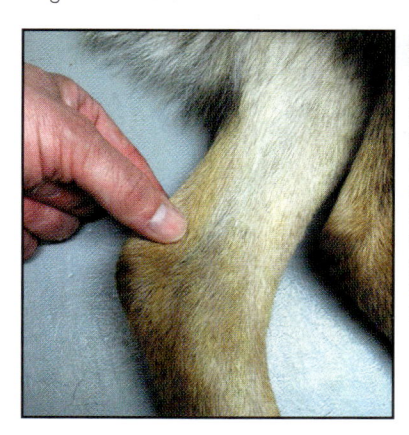

23.5 Palpation of the distal Achilles tendon. The tendon should be examined for thickness, tautness and any pain on palpation. This is best done during weightbearing.

Chapter 23 The tarsus

> **PRACTICAL TIP**
> The lame and sound limbs should always be compared during the physical examination, although it must be borne in mind that some conditions (e.g. OCD) are commonly bilateral.

Ancillary aids to diagnosis

Radiography
The osseous anatomy of the tarsus is complex and it is important that the viewer is familiar with the normal appearance, or has access to textbooks of radiology or to anatomical specimens. Radiography of the tarsus should include, as a minimum, mediolateral and extended dorsoplantar (or plantarodorsal) projections (Figure 23.6). It is occasionally helpful to take oblique views or flexed dorsoplantar (Figure 23.7) views as well. Stressed radiographs can be helpful in documenting joint instability. Radiographic positioning is described in Chapter 2.

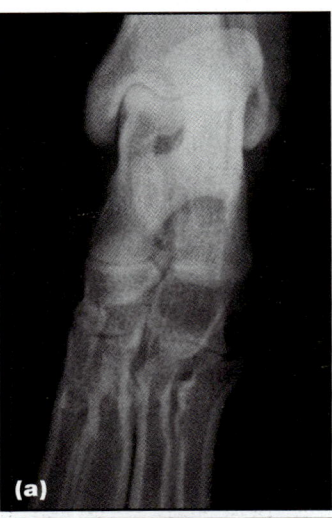

23.6 (a) Dorsoplantar radiograph of the normal canine tarsus. Note the uniformly narrow talocrural joint space and the superimposition of the calcaneus over the lateral talocrural joint space. (b) Lateral radiograph of the normal canine tarsus. Note the limits of the calcaneoquartal joint (arrowed).

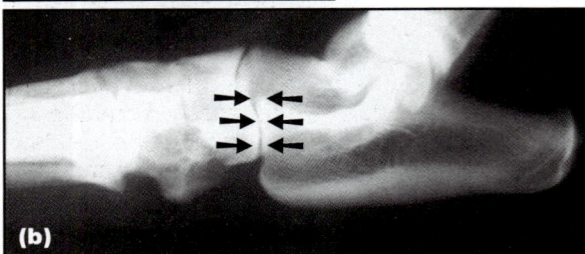

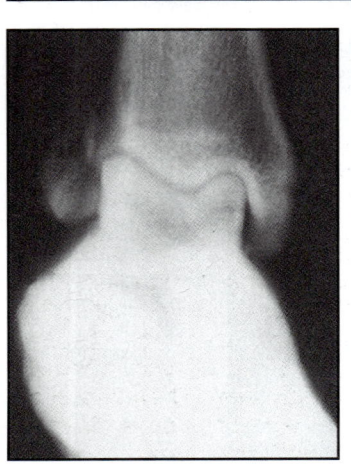

23.7 Flexed dorsoplantar radiograph of the normal canine tarsus. Note the increased visibility of the lateral aspect of the talocrural joint space.

Synovial fluid analysis
This can be very helpful, particularly in the diagnosis of inflammatory joint disease. Sampling technique is described in Chapter 3.

Arthroscopy and computed tomography scanning
These techniques are becoming increasingly available.

Surgical approaches

A number of surgical approaches to the talocrural joint have been described. Exposure is limited by interdigitation of the trochlear joint and collateral ligamentous stability. Maximum exposure is offered by medial malleolar osteotomy (Sinibaldi, 1979) (see Operative Technique 23.1) or collateral desmotomy. However, such techniques have been associated with complications such as prolonged morbidity, failure of orthopaedic implants, joint instability, inaccurate articular reconstruction, iatrogenic cartilage trauma and subsequent osteoarthritis (Smith and Vasseur, 1985; Beale et al., 1991). Approaches that do not involve an osteotomy or desmotomy are preferred, but access is limited (Beale and Goring, 1990; Goring and Beale, 1990) and accurate localization of lesions is essential before surgery is undertaken.

OCD of the medial or lateral trochlear ridges of the talus is the most common indication for talocrural arthrotomy. Plantaromedial (see Operative Technique 23.2), dorsomedial, plantarolateral and dorsolateral approaches which conserve the collateral ligaments have been described in detail (Beale and Goring, 1990; Goring and Beale, 1990). Dorsal and plantar approaches may be combined via a single incision. Conservation of the collateral ligaments reduces postoperative morbidity, and while exposure of the trochlear ridges, particularly the medial ridge, is limited, these approaches are usually adequate for recovery of osteochondral fragments. Tenosyntharthrotomy of the lateral head of the deep digital flexor tendon to give improved plantar access has also been described (Dew and Martin, 1993). Surgical approaches to the bones and other joints of the tarsus are simple and direct as there is little intervening soft tissue. Tendinous and neurovascular structures are retracted as appropriate.

Arthroscopy of the tarsus

This is described in detail in Operative Technique 23.3.

Indications
The tarsal joint is difficult to treat arthroscopically, even for the experienced surgeon. For this reason, the surgeon must be prepared to convert the arthroscopic procedure into an open arthrotomy. Early arthroscopic intervention is recommended because imaging becomes more difficult as joint capsule fibrosis and synovial proliferation advance with articular disease. Although used sparingly, arthroscopy of the tarsus is likely to become more common as future applications, expertise and experience are gained. Currently the indications for arthroscopy of the tarsus include:

- Diagnosis and treatment of OCD of the medial ridge of the talus
- Diagnosis and treatment of OCD of the lateral ridge of the talus
- Synovial biopsy
- Treatment of infective arthritis.

The tarsus should be divided into four quadrants for evaluation: dorsomedial, dorsolateral, plantaromedial, and plantarolateral. Once a lesion is localized to a specific region of the tarsus, the surgical approach or arthroscopic portal that gives best access to the area of interest can be selected. If the dorsal aspect of the joint is to be approached, the dog is positioned in dorsal recumbency with the pelvic limbs extended. If the plantar aspect of the joint is to be approached, the patient can be best assessed in sternal recumbency, again with the pelvic limbs extended.

The talocrural joint is the only site where arthroscopy is possible within the tarsus (Figure 23.8). When evaluating the tarsus arthroscopically, it is often useful to utilize multiple portals to allow thorough examination of the joint. Hyperflexion and hyperextension may improve inspection of the articular surfaces, by separating the joint surfaces and increasing the amount of articular surface visible from each portal.

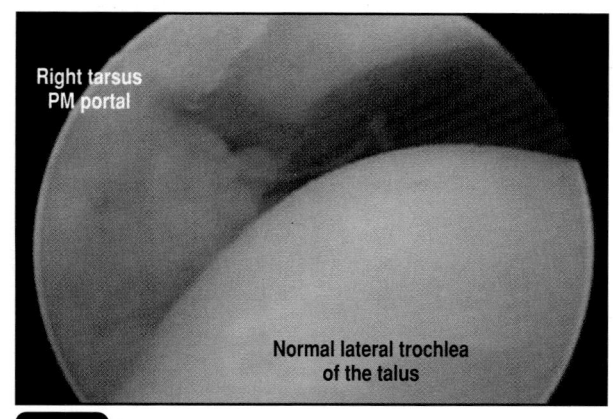

23.8 Arthroscopic view of the normal tarsal joint.

When viewing the dorsal aspect of the talocrural joint, the tarsus should be positioned in extension. While maintaining the position of the camera head, the light post is rotated to the side to view other regions of the trochlear ridges, the trochlear sulcus, synovial membrane and collateral ligaments. The articulation of the tibia, fibula and talus is also visible. As the light post is rotated to the 6 o'clock (distal) position, the articular surface of the distal tibia can be seen.

When viewing the plantar aspect of the tibiotarsal joint, the tarsus should be positioned in flexion. While maintaining the position of the camera head, the light post is rotated to the side to view other regions of the trochlear ridges, trochlear sulcus, flexor hallucis longus tendon, synovial membrane and collateral ligaments. The articulation of the tibia, fibula and talus is also visible. As the light post is rotated to the 6 o'clock (distal) position, the articular surface of the distal tibia can be seen. The medial and lateral collateral ligaments are also visible.

Portal location

The number of portal sites varies, depending on the objective of the procedure. If joint exploration is the goal of the surgery, an arthroscope portal and egress portal are all that are required. If tissue biopsy or treatment is required, the egress portal is converted to an instrument portal. Ancillary instrument portal sites can be triangulated to a region as needed. The most commonly used portal sites are plantarolateral and plantaromedial; however, dorsal sites are also used if lesion access is better achieved by this route. The arthroscope portal is located medially if the lateral aspect of the joint is to be viewed and laterally if the medial aspect of the joint is to be viewed. The surgeon should be familiar with all of the arthroscopic portals of the tarsus because complete inspection and access to the joint may require use of multiple portals. The surgeon should not hesitate to change to a new portal if the field of view is inadequate or if the scope is difficult to maintain in an intra-articular position.

Dorsomedial portal

The dorsomedial arthroscope portal is commonly used to assess the dorsolateral joint compartment, the dorsal aspect of the lateral trochlear ridge and the trochlea of the talus. The dorsal aspect of the medial trochlear ridge can also be evaluated, but inadvertent dislodgement of the arthroscope tip is more likely. The arthroscope cannula and blunt obturator are introduced medial to the extensor tendons just over the palpable medial trochlear ridge, cranial to the medial malleolus. The cannula is directed laterally, below the extensor tendons, directing the tip into the dorsolateral compartment.

Dorsolateral portal

The dorsolateral 'scope portal is commonly used to assess the dorsomedial joint compartment, the dorsal aspect of the medial trochlear ridge and the trochlea of the talus. The dorsal aspect of the lateral trochlear ridge can also be evaluated, but inadvertent dislodgement of the arthroscope tip is more likely. The arthroscope cannula and blunt obturator are introduced lateral to the extensor tendons just over the palpable lateral trochlear ridge, cranial to the lateral malleolus. The cannula is directed medially, below the extensor tendons, directing the tip into the dorsomedial compartment.

Plantaromedial portal

The plantaromedial 'scope portal is commonly used to assess the plantarolateral joint compartment, the plantar aspect of the lateral trochlear ridge and the trochlea of the talus. The arthroscope cannula and blunt obturator are introduced medial to the flexor tendons just over the palpable medial trochlear ridge, caudal to the medial malleolus. The plantar aspect of the medial trochlear ridge can also be evaluated, but inadvertent dislodgement of the arthroscope tip is more likely. This portal is used to view lesions associated with OCD, especially if an adequate view cannot be obtained using a plantarolateral portal due to synovial hyperplasia and loss of range of joint motion. The arthroscope is directed laterally, below the flexor tendons, directing the tip into the plantarolateral compartment.

Chapter 23 The tarsus

Plantarolateral portal
The plantarolateral 'scope portal is commonly used to assess the plantaromedial joint compartment, the plantar aspect of the medial trochlear ridge and the trochlea of the talus (Figure 23.9). The plantar aspect of the lateral trochlear ridge can also be evaluated, but inadvertent dislodgement of the arthroscope tip is more likely. The arthroscope cannula and blunt obturator are introduced lateral to the flexor tendons just over the palpable lateral trochlear ridge, caudal to the lateral malleolus. The 'scope is directed medially, below the flexor tendons, directing the tip into the plantaromedial compartment.

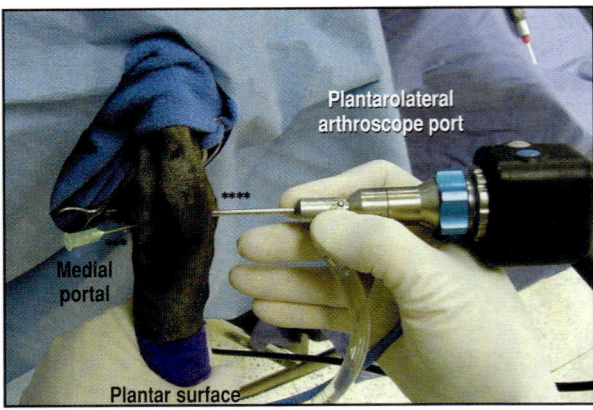

23.9 Positioning of the plantarolateral portal for arthroscopy of the tarsus.

Congenital conditions of the tarsus

Congenital anomaly of the central tarsal bone
A congenital anomaly of the central tarsal bone is not uncommon, especially in large and giant breeds of dog. This consists of medial osseous 'spurs' of variable size that project beyond the proximal and distal extremities of the bone. This anomaly is usually an incidental radiographic finding and does not appear to be associated with lameness (Figure 23.10).

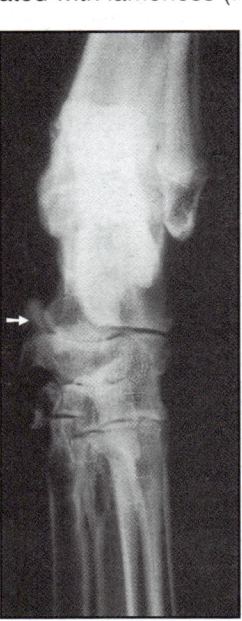

23.10 Dorsoplantar radiograph of a Newfoundland with congenital medial 'spur' formation affecting the central tarsal bone (arrowed). There is also marked rotation of the tarsus and metatarsus in relation to the distal tibia and fibula. There was no lameness related to these abnormalities.

Torsion of the tarsus
Many large and giant breeds of dog also have abnormal external rotation of the limb distal to the tarsus. This rotation appears to originate within the tarsal region and can result in significant external rotation of the foot. Again, lameness does not appear to be associated with this abnormality.

Hyperextension of the tarsus
The tarsus is occasionally seen to 'pop' forwards into over-extension, usually at rest. Larger breeds of dog are more commonly affected. This does not appear to be a cause of lameness in its own right but it can be associated with more significant abnormalities more proximally, e.g. hip dysplasia and cranial cruciate ligament problems.

Angular deformity of the distal tibia/fibula
Angular deformities of the distal crus occur far less commonly than in the distal antebrachium and are usually apparently spontaneous, presumably related to asynchronous premature closure of the distal growth plates. Lateral angulation (pes valgus) may be seen in Collies, Shetland Sheepdogs (McCarthy, 1998) and large breeds (Figure 23.11) and medial angulation (pes varus) has been described in Dachshunds (Johnson et al., 1989). Diagnosis should be straightforward upon inspection and easy to confirm radiographically. Treatment is by corrective osteotomy if the degree of angulation is severe enough to cause lameness.

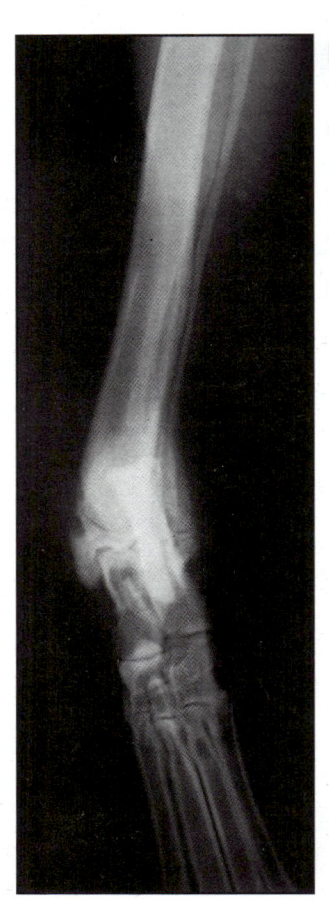

23.11 Valgus deviation of the tarsus and foot (pes valgus) in a juvenile Newfoundland. This deviation was causing lameness and was corrected by a medially based closing wedge osteotomy. The opposite limb was less severely affected.

Chapter 23 The tarsus

Developmental conditions of the tarsus

Osteochondritis dissecans of the medial ridge of the talus

OCD of the tarsus most commonly involves the caudomedial ridge of the talus, with Labrador Retrievers, Rottweilers and Bull Terriers most commonly affected. Most dogs are presented at 5–9 months of age, although later presentation can occur. Physical signs may be bilateral, which can complicate diagnosis. Affected animals tend to have a hyperextended tarsal posture and careful inspection or palpation will reveal swelling of the caudomedial talocrural joint. Flexion is significantly restricted compared to normal and, if forced, causes pain.

> **PRACTICAL TIP**
> A key clinical feature is that the caudal medial ridge of the talus cannot be palpated readily on flexion of the joint.

A diagnosis of OCD of the medial ridge of the talus can usually be confirmed radiographically. On a mediolateral view, flattening of the trochlear ridge can be seen and there will often be marginal osteophyte formation at the caudal aspect of the distal tibia, as secondary osteoarthritis tends to develop early and progress rapidly (Figure 23.12a). A mineralized fragment may be seen caudal to the talus if the OCD lesion has detached. On the plantarodorsal view, there is flattening of the medial trochlear ridge, with an increased medial talocrural joint space (Figure 23.12b). A mineralized fragment may be seen proximal to the trochlear ridge and there will usually be osteophyte formation along the medial aspect of the talus. The diagnosis can be confirmed by arthroscopy (Figure 23.13).

Most affected dogs under 10–12 months of age appear to benefit from surgical removal of the OCD lesion via a plantaromedial arthrotomy or arthroscopy. Surgery is less helpful in older dogs. Bilateral surgeries can be done simultaneously.

The majority of tarsal OCD lesions are located at the plantaromedial aspect of the trochlea and the location of the lesion should guide the surgeon's approach. For example, the most common arthroscopic portal is the plantarolateral position.

A soft support bandage is applied for 4–5 days postoperatively and exercise is restricted to short walks on a lead only for 4 weeks, with a phased increase in the lengths of walks after that period.

Most owners feel that their pet's comfort, exercise tolerance and quality of life are improved by surgery. The hyperextended joint posture and periarticular thick-

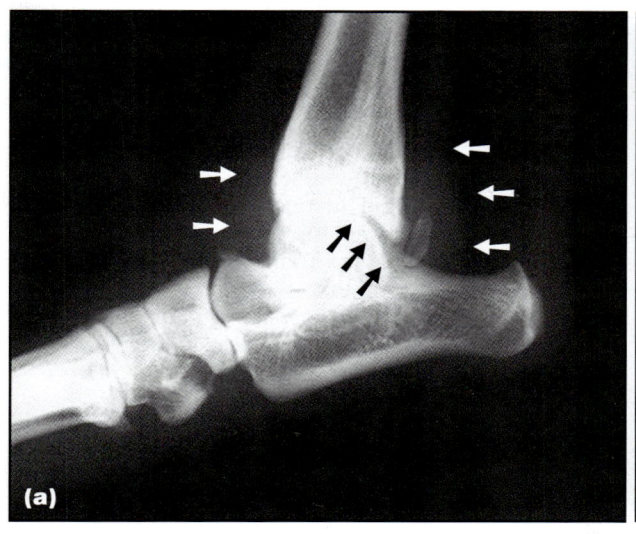

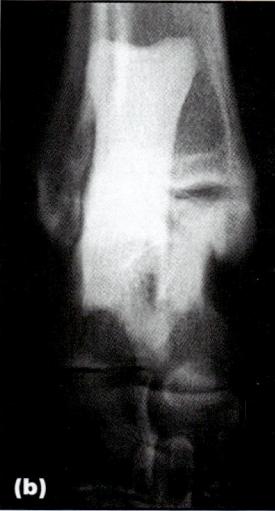

23.12 **(a)** Mediolateral radiograph of OCD of the hock. There is periarticular soft tissue swelling (white arrows) and the talocrural joint space is widened caudally. Flattening of the trochlear ridge is evident (black arrows) and the caudal edge of the distal tibia appears extended by marginal osteophyte formation. There is a free mineralized body (the OCD lesion) caudal to the trochlear ridge. **(b)** Plantarodorsal radiograph of OCD of the medial trochlear ridge. The medial joint space is abnormally widened (compare to Figure 23.6a).

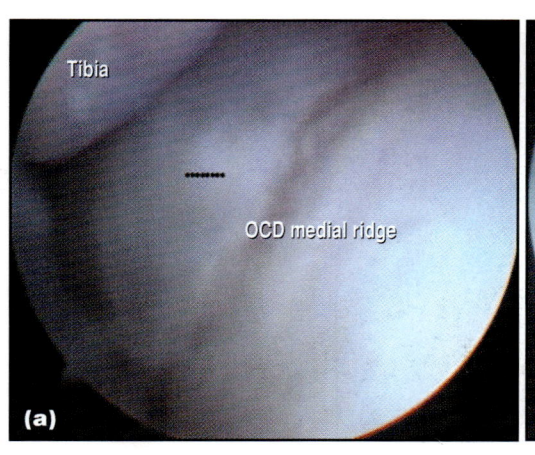

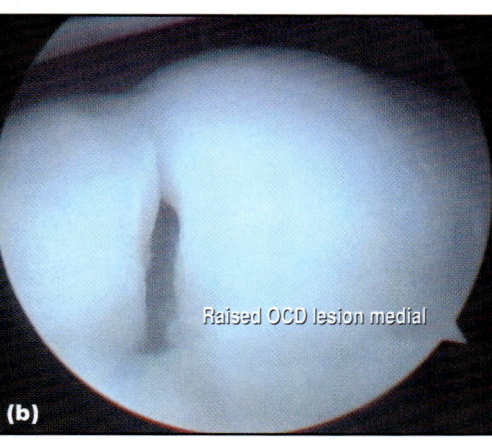

23.13 Arthroscopic diagnosis of OCD of the tarsus. **(a)** OCD of the medial ridge of the talus. **(b)** Raised OCD lesion of the medial ridge of the talus.

Chapter 23 The tarsus

ening may persist and osteoarthritis progresses despite surgery. Some dogs may remain lame despite removal of the OCD lesion, or lameness may recur in the future. If lameness cannot be controlled by conservative means, pantarsal arthrodesis is available as a salvage procedure.

Osteochondritis dissecans of the lateral ridge of the talus

OCD occasionally affects the lateral trochlear ridge of the talus (Robins *et al.*, 1983). Physical signs are similar to lesions of the medial ridge, although periarticular swelling is more evident laterally. The lesion may be located caudally or more cranially on the trochlear ridge. The radiographic signs are the same as in medial ridge lesions, although diagnosis is more difficult due to superimposition of the calcaneus and lateral trochlear ridge on the plantarodorsal projection. Oblique views or a flexed dorsoplantar view may be more helpful.

Treatment options are similar to those for medial ridge OCD, although a craniolateral surgical approach can be advantageous for treatment of more cranially positioned lesions.

Acquired conditions of the tarsus

Fractures

Fractures involving the tarsus are covered in detail within the *BSAVA Manual of Small Animal Fracture Repair and Management*. Most commonly, they involve the calcaneus, the talus, the central tarsal and the numbered tarsal bones. They are generally closed, comminuted and due to indirect trauma. They are generally seen in working dogs, although calcaneal fractures can also occur in the pet animal.

Collateral ligament injury

Injuries to the tarsal collateral ligaments are usually associated with acute trauma, either closed (e.g. a fall or twisting injury) or in association with open or shearing injuries (e.g. road traffic accident). Diagnosis is easy in shearing injuries and can usually be made by palpation or by the use of stress radiography in closed injuries. Radiography is also helpful in identifying avulsion fractures of ligamentous attachment points.

Talocrural collateral ligament injury

Most cases of talocrural collateral ligament injury involve complete injury to the medial and/or lateral collateral ligament complex, although injury to the short component of the lateral collateral has been described as a cause of lameness (Sjöstrom and Hakanson, 1994).

Shearing injuries can affect the medial or lateral aspect of the joint. In addition to loss of collateral support there will be loss of varying amounts of bone and overlying soft tissues. These injuries are best managed initially using transarticular external skeletal fixation and appropriate open wound management. Soft tissue defects can be allowed to heal by secondary intention or treated by delayed primary closure or skin grafting techniques. Where there is loss of collateral ligaments, their replacement using ligament prostheses is advisable to restore joint stability, although sufficient joint stability can return following healing of the soft tissues in some small and medium-sized dogs. If there has been significant loss of bone beyond the axial margin of the malleolus, or joint stability cannot be restored, pantarsal arthrodesis (see Operative Technique 23.6) should be considered from the outset.

Malleolar avulsion fractures are best treated by open reduction and internal fixation using pin(s) and a tension band wire.

When planning prosthetic replacement of the talocrural collateral ligaments, it is essential to mimic as closely as possible the normal anatomy so that the joint can be stabilized throughout its full range of movement (Aron and Purinton, 1985). Two prosthetic ligaments need to be inserted, with a single anchor point proximally but two distinct points distally (Figure 23.14). The proximal anchor point is usually a bone

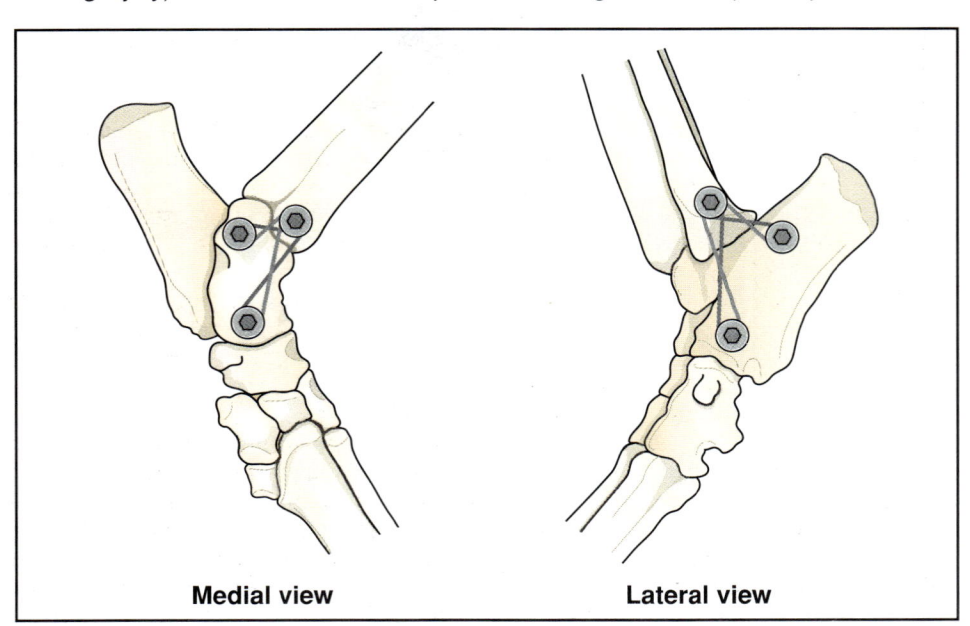

23.14 Positioning of anchorage points for prosthetic talocrural collateral ligaments.

Medial view   Lateral view

402

screw with a washer; the distal anchor points may also be small screws with washers, although the insertion of the short component of the medial collateral is on the abaxial aspect of the medial trochlear ridge of the talus. A protruding screw head at this point may impinge on the medial malleolus when the joint extends. A suture anchor (see Chapter 14) recessed beneath the bone surface is probably more appropriate in this location.

> **PRACTICAL TIP**
> Consider the use of suture anchors for prosthetic ligament replacement: this avoids interference with joint motion and facilitates wound closure.

Depending upon the size of the patient, braided non-absorbable material or monofilament nylon leader line are suitable materials for the ligament prosthesis. Leader line tends to result in a bulkier knot. The long component should be tightened with the joint extended and the short component with the joint flexed to recreate the correct combination of joint stability without interfering with normal mobility.

> **PRACTICAL TIP**
> In cats, imbrication of the local soft tissues (if present) or periarticular fibrosis associated with open wound healing in shearing injuries usually seems to provide sufficient stability without the need for prosthetic ligaments.

Following surgery the tarsus should be supported in a splint or cast for 6–8 weeks, followed by a further 4–6 weeks of restricted exercise. Most dogs seem to have a favourable result, although some degree of joint stiffness, lameness or osteoarthritis may result.

Intertarsal and tarsometatarsal collateral ligament injury

Loss of collateral support at the intertarsal or tarsometatarsal joints can be seen in isolation or as part of a more complex soft tissue injury. In either event, intertarsal or tarsometatarsal arthrodesis usually represents the best treatment. This is typically best performed using a plate and screws located medially or laterally (Dyce *et al.*, 1998), depending upon the joint involved and the location of the major soft tissue injury. Standard compression plates, hybrid 3.5/2.7 mm or 2.7/2.0 mm pancarpal arthrodesis plates or sections of cuttable plate can be used, depending upon patient size (Figure 23.15). Alternatively, in cats, fine pins may be introduced into the distal metatarsal bones via dorsal cortical slots and driven across the tarsometatarsal joint into the tarsal bones.

Whatever technique is used, standard principles of arthrodesis, i.e. removal of articular cartilage, insertion of a cancellous bone graft and additional external support following surgery, should always be adhered to. Intertarsal and tarsometatarsal fusions usually provide good results.

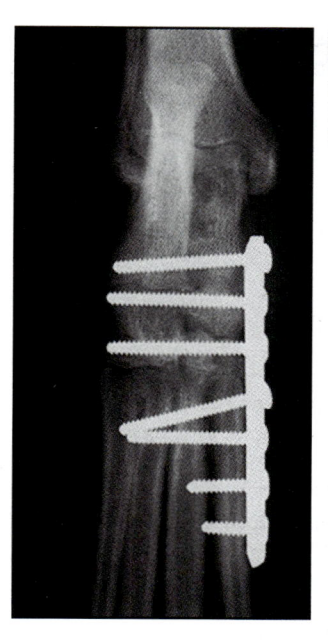

23.15 Tarsometatarsal arthrodesis using a section of 2.7/2.0 mm veterinary cuttable plate applied medially.

Plantar ligament degeneration

Idiopathic degeneration of the plantar supporting structures of the calcaneoquartal or proximal intertarsal joint is seen commonly, notably in middle-aged Shetland Sheepdogs. Affected individuals are typically overweight and usually have a sedentary lifestyle. Progressive ligament degeneration allows hyperextension of the proximal intertarsal joint, causing a plantigrade posture and lameness. Such changes may be bilateral; if not, soft tissue swelling can often be detected on the plantar surface of the contralateral proximal intertarsal joint and this frequently indicates incipient plantar ligament degeneration.

Affected dogs may be lame if there is unilateral hyperextension or exercise intolerant if bilateral. The affected tarsus (tarsi) will be dropped and the calcaneus will be rotated proximally by the Achilles tendon. There is usually palpable instability (hyperextension) of the proximal intertarsal joint but manipulation appears to cause little discomfort.

A mediolateral radiograph of the affected tarsus (tarsi) will confirm the diagnosis, although stressed films, with hyperextension of the proximal intertarsal joint, will facilitate this (Figure 23.16). Periarticular new bone formation/enthesopathy, indicating chronic pathology, is usually seen on the plantar aspect of the distal calcaneus, and this can also be seen as a sign of impending plantar ligament failure in the contralateral limb (Figure 23.17).

Any type of dog can also suffer traumatic injury to the plantar ligamentous support, usually with obvious local swelling and visible or palpable instability.

The treatment in either case is arthrodesis of the calcaneoquartal joint (Allen *et al.*, 1993). Several techniques have been described to achieve this and the most popular are a pin and plantar wire loop, a lag screw (± plantar wire loop) or a compression plate applied laterally) (see Operative Technique 23.4). In each case articular cartilage should be completely removed from the joint surfaces, a cancellous bone graft should be used and external support should be

Chapter 23 The tarsus

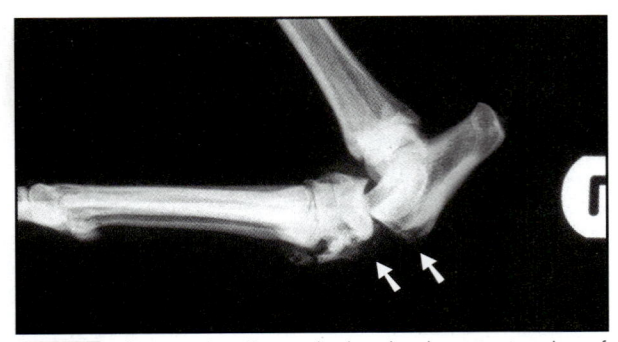

23.16 Stressed radiograph showing hyperextension of the proximal intertarsal joint due to plantar ligament degeneration in a Shetland Sheepdog. There is enthesophyte formation on the plantar aspect of the calcaneoquartal joint (arrows) and new bone formation dorsal to the centrodistal joint.

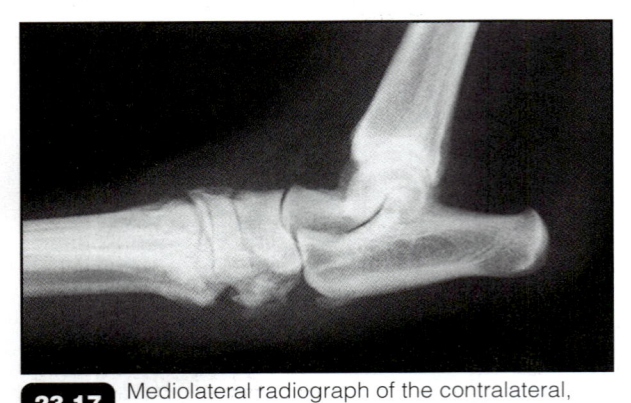

23.17 Mediolateral radiograph of the contralateral, apparently normal limb in a dog with subluxation of the proximal intertarsal joint. There is periarticular soft tissue swelling and plantar enthesophyte formation adjacent to the calcaneoquartal joint. These changes signify ongoing degenerative changes that may lead to failure of plantar ligament support.

applied for 6–8 weeks, or until signs of osseous fusion are visible radiographically. In bilateral cases, surgeries should be staged if possible, with an interval of 4–6 weeks between operations.

If a successful arthrodesis can be achieved, the vast majority of dogs will return to a good level of function. The most common complication is failure to achieve arthrodesis and subsequent fixation failure, especially in dogs affected bilaterally. Prolonged external support prior to surgery seems to be associated with a greater risk of postoperative complications, so surgery should normally be undertaken as soon as possible after diagnosis.

Dorsal ligament rupture

Rupture of dorsal intertarsal ligaments occurs sporadically, usually following traumatic hyperflexion of the involved intertarsal or tarsometatarsal joint. Instability can be detected by palpation and stressed radiography.

Isolated dorsal ligament rupture can be managed non-surgically, by external support for 4–6 weeks, as weightbearing automatically holds the affected joint in reduction. If there is gross instability, imbricating the ruptured dorsal soft tissues using polydioxanone can be helpful. Arthrodesis should be required only in extremely unstable joints.

Achilles tendon injuries

Injury to the Achilles mechanism encompasses complete ruptures, partial ruptures and avulsion/enthesopathy of the insertion on the calcaneus. Injury can be due to acute trauma, sometimes with a penetrating wound, or be more chronic in nature. Achilles tendon injuries have been classified into three main types by Meustege (1993). Physical signs vary depending upon the severity of injury and may be bilateral in chronic cases.

- Complete ruptures result in a plantigrade tarsal posture or severely dropped tarsus (Figure 23.18). The tarsus can be manually hyperflexed if the stifle is fixed in extension and there may be a palpable defect in the substance of the tendon in acute rupture. There may be no palpable defect in long-standing injuries.
- Partial ruptures (e.g. injury to the gastrocnemius tendon in isolation) may result in a partially dropped tarsus with hyperflexion ('clenching') of the digits on weightbearing or manual flexion of the tarsus (Figure 23.19). The appearance of the digits is due to the superficial digital flexor tendon remaining intact and being tensioned as the tarsus hyperflexes. This appearance is particularly common in middle-aged Dobermanns affected by gastrocnemius enthesopathy (Bonneau et al., 1982; Butterworth, 1995). In these cases there is also palpable swelling of the tendon insertion on the calcaneus and pain upon digital pressure.
- So-called tendinosis/peritendinitis may cause palpable thickening of the Achilles mechanism without any alteration in joint posture.

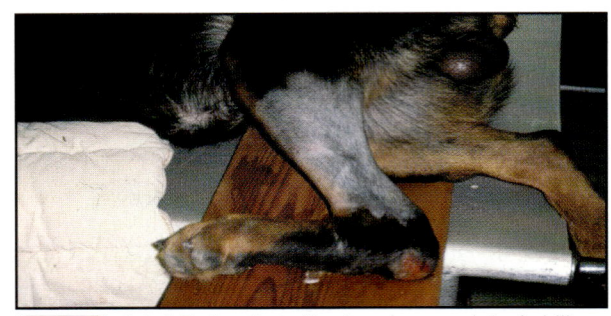

23.18 Adult Rottweiler with chronic complete Achilles tendon rupture. There is a pressure sore on the plantar aspect of the calcaneus and thickening of the distal Achilles tendon. The hock is hyperflexed.

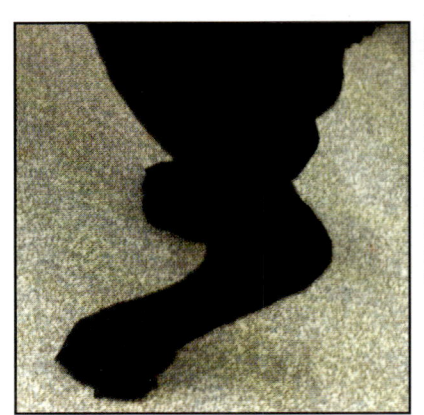

23.19 Gastrocnemius avulsion in a Labrador. Note the partially 'dropped' hock posture with hyperflexion ('clenching') of the digits.

Radiography (mediolateral view) will reveal soft tissue swelling. Cases of chronic gastrocnemius avulsion/enthesopathy may show small islands of mineralization proximal to the insertion of the tendon and new bone formation ('capping') around the free end of the calcaneus (Figure 23.20).

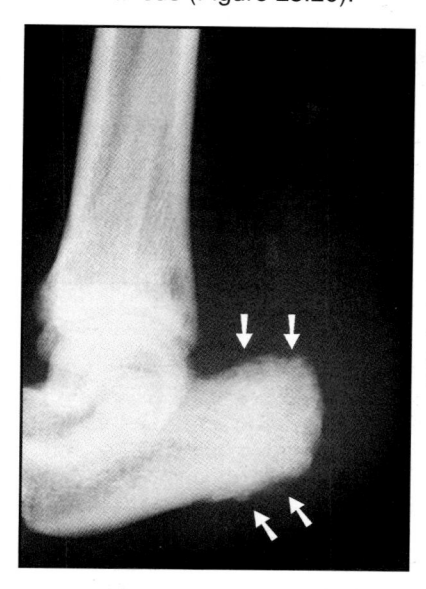

23.20 Mediolateral radiograph of gastrocnemius avulsion. Note the small areas of mineralization proximal to the calcaneus and the 'capping' of the tip of the calcaneus by new bone formation (arrows).

Treatment of Achilles tendon ruptures may be conservative or surgical, depending upon presentation. Dogs with normal joint and digital posture and mild lameness may be suitable for non-surgical management. Restriction to leash exercise for 6–8 weeks and use of non-steroidal anti-inflammatory drugs, if required, may allow resolution of lameness. If not, or if progressive postural changes develop, surgery is indicated (see Operative Technique 23.5).

As a salvage procedure, pantarsal arthrodesis is possible (see Operative Technique 23.6).

Superficial digital flexor tendon luxation

Lateral luxation of the superficial digital flexor tendon from the calcaneus as a result of rupture of its medial retinacular attachment occurs sporadically in Shetland Sheepdogs and racing Greyhounds (Vaughan, 1987). The luxation can be palpated as a slipping of the tendon on and off its normal location in acute cases, although it may become more fixed laterally in time, in which case there will only be local swelling.

Surgical repair of the torn retinaculum via a plantaromedial incision is best. The torn or stretched retinaculum is sutured directly or overlapped using polydioxanone mattress sutures. In chronic cases, or if primary repair fails, revision surgery using polypropylene mesh to reinforce the repair has been described (Houlton and Dyce, 1993).

References and further reading

Allen MJ, Dyce J and Houlton JEF (1993) Calcaneoquartal arthrodesis in the dog. *Journal of Small Animal Practice* **34**, 205–210
Aron DA and Purinton PT (1985) Replacement of the collateral ligaments of the canine tarsocrural joint – a proposed technique. *Veterinary Surgery* **14**, 178–184
Beale BS and Goring RL (1990) Exposure of the medial and lateral trochlear ridges of the talus in the dog. Part I. Dorsomedial and plantaromedial surgical approaches to the medial trochlear ridge. *Journal of the American Animal Hospital Association* **26**, 13–18
Beale BS, Goring RL *et al.* (1991) A prospective evaluation of four surgical aproaches to the talus of the dog used in the treatment of osteochondritis dissecans. *Journal of the American Animal Hospital Association* **27**, 221–229
Bonneau NH, Olivieri M and Breton L (1982) Avulsion of the gastrocnemius tendon in the dog causing flexion of the hock and digits. *Journal of the American Animal Hospital Association* **19**, 717–722
Braden TD (1976) Fascia lata transplant for repair of chronic Achilles tendon defects. *Journal of the American Animal Hospital Association* **12**, 800–805
Butterworth SJ (1995) Gastrocnemius enthesiopathy. *Veterinary Practice* **1**, 8
Dew TL and Martin RA (1993) A caudal approach to the tibiotarsal joint. *Journal of the American Animal Hospital Association* **29**, 117–121
Dyce J, Whitelock RG, Robinson KV, Forsythe F and Houlton JEF (1998) Arthrodesis of the tarsometatarsal joint using a laterally applied plate in 10 dogs. *Journal of Small Animal Practice* **39**, 19–22
Goring RL and Beale BS (1990) Exposure of the medial and lateral trochlear ridges of the talus in the dog. Part II. Dorsolateral and plantarolateral surgical approaches to the lateral trochlear ridge. *Journal of the American Animal Hospital Association* **26**, 19–24
Guilliard MJ (2005) Centrodistal joint lameness in dogs. *Journal of Small Animal Practice* **46**, 199–202
Houlton JEF and Dyce J (1993) The use of polypropylene mesh for revision of failed repair of superficial digital flexor tendon luxation on three dogs. *Veterinary and Comparative Orthopaedics and Traumatology* **6**, 129–130
Jenkins DHR, Forster IW, McKibbin B and Ralis ZA (1977) Induction of tendon and ligament formation by carbon implants. *Journal of Bone and Joint Surgery* **59B**, 53
Johnson SG, Hulse DA, Vangundy TE and Green RW (1989) Corrective osteotomy for pes varus in the dachshund. *Veterinary Surgery* **18**, 373–379
McCarthy PE (1998) Bilateral pes valgus deformity in a Shetland Sheepdog. *Veterinary and Comparative Orthopaedics and Traumatology* **11**, 197–199
Meustege FJ (1993) The classification of canine Achilles tendon lesions. *Veterinary and Comparative Orthopaedics and Traumatology* **6**, 53–55
Moores AP, Owen MR and Tarlton JF (2004) The three-loop pulley suture versus two locking-loop sutures for the repair of canine Achilles tendons. *Veterinary Surgery* **33**, 131–137
Robins GM, Read RA, Carlisle CH and Webb SM (1983) Osteochondritis dissecans of the lateral ridge of the trochlea of the tibial tarsal bone in the dog. *Journal of Small Animal Practice* **24**, 675–685
Sinibaldi KR (1979) Medial approach to the tarsus. *Journal of the American Animal Hospital Association* **15**, 77
Sjöstrom L and Hakanson N (1994) Traumatic injuries associated with the short lateral collateral ligaments of the talocrural joint of the dog. *Journal of Small Animal Practice* **35**, 163–168
Smith MM and Vasseur PB (1985) Clinical evaluation of dogs after surgical and non surgical management of osteochondritis dissecans of the talus. *Journal of the American Veterinary Medical Association*, **187**, 31–35
Vaughan LC (1987) Disorders of the tarsus in the dog parts 1 and 2. *British Veterinary Journal* **143**, 388–498

Chapter 23 The tarsus

OPERATIVE TECHNIQUE 23.1
Medial malleolar osteotomy and repair

WARNING
Osteotomy of the medial malleolus is not a low morbidity procedure and it should be avoided unless extensive exposure of the joint is necessary.

Positioning
Lateral recumbency on the affected side with the unaffected limb abducted and drawn cranially and the affected limb suspended to allow free limb draping.

Assistant
Not essential.

Tray extras
Powered sagittal or reciprocating saw, or osteotome and mallet if preferred; standard and small Gelpi self-retaining retractors; pointed reduction forceps; powered drill and range of arthrodesis pins; pin benders and cutters; orthopaedic wire and twisters.

Surgical approach
A medial skin incision is made over the malleolus extending proximally to the distal third of the tibia and distally to the level of the tarsometatarsal joint. The malleolus, collateral ligaments and caudal tendons (tibialis caudalis and deep digital flexor) are identified.

Surgical technique
The tendons are retracted caudally and the malleolus isolated by making small arthrotomies cranial and caudal to the collateral ligament complex (Figure 23.21). Holes slightly smaller than the fixation pins to be used in repair of the malleolar osteotomy can be drilled at this stage. The drill holes should be angled sufficiently proximally to avoid entering the joint; joint mobility should be checked with the drill bit in place as each hole is drilled to check this.

The osteotomy should be angled sufficiently to produce a large enough fragment for repair but not so angled that the cut violates the weightbearing articular surface of the distal tibia. The cut portion of the malleolus is retracted distally and the arthrotomy is extended transversely as far as necessary to complete the exposure.

The osteotomy is reduced using pointed reduction forceps and repaired using two pins inserted into the holes previously prepared. The pin ends are bent over to prevent migration and a tension band wire is secured around them and through a transverse bone tunnel drilled proximally in the tibia.

Alternative technique
The pins used to repair the osteotomy may be inserted directly through the malleolus at the time of repair rather than using pre-drilled tunnels if a small enough drill bit is not available. Arthrodesis pins are superior to Kirschner wires in this event, as they have a cutting trocar tip at each end.

PRACTICAL TIP
When drilling fine pins into bone it is important that only a short portion of the pin protrudes from the chuck, otherwise the pin will be too flexible. This may necessitate several pauses to adjust pin length while drilling.

→

OPERATIVE TECHNIQUE 23.1 *continued*
Medial malleolar osteotomy and repair

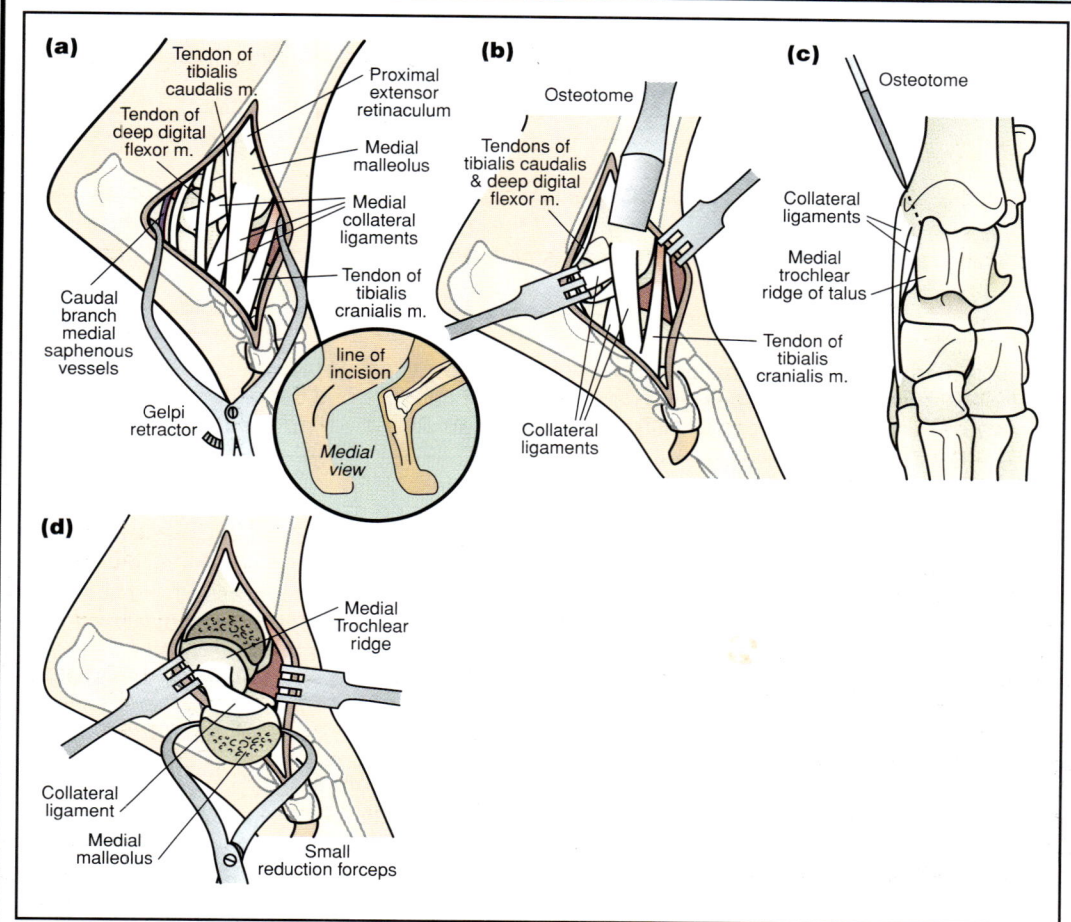

23.21 Medial talocrural arthrotomy by osteotomy of the medial malleolus. **(a)** Exposure of the medial aspect of the tarsus. **(b)** Retraction of caudal tendons prior to osteotomy. **(c)** Position of osteotomy. **(d)** Distal reflection of medial malleolus to expose the medial trochlear ridge.

Closure
The arthrotomy incisions are closed using a fine synthetic absorbable material of the surgeon's preference. The remainder of the closure is routine.

Postoperative care
A postoperative radiograph should be taken to assess reduction of the osteotomy and implant positioning. A padded support bandage should be applied for 2 weeks and activity restricted to short walks on a leash only for 4 weeks after that. Analgesia should be provided for as long as necessary. Follow-up radiographs should be taken after 6 weeks to assess healing of the osteotomy and check for any implant migration. Implants are not removed routinely.

Chapter 23 The tarsus

OPERATIVE TECHNIQUE 23.2
Medial arthrotomy for osteochondritis dissecans of the medial ridge of the talus

Positioning
Lateral recumbency on the affected side with the unaffected limb abducted and drawn cranially and the affected limb suspended to allow free limb draping.

Assistant
Not essential.

Tray extras
Small Gelpi self-retaining retractors; small grasping forceps; small spoon or OCD curette; electrocautery very helpful if available.

Surgical approach
A medial skin incision is made caudal to the malleolus extending proximally to the tibial metaphysis and distally to the level of the talocentral joint. The tendons lying caudally (tibialis caudalis and deep digital flexor) should be identified and retracted caudally. This can be difficult due to periarticular swelling in cases of OCD.

Surgical technique
A vertical arthrotomy is made between the collateral complex and retracted caudal tendons (Figure 23.22). Commonly this corresponds with the area of greatest swelling. The arthrotomy is opened using small Gelpi retractors and the medial ridge of the talus can be seen. The caudal end of an OCD lesion is usually easy to see but full flexion of the tarsus is necessary for a more cranial exposure. The OCD flap is grasped and removed. The edges of the defect are inspected and any remaining loose osteochondral fragments are removed by gentle curettage. More vigorous curettage should be avoided as this only increases what may already be substantial loss of the medial ridge of the talus and could contribute to joint instability. The joint should be lavaged using sterile lactated Ringer's solution or saline prior to closure.

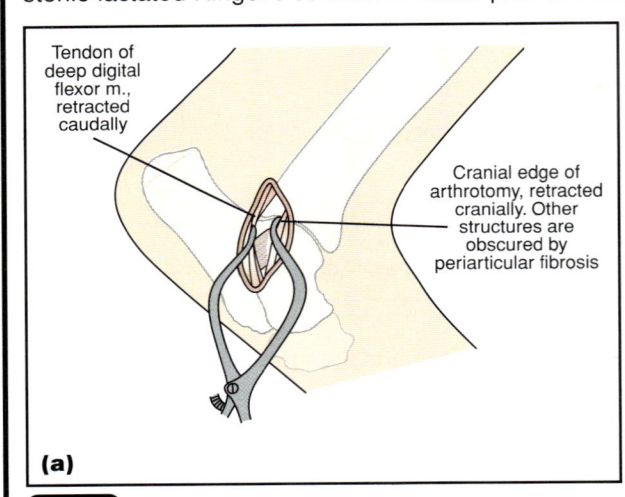

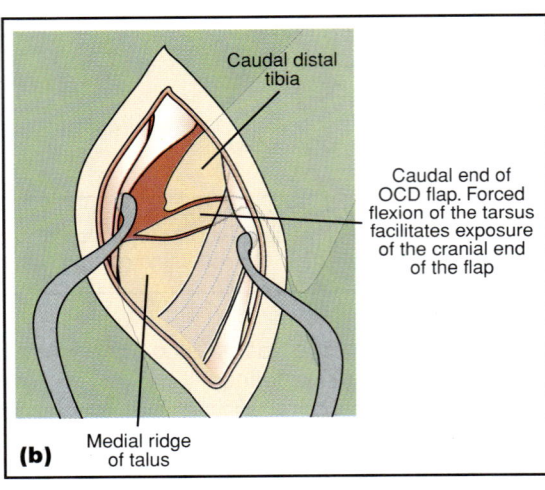

23.22 **(a)** Vertical arthrotomy between tendons. **(b)** Exposure of the medial ridge of the talus.

PRACTICAL TIP
Haemorrhage from periarticular tissues can reduce visibility, and electrocautery, if available, is very helpful. Full flexion of the tarsus is necessary for inspecting the cranial end of the lesion so a tourniquet cannot be used.

OPERATIVE TECHNIQUE 23.2 *continued*
Medial arthrotomy for osteochondritis dissecans of the medial ridge of the talus

Alternative technique
Attempts at reattaching large osteochondral fragments in OCD have been made. In that event, or in other situations where a more extensive exposure is required, osteotomy of the medial malleolus (see Operative Technique 23.1) is necessary.

Closure
The arthrotomy is closed using a fine synthetic absorbable material of the surgeon's preference. The remainder of the closure is routine.

Postoperative care
A padded bandage should be applied for 4 or 5 days and analgesics used for as long as necessary. Exercise is restricted to short (10–15 minute) bouts of lead walking for 4 weeks with a phased increase in the level of activity after that.

Chapter 23 The tarsus

OPERATIVE TECHNIQUE 23.3
Arthroscopy of the tarsus

Positioning
The imaging tower is positioned at the head of the patient or opposite the surgeon. The limb is prepared as for an open arthrotomy. Best results will be obtained through a hanging limb preparation. The dog is positioned in dorsal or ventral recumbency depending on the location of the arthroscope and instrument portals.

Assistant
Not necessary for diagnostic arthroscopy. Desirable for operative arthroscopy.

Tray extras
Arthroscopy tower with light source, camera unit, monitor; 1.9 or 2.4 mm 30 degree arthroscope with sleeve and blunt obturator (2.7 mm arthroscope in giant-breed dogs); two 25–37 mm (1–1.5 inch) 20 gauge needles; two 10 ml hypodermic syringes; giving set; sufficient quantity of Hartmann's solution (usually 1l); an assortment of hand instruments is necessary for examination, biopsy or treating pathological lesions. Recommended are appropriately sized cannulae; switching stick; small probe; small joint graspers; small joint curette; small joint hand burr; small joint biopsy forceps.

Optional but useful instrumentation includes a small joint motorized shaver and/or radiofrequency ablation unit. Often synovial proliferation is such that in the small joint space the viewing field is obscured. A small joint motorized shaver or ablation unit is helpful in removing synovial villi to create a viewing window.

Clipping and draping
A hanging limb preparation is preferred with the clip extending from just distal to the stifle to just proximal to the tarsal pad. Four field drapes and a foot drape are used and covered by a sterile impervious transparent adhesive disposable drape.

Surgical technique
To begin, a 20 gauge needle (25 mm, 1 inch) is inserted and the joint is distended with fluid. The needle can be inserted in the same location as the intended egress portal or alternatively opposite the side of the intended portals. Portals may be dorsal or plantar, medial or lateral. The arthroscope portal is typically located opposite the site of the lesion to be viewed. For example, with an OCD of the medial ridge of the talus, the arthroscope portal is located plantarolaterally. A guide needle (22 gauge) is inserted at the intended site and direction of the 'scope portal. Fluid should leak from the hub of the needle if it is positioned correctly. The needle is removed and a small entry incision is made with a no. 11 blade through the skin and superficial soft tissues; the same direction as the guide needle is followed. The arthroscope sheath and obturator are inserted through the entry wound into the joint. Next, egress flow is established by inserting a 20 gauge needle into the joint at the intended site of the instrument portal. The arthroscope and light post are positioned to view the area of interest. Then the egress needle is inserted so as to triangulate the tip of the needle directly into the viewing window of the arthroscope. Once it is in place, fluid ingress is increased to establish flow.

> **WARNING**
> **Manipulation of the arthroscope should be kept to a minimum to avoid inadvertent damage to the cartilage surface and reduce the chance of accidental dislodgement of the arthroscope.**

If visualization of the cartilage surface is difficult due to synovial proliferation, the joint should be distended further by temporarily occluding egress of fluid. If the view remains obstructed, an instrument portal is established (see below) and a mini-motorized shaver blade is inserted to perform a synovectomy. Haemorrhage is controlled by ingress fluid pressure for tamponade, electrocoagulation or ablation with a radiofrequency unit.

An instrument portal is established if the viewing window is obscured by synovial villi, a biopsy of intra-articular tissue is desired or if treatment of joint pathology is required. The egress site is easily converted to an open instrument portal by advancing a no. 11 blade adjacent to the needle. Once the scapel blade appears in the viewing window, the needle and blade are withdrawn from the joint. A blunt obturator is inserted into the incision to widen the portal. Hand instruments, a shaver blade (motorized shaver) or radiofrquency probe can now easily be inserted, withdrawn and re-inserted into the joint space.

→

OPERATIVE TECHNIQUE 23.3 *continued*
Arthroscopy of the tarsus

PRACTICAL TIP
All portals are interchangeable if necessary.

Removal of tarsal OCD lesions
The arthroscope and instrument portal are located appropriately. If the osteochondral tissue is still attached at one or more sites, a probe or small elevator is inserted to free partially the edge of the flap. The osteochondral flap is not freed completely but is left attached at one site. Depending upon the size of free osteochondral tissue, the instrument portal (joint capsule and soft tissue tunnel) may need to be dilated. The portal is dilated with a series of increasing diameter obturators or small scissors. Increasing sized obturators are inserted through the soft tissue tunnel into the joint and rotated gently. If scissors are used, the tip of the scissors is inserted into the joint and the joint capsule and soft tissue are spread by opening the scissors.

Grasping forceps are inserted and the free osteochondral flap removed. The cartilage flap may be removed as a single large fragment or, as is often the case, in two to three smaller pieces. It is often helpful to hyperflex the joint in cases of plantaromedial OCD lesions to separate the joint surfaces and improve access. A curette is used to debride the edges of the lesion. The subchondral bone surface of the lesion is abraded using a hand-held curette, hand-held burr or motorized shaver. The surface is lightly abraded until the underlying bone bleeds freely. The surgeon should stop ingress fluid flow to observe the extent of bleeding bone. Abrasion arthroplasty should be halted once multifocal pinpoint bleeding is observed. Further abrasion leads to a deepening of the defect, which may increase instability. Upon completion of surface abrasionplasty or microfracture, small bone or cartilage fragments are flushed from the joint by increasing the ingress flow. The joint is inspected for remaining bone or cartilage fragments, the arthroscope is removed and the portals are sutured with non-reactive, non-absorbable suture.

Closure
Single skin sutures are placed in the portal sites.

Postoperative care
See appropriate Operative Technique. Generally 48 hours' rest is needed following diagnostic arthroscopy. If operative procedures are used, the period of rest is extended as appropriate to each individual procedure.

Complications
Accumulation of subcutaneous fluid can occur during the procedure; this can cause some joint space collapse. It resolves within 48–72 hours.

Chapter 23 The tarsus

OPERATIVE TECHNIQUE 23.4
Calcaneoquartal arthrodesis using a lag screw or bone plate

Preoperative planning
The most common indication for calcaneoquartal arthrodesis is plantar ligament degeneration and hyperflexion of the joint, so considerable periarticular fibrous reaction should be anticipated. Intra-operative haemorrhage may hamper visibility and diathermy, if available, is very helpful. A tourniquet can be used but compromises manipulation of the tarsus during surgery. Reference should be made on preoperative radiographs to the amount of new bone formation on the plantar surface of the calcaneoquartal joint and the location of the joint proper, which can be more dorsal than anticipated in relation to this. A donor site for harvesting cancellous bone graft must be prepared. This can be the ipsilateral tuber coxae or proximal humeral metaphysis (recommended) or, if preferred, the contralateral proximal tibial metaphysis.

Positioning
Lateral recumbency with the affected limb uppermost and suspended for free limb draping. If the ipsilateral proximal humerus is to be the source of cancellous bone for grafting it is helpful to have this limb drawn caudally.

Assistant
Helpful but not essential.

Tray extras
Standard and small Gelpi self-retaining retractors; appropriately sized drill bit and spoon curette for harvesting cancellous bone; small curette or high-speed burrs for removal of articular cartilage; small rongeurs; appropriately sized drills, depth gauge, tap etc. for insertion of lagged bone screw or plate and screws; orthopaedic wire and instrumentation for its insertion (if desired).

Surgical approach
A skin incision is made along the plantarolateral edge of the calcaneus and extended proximally 2–3 cm beyond the tip of the calcaneus and distally 2–6 cm beyond the tarsometatarsal joint, depending upon size of patient and technique selected. The superficial digital flexor is reflected medially from the calcaneoquartal joint and calcaneus.

Surgical technique

Lag screw
Reactive soft tissue and new bone formation are removed as required from the plantar aspect of the calcaneoquartal joint to allow inspection of the articular surfaces. The joint is forcibly hyperextended and articular cartilage is removed from the joint surfaces using a sharp curette or high-speed burr. A gliding hole is drilled from the calcaneal articular surface proximally to emerge through the superficial digital flexor. An insert guide is placed into the proximal end of this drill hole and cancellous bone graft is packed into the calcaneoquartal joint. The joint is then forcibly hyperflexed to ensure proper alignment of the calcaneoquartal articular surfaces. A pilot hole is drilled through the insert guide into the fourth tarsal bone and proximal metatarsus. The drill hole is measured and tapped and an appropriately sized bone screw, 2 mm shorter than the measured depth, is inserted and tightened to produce compression of the joint space (Figure 23.23). If desired, orthopaedic wire can now be placed in a figure-of-eight pattern through bone tunnels in the calcaneus and proximal end of metatarsal bone V.

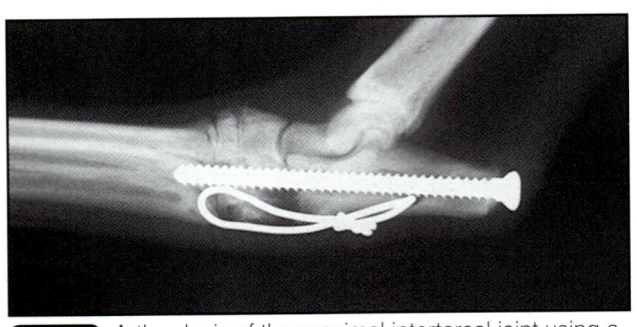

23.23 Arthrodesis of the proximal intertarsal joint using a lag screw. The superficial digital flexor tendon is retracted medially and the joint is forcibly hyperextended to allow removal of articular cartilage and drilling a gliding hole retrograde in the calcaneus. The joint is reduced and a pilot hole is drilled through the fourth tarsal bone for insertion of a lag screw. Note that the screw is well seated in the fourth tarsal bone and the distal end of the wire is anchored in the proximal metatarsal bones.

OPERATIVE TECHNIQUE 23.4 *continued*
Calcaneoquartal arthrodesis using a lag screw or bone plate

This is intended to act as a prosthetic plantar ligament and helps protect the screw from bending. Further cancellous bone graft is then packed into the plantar aspect of the joint.

> **WARNING**
> **A common mistake is to fail to identify the distal articular surface of the calcaneus properly and start the gliding hole too far plantar. This directs the pilot hole and consequently the lag screw into the fibrocartilage plantar to the fourth tarsal bone rather than into its proper location within the bone.**

Bone plate
Reactive soft tissue and new bone formation are removed as required from the plantar aspect of the calcaneoquartal joint to allow inspection of the articular surfaces. The joint is forcibly hyperextended and articular cartilage is removed from the joint surfaces using a sharp curette or high-speed burr. The lateral tarsometatarsal joint is exposed and articular cartilage is drilled out using a drill bit or side-cutting burr. The lateral prominence of the proximal end of metatarsal bone V can be removed using rongeurs. Cancellous bone is packed into the joint spaces and the calcaneoquartal joint is reduced and held in position. A temporary transarticular pin can be placed to assist in controlling the proximal intertarsal joint and, if wished, this can be used to form a plate–rod combination. An appropriately sized plate is contoured to fit the lateral aspect so that three to four screws can be placed in the calcaneus and metatarsal bones (Figure 23.24). Hybrid 2.7/2.0 mm pancarpal arthrodesis plates or veterinary cuttable plates (see Figure 23.15) fit this location well. 2.7 mm dynamic compression plates are also suitable in larger dogs. The proximal two metatarsal screws should engage as many metatarsal bones as possible. More distal screws should only engage one or two metatarsal bones.

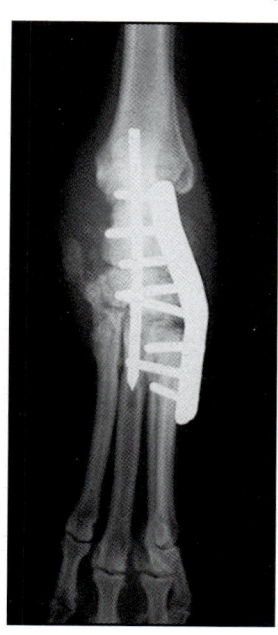

23.24 Arthrodesis of the proximal intertarsal joint using a lateral plate. A plate–rod combination has been utilized in this dog, an obese Shetland Sheepdog with bilateral proximal intertarsal joint hyperextension.

Closure
The superficial digital flexor tendon is apposed to the lateral periarticular soft tissues using fine polydioxanone sutures to help in retaining the ventral cancellous bone graft. The remainder of the closure is routine.

Postoperative care
Postoperative radiographs should be taken to assess alignment and implant positioning. External support should be applied postoperatively and this may be a cast or splint, depending upon patient size. It is not necessary to immobilize the talocrural joint. Follow-up radiographs should be taken after 6 or 8 weeks and, assuming there is sufficient evidence of healing, external support can usually be discarded at that time.

Chapter 23 The tarsus

OPERATIVE TECHNIQUE 23.5
Repair of Achilles tendon rupture

Preoperative planning
Treatment of Achilles tendon ruptures may be conservative or surgical, depending upon presentation. Surgery is indicated in dogs with abnormal joint and digital posture and/or obvious lameness.
  A tourniquet cannot be used since it compromises manipulation of the tarsus during surgery.

Positioning
Sternal recumbency with the affected limb extended caudally and suspended for free limb draping.

Assistant
Helpful but not essential.

Tray extras
Standard Gelpi self-retaining retractors; appropriately sized drill, depth gauge, tap etc. for insertion of positional calcaneotibial bone screw; appropriately sized drill for creation of bone tunnel in calcaneus (if necessary).

Surgical approach
With the patient in sternal recumbency and the affected limb extended caudally, the calcaneus is exposed via a plantarolateral approach. The superficial digital flexor tendon is reflected medially after sectioning its lateral retinaculum and the tarsus is maximally extended using pointed reduction forceps applied to the tip of the calcaneus and the cranial tibia. This permits fixation of the tarsus in extension using an appropriately sized calcaneotibial screw.

Surgical technique

Positional calcaneotibial screw
The tarsus is fixed in extension using an appropriately sized calcaneotibial screw (e.g. 4.5 mm diameter screw in a Dobermann or large Labrador Retriever).
  With the joint hyperextended, a pilot hole is drilled in a plantarodorsal direction through the proximal aspect of the calcaneus to emerge at the cranial aspect of the tibia. The length of the entire drill hole is measured and the calcaneus and tibial holes tapped. An appropriately sized bone screw, 2–4 mm longer than the measured depth, is inserted and tightened. The screw should be inserted in a positional fashion (Figure 23.25).

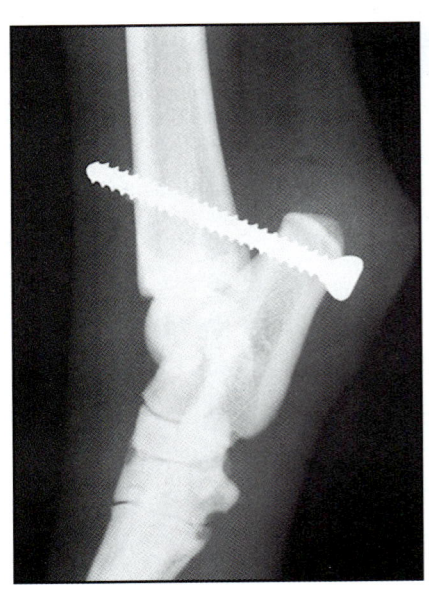

23.25 Positioning of calcaneotibial screw. The screw tip should protrude sufficiently from the cranial cortex of the tibia so that each part can be removed if the screw breaks.

> **CLINICAL TIP**
> Fixing the tarsus in extension with a pair of pointed reduction forceps during the entire procedure will simplify lining up the bone tunnel in the calcaneus with that in the tibia.

> **WARNING**
> The screw tip should extend 3–4 mm beyond the cranial cortex of the tibia so that, if it breaks postoperatively, both ends can be removed if required.

→

414

OPERATIVE TECHNIQUE 23.5 continued
Repair of Achilles tendon rupture

Repair of the tendon injury
In acute, complete injuries it should be easy to identify the gastrocnemius and superficial digital flexor components and, if both are lacerated, these should be repaired separately using polydioxanone or monfilament nylon. A modified Kessler locking-loop or a three-loop pulley suture pattern (Moores *et al.*, 2004) is recommended. In longer-standing injuries, muscle contracture may create difficulties in reapposing the tendon ends, in which case strands of carbon fibre or polyester (Jenkins *et al.*, 1977) or fascia lata grafts (Braden, 1976) can be used to fill the defect.

Repair of gastrocnemius tendon avulsion
Gastrocnemius tendon avulsions should be reattached via one or two bone tunnels drilled transversely across the tip of the calcaneus to act as distal anchorage points for sutures.

If primary treatment of Achilles mechanism injuries fails, pantarsal arthrodesis (Operative Technique 23.6) can be considered to salvage limb function. This may also be a valid consideration from the outset in bilateral chronic tendon avulsions.

Closure
The lateral retinaculum of the superficial digital flexor should be repaired using polydioxanone sutures. The remainder of the closure is routine.

Postoperative care
Postoperative radiographs should be taken to assess alignment and implant positioning. A padded splint or cast is applied for 3–4 weeks to protect the calcaneotibial screw. The screw is removed after 6–8 weeks and exercise restricted to lead walking for a further 4–6 weeks.

Chapter 23 The tarsus

OPERATIVE TECHNIQUE 23.6
Pantarsal arthrodesis

Preoperative planning
Pantarsal arthrodesis is a technically demanding procedure and should never be undertaken lightly. A tracing of a mediolateral projection radiograph taken with the tarsus at a normal standing angle for the patient in question is used to design a custom-made angled plate. Depending on patient size, this will be either a hybrid 3.5/2.7 mm or 2.7/2.0 mm plate. The angle is typically around 135 degrees. Location of screw holes and designation as load or neutral holes is made at this stage. Depending upon surgeon preference, the plate can be positioned medially (the author's preference) or laterally. Consideration must also be given to harvesting cancellous bone for grafting. For a medial approach the contralateral proximal humeral metaphysis is advised.

Positioning (for medial approach)
Lateral recumbency on the affected side with the unaffected limb abducted and drawn cranially and the affected limb suspended to allow free limb draping. The cancellous bone graft donor site selected should be readily accessible.

Assistant
Helpful but not essential.

Tray extras
Custom-made angled hybrid compression plate; appropriate bone plate and screw instrumentation, i.e. drills, depth gauges, taps, screwdrivers etc.; plate bending instruments; appropriately sized drill bit and curette for harvesting cancellous bone; Gelpi self-retaining retractors (standard and small); rongeurs; powered bone saw, or (if preferred) osteotome/bone chisel and mallet; high-speed burr or small curette for removal of articular cartilage. Tourniquet is inappropriate but electrocautery is very helpful.

Surgical approach
An angled skin incision is made medially from the mid tibia to the level of the second metatarsophalangeal joint.

Surgical technique
A suitable volume of cancellous bone for grafting is harvested from the selected site. An osteotomy of the medial malleolus is performed in such a way that the osteotomy site, distal tibia and tarsal/metatarsal bones are flush. The osteotomized malleolus is discarded and the articular surfaces of the talocrural joint are thoroughly debrided of articular cartilage. The talocentral, centrodistal and medial tarsometatarsal joints are opened and the articular cartilage and dense subchondral bone plate are removed using a drill or (ideally) a high-speed burr. Preserving the normal contour of the talocrural joint facilitates reduction and stabilization. The proximal metatarsal prominence is removed using rongeurs. The exposed joint spaces are lavaged using sterile lactated Ringer's solution or saline, and cancellous bone is packed into the joint spaces. The tarsus is positioned at the appropriate angle and the plate is contoured to fit the limb perfectly. The first screw to be placed is inserted into the talus; this is a neutral screw. Load screws are then placed into the distal tibia and proximal metatarsus. Subsequent screws are inserted sequentially proximally and distally. In the proximal metatarsus, two screws should engage three or four metatarsal bones. The distal plate screws should engage one or two metatarsal bones only (Figure 23.26). The most proximal screw in the tibia should be monocortical. Once the plate has been applied, a calcaneotibial position screw can be placed to help protect the plate from bending in the sagittal plane.

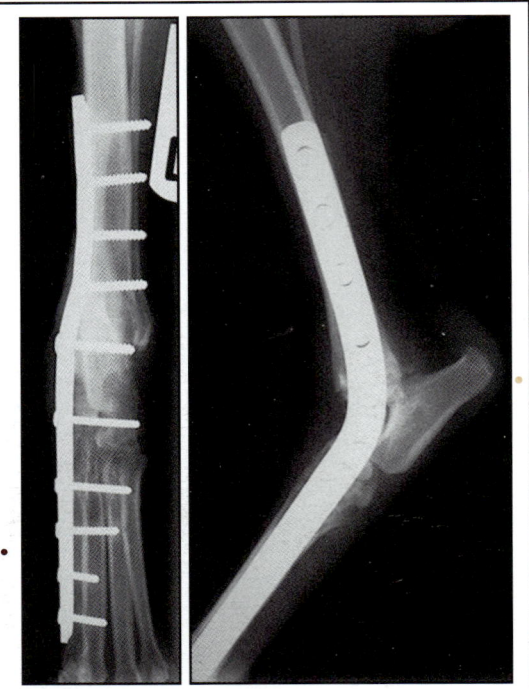

23.26 Pantarsal arthrodesis using a custom-made angled hybrid 3.5/2.7 mm plate applied medially.

OPERATIVE TECHNIQUE 23.6 continued
Pantarsal arthrodesis

Alternative techniques
- The talocrural articular surfaces can also be removed using a saw. This involves a transverse cut across the distal tibia and an appropriately angled cut across the talus. Calculating the angle of the talar cut is challenging but this method does produce a substantial area of cancellous bone-to-bone contact at the arthrodesis site
- An angled plate may also be applied laterally, although the plate and screws can be more awkward to seat satisfactorily on that side. Dorsal or plantar application of straight plates is also possible, but more difficult
- Arthrodesis of the talocrural joint alone has been done using multiple screw techniques but is not advised due to a significant failure rate.

Closure
Routine.

Postoperative care
A postoperative radiograph should be taken to assess reduction and alignment of the arthrodesis as well as implant positioning. External support for around 6 weeks in a cast is necessary, although it is preferred to apply a padded support bandage for the first week to allow postoperative swelling to subside prior to cast application. Analgesia should be provided for as long as necessary.

Follow-up radiographs should be taken 6 weeks postoperatively and, typically, advanced fusion of the arthrodesis should be seen at that time. In that event, external support can be discarded and a phased increase in lead exercise allowed. Off-lead exercise should not be permitted for 6 weeks after cast removal. Pantarsal arthrodesis, if well executed, should give good results in the majority of cases, although angular or rotational deformities can be created by surgery and some dogs will be lame despite successful arthrodesis.

24

The temporomandibular joint

Colin Stead

Clinical and surgical anatomy

The temporomandibular joint (TMJ) is a hinge joint formed by the articular process or condyle of the mandible and the retroarticular process of the temporal bone. The condyle is quite wide in a lateromedial direction. The joint contains a fibrocartilaginous meniscus. Important structures close to the TMJ include the palpebral nerve and the dorsal buccal branch of the facial nerve. The palpebral nerve runs across the face parallel to and dorsal to the zygoma but it should not be a problem to the surgeon unless an incision is made too high. The dorsal buccal branch of the facial nerve crosses the masseter muscle horizontally a few millimetres below the zygoma.

Diagnostic imaging

Plain radiography

For details on imaging the TMJ, the reader is referred to the *BSAVA Manual of Canine and Feline Musculoskeletal Imaging*. Imaging of the TMJ is best performed under general anaesthesia. A dorsoventral (DV) view is most useful, taken with the beam centred in the midline at the level of the cranial border of the orbits. The skull must be positioned straight; a sandbag placed across the neck can be used to stabilize it so that the two TMJs are symmetrically placed for comparison. This view is relatively easy to produce.

Conventional lateral views are not useful due to superimposition, so oblique views are normally taken to project the joints without superimposition of other parts of the skull. This can be difficult because different skull shapes require different positioning. Lateral oblique views are best taken by placing the skull in a lateral position and then tilting the nose upwards by approximately 5–25 degrees. This avoids superimposition by projecting each TMJ separately. It may be necessary to rotate the median axis of the skull about 10 degrees to avoid superimposition of the base of the skull across the lower TMJ. The angle of tilt may need to be varied slightly with different skull shapes to obtain the optimal projection. The X-ray beam is centred to the lower TMJ. With the left side down, this could be a Rt15°R–LeCdO projection (Figure 24.1) or, with median rotation, a Rt15°R10°V–LeCdDO projection. Figure 24.2 illustrates a similar view in a cat with only 5 degrees of tilt (Rt5°R–LeCdO view). Use of an image intensifier may simplify correct positioning.

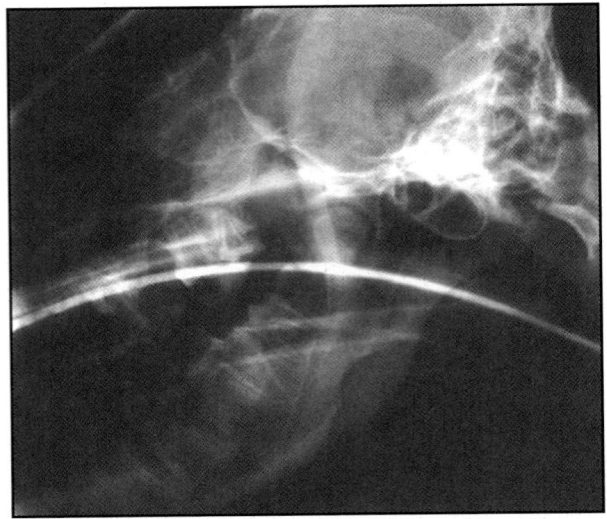

24.1 Rt15°R–LeCdO view of a normal left TMJ in a 7-month-old German Shepherd Dog. Note the line of the base of the skull crossing just dorsal to the joint.

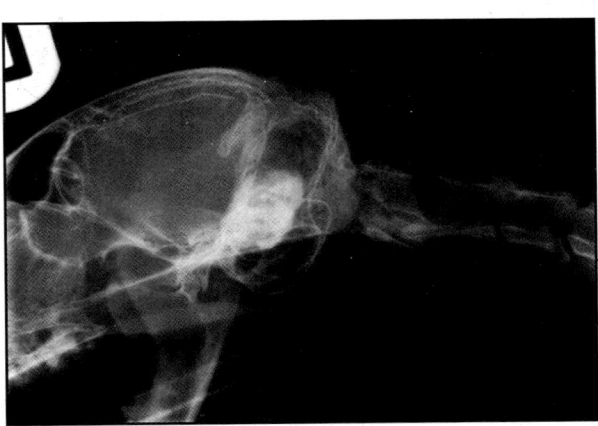

24.2 Rt5°R–LeCdO view of a normal left TMJ of a cat. Note the base of the skull just dorsal to the joint.

An alternative radiographic view for cats and small dogs, which allows both TMJs to be imaged in lateral oblique projection on the same film, has been described by Schwarz *et al.* (2002). This requires the animal in lateral recumbency with the head and neck extended and the beam, at 100 cm focus–film distance, to be centred on the third cervical vertebra at the level of the joints with the collimation to include both joints. The lower TMJ will be most caudal on the film. This is an RtCd–LeRO projection.

Chapter 24 The temporomandibular joint

Advanced imaging

The use of computed tomography (CT) and magnetic resonance imaging (MRI) is becoming more common in veterinary imaging. Schwarz *et al.* (2002) have shown the value of high-resolution, thin-slice, transverse CT scans for imaging the TMJ in both cats and dogs, particularly for showing articular fractures (Figure 24.3). Other lesions, such as neoplastic change, may also be shown by CT (Figure 24.4).

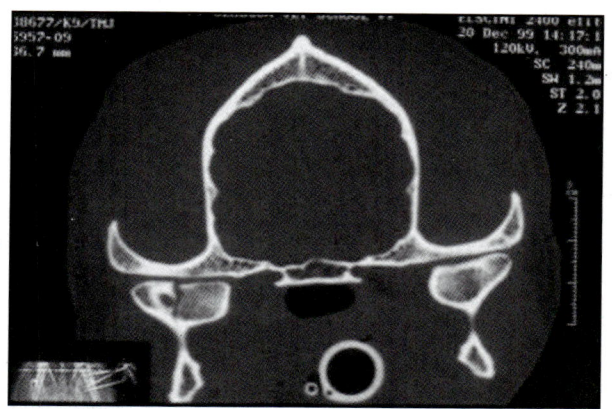

24.3 Transverse CT scan of the right TMJ of a 3-year-old Border Collie with a fracture across its mandibular condyle. (Courtesy of T. Schwarz)

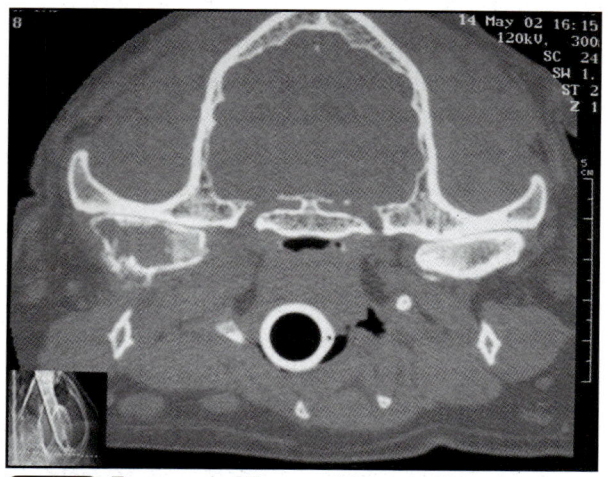

24.4 Transverse CT scan of the right TMJ of a dog with a tumour affecting its mandibular condyle. The architecture of the condyle is extensively destroyed. (Courtesy of T. Schwarz)

Conditions of the temporomandibular joint

Conditions affecting the TMJ are not common and are mostly traumatic or developmental in origin; they normally present with the animal having difficulty in opening or closing its mouth.

Luxation

This condition arises through trauma, mostly road traffic accidents, and is more common in cats than in dogs. The mandibular condyle will displace cranially and slightly dorsally. An animal with a luxation is unable to close its mouth, due to malocclusion of its teeth. The lower jaw will deviate towards the *normal* side in a unilateral case. If both condyles are dislocated, the mandible displaces *cranially*. Radiography under general anaesthesia will reveal cranial displacement of the affected condyle; luxation is best appreciated on a dorsoventral view (Figure 24.5).

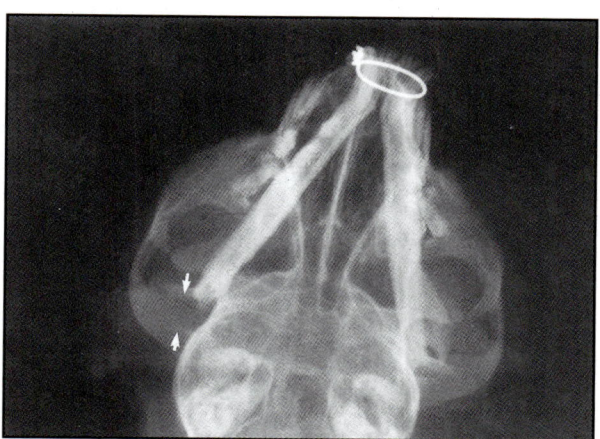

24.5 DV view of the skull of a cat with cranial dislocation of its right TMJ. The right mandibular condyle is displaced cranially from its retroarticular process (arrowed). Compare the normal position of the left TMJ. The jaw is deviated toward the normal left side. A symphyseal separation of the mandibular symphysis has been wired.

> **PRACTICAL TIP**
> Examine radiographs very carefully to ensure that there are no associated fractures; these can be difficult to identify, especially in cats.

Conservative treatment

Reduction of a luxation, whether unilateral or bilateral, is normally possible by manipulation under general anaesthesia with the aid of a wooden or soft plastic rod (to protect the teeth) as a fulcrum. The rod is placed horizontally across the mouth as far back as possible and an attempt made to close the mouth while pushing the mandible caudally. The condyle should click back into place and dental occlusion should be normal. Joint movement should be free and smooth and the jaw should be straight.

Surgical treatment

In the event of a failed closed reduction, open reduction is required to remove any debris or fibrosis from in and around the joint (see Operative Technique 24.1). Normally, additional measures to maintain the joint reduction following capsular closure are unnecessary. If required, a wire loop can be inserted through a hole drilled dorsoventrally through the distal temporal part of the zygoma and craniocaudally through the neck of bone just distal to the condyle; the loop is tightened sufficiently to allow normal joint movement (Figure 24.6). Postoperative care involves soft feeding for 4 weeks and the application of a loose-fitting tape or 'Mikki' muzzle for the first week to restrict mouth opening but to allow feeding and drinking. Use of the muzzle is discretionary.

419

Chapter 24 The temporomandibular joint

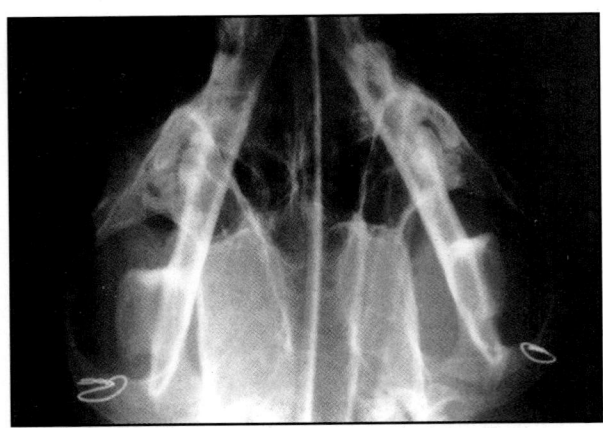

24.6 DV view of the TMJs of a Boxer that had undergone wiring of both joints to stabilize them following episodes of open-mouth jaw locking unassociated with the zygomatic arch.

Ankylosis

Fracture callus of the zygomatic process or the temporal bone
A fracture of the zygomatic process of the temporal bone or vertical ramus close to the TMJ may, if not recognized or diagnosed, produce a callus that progressively restricts the ability of the animal to open its mouth and eat. These injuries are more common in cats than in dogs, but still rare. Treatment requires a surgical approach to the TMJ (see Operative Technique 24.1) and removal of the callus with small bone rongeurs. If joint movement cannot be restored by these means, an excision arthroplasty should be performed (see Operative Technique 24.1).

Masticatory muscle myopathy
Masticatory muscle myopathy gives a non-painful, progressive ankylosis of the TMJ due to severe atrophy and fibrosis of the muscles of mastication. It is believed to be immune-mediated but some cases develop after trauma. The muscles are severely atrophied and mouth opening is restricted; the TMJs are normal on radiography. Treatment is non-surgical and involves immunosuppressive doses of corticosteroids, reducing the dose to zero over 3 months, plus supportive therapy if necessary.

Craniomandibular osteopathy
Craniomandibular osteopathy occasionally produces ankylosis of the TMJs in young dogs, particularly West Highland White Terriers, due to proliferative bone formation. This is normally treated with corticosteroids, initially at immunosuppressive doses and gradually reducing or stopping therapy over 3 months, plus supportive therapy.

Osteomyelitis
Osteomyelitis may occasionally spread to the TMJ from the osseous bulla, possibly following bulla osteotomy. Affected animals have difficulty in eating and have pain on opening the mouth. Destructive changes in and around the joint are seen on radiography. If the condition does not resolve with antibiotic therapy and possible joint drainage, an excision arthroplasty may be indicated (see Operative Technique 24.1).

Neoplasia
Neoplasia in the region of the TMJ, particularly osteochondrosarcoma arising from the vertical rami of the mandible in dogs, may produce a progressive ankylosis of the TMJ as well as an exophthalmos. Surgical removal is indicated, requiring ostectomy of part of the zygoma for access to the site (see Operative Technique 24.2). These tumours are difficult to remove in their entirety and tend to regrow in a matter of months, although occasional cases may have a good outcome. There is no consensus on the best treatment for these rare tumours.

Open-mouth jaw locking (TMJ dysplasia)
This is a rare condition which principally affects dogs but has been recorded in one cat (Lantz, 1987). It is presumed to be developmental or congenital in origin. It usually presents in young animals that show incongruity of the TMJ articular surfaces and sometimes osteophytes indicative of secondary osteoarthritis. The condition has been identified in several dog breeds, including Basset Hounds, Irish Setters, Boxers, Labrador and Golden Retrievers, American Cocker Spaniels and Bernese Mountain Dogs. The condition may be bilateral. There appear to be two types of jaw locking:

- The more frequent type involves cranial displacement of a dysplastic articular process, deviation of the mandible to the contralateral side and locking of its coronoid process on or lateral to the zygomatic arch
- In the second type, the jaw locking is not associated with impingement of the coronoid process on the zygoma. Animals present with a history of open-mouth jaw locking following eating, play or yawning. This may cause considerable distress and pawing at the face. Some owners become quite adept at reducing these by massage or medially directed pressure on the affected side of the face or by opening the mouth further and twisting the mandible slightly. Some cases of this type will reduce spontaneously.

Diagnosis
Examination of the mouth is carried out under general anaesthesia. The mouth must be examined carefully to rule out any oral or dental pathology that could be associated with jaw locking. Attempts to dislocate the jaw should be made by opening the mouth fully and moving the TMJs lateromedially. Radiography of the TMJs using oblique lateral views will show whether there is incongruity or osteophytic reaction. With the mouth open, an attempt should be made to dislocate the jaw and obtain a radiograph in the dislocated position to show any zygomatic impingement (Figure 24.7). With non-zygomatic involvement, inducing a dislocation may not be so easy.

Chapter 24 The temporomandibular joint

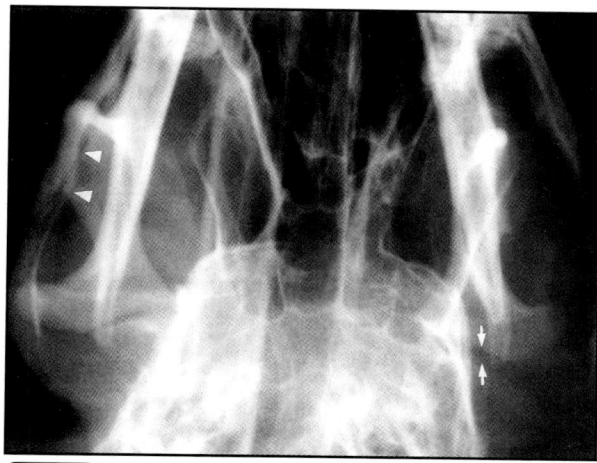

24.7 DV view of the TMJs of a Basset Hound with open-mouth jaw locking due to TMJ dysplasia. The left TMJ is cranially displaced with a widened joint space (arrows) and the right coronoid process is impacting the right zygomatic arch (arrow heads).

Treatment

If there is zygomatic involvement in the jaw locking, part of the zygomatic arch is removed, probably bilaterally (see Operative Technique 24.2). Attempts to plicate the joint capsule of the TMJ are normally unsuccessful. If the jaw locking is not associated with the zygomatic arch, an excision arthroplasty is performed on the affected joint or joints (see Operative Technique 24.1). As an alternative to excision arthroplasty, the author has successfully used 0.8 mm wire loop stabilization of the TMJs in two dogs where open-mouth jaw locking occurred unassociated with the zygomatic arch, with follow-up times of 1 year and 6 months (see Figure 24.6). It is too early to say whether this approach will ensure long-term correction of the problem because the wire loops will eventually 'fatigue' and break.

References and further reading

Barr F and Kirberger R (eds) (2006) *BSAVA Manual of Canine and Feline Musculoskeletal Imaging.* BSAVA Publications, Gloucester

Bennett D and Campbell JR (1976) Mechanical interference with lower jaw movement as a complication of skull fractures. *Journal of Small Animal Practice* **17**, 747–751

Bennett D and Prymak C (1986) Excision arthroplasty as a treatment for temporomandibular dysplasia. *Journal of Small Animal Practice* **27**, 361–370

Hoppe F and Svalastoga E (1980) Temporomandibular dysplasia in American Cocker Spaniels. *Journal of Small Animal Practice* **21**, 675–678

Johnson KA (1979) Temporomandibular dysplasia in an Irish Setter. *Journal of Small Animal Practice* **20**, 209–218

Lane JG (1982) Disorders of the canine temporomandibular joint. *Veterinary Annual* **22**, 175–187

Lantz GC, Cantwell GO, Van Vleet SF and Cechner RE (1982) Unilateral mandibular condylectomy: experimental and clinical results. *Journal of the American Animal Hospital Association* **18**, 883–889

Lantz GC (1985) Temporomandibular joint ankylosis: surgical correction of three cases. *Journal of the American Animal Hospital Association* **22**, 173–177

Lantz GC (1987) Intermittent open-mouth locking of the temporomandibular joint in a cat. *Journal of the American Veterinary Medical Association* **190**, 1574

Lantz GC and Cantwell HD (1986) Intermittent lower mouth open jaw locking in five dogs. *Journal of the American Veterinary Medical Association* **188**, 1403–1405

Piermattei DL and Johnson KA (2004) *An Atlas of Surgical Approaches to the Bones and Joints of the Dog and Cat,* 4th edn. WB Saunders, Philadelphia

Robins G and Grandage J (1977) Temporomandibular joint dysplasia and open mouth jaw locking in the dog. *Journal of the American Veterinary Medical Association* **171**, 1072–1076

Schwarz T, Weller R, Dickie AM, Konar M and Sullivan M (2002) Imaging of the canine and feline temporomandibular joint: a review. *Veterinary Radiology and Ultrasound* **43**, 85–97

Stead AC (1994) The temporomandibular joint. In: *BSAVA Manual of Small Animal Arthrology,* ed. JEF Houlton and RW Collinson, pp. 325–336. BSAVA Publications, Cheltenham

Straw RC, Le Couteur RA, Powers BE and Withrow SJ (1989) Multilobular osteochondrosarcoma of the canine skull; 16 cases. *Journal of the American Veterinary Medical Association* **195**, 1764–1769

Thomas RE (1979) Temporomandibular dysplasia and open mouth jaw locking in a Basset Hound: a case report. *Journal of Small Animal Practice* **20**, 697–701

Thomlinson J and Presnell K (1983) Mandibular condylectomy: effects in normal dogs. *Veterinary Surgery* **12**, 148

Ticer JM and Spencer CP (1978) Injury of the feline temporomandibular joint: radiographic signs. *Journal of the American Veterinary Radiology Society* **19**, 146

Chapter 24 The temporomandibular joint

OPERATIVE TECHNIQUE 24.1
Approach to the temporomandibular joint

Indications
Examination of joint; open reduction of dislocation; excision arthroplasty.

Positioning
Lateral recumbency with the affected joint uppermost.

> **WARNING**
> Beware of the eye when positioning towel clips!

Assistant
Desirable.

Tray extras
Gelpi self-retaining retractors; small Langenbeck retractors; small periosteal elevator. For excision arthroplasty, a small scalpel blade (size 15 or less); high speed air drill and 2 mm round burrs; mallet and small osteotome; duckbill rongeurs.

Surgical technique

> **WARNING**
> The palpebral nerve runs across the face parallel to and dorsal to the zygoma. It should not be a problem unless the incision is made too high.
>
> The dorsal buccal branch of the facial nerve crosses the masseter muscle horizontally a few millimetres below the zygoma. It should be protected by the retraction of the masseter unless the initial incision is made too low.

The TMJ lies distal to the caudal part of the zygoma. An incision is made following the curve of the caudal third of the zygoma just above its ventral border, curving distally (Figure 24.8). The thin platysma muscle is incised to expose the zygoma and the masseter muscle. An incision is made through the origin of the masseter muscle which attaches to the ventral border of the zygoma. Subperiosteally the masseter is reflected distally to expose the TMJ joint capsule. This is incised horizontally to expose the mandibular condyle and the meniscus (Figure 24.9). Having entered the joint, the capsule is incised lateromedially along its full length at its distal margin to avoid meniscal damage. The small blade is used and the capsule is scraped distally to clear the neck of the condyle and visualize the mandibular notch. The meniscus is preserved.

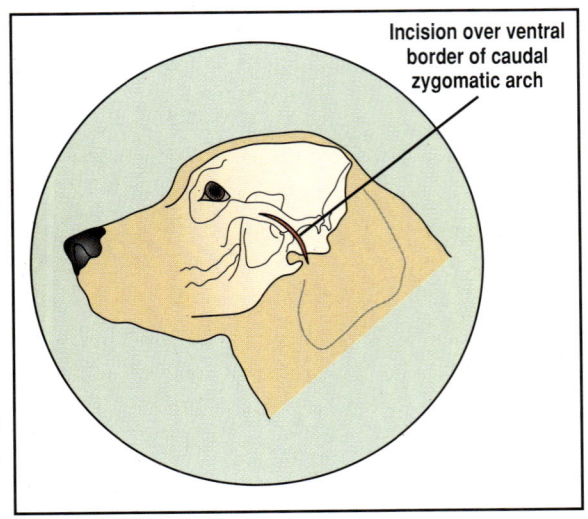

24.8 Landmarks for the approach to the TMJ.

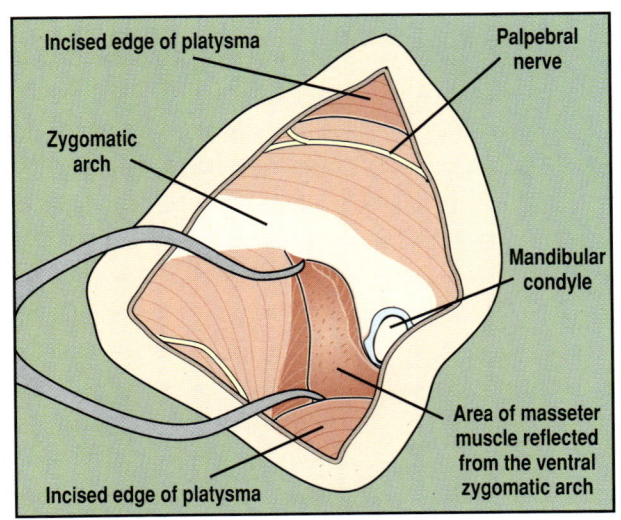

24.9 The joint capsule has been incised horizontally to expose the mandibular condyle and the meniscus.

Chapter 24 The temporomandibular joint

OPERATIVE TECHNIQUE 24.1 *continued*
Approach to the temporomandibular joint

Excision arthroplasty
The air drill and burr are used to make a slightly curved incision from the neck of the condyle to the mandibular notch. The notch is nearly cut through with the burr (Figure 24.10). The incision through the neck of the condyle is completed *gently* using the osteotome and mallet. The rongeurs may be used if necessary to tidy up the osteotomy. The remains of the medial and caudal joint capsule are carefully incised to free and remove the condyle. The meniscus can be left *in situ*. It is important to ensure removal of the entire condyle, whose medial extension is quite extensive.

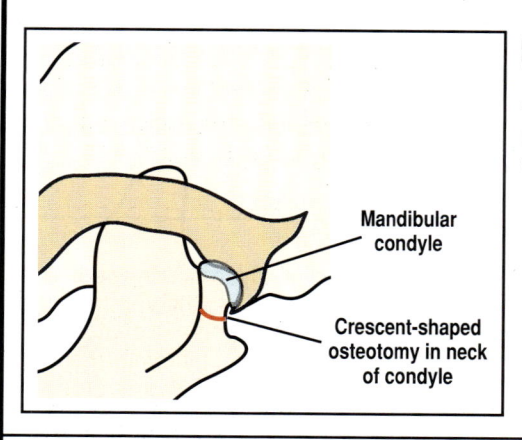

24.10 Excision arthroplasty. The crescent-shaped line of the osteotomy is depicted.

Closure
No attempt is made to close the joint capsule. The masseter muscle is reattached to the dorsal fascia and the platysma and skin are closed.

Postoperative care
For reduced luxations, a tape muzzle should be applied for 7–10 days to limit jaw movement but allow intake of sloppy food. After excision arthroplasty, jaw movement should be encouraged to maintain range of motion.
   Appropriate analgesia should be provided and within a few days of surgery, normal feeding should be encouraged, including hard food and chews to encourage jaw movement.

Chapter 24 The temporomandibular joint

OPERATIVE TECHNIQUE 24.2
Zygomatic ostectomy for jaw locking

Positioning
Lateral recumbency with contralateral zygomatic arch uppermost.

> **WARNING**
> **Beware the eye position when placing towel clips.**
>
> **The dorsal buccal branch of the facial nerve lies a few millimetres below the ventral edge of the zygoma and should be protected.**

Assistant
Unscrubbed assistant useful to manipulate the jaw.

Tray extras
Small bone-cutting forceps; duckbill rongeurs; small periosteal elevator.

Surgical technique
A skin incision is made along the middle ventral portion of the zygomatic arch. The platysma is incised. The periosteum is incised and the origin of the masseter muscle is detached subperiosteally from the ventral edge of the bone. It is carefully cleared from the medial aspect of the zygoma using the small periosteal elevator. The non-scrubbed assistant should dislocate the jaw to allow the surgeon to identify the area of impingement or overlap of the coronoid process of the mandible on the zygomatic arch. The ventral part of the zygomatic arch in the area of impingement is carefully removed using the bone-cutting forceps and rongeurs until the coronoid process no longer contacts the zygomatic arch when the non-scrubbed assistant opens and closes the mouth, to ensure that locking no longer occurs on that side (Figure 24.11). It is often possible to preserve the dorsal border of the zygomatic arch but occasionally total removal of an entire section is required.

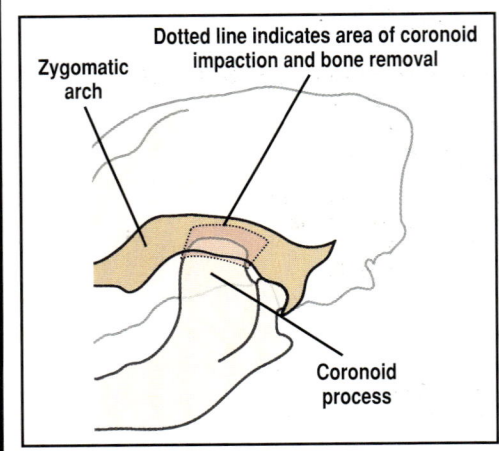

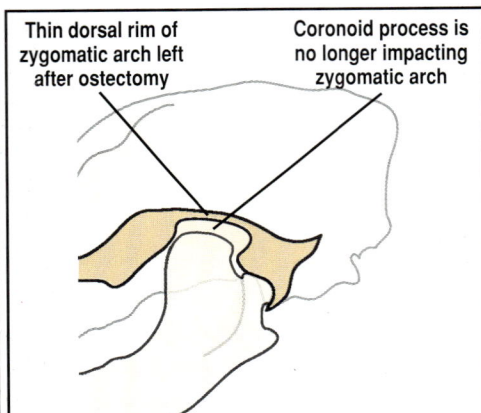

24.11 Technique for zygomatic ostectomy. The ostectomy is of sufficient size to ensure that the coronoid process of the mandible no longer impacts on the zygomatic arch.

Closure
The masseter origin is sutured to the dorsal fascia. The remaining closure is routine.

Postoperative care
Approriate analgesia along with soft food are provided for a few days postoperatively. The animal should be able to return to a normal diet after this period.

Index

Page numbers in *italics* refer to illustrations. Page numbers in **bold** indicate Operative Techniques.

Abductor pollicis longus tendon
  sprain 283
  stenosing tenosynovitis 283
Abyssinian cat, hypothyroid dwarfism 64
Accessory carpal bone luxation/subluxation 284–5
Acepromazine 193
Achilles tendon
  palpation *397*
  rupture 404–5
    repair **414–15**
  tendinitis/peritendinitis 404
Achondroplasia *59*, 60
Actinomyces bovis 42
Acute canine polyradiculoneuritis *138*
Adson suction tip *167*
Age, effects on healing 149–50
Akita
  glycogenosis 124
  juvenile-onset polyarthritis *89*, 95, *97*
Alaskan Malamute, osteochondrodysplastic dwarfism 58, *59*
Allis tissue forceps *161*, *162*
American Cocker Spaniel
  glycogenosis 124
  open-mouth jaw locking 420
Amoxicillin 154
Amoxicillin/clavulate 102
Ampicillin 154
Amputation
  digital 297
  phalangeal, complications 295
Anaesthesia for arthroscopy 185
Analgesia *see* Pain management
Angiography 9
Ankylosis
  in infective arthritis 100
  temporomandibular joint 420
Antibacterial agents
  and PMMA 174
  and surgery 154
Antinuclear antibody 25, 92, 94
Apodia 62
Artery forceps *162*
Arthritis
  classification *81*, *89*
  clinical approach 81–2
  diagnostic imaging 82
  immune-mediated
    aetiopathogenesis 89–90
    classification *89*, 91–5
    cytology *24*
    diagnosis 90–1
    prognosis 96–7
    treatment 95–9
  infective
    autoantibodies *25*
    bacterial
      clinical features 98–9
      diagnosis 99–102
      infected prostheses 104
      L-forms 105
      MRSA 103–4
      pathogenesis 98
      prognosis 103
      radiology 99–100
      route of infection 97–8
      treatment 102–3
    borrelial 104–5
    cytology *24*
    fungal 105–6
    mycoplasmal 105
    proteins in synovial fluid *25*
    protozoal 106
    rickettsial 105
    viral 106
  osteoarthritis
    clinical signs 83–4
    diagnosis 84
    management 84–9
    pathogenesis 83
  physical examination 82
  rheumatoid
    anti-canine distemper virus antibodies 25
    autoantibodies *25*, 92
    clinical signs 91
    diagnosis *89*, 91–2
    prognosis *96*
    proteins in synovial fluid *25*
    rheumatoid factor role 92
  synovial biopsy 82
  synovial fluid analysis 82
Arthrocentesis 21–3
  carpus 282
Arthrodesis 158–9
  carpus 286, 287
    pancarpal **289–90**
    partial **291**
  elbow 260
  metacarpophalangeal joint 297, **302**
  proximal interphalangeal joint 299, **306**
  shoulder 228, **246–8**
  stifle 373
  tarsus **412–13, 416–17**
  wire 166
Arthrography 9, 115
  biceps tendon *223*
  shoulder 217
Arthroplasty
  elbow 173
  hip 173, 317–18, **338–46**
  implant failure 173–4
Arthroscopy 151, 158
  advantages 184
  biopsy *184*

Index

carpus *189*
cartilage 187–8
complications 191
draping 185–6
elbow *184, 185, 187, 188, 189, 190,* 250–1, **262–3**
    FCP 257
    OCD *258*
    UAP 255
equipment
    aiming device 182
    arthroscope 177–8
    camera 179
    care 182
    instruments 180–2
    light source 178–9
    monitor 179
    sterilization 182
general procedure 186
hip 311, **325–6**
indications 191
joint distension and irrigation 182–3
ligaments/tendons 189–90
limitations 191
menisci 191
osteoarthritis 84
osteophytes 188
patient preparation 185, 186
postoperative care 186
principles 184–92
recording 179–80
shoulder *184, 187, 188, 189, 190,* 214–15, *217,* 218, 223, *225, 226,* **237**
stifle *187, 188, 189,190,* 350–1, *352, 362,* **378–9**
subchondral bone 190–1
synovial membrane 188–9
tarsus 398–400, *401,* **410–11**
Arthrotomy 151, 156
    in infective arthritis 103
    shoulder 218, **238–9**
    tarsus **408–9**
Articular surgery
    antimicrobial prophylaxis 154
    asepsis 154
    assistants 153
    bandaging 159, 195, 196
    biomaterials 168–76
    cement 174
    closure 157
    draping 154–5
    dressings 159
    goals 151–2
    haemostasis 156
    instrumentation 153
    operating theatre 151–3, 158
    pain management 193–5
    patient evaluation 151
    patient positioning 154
    patient preparation 153–5, 158
    physical rehabilitation 196–9, 202–11
    postoperative management 159, 193–211
    prostheses 171–4
    surgeon preparation 153
    surgical approaches 156–7
    suture anchors 169–71
    suture materials/patterns 157, 168–9
    techniques 156–9
    (*see also* specific procedures)
Aspergillus
    arthritis 105
    fumigatus 43
        arthritis 106
Aspirin 194

Australian Cattle Dog, sesamoid disease 298
Australian Kelpie, sesamoid disease 298
Australian Shepherd Dog, osteopetrosis 61
Autoantibodies
    in arthritis 25
    in myasthenia gravis 127
    (*see also* Antinuclear antibody; Rheumatoid factor)
Azathioprine 95

Backhaus towel clips *161*
Bacterial arthritis *see* Arthritis, infective
Bacteroides 97
Bandaging 159
    postoperative 195–6
    technique 202–3
Barden test 310
Barlow test 310
Bassett Hound
    chondrodysplasia 58
    elbow subluxation 53
    open-mouth jaw locking 420
    panosteitis 34
    un-united anconeal process 254
Beagle, chondrodysplasia punctata *59*
Bearded Collie, radial head luxation 252
Bell–Tawse procedure 253
Bernese Mountain Dog
    fragmented medial coronoid process 255
    open-mouth jaw locking 420
    polyarthritis/meningitis syndrome 94
    shoulder osteochondrosis 216
Biceps tendon
    arthroscopy *190,* 224, *227*
    avulsion *227*
    diagnostic imaging 223
    disorders *115*
    medial luxation 221
    rupture *190,* 224
    tendinitis/tenosynovitis 222–4
    tenotomy/tenodesis **244–5**
Biomaterials
    joint prostheses 173–4
    joint stabilization 171–2
    ligament prostheses 171
    polymethylmethacrylate 174
    porcine SIS 175
    prospects 175
    suture 168–9
    suture anchors 169–71
    toggle pins 171
Biomechanics of joints 147–8
    effects on healing 149
    stifle 353, 357–8
Biopsy
    bone *130*
    nerve 137
    synovial 7, 25, 82, 91
Bisection technique
    radius/ulna **71**
    tibia **79**
Blastomyces dermatitidis 42
    arthritis 106
Block vertebrae 62
Bone
    allograft *131*
    biopsy *130*
    cement 174
    cutters 165
    cysts *129*
        aneurysmal 47–8
        unicameral 47

Index

diseases and disorders 34–49, 50–80
    genetically determined 58–64
    growth plate injuries 50–8
    hyperostotic 34–43
    osteopenic 43–8
growth plates, premature closure 50–7
medullary infarcts 40
radiographic changes 19–20
rasps 165
scoops 165
subchondral, arthroscopy 190–1
tumours in dogs *128–9*
(see also specific bones and disorders)
Border Collie
    metaphyseal osteopathy 36
    shoulder osteochondrosis 216
Borrelia burgdorferi 24, 92
    arthritis 104
Boston Terrier
    craniomandibular osteopathy 38
    humeroulnar luxation 251
Boxer
    cranial cruciate ligament disease 359
    hypertrophic osteopathy 39
    hypothyroid dwarfism 64
    metaphyseal osteopathy 36
    open-mouth jaw locking 420
    polyarthritis/meningitis syndrome 94
    radial head luxation 252
    stifle osteochondrosis 351
Brachial plexus
    avulsion 141
    neuritis 141
    tumours 141, 228
Brucella 92
    abortus, arthritis 101
Bull Terrier
    multiple enchondromatosis 61
    radial head luxation 252
Bulldog
    achondroplasia 60
    humeroulnar luxation 251
    medial patellar luxation 354
    radial head luxation 252
Bullmastiff, radial head luxation 252
Bupivacaine 186, 194
Burmese cat, osteochondroma 60
Burrs 165
Butorphanol 193, 194
BVA/KC hip dysplasia scheme 314

Cairn Terrier
    craniomandibular osteopathy 38
    Legg–Calvé–Perthes disease 318
Calicivirus arthritis 106
Canine distemper virus 25, 34, 36
Capsulorrhaphy 168–9
    hip 321, **347**
    thermal, shoulder 226
Carbocaine 194
Carboplatin *131*
Carnelian Bear Dog, pituitary dwarfism 64
Carpal valgus *53*, 58, *59, 70, 73*
    surgery 54, **69–70**
Carprofen *86*, 87, 193, 195
Carpus
    abductor pollicis longus tendon injury 283
    accessory carpal bone luxation/subluxation 284–5
    anatomy 281
    arthrocentesis 282
    arthrodesis *158*, 286, 287
        pancarpal **289–90**
        partial **291**
    arthroscopy 22, *189*
    developmental disorders 282
    dorsal radiocarpal ligament sprain 283
    flexor carpi ulnaris tendon strain 284
    flexural deformity *116,* 282
    fractures 287
    growth plate disorders 282
    hyperextension 116, 282, 286
    lameness diagnosis 282
    luxation/subluxation 283–4, 285–6, *287*
    radial collateral ligament rupture 285
    radiographic views, stressed 11
    shearing injuries 287
    short radial collateral ligament
        enthesopathy 283
        sprain 283
    soft tissue injuries 282–4
    sprains 283, 284
    superficial palmar fascia tears 284
Cartilage
    arthroscopy 187–8
    composition 145–6
    healing and remodelling 148
    metabolism 83
    microstructure 146–7
    proteins in arthritis 24–5
    retained cores 52
    synthesis 147
Caudal cruciate ligament rupture 367
Cavalier King Charles Spaniel, syringomyelia 137
Cefazolin 174
Central tarsal bone anomaly 400
Cerclage wire 166
Cervical spondylopathy and nerve root compression 139
Chemotherapy for osteosarcoma *131, 132*
Chihuahua, humeroulnar luxation 251
Chisels 165
Chlamydia 92
    arthritis 97, 105
    trachomatis 93
Chloramphenicol 105
Chondrodysplasia 58
Chondrodysplasia punctata *59*
Chondroitin sulphate 88
Chondromalacia *187*
Chondrosarcoma
    in cats 134
    in dogs *128*, 132
    and osteochondromatosis 60
Chow Chow
    cranial cruciate ligament disease 359
    fragmentation of the medial coronoid process 255
    myotonia congenita 125
Ciclosporin 95
Cisplatin *131*
Clindamycin 105, 142
Clumber Spaniel
    osteochondrodysplastic dwarfism 58
    pyruvate dehydrogenase deficiency 125
Coaptation 195–6
Coccidioides immitis 42
    arthritis 106
Cocker Spaniel, humeroulnar luxation 251
Codeine 194
Codman's triangle 20
Colchicine 95
Collagen, autoantibodies 25
Compound muscle action potential (CMAP) 137
Computed tomography 27–8
    elbow 255

Index

infective arthritis 100
lung metastases 131
osteoarthritis 84
temporomandibular joint 419
Corn 294
Coxofemoral joint see Hip
Cranial cruciate ligament
  anatomy and function 357
  arthroscopy 190, 362
  biomechanics 357–8
  disease
    aetiopathogenesis 358
    in cats 366–7
    clinical examination 359–60
    clinical features 359
    complications 366
    diagnostic imaging 360–3
    postoperative rehabilitation 366
    prognosis 366
    prostheses 171
    synovial fluid analysis 362
    treatment 363–5
  rupture 190, 358, 366
    and patellar luxation 356
Cranial draw test 5, 360
Cranial tibial thrust 357–8
Craniomandibular osteopathy 37–9, 420
Crepitus 5
Crimp clamping 172
Crucial ligaments see Caudal crucial ligament; Cranial crucial ligament
Cryotherapy 194, 195
Cryptococcus neoformans 43
  arthritis 106
Cubital varus 58, 59
Curettes 165
Cyclophosphamide 95, 106
Cysts
  bone 47–8, 129
  extradural 139
Cytokines 148
Cytology, synovial fluid 23–4

Dachshund
  chondrodysplasia 58
  hypochondroplasia 59
  metaphyseal chondrodysplasia 59
  osteopetrosis 61
  tarsal varus 57
DeBakey dissecting forceps 161, 162
Deep digital flexor tendon failure 300
Deformities in lameness 3
Denervation of the hip 317
Deracoxib 86, 193
Digits
  amputation 297
  examination 295–6
  radiographic views, dorsopalmar/dorsoplantar 11
  (see also Distal limb; Toes)
Disarticulators 164
Discospondylitis 140
Dissecting forceps 162
Distal denervating disease 138
Distal interphalangeal joint
  collateral ligament repair **307–8**
  deep digital flexor tendon failure 300
  luxation 299–300
Distal limb
  anatomy 292–3
  clinical examination 293–6
  joint luxations 297, 299–300

radiography 296
sesamoid disease 298–9
surgery 297, **301–8**
Dobermann
  bone cysts 47
  craniomandibular osteopathy 38
  flexor carpi ulnaris contracture 116
  osteosarcoma 129
  panosteitis 34
Dorsal radiocarpal ligament sprain 283
Doxorubicin 131
Doxycycline 105
Drainage of infected joints 102–3
Dressings 159
Drills 165
'Dropped toe' 296, 299
Dwarfism 52, 58–60, 64
Dysostoses 62–3

Ectrodactyly 62
Ehmer sling 195, 196, 320–1
Ehrlichia 92
  arthritis 105
Elbow
  anatomy 249–50
  arthrodesis 158, 260
  arthroscopy 22, 184, 185, 187, 188, 189, 190, 250, 257, 259, **262–3**
  collateral ligament repair **274**
  computed tomography 28
  degenerative changes 27
  dysplasia
    FCP 255–8, **279–80**
    OCD 258–9, **279–80**
    UAP 254–5, **275–6, 277**
  fragmented coronoid process 28
  incongruity from growth plate damage 259–60
  ligaments 249–50
  luxation 60, 62
    closed reduction **273**
    congenital 251–3
    traumatic 253
  nerves 250
  osteochondritis dissecans 28
  osteochondroma 60
  panosteitis 35
  postoperative care 200
  prostheses 173, 260
  radiographic views
    caudocranial/craniocaudal 11
    flexed lateral 10
  replacement 260
  subluxation 55, 56, 57, 58–9, 62, 75, 259
  surgery 54
  surgical approaches 156, 251
    caudal **269–70**
    caudolateral **264–6**
    medial **267–8**
    'open-book' **271–2**
    transolecranon **269–70**
Electromyography 136
Electrosurgery 167
Enchondrodystrophy 59, 60
Endocrine disorders and muscle disease 123
Endosteal osteosarcoma 128
English Pointer, enchondrodystrophy 59, 60
Enthesophytes, stifle 361
Epidural analgesia 194
Epiphysiolysis 319
Erosive feline chronic progressive polyarthritis 89, 96
Erosive polyarthritis of Greyhounds 89, 92, 96

Index

Erysipelothrix rhusiopathiae arthritis 100, 101
Erythromycin 93, 105
Escherichia coli in surgical wounds 154
Esmarch bandage *159*
Essential fatty acids in osteoarthritis 88
Etodolac *86*
Excision arthroplasty rasp *165*
Exercise, control in osteoarthritis 85, 315
    (*see also* Physical rehabilitation)
Extensor carpi radialis avulsion 115–16
External skeletal fixation
    and ostectomy **71, 72**
    and osteotomy **77–8, 79–80**
    for stifle luxation 370–1

FCP *see* Fragmentation of the medial coronoid process
Feline chronic progressive polyarthritis *89,* 92, 93, *96*
Feline infectious peritonitis 106
Feline leukaemia virus 60, 62, 93, 106, 133
Feline metaphyseal osteopathy 319
Feline syncytium-forming virus 93, 106
Femoral head and neck excision (FHNE) arthroplasty 317, **338**
Femorotibial joint *see* Stifle
Femur, horizontal beam view 12
Fentanyl *121,* 193
Fibrosarcoma
    in cats 134
    in dogs *129,* 132
Fibula *see* Tibia/Fibula
Firocoxib *86*
Flexor carpi ulnaris
    contracture 116
    laceration 116
    tendon strain 116, 284
Foot
    conditions affecting 294
    surgical considerations 297
Foot bag *155*
Foot pad, conditions 294–5
Forceps 162
Fractures
    carpus 287
    sesamoids 298
    tarsus 402
Fragmentation of the medial coronoid process (FCP)
    aetiology and pathogenesis 255–6
    arthroscopy 257, **263**
    clinical signs 256
    pathology 256
    radiography 256–7
    surgery 258, **279–80**

Gait analysis 5–6, 31–3
Gastrocnemius muscle avulsion 118, 372, *404, 405*
Gelpi retractors *153,* 163
Gentamicin-impregnated beads/sponges 102
Genu recurvatum 57–8
Genu valgum 57, 356
Genu varum 57
German Shepherd Dog
    bone cysts 47
    carpal hyperextension 282
    fragmented medial coronoid process 255
    glycogenosis 124
    osteochondrodysplastic dwarfism 58
    osteosarcoma 129
    panosteitis 34
    pituitary dwarfism 64
    stifle osteochondrosis 351
    un-united anconeal process 254

German Short-haired Pointer, polyarthritis/meningitis syndrome 94
Giant Schnauzer, hypothyroid dwarfism 64
Gigli saw 164
Glenohumeral ligament, rupture *190*
Glucocorticoid excess and myopathy *124*
Glucosamine 87–8
Glycogenosis 124
Gold aurothiomalate 95
Golden Retriever
    cranial cruciate ligament disease 359
    fragmentation of the medial coronoid process 255
    open-mouth jaw locking 420
    osteochondritis dissecans 258
    osteosarcoma 129
    panosteitis 34
    shoulder osteochondrosis 216
    stifle osteochondrosis 351
Gracey-type scaler *165*
Gracilis muscle
    contracture 118
    injuries 117–18
Graft passers 163–4
Great Dane
    angular limb deformity 53
    bone cysts 47
    cranial cruciate ligament disease 359
    craniomandibular osteopathy 38
    genu valgum 57
    metaphyseal osteopathy 36
    osteosarcoma 129
    panosteitis 34
    shoulder osteochondrosis 216
    stifle osteochondrosis 351
    un-united anconeal process 254
Great Pyrenees, osteochondrodysplastic dwarfism 58
Greyhound
    carpal sprain injury 284
    carpal subluxation 283
    digital amputation 297
    distal interphalangeal joint luxation 299, 300
    dorsal radiocarpal ligament sprain 283
    extensor carpi radialis avulsion 115
    flexor carpi ulnaris tendon strain 284
    gracilis muscle injury 117
    palmar fascial tears 284
    papilloma 295
    sesamoid disease 298
    short radial collateral ligament enthesiopathy 283
    tensor fasciae latae injury 116
    toe injuries 295
    triceps rupture 113

Hacksaws 164
Haemangiosarcoma
    in cats 134
    in dogs *128, 129,* 132
Haemarthrosis, cytology 24
Haemostasis
    in arthrotomy 156
    electrosurgical 167
Halsted artery forceps *161,* 162
Hatt spoon *164*
Heat therapy 198
Hemiatrophy 62
Hemimelia 62
Hemivertebrae 60, 62
Hereditary myopathy of Labrador Retrievers 125–6
Hip
    anatomy 309
    arthroscopy 22, 311, **325–6**

Index

dysplasia 58
    aetiopathogenesis 311–12
    clinical signs 312
    differential diagnoses *312*
    management
        diet 315
        drugs 315
        exercise 315
    radiography 12, 312–13
    screening programmes
        BVA/Kennel Club 314
        hip laxity 314
        OFA 314
        Penn-Hip 314
    surgery
        denervation 317
        femoral head and neck excision arthroplasty 317, **338**
        juvenile pubic symphysiodesis 315–16, **333–4**
        palliative 317
        total hip arthroplasty 317–18, **339–46**
        triple pelvic osteotomy 316–17, **335–7**
    ultrasonography 313
epiphysiolysis 319
feline metaphyseal osteopathy 319
Legg–Calvé–Perthes disease 318–19
luxation
    clinical signs 319
    diagnosis 320
    physical examination 319
    prognosis 322
    repair *170*
    treatment
        capsulorrhaphy 321, **347**
        closed reduction 320–1
        hip toggle 322, **349**
        transarticular pinning 321, **348**
manipulation 5, 309–10, 319
palpation 309
postoperative care 200
prostheses 173
radiographic views
    distraction 12
    dorsal acetabular rim 11
    extended/flexed ventrodorsal 310–11
range of motion 5
surgical approaches *156*
    caudal 311, **331–2**
    craniodorsal 311, **327–8**
    dorsal 311, **329–30**
    ventral 311
von Willebrand's heterotopic osteochondrofibrosis 322
Histiocytic sarcoma *128,* 132
Histoplasma capsulatum 42
Hock *see* Tarsus
Hohmann retractors 163
Humeroradial joint *see* Elbow
Humeroulnar joint *see* Elbow
Humerus
    osteochondritis dissecans 258–9
    panosteitis 35
    radiographic views, horizontal beam 10
    (*see also* Elbow)
Hydrotherapy 199
    underwater treadmill technique 210–11
Hydroxychloroquine 95
Hyperinsulinism and myopathy *124*
Hyperparathyroidism
    primary 45
    secondary
        nutritional 43–4, 282
        renal 44–5
Hyperthyroidism in cats and myopathy *124*
Hypertrophic osteodystrophy *see* Metaphyseal osteopathy
Hypertrophic osteopathy 39–40
Hypervitaminosis A in cats 39
Hypoadrenocorticism and myopathy *124*
Hypochondroplasia 59
Hypothyroidism
    and myopathy *124*
    and skeletal abnormalities 64

Iliopsoas muscle injury 117
Imaging in lameness 7, 27–31
    (*see also specific techniques*)
Immune-mediated polyarthritis (IMPA) *see* Arthritis, immune-mediated
Immunofluorescence in muscular dystrophy *122*
Implants 166
    (*see also* Prostheses)
Infantile scurvy *see* Metaphyseal osteopathy
Infraspinatus muscle
    bursal ossification 114, 224–5
    contracture 113–14, 221–2
Inherited myopathy of the Great Dane 126
Instruments *see* Surgical instrumentation *and specific instruments*
Insulin-like growth factor-1, role in cartilage metabolism 148
Interdigital webbing, clinical examination 294–5
Interleukin-1 antagonists 96
Interphalangeal joints
    anatomy 293
    arthroscopy 22
    distal
        deep digital flexor tendon failure 300
        examination 296
        ligament repair **307–8**
        luxation 299–300
    proximal
        arthrodesis **306**
        examination 296
        ligament repair **305**
        luxation 299
Intervertebral disc disease
    magnetic resonance imaging *29*
    treatment/prognosis 139
Irish Setter
    canine leucocyte adhesion deficiency 38
    hypochondroplasia *59*
    metaphyseal osteopathy 36
    open-mouth jaw locking 420
    osteosarcoma 129
Irish Wolfhound
    angular limb deformity 53
    bone cysts 47
    metaphyseal osteopathy 36
    osteosarcoma 129
    shoulder osteochondrosis 216

Jack Russell Terrier, elbow subluxation 53
Jaquette-type scaler *165*
Jaw locking 420–1
Joint capsule
    anatomy and physiology 144, *145*
    closure 157, 168–9
    imbrication 169
    surgical approaches 156–7
    suture materials/patterns 157, 168–9
Joint distractors 164
'Joint mice'
    arthroscopy *184,* 187
    shoulder 216

Index

Joints
    anatomy and physiology 144–8
    biomechanics 147–8
    disease types *18*
    healing and remodelling 148–50
    innervation 138
    lubrication 138
    manipulation 4–5
    prostheses, infection 104
    radiographic changes 18–19
    range of motion 4–5
    salvage 152
    stabilization 152, 171–2
    surgical principles 151–60
    tumours in dogs *128*
    (see also specific joints and procedures)
Juvenile pubic symphysiodesis 315–16, **333–4**
Juxtacortical osteosarcoma *128*

Ketamine 195
Ketoprofen *86*
Kirchner wires 166
'Knocked up' toe *295*, 300

Labrador Retriever
    craniomandibular osteopathy 38
    fragmentation of the medial coronoid process 255
    medial patellar luxation 354
    mucopolysaccharidosis II 64
    open-mouth jaw locking 420
    osteochondritis dissecans 258
    osteochondrodysplastic dwarfism 58, 59
    panosteitis 34
    short radial collateral ligament enthesiopathy 283
    shoulder osteochondrosis 216
    stifle osteochondrosis 351
    supraspinatus mineralization 114
Lameness
    in arthritis 81
    behavioural changes 135
    in chondrodysplasia 58
    clinical approach 1–7
    carpus 282
    in cranial cruciate ligament disease 359, 366
    diagnosis
        electromyography 136
        magnetic resonance imaging 136
        nerve conduction studies 137
    in elbow luxation 55, 60
    in fragmentation of the medial coronoid process 256
    gait analysis 5–6, 293
    history-taking 1–2, 151
    imaging 7
    infra/supraspinatus contracture 113
    in multiple enchondromatosis 61
    neurological causes 135–43
    neurological examination 6
    observation 3
    in osteodystrophy 60
    in osteosarcoma in cats 133
    pain 4
    in patellar luxation 57, 60
    physical examination 2–5
        distal limb 293–4
        manipulation 4
        palpation 3–4, 135
        restraint 2
    in premature growth plate closure 52, 259
    in shoulder problems 213, 216, 222, 227
    supporting leg 6
    swinging leg 6
    in syndactyly 63
    tarsal 397
    treatment planning 7
Langenbeck retractor 163
Lapland Dog, glycogenosis 124
Lateral collateral ligament integrity testing *253*
Lateral/medial collateral ligament repair **274**
Leflunomide 95
Legg–Calvé–Perthes disease 18, 318–19
Leishmania donovani arthritis 106
Lempert rongeurs *165*
Lhaso Apso, achondroplasia 60
Ligaments
    anatomy and physiology 144
    arthroscopy 189–90
    avulsion 157
    elbow 249–50
    healing and remodelling 148
    prostheses 171–3, 402
    repair 157, 285, **274, 301, 305, 307–8**, 402–3
    surgical exposure *156*
    suture materials/patterns 157
    tarsal *396*
    (see also specific ligaments and joints)
Limb
    deformity 362
    hypoplasia 62
    length discrepancy 50, 52, 55, 56, 57,
    -sparing surgery for osteosarcoma *131, 132*
Lincomycin 93, 105
Lining technique
    radius/ulna **71**
    tibia **79**
Lion jaw *see* Craniomandibular osteopathy
Local anaesthetics in joint surgery 194
Long digital extensor tendon avulsion 372
Lower motor neuron (LMN) disease 135, 142
Lung, metastases from osteosarcoma 131
Lyme disease 24, 104–5
Lymphangiography 9
Lymphoma 132

Mach lines 296
Magnetic resonance imaging 28–9
    infective arthritis 100
    meniscal injuries 363
    neurological lameness 136
    osteoarthritis 84
Malignant peripheral nerve sheath tumours 140, 141
Manchester Terrier, Legg–Calvé–Perthes disease 318
Mandible
    hypoplasia 62
    periostitis *see* Craniomandibular osteopathy
    prognathism 60
Mannosidoses 64
Marie's disease *see* Hypertrophic osteopathy
Massage therapy 196–7
Masticatory muscle myopathy 420
Mastiff
    cranial cruciate ligament disease 359
    genu valgum 57
    medial patellar luxation 354
    stifle osteochondrosis 351
Matrix metalloproteinases (MMPs) 148
    in arthropathies 25
Mayo scissors *161*, 162
Mayo–Hegar needle holder *161*, 162
Medial glenohumeral ligament, tear *188*

Index

Medial meniscus luxation *191*
Meglumine antimonate 106
Meloxicam *86*, 193, 195
Meninigitis and immune-mediated polyarthritis *89*, 94
Menisci *see* Stifle
Metacarpals, hypertrophic osteopathy 40
Metacarpophalangeal joint
   anatomy 292–3
   arthrodesis **302**
   arthroscopy 22
   examination 296
   ligament repair **301**
   luxation 297
   range of motion 5
Metaphyseal chondrodysplasia *59*
Metaphyseal dysplasia *see* Metaphyseal osteopathy
Metaphyseal osteopathy 36–7, 52
Methadone 193, 194
Methicillin-resistant *Staphylococcus aureus* infection (MRSA) 103–4
Methotrexate 95
Methylprednisolone 222
Metzenbaum scissors 162
Miniature Pinscher, humeroulnar luxation 251
Miniature Poodle
   chondrodysplasia punctata *59*
   humeroulnar luxation 251
   Legg–Calvé–Perthes disease 318
   medial patellar luxation 354
   osteochondrodysplastic dwarfism 58
   pseudochondroplasia *59*
Miniature Schnauzer
   medullary bone infarcts 40
   myotonia congenita 125
Minocycline 105
Mitochondrial myopathy 125
Möller Barlow's disease *see* Metaphyseal osteopathy
Morphine 193, 194
MRSA 103–4
Mucin clot test 24
Mucolipidosis 64
Mucopolysaccharidoses 63–4
Multilobular osteochondrosarcoma *129*
Multiple cartilaginous exostoses
   in cats *129*, 133–4
   in dogs *129*
Multiple enchondromatosis 61
Muscle(s)
   anatomy and physiology 110
   biopsy 121
   changes in lameness 3
   contracture 111
   contusion 111
   diseases/disorders
      clinical signs 120
      diagnosis 120
      myopathies 120–6
      neuromuscular transmission disorders 126–7
      pelvic limb 116–18
      thoracic limb 113–16
   elbow 250
   injury classification 111
   laceration 111
   response to injury 111
   rupture 111
   strains 111
   surgical principles 111–12
   suture patterns *112*
   tumours in dogs *128*
   (*see also specific muscles and conditions*)
Muscular dystrophies 121–3
Myasthenia gravis 126–7

Mycoplasma
   gateae, arthritis 105
   spumans, arthritis 105
Myelography 138, *139*
Myeloma 132
Myerding retractor 163
Myopathies
   inflammatory 120–1
   non-inflammatory
      in endocrine disorders 123–4
      hereditary myopathy of Labrador Retrievers 125–6
      inherited myopathy of the Great Dane 126
      metabolic disorders 124–5
      muscular dystrophies 121–3
      myotonia 125
Myotatic reflexes 6
Myotonia 125
Myotonia congenita 125

Needle holders 162
Neoplasia *see* Tumours
Neospora 117
   caninum 121, 142
Neostigmine 126
Nerve
   biopsy 137
   conduction studies 137
   entrapment
      clinical signs 138
      diagnosis 138–9
      pain management 139
      treatment/prognosis 139–40
   tumours 140
Nerve root signature *135*
Neuritis 141–2
Neurological examination in lameness 6, 214
Neuromuscular electrical stimulation (NMES) 197–8
   technique 206–7
Neuromuscular junction disease 120, 126–7
Newfoundland
   fragmentation of the medial coronoid process 255
   osteochondrodysplastic dwarfism 58
   stifle osteochondrosis 351
NMES *see* Neuromuscular electrical stimulation
Nocardia 42
   asteroides, arthritis 101, 105
Norberg–Olsson angle *313*
Norwegian Elkhound, osteochondrodysplastic dwarfism 58, 59
Norwegian Forest cat, glycogenosis 124
Nuclear scintigraphy 29–30
   in panosteitis 35
Nutritional supplementation in osteoarthritis 87–9

Obesity, effects on healing 149
OCD *see* Osteochondritis dissecans
OFA hip dysplasia scheme 314
Old English Sheepdog
   mitochondrial myopathy 125
   radial head luxation 252
Operating theatre 152–3
Operative Techniques
   Carpus
      pancarpal arthrodesis **289–90**
      partial arthrodesis **291**
   Distal limb
      DIPJ ligament repair **307–8**
      MCPJ
         arthrodesis **302**
         ligament repair **301**
      PIPJ
         arthrodesis **306**

        ligament repair **305**
        sesamoidectomy **303–4**
   Elbow
        arthroscopy **262–3**
        caudal approach **269–70**
        caudolateral approach **264–6**
        closed reduction of luxations **273**
        collateral ligament repair **274**
        dynamic ulnar osteotomy/ostectomy **277–8**
        FCP and OCD **279–80**
        medial approach **267–8**
        'open-book' approach **271–2**
        transolecranon approach **269–70**
        un-united anconeal process **275–6**
   Hip
        arthroscopy **325–6**
        capsulorrhaphy **347**
        caudal approach **331–2**
        craniodorsal approach **327–8**
        dorsal approach **329–30**
        juvenile pubic symphysiodesis **333–4**
        toggle **349**
        total arthroplasty
            cemented **339–42**
            non-cemented **343–6**
        transarticular pinning **348**
        triple pelvic osteotomy **335–7**
   Radius/ulna
        distal ulnar osteotomy/segmental ostectomy **67–8**
        dynamic lengthening of the radius **77–8**
        dynamic proximal ulnar osteotomy/segmental ostectomy **74–5**
        radius and ulna osteotomy **71–3**
        resection of a partially closed distal radial physis **76**
        stapling the distal radial growth plate **69–70**
   Shoulder
        arthrodesis **246–8**
        arthroscopy **237**
        arthrotomy **238–9**
        caudolateral approach **235–6**
        craniolateral approach **233–4**
        craniomedial approach **231–2**
        lateral stabilization **240–2**
        medial stabilization **243**
        tenotomy/tenodesis of biceps tendon **244–5**
   Stifle
        arthroscopy **378–9**
        lateral fabellotibial suture with self-locking knot **389–90**
        lateral parapatellar approach **375**
        limited medial approach **377**
        medial meniscal release **388**
        medial parapatellar approach **376**
        meniscal inspection **387**
        over-the-top graft **388**
        partial meniscectomy **387**
        rectangular recession trochleoplasty **381–2**
        tibial plateau levelling osteotomy **394–5**
        tibial tuberosity transposition **385–6**
        tibial wedge osteotomy **391–3**
        wedge recession trochleoplasty **383–4**
   Tarsus
        Achilles tendon repair **414–15**
        arthrodesis **416–17**
        arthroscopy **410–11**
        calcaneoquartal arthrodesis **412–13**
        medial arthrotomy **408–9**
        medial malleolar osteotomy and repair **406–7**
   Temporomandibular joint
        surgical approach **422–3**
        zygomatic ostectomy **424**
   Tibia
        osteotomy for tarsal varus/valgus **79–80**
        plateau levelling osteotomy **394–5**

        tuberosity transposition **385–6**
        wedge osteotomy **391–3**
Ortolani test 310
Ostectomy
   for carpal valgus 54
   segmental (partial) 51, 52, **67–8, 74–5**
   ulnar *277*
   zygomatic arch **424**
Osteoarthritis
   arthroscopy 84
   autoantibodies *25*
   cartilage metabolism 83
   clinical signs 83–4
   computed tomography 84
   diagnostic imaging 84
   and fragmentation of the medial coronoid process 256, 258
   hip 311, 312, *313*, 315
   lameness 2
   magnetic resonance imaging 84
   management 84–9
      client education 85
      clinical monitoring 85
      drug treatment 85–7
      exercise control 85
      nutritional supplementation 87–9
      physiotherapy 85
      weight control 85
   in metacarpophalangeal joint 297
   and osteochondritis dissecans 259
   osteophytes 84
   pathogenesis 83
   postoperative exercise 199
   proteins in synovial fluid *25*
   retardation 365
   return to function 201
   scintigraphy 84
   stifle *368*
   synovial fluid 84
   and un-united anconeal process 255
Osteochondritis dissecans (OCD)
   arthroscopy *187, 190, 217, 259,* **263**
   curette *165*
   elbow *28, 190*
      medial humeral condyle 258–9
   and fragmentation of the medial coronoid process 256
      surgery **279–80**
   shoulder *216, 217*
      surgery **238–9**
   talus *397,* 399, 401–2
      surgery **408–9**
Osteochondrodysplasias 58–62
Osteochondrodysplastic dwarfism 58–60
Osteochondroma in cats 60–1
Osteochondromatosis 60, 133
Osteochondrosarcoma 420
Osteochondrosis
   shoulder 215–18
   stifle 351–3
Osteodystrophy II *see* Metaphyseal osteopathy
Osteogenesis imperfecta 61
Osteolysis *30*
Osteoma
   in cats 134
   in dogs *129*
Osteomalacia 19
   in rickets 46
Osteomyelitis 40–3
   acute haematogenous 40–1
   acute post-traumatic 41
   chronic post-traumatic 41–2
   fungal 42–3, 105
   in infective arthritis 100
   temporomandibular joint 420

Index

Osteopenia
    causes *19*
    in mannosidosis 64
    in osteogenesis imperfecta 61
    in rickets 46
    in secondary hyperparathyroidism 44, 45
Osteopetrosis 19, 61–2
Osteophytes
    arthroscopy 188
    elbow *188*
    in fragmentation of the medial coronoid process 255
    in osteoarthritis 84, 313
    removal 157
    shoulder *188*
    stifle *188*, 361
Osteoporosis 19
Osteosarcoma
    in cats *129*, 133
    in dogs
        and osteochondromatosis 60
        breeds affected 129
        diagnosis 129–30
        differential diagnoses 130
        metastases 130
        radiographic appearance 129, *130*
        staging 130
        treatment/prognosis 131–2
    shoulder 227
Osteosclerosis fragilis *see* Osteopetrosis
Osteotomes 165
Osteotomy 51–2
    for carpal valgus 54
    cuneiform 51
    distal ulnar **67–8**
    for fragmentation of the medial coronoid process 258, *279*
    hip 151
    ilial **336**
    ischial **335**
    to lengthen radius 56
    for ligament/tendon exposure *156*
    medial malleolar **406–7**
    oblique 51
    opening wedge 51, 57, **80**
    proximal ulnar **74–5**
    pubic **335**
    radial and ulnar **71–3**, 152
    for radial head luxation 252
    repair *272*
    for stifle instability 355
    for tarsal valgus/varus 57
    tibial **79–80**, 368, **391–5**
    transverse 51
    triple pelvic 316–17, **335–6**
    for un-united anconeal process 255, **275–6**, *277*
Oxacillin 154

Pain
    in hip dysplasia 311
    in lameness 4, 6, 135
    management
        in cats 195
        in nerve entrapment 132
        in osteosarcoma *131*
        postoperative 194
        preoperative 193–4
Palmar fascial tears 284
Pannus 187, *188*
Panosteitis
    aetiology/pathogenesis 34
    breeds associated 34
    diagnostic imaging 35

differential diagnoses 35
    history/clinical signs 34–5
    treatment/prognosis 36
Papilloma in foot webbing 295
Paracetamol 194
    plus codeine 86
Paraneoplastic neuropathy 137–8
Parosteal osteosarcoma *128*
Pasteurella multocida
    arthritis 97, 101
Patella
    anatomy/biomechanics 353
    luxation 57, 58, 60
        aetiopathogenesis 353–4
        lateral 356
        medial
            in cats 356
            diagnostic imaging 354
            grading 354
            prognosis 356
            surgery 354–6, **381–6**
Patellar tendon rupture 371
Patellectomy 355
Pekingese
    achondroplasia *59*, 60
    humeroulnar luxation 251
    radial head luxation 252
D-Penicillamine
Penn-Hip scheme 314
Penrose drains 163
Pentosan polysulphate 87
Peptostreptococcus arthritis 101
Periosteal osteosarcoma *128*
Persian cat, mannosidosis 64
Pes varus, osteotomy **80**
Phenylbutazone 86
Phocomelia 62
Physes *see* Bone, growth plates
Physical rehabilitation 196–9
    in arthritis 85, 103
    heat 198
    hydrotherapy 199
        technique 210–11
    massage 196–7
    neuromuscular electrical stimulation 197–8
        technique 206–7
    ROM exercises 195, 197
        technique 204–5
    stretching exercises 195, 197
    walks 198–9
    weightshifting exercises, technique 208–9
Pituitary dwarfism 64–5
Plantar ligament degeneration 403–4
PMMA *see* Polymethylmethacrylate
Polyarteritis nodosa *89*, 94, 97
Polyarthritis *see* Arthritis *and specific conditions*
Polyarthritis/meningitis syndrome *89*, 94, 97
Polyarthritis/polymyositis syndrome *89*, 94, 97
Polydactyly 62–3
Polymethylmethacrylate (PMMA)
    antibiotic-impregnated beads 102, 174
    cement 174
Polymyositis *89*, 94
Pomeranian
    humeroulnar luxation 251
    radial head luxation 252
Popliteal tendon avulsion 372
Popliteus muscle avulsion 118
Porcine SIS 173, 175
Postoperative care
    after arthroscopy 186, 218
    bandaging 159, 196, 202–3
    chronic management 199

Index

coaptation 195
cryotherapy 194
dressings 159
after elbow surgery 200
after hip surgery 200, 318
muscle repair 112
pain management 194
  in cats 195
patient follow-up 196
physical rehabilitation 196–9
  after cranial cruciate ligament surgery 366
  heat 198
  hydrotherapy 199, 210–11
  massage 196–7
  neuromuscular electrical stimulation 197–8, 206–7
  ROM exercises 195, 197, 204–5
  stretching exercises 195, 197
  walks 198–9
  weightshifting exercises 208–9
principles 159
return to function 201
after shoulder surgery 218, 220
slings 195, 196
after stifle surgery 200
after temporomandibular joint luxation 419
(see also within individual Operative Techniques)
Power tools 166
Prednisolone 95, 106, 121, 139
Premedication 193-194
Proprioception 6
Proprionibacterium arthritis 101
Prostheses
  elbow 173
  failure 173–4
  hip 173, 317
  ligaments 171–3
  stifle extracapsular 171
  (see also Implants)
Proteus arthritis 101
Proximal interphalangeal joint
  arthrodesis 299, **306**
  ligament repair **305**
  luxation 299
Pseudochondroplasia 59
Pseudomonas aeruginosa arthritis 101
Pug
  achondroplasia 59
  humeroulnar luxation 251
Pyrenean Mountain Dog
  polydactyly 62–3
  shoulder osteochondrosis 216
Pyridostigmine 126
Pyrimethamine 142
Pyruvate dehydrogenase deficiency 125

Quadriceps contracture 117
  prevention 195

Radial collateral ligament rupture 285
Radiography 8–20
  in arthritis 99
  contrast 9
  distal limb 296
  equipment 8
  hip 310–11, 312–13
  indications 9
  interpretation 13–20
    bone 19–20
    joints 18–19
    soft tissue 17–18

safety 9–10
  terminology 15–17
stifle 360–1
temporomandibular joint 418
views 9–12
Radiotherapy for osteosarcoma *131, 132*
Radius/Ulna
  anatomy 249–50
  bone cyst *47*
  bone graft *131*
  dynamic lengthening **77–8**
  fracture 286
  growth plates 52
    partially closed, resection **76**
    premature closure 52–4, 255, 259–60
    stapling **69–70**
  limb-sparing surgery *131*
  metaphyseal osteopathy 37
  ostectomy 56
    segmental ulnar **67–8, 74–5**
    for UAP *277*
  osteotomy 56, **71–3**, 252
    distal ulnar **67–8**
    dynamic **277–8**
    for FCP 258
    proximal ulnar **74–5**, 255
    repair *272*
    for UAP **275–6**, *277*
  radius curvus 52–3
  retained cartilaginous cores 52, 54–5
  synostosis 56–7
Range of motion (ROM) *see* Joints; Physical rehabilitation
Rat-tooth dissecting forceps *161, 162*
Rectus femoris muscle transplantation 355
Rehabilitation *see* Physical rehabilitation
Resectors 164
Retractors 162–3
Rhabdomyosarcoma *128*
Rheumatoid arthritis *see* Arthritis, rheumatoid
Rheumatoid factor 25, 92
Rhodesian Ridgeback, fragmentation of the medial coronoid process 255
Rickets 45–7
  comparison with enchondrodystrophy 60
Rickettsia 92
Robinson sling 195
Rongeurs 165
Rottweiler
  cranial cruciate ligament disease 359
  fragmentation of the medial coronoid process 255
  sesamoid disease 298
  supraspinatus mineralization 114
  un-united anconeal process 254
Rough Collie
  carpal hyperextension injury 286
  radial head luxation 252

Salmonella 93
Samoyed
  osteochondrodysplastic dwarfism 59
  stifle osteochondrosis 351
'Sand ulcers' 295
Sarcoma
  histiocytic *128, 132*
  synovial cell, in dogs *128, 132*
Saws 164
Scalpels 161, *162*
Scapula, luxation 221
  (*see also* Shoulder)
Scapulohumeral joint *see* Shoulder

435

Index

Scintigraphy
    bone tumours 131
    fragmentation of the medial coronoid process 258
    infective arthritis 100
    osteoarthritis 84
    osteochondritis dissecans 259
Scissors 162
Scottish Deerhound
    hypothyroid dwarfism 64
    osteochondrodysplastic dwarfism 58
    osteosarcoma 129
Scottish Fold cat osteodystrophy 60
Scottish Terrier
    craniomandibular osteopathy 37
    hypochondroplasia *59*
Semitendinosis muscle contracture 118
Senn retractor 163
Sequestra in chronic post-traumatic osteomyelitis 41
Serratus ventralis muscle, rupture 113
Sesamoidectomy 299, **303–4**
Sesamoids
    anatomy 292–3
    bipartite 298
    disease in young dogs 298
    fractures 298
    radiographic changes 18
    removal **303–4**
    tripartite 298
Shar Pei
    familial amyloidosis *89, 97*
    'fever' 95
    flexor carpi ulnaris contracture 116
Shetland Sheepdog
    humeroulnar luxation 251
    shoulder luxation 215
    tarsal valgus 57
Shigella 93
Shih Tzu, achondroplasia *59, 60*
Short radial collateral ligament
    enthesiopathy 283
    sprain 283
Short radius syndrome *256*
Shoulder
    anatomy 212–13
    arthrodesis *158*, 228, **246–8**
    arthroscopy 21–2, *184, 187, 188, 15b.6, 190*, 214–15, 223, **237**
    arthrotomy **238–9**
    capsulorrhaphy 226
    clinical examination 213–14
    dysplasia 215
    instability 225–6
    luxation 215
        biceps brachii tendon 221
        scapula 222
        scapulohumeral 218–20
    muscle disease
        infraspinatus/supraspinatus contracture 221–2
        teres minor myopathy 222
    neoplasia 227–8
    osteochondritis dissecans **238–9**
    osteochondrosis
        diagnostic imaging 216–17
        history-taking 216
        treatment 217–18
    osteosarcoma *133*
    radiographic views
        fractures 10
        skyline 10
    range of motion *248*
    stabilization
        lateral **240–2**
        medial **243**

    surgical approaches 214
        caudolateral **235–6**
        craniolateral **233–4**
        craniomedial **231–2**
    surgical exposure *156*
    tendon/ligament disease
        biceps tendon
            rupture/avulsion 226–7
            sheath rupture 224
        bicipital tendinitis/tenosynovitis 222–4
        infraspinatus bursal ossification 224–5
        scapulohumeral instability 225–6
        supraspinatus mineralizing tendinopathy 224
    tenotomy/tenodesis **244–5**
    un-united caudal glenoid 218
Siamese cat, osteochondroma 60
Sinography/fistulography 9
Sjögren's syndrome 94
Skeletal maturity and age 52
Skeletal scurvy *see* Metaphyseal osteopathy
Skin clipping for surgery 154
Skye Terrier, dwarfism 52
Slings 195
    Ehmer *195*, 196, *320–1*
    for shoulder luxation 219, *220*
    Velpeau 196, *220, 226*
Sodium stilbogluconate 106
Soft tissues, radiographic changes 17–18
    (*see also* Ligaments; Muscle; Tendons)
Spencer Wells artery forceps *161*, 162
Spine
    cysts 139
    fractures/luxations 139
    (*see also* intervertebral disc disease)
Spiramycin 105
Spitz, pituitary dwarfism 64
Spondylosis *39*, 139
Sporothrix schenkii, arthritis 106
Springer Spaniel, glycogenosis 124
St Bernard
    cranial cruciate ligament disease 359
    fragmentation of the medial coronoid process 255
    genu valgum 57
    metaphyseal osteopathy 36
    osteochondrodysplastic dwarfism 58
    osteosarcoma 129
    un-united anconeal process 254
Staffordshire Bull Terrier
    medial patellar luxation 354
    sesamoid disease 298
Staphylococcus 100
    aureus
        arthritis 101
        methicillin-resistant 103–4
    intermedius, arthritis 97, 101
    in surgical wounds 154
Stapling
    for carpal valgus 54, **69–70**
    distal radial growth plate **69–70**
Stifle
    anatomy 353, 357, 358–9
    arthrodesis 117, *158*, 373
    arthroscopy 22–3, *187, 188, 189, 190*, 350–1, **378–9**
    biomechanics 353, 357–8
    caudal cruciate ligament disease 367
    collateral ligament rupture 368–9
    cranial cruciate ligament disease 357–67
    cranial tibial thrust reduction 365
    gastrocnemius muscle avulsion 372
    infection 98, 99, 103
    long digital extensor tendon avulsion 372
    luxation 369–71
    magnetic resonance imaging 29

Index

manipulation 5
menisci 144
    anatomy 358–9
    arthroscopy 191
    injury 365
    surgery **387–8**
nuclear scintigraphy *30*
osteochondrosis
    aetiopathogenesis 351
    clinical findings 351
    diagnostic imaging 351–2
    prognosis 353
    treatment 352
patellar luxation 353–7
patellar tendon rupture 371
popliteal tendon avulsion 372
postoperative care 200
    ROM exercises *204*
radiographic views, tibial plateau angle 12
stabilization
    materials *172*
    techniques 365, **384–90**
    surgical approaches *156*
        lateral parapatellar **375**
        limited medial **377**
        medial parapatellar **376**
tibial deformity 367–8
tibial plateau levelling osteotomy 365, **394–5**
tibial tuberosity transposition 355, **385–6**
tibial wedge osteotomy 365, **391–3**
trochleoplasty 355, **381–4**
Strains 111, 116
Streptococcus
    arthritis 100
    pneumoniae, arthritis 97
Suction 167
Sulfasalazine 95
Superficial digital flexor tendon luxation 405
Supraspinatus muscle
    contracture 113–14
    mineralization 114–15, 224
Surgical draping 154–5
Surgical instrumentation 153
    basic kit 161–2
    electrosurgery 167
    lighting 166
    periarticular implants 166
    retractors 162–3
    specialist orthopaedic 163–6
    suction 167
    (*see also* specific instruments)
Sussex Spaniel, pyruvate dehydrogenase deficiency 125
Suture anchors 169–71
    (*see also* Tissue anchors)
Suture materials *168*
    failure 172
    joint capsule closure 157, 168–9
    ligament repair 157
    sterilization 171–2
    stifle stabilization 171–2
    tendon repair 112
Suture patterns
    for muscle *112*
    for tendons *113*, 168
Swellings in lameness 3–4
Syndactyly 63
Synostosis
    radius/ulna 56–7
Synovial cell sarcoma
    arthroscopy *187*
    in cats 134
    in dogs *128*, 132
Synovial effusion in lameness 3–4

Synovial fluid
    assessment 7, 362
        appearance 23
        biochemistry 24–5
        cytology 23–4
        immunology 25
        microbiology 24
    collection 21–3
    composition 144–5
    in infective arthritis 100–1
    in osteoarthritis 82, 84
    sample handling 23
Synovial membrane 144
    arthroscopy 188–9
    biopsy 7, 25, 82, 91
    healing and remodelling 148
    histology in arthritis 1–2
    myxoma *128*, 132
    sarcoma 228
Synoviocytes 144, 145
Synovium *see* Synovial membrane
Syringomyelia 137
Systemic lupus erythematosus
    clinical signs 94
    diagnosis *89*, 94
    prognosis *96*

Talus *396*
    osteochondritis dissecans *397*, 399, 401–2
    surgery **408–9**
Tarsal valgus 57
Tarsal varus 57, 58
Tarsus
    Achilles tendon injuries 404–5
        rupture repair **414–15**
    anatomy 396–7
    arthrodesis *158*, **412–13, 416–17**
    arthroscopy *22*, 23, 398–400, **410–11**
    arthrotomy **408–9**
    central tarsal bone anomaly 400
    collateral ligament injury 402–3
    congenital conditions 400
    developmental conditions 401–2
    diagnostic imaging 398
    dorsal ligament rupture 404
    fractures 402
    hyperextension 400
    medial malleolar osteotomy and repair **406–7**
    osteochondritis dissecans 399, 401–2
    physical examination 397–8
    plantar ligament degeneration 403–4
    radiographic views
        dorsoplantar 12
        plantarodorsal 12
    superficial digital flexor tendon luxation 405
    surgical approaches 352
    torsion 400
Temporomandibular joint
    anatomy 418
    ankylosis 420
    craniomandibular osteopathy 37–9, 420
    diagnostic imaging 418–19
    fracture callus 420
    jaw locking 420–1
    luxation 419
    masticatory muscle myopathy 420
    neoplasia 420
    osteomyelitis 420
    surgical approach **422–3**
    zygomatic ostectomy **424**

Index

Tendons
    anatomy and physiology 110, 144
    arthroscopy 189–90
    elbow 250
    healing 112
    injuries 112
    surgical exposure *156*
    surgical principles 112–14
    suture materials 112
    suture patterns *113*, 168
    (see also specific tendons and joints)
Tenotomy/tenodesis of biceps brachii tendon **244–5**
Tensor fasciae latae muscle injuries 116
Tepoxalin *86*
Teres minor myopathy 222
Tetracycline 105
Thermal capsulorrhaphy, shoulder *226*
Tiamulin 105
Tibia/Fibula
    deformity 367–8, 400
    infarcts *40*
    osteomyelitis *41*
    osteotomy **79–80, 391–5**
    premature growth plate closure 57
Tibial compression test 360
Tibial drift 57
Tibial plateau angle 57
    measurement *12*, 361–2
Tibial tuberosity transposition 355, **385–6**
Tibial valgus/varus, surgery *54*
Tissue anchors 166
Tissue forceps 162
Toenails, clinical examination 295
Toes
    'bunched' 293
    'dropped' *296*, 299
    'knocked-up' *295*, 300
Toggle pins *170*, 171
Tolfenamic acid *86*
Total joint arthroplasty
    elbow 173
    hip 173, 317–18, **339–46**
    implant failure 173–4
Towel clamps 161
Toxoplasma 117
    gondii 121
Toy Pinscher, pituitary dwarfism 64
Toy Poodle
    multiple enchondromatosis 61
    shoulder luxation 215
Tramadol 194
Transarticular pinning for hip luxation 321, **348**
Travers retractor 162
Triceps muscle, rupture 113
Trimethoprim/sulphonamide 142
Triple pelvic osteotomy 316–17, **335–6**
Trochleoplasty
    rectangular recession 355, **381–2**
    trochlear chondroplasty 355
    wedge recession 355, **383–4**
Tumour necrosis factor antagonists 96

Tumours
    bone 128–32, 133–4
    cats *129*
    dogs *128–9*
    joints *128*, 132
    muscle *128*
    nerve 140, 141
    shoulder 227–8
    spine 140
    temporomandibular joint 420
    (see also specific tumour types)
Turmeric extract 88–9
Tylosin 105

Ulna *see* Radius/Ulna
Ultrasonography 30–1
    hip dysplasia 313
Ultrasound heat therapy 198
Un-united anconeal process (UAP) 254–5
    surgery **275–6, *277***
Un-united caudal glenoid 218

Vaccination-associated immune-mediated polyarthritis 93, *96*
Vedaprofen *86*
Velpeau sling 195, 196, *220*, *226*
Vertebral tumours 140
Vitamin D metabolism *46*
von Willebrand's heterotopic osteochondrofibrosis 322

Walks 198–9
Weight control
    in hip dysplasia 315
    in osteoarthritis 85
Weimaraner
    bone cysts 47
    metaphyseal osteopathy 36
    pituitary dwarfism 64
    polyarthritis/meningitis syndrome 94
Weitlander retractor *162*, 163
Welsh Corgi, hypochondroplasia *59*
West Highland White Terrier
    craniomandibular osteopathy 37
    Legg–Calvé–Perthes disease 318
West retractor *162*, 163
Wire drivers and benders *166*
Wirehaired Dachshund, mucoploysaccharidosis IIIA 64

Yorkshire Terrier
    humeroulnar luxation 251
    Legg–Calvé–Perthes disease 318
    medial patellar luxation 354
    radial head luxation 252

Zygomatic arch, ostectomy **424**

BSAVA Manuals
Best for Orthopaedics

Available Spring 2006

BSAVA Manual of Canine and Feline Musculoskeletal Imaging

Edited by Frances J. Barr and Robert M. Kirberger

- Brand new manual
- Focus on radiology
- Radiographic features of bone and joint disorders
- Normal films for comparison
- High quality illustrations

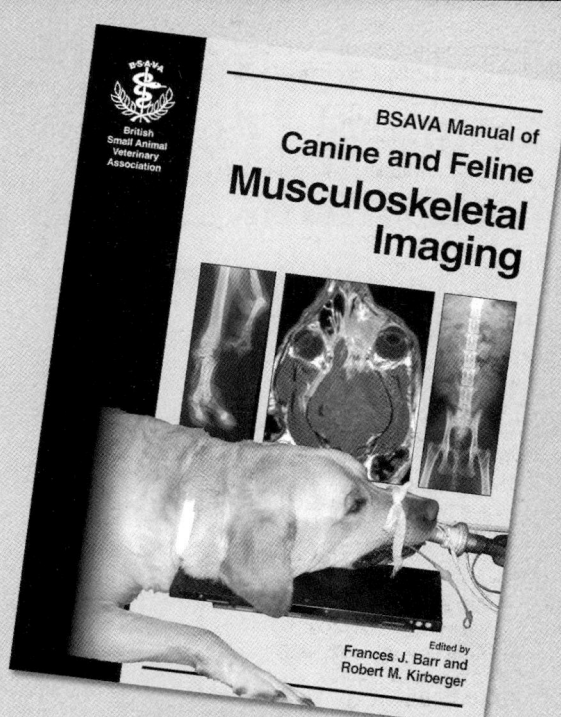

BSAVA Manual of Small Animal Fracture Repair and Management

Edited by Andrew Coughlan and Andrew Miller

- Revised reprint
- Key concepts in fracture fixation and healing
- Emphasis on decision-making and practical advice
- Treatment and prevention of complications
- Specially commissioned drawings in full colour

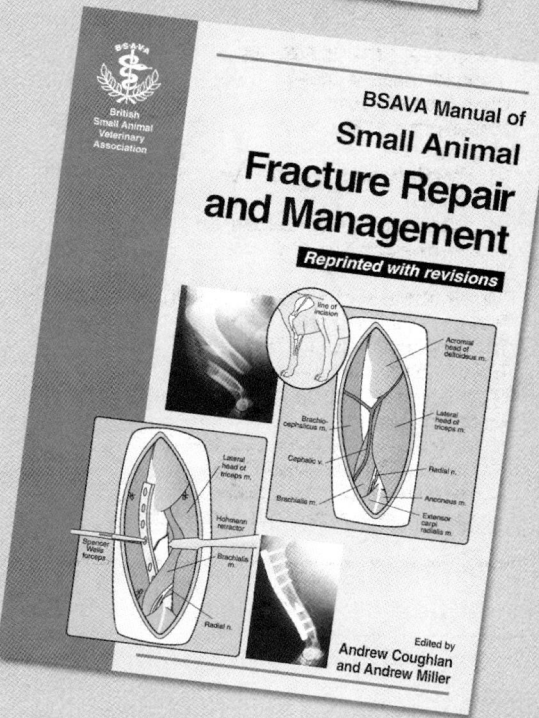

For information and to order please contact us at:
British Small Animal Veterinary Association • Woodrow House
1 Telford Way • Waterwells Business Park • Quedgeley • Gloucester • GL2 2AB
Tel: 01452 726700 • e-mail: customerservices@bsava.com • www.bsava.com

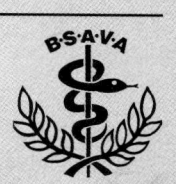

BSAVA Manuals
Best for Soft Tissue Surgery

Brand new titles

BSAVA Manual of Canine and Feline Abdominal Surgery

Edited by John M. Williams and Jacqui D. Niles

- Introductory chapters in Principles of abdominal surgery and Equipment and instrumentation
- System and organ oriented approach
- Step-by-step Operative Techniques
- Chapters on Gastric dilatation and volvulus and Peritonitis
- Specially commissioned full colour illustrations throughout

BSAVA Manual of Canine and Feline Head, Neck and Thoracic Surgery

Edited by Daniel J. Brockman and David E. Holt

- Demystifies common surgical techniques
- System and organ oriented approach
- Step-by-step Operative Techniques
- Focus on most common conditions encountered in practice
- Specially commissioned full colour illustrations throughout

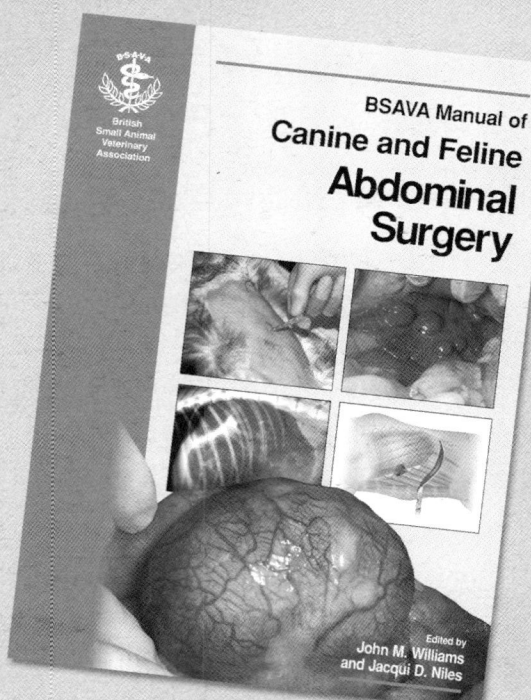

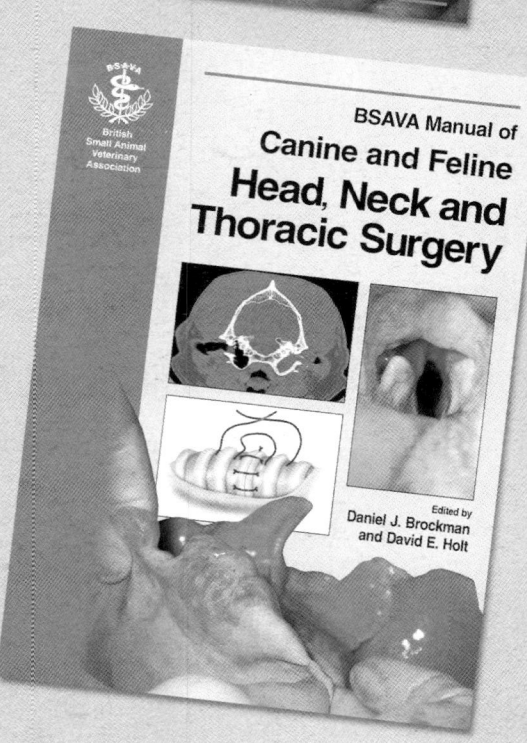

For information and to order please contact us at:
British Small Animal Veterinary Association • Woodrow House
1 Telford Way • Waterwells Business Park • Quedgeley • Gloucester • GL2 2AB
Tel: 01452 726700 • e-mail: customerservices@bsava.com • www.bsava.com

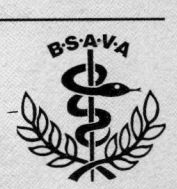